KINN'S
THE Administrative
Medical
Assistant

AN APPLIED LEARNING APPROACH

FIFTH EDITION

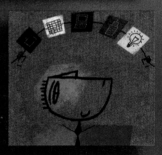
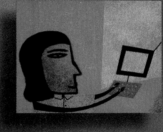

KINN'S
THE Administrative
Medical
Assistant

AN APPLIED LEARNING APPROACH

FIFTH EDITION

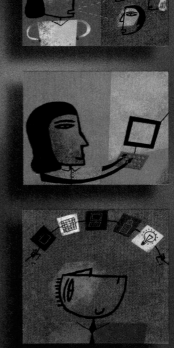

Alexandra Patricia Young, BBA, RMA, CMA

Director of Admissions
Parker College of Chiropractic
Dallas, Texas;
Former Program Director, Health Information Specialist Division
Former Lead Medical Assisting Instructor
Ultrasound Diagnostic School
Dallas, Texas

with more than 270 illustrations

SAUNDERS
An Imprint of Elsevier Science

SAUNDERS

An Imprint of Elsevier Science

11830 Westline Industrial Drive
St. Louis, Missouri 63146

Kinn's The Administrative Medical Assistant:
An Applied Learning Approach

ISBN 0-7216-9102-1

NOTICE

Medical assisting is an ever-changing field. Standard safety precautions must be followed, but as
new research and clinical experience broaden our knowledge, changes in treatment and drug
therapy may become necessary or appropriate. Readers are advised to check the most current
product information provided by the manufacturer of each drug to be administered to verify the
recommended dose, the method and duration of administration, and contraindications. It is the
responsibility of the licensed medical assistant, relying on experience and knowledge of the patient,
to determine dosages and the best treatment for each individual patient. Neither the publisher nor
the author assumes any liability for any injury and/or damage to persons or property arising from
this publication

Previous editions copyrighted 1999, 1993, 1988, 1982 by W.B. Saunders Company.

International Standard Book Number 0-7216-9102-1

Executive Editor: Adrianne Cochran
Associate Developmental Editor: Beth LoGiudice
Publishing Services Manager: Pat Joiner
Project Manager: David Stein
Senior Designer: Mark A. Oberkrom
Designer: Bill Donnelly

RT/QWK
Printed in the United States of America

Last digit is the print number: 9 8 7 6 5 4 3 2 1

Dedication

It is with great honor that the publisher and authors dedicate the ninth edition of this textbook, and its Administrative and Clinical spin-off publications, to Mary E. Kinn, CPS, CMA-A. Mary's contribution to quality medical assisting education spans nearly half a century, starting in 1954 with a telephone crusade to bring medical office "girls," as they were then called, together to create a local medical assistant's association in Southern California. Her contribution continued right through the publication of this edition, with Mary's oversight and review of the text and supplement manuscripts.

A devoted wife and mother, Mary gave generously of her time to furthering the professionalism of her chosen career. She provided leadership and vision to every organization in which she became involved, first as president of a local medical office worker's organization in Southern California, to the second president of the California Medical Assistant's Association, to helping establish a national association, the American Association of Medical Assistants and serving as its president from 1958 to 1959, and finally in 1959 to helping establish a certifying program for members, and serving as its first chairman.

During her time as chairman of the Certifying Board of AAMA, from 1959 to 1967, Mary also became active in the California Association of Medical Assisting Instructors (CAMAI) because of her keen interest in the training and competency of medical assisting instructors. Her work within that organization led her to be hand-selected by the publisher of Frederick and Towner's *The Office Assistant in Medical Practice* in 1967 to replace Carol Towner, who was an executive assistant at the American Medical Association, and who was retiring from the project. Mary's classroom experience, combined with her work on the state and national level to further the interests of the medical assisting profession, made her an ideal choice to co-author this textbook for WB Saunders, and she applied her classroom experience into infusing the text with the sound educational principles of competency-based learning, together with a real-world approach to the presentation of material.

In over six editions and 32 years, Mary Kinn's contribution to both the textbook and her profession would have a profound impact on the training of several generations of medical office personnel. Today, there are nearly 350,000 medical assistants, many of whom have Mary Kinn to thank for paving the way for them to enjoy a career with unlimited possibilities due to the professional recognition of the certification credential, as well as the breadth of skills that have all become part of the medical assisting curriculum. Medical assisting is a viable career for the thousands of women and men who have entered it, and it provides a solid springboard from which to launch a career in medical office management, insurance billing and coding, phlebotomy, medical laboratory technician, and even nursing.

It is therefore both fitting and right that the ninth edition of Mary Kinn's textbook, as well as its Administrative and Clinical spin-off publications, bear her name from this edition forward. Few have earned that honor, but then few have provided so much to so many for so long as has Mary Kinn. The new author team of Alexandra Patricia Young and Deborah B. Kennedy, the publisher, particularly Mary's editors Adrianne Cochran, Andrew Allen, and Helaine Tobin, and the thousands of instructors and students whose lives Mary has affected over the years thank her for all her years of dedication to quality medical assisting education. Enjoy your well-deserved retirement, Mary, but know you will be greatly missed.

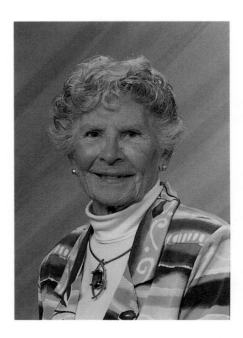

Foreword

(Publisher's Note To The Reader: The following is the Foreword to Kinn's The Medical Assistant: An Applied Learning Approach, Ninth Edition, from which this Administrative textbook has been created. Because it offers the reader a glimpse into the history behind the parent textbook, it is reprinted here in its entirety for interest's sake.)

Medical assisting as a profession has changed dramatically in the 36 years since I became involved as co-author with Portia Frederick of the third edition of *The Office Assistant in Medical Practice* in 1967. That was a time of tremendous change, both for our nation, and for the field of medical assisting. John Dusseau, our editor at WB Saunders, was the chief medical editor and a most remarkable individual. It was John who encouraged me to become involved in this project, and who nurtured me as a fledgling author through that first edition. At that time, WB Saunders had no Health-Related Professions publishing department as it does today, and the Nursing department wanted nothing to do with medical assistants. John lobbied the medical editorial staff at the publishing house to continue supporting this book in its third edition because he knew as Portia and I did that properly trained medical assistants can "make or break" a medical office.

My first professional career started as a legal assistant. I had no interest in the medical field, and no inclination to even explore it as a potential profession. But in 1950, after my children reached school age, and with legal support positions limited, I took a job as an office manager, working for a young surgeon in Southern California who had just opened his first solo medical practice. Office management, I figured, was something I could do, a piece of cake. My first professional shock was discovering that if you worked in a medical practice back then, but were not the nurse, you were simply referred to as "the girl." My second shock was discovering there were no textbooks or reference manuals to guide me, and no educational opportunities in this area. It was all on-the-job training; we "girls" learned as we gained experience, and we learned from one another.

It was out of that dearth of training materials that in 1954, with the encouragement of the local medical society, a few of us "girls" who had become acquainted by telephone, got together and developed a countywide medical assistant's association. Our initial membership of 200 medical assistants met with opposition from some physicians, who were afraid we were trying to unionize. As the group's first president, it was my job to change that attitude, which eventually happened over the course of several subsequent and rocky years. Concurrently, there was action taking place on the state level in California, and I became the second president of the California Medical Assistant's Association.

It was through these activities that I became acquainted with Portia Frederick, the daughter of a physician who had developed a course for medical assistant training in a nearby community college. Portia had been requested by an official of the American Medical Association to co-author a textbook with Carol Towner, an executive assistant in the AMA's Department of Public Relations. The result of their efforts was the first edition of *The Office Assistant in Medical and Dental Practice,* published in 1956 by WB Saunders, which was the forerunner of today's *Kinn's The Medical Assistant: An Applied Learning Approach, Ninth Edition.* Simplistic and chatty, that first edition had a few poorly drawn illustrations and no color. The entire book, including the index, contained 351 pages, but it covered the necessary information and was the best and only book to address the training needs of medical office supportive personnel. The Foreword, written by George F. Lull, MD, then the secretary and general manager of the AMA, stated *"The modern day physician runs a constant race against the clock. As his practice grows, the demands of his patients for medical services increase. In order to make the best use of his time, he continually seeks ways to run his practice more efficiently. At least 75% of all practicing physicians in this country have found that one logical answer is to employ a girl in the office to whom many routine duties can be delegated...it is becoming quite apparent that the ideal assistant should be trained to handle efficiently both medical assisting and medical secretarial duties in the office."*

At about the time of the second edition of this text, which was retitled *The Office Assistant in Medical Practice,* I had become involved with others in establishing a national association, the American Association of Medical Assistants, and served as its president in 1958-1959. At the 1959 AAMA meeting in Philadelphia, at the end of my term, a resolution was adopted to establish a certifying program for our members, and I was appointed its first chairman. I served as founding chairman of the Certifying Board from 1959 through 1967, and became deeply interested in the training and competency of medical assistants.

About that time, a new organization for instructors was coming to life, named California Association of Medical Assisting Instructors (CAMAI), and Portia Frederick invited me to attend the early informal meetings. The contacts I met at that meeting increased my interest in medical assistant training, and I was thrilled to be asked to co-author the next edition of the text, to replace Carol Towner who had answered the call to motherhood. I began my teaching career in 1970 using the third edition that John Dusseau had so clairvoyantly lobbied to preserve, and began to realize how the book could be enlarged and improved as a teaching tool and a reference. As an instructor, I was eligible to become a full-fledged member of CAMAI, and I jumped in with both feet. Because of my involvement in that organization, this third edition had more information about medical assisting associations, and of course the certified medical assistant credential. Management, medical ethics, and law were also expanded and given more attention, and a chapter on medical emergencies was added.

The fourth edition, published in 1974, was retitled *The Medical Office Assistant: Administrative and Clinical,* and the book was reorganized into its three sections of general, administrative, and clinical. Government-sponsored health insurance was dominating office practice, and we greatly expanded this section of the book to reflect the impact of Medicare and Medicaid. Nutrition and diet therapy and microbiology were added, the clinical section was divided into the various medical specialties, now a hallmark of the text. Still no color was added, but the book topped out at 742 pages and was a vast improvement over the previous edition in terms of its integration in the training program.

The fifth edition, in 1981, is still my favorite edition because the manuscript was updated and enlarged to better reflect the changing face of the profession. Different print font and margin width, as well as thinner paper, allowed for the inclusion of extended content without requiring more pages. Color was used for marginal paragraph headings, and many photographs appeared throughout the text. But the joy of achievement in that edition was overshadowed by the sudden and unexpected death of my friend, Portia Frederick, before the new edition had gone to press.

Major changes were taking place within the medical assisting profession at that time. The 1984 DACUM Analysis of the Medical Assisting Profession had been circulated. More and more physicians were using computers in their practice. The sixth edition of the text brought in Eleanor Derge to help completely update the content and format, which included a vocabulary list at the beginning of each chapter, learning objectives for both didactic and practical application, and step-by-step procedures covering all essential entry-level skills, including terminal performance objectives and current safety precautions for the prevention of AIDS transmission. This edition also saw the debut of the first *Student Review and Activities Manual* and an instructor's manual added to the package.

The seventh edition, authored by Kinn, Derge, and Dr. MaryAnne Woods, was published in 1993 and topped out over 900 pages. The book had a whole new look and a fresh approach. Personal communication, dictation, and transcription were added to the Administrative section. More color was used, and more emphasis was placed on personal communications and the medical specialty chapters. The accompanying ancillaries were updated and improved to reflect the expanded text content.

When the eighth edition of Kinn and Woods published in 1999, I turned to my editor, Adrianne Cochran, and announced that I was done. It had been a long road from the time John Dusseau had flown to San Francisco in 1965 to meet with Portia Frederick and me, to "look me over" as a suitable candidate for co-authoring this text. In the ensuing years, the book had grown to 1144 pages, had collected a student workbook, instructor's manual, text software, and a dedicated website. I felt I'd made a real contribution to the text at the publication of the eighth edition, and had made a difference in the training of thousands of medical assistants over the 22 years in which I was involved. But I had things I still wanted to do in life, I'd retired from teaching, and I felt it was time to pass along the torch to others with a similar devotion to quality medical assisting education.

I feel that the publisher has found those individuals in Tricia Young and Debby Kennedy, and it was with a mix of nostalgia, sadness, and excitement that I relinquished my participation in the future of this text and turned it over to these two very capable and dedicated medical assisting instructors.

Alexandra Patricia Young, BBA, CMA, RMA, is the former program director of the Health Information Specialist program and the former lead instructor for the Medical Assisting program at Ultrasound Diagnostic School, a large vocational chain of schools with campuses all over the country. She was also the director of education for allied health for Bryan Institute. Tricia's natural writing gift, her love of the subject material, and her devotion to medical assisting training have infused the Administrative section of this textbook with a brilliance that reflects current practice and a sensitivity to topics that are crucial to quality medical assisting education. Tricia has done a wonderful job of updating the material and bringing together both her mastery of current information and her creative instincts. As this was the section for which I was responsible for so many years, I feel particularly good about the chapters I reviewed that Tricia authored.

Deborah B. Kennedy, EdD, RN, CMA, the new author of the clinical section, is the Director and Associate Professor of the Medical Assistant Program at Butler County Community College, in Butler, PA. Debby brings particularly excellent credentials to the half of the book that requires a keen knowledge of patient interaction, current medical diagnostic and therapeutic practice, and instructional expertise in order to convey particularly difficult subjects in a straightforward, retainable way. This is not an easy task given how complicated the clinical portion of the medical assisting curriculum has become today. Medical assistants are now the primary patient educators. They must reason, problem-solve, and react to patients during sometimes difficult and trying times in the patients' lives with a sensitivity and grace that is often difficult to convey in a textbook. From the chapters I reviewed of Debby's work, I was extremely pleased to see she has raised the level of the clinical chapters to a quality of training that is not just nice to have, but required in today's demanding medical office.

Although it was over 36 years ago, I well remember the anticipation of that first publication and seeing the cover on which my name would be listed as a co-author. Students were going to read what I wrote, and that both thrilled and intimidated me, but as Tricia and Debby have discovered, it's an experience of a lifetime to be involved in a project with such a worthy cause. Tricia and Debby have done an exemplary job at completely rewriting the entire textbook; reorganizing chapters; adding new chapters, photos, and illustrations; and integrating an innovative new "applied" approach; and have taken the training a step beyond with the new Study Skills and Career Development and Life Skills chapters that bookend the primary material.

Tammy B. Morton, MS, RN, CS, CMA, has also written the revision of the *Student Study Guide* and *Instructor's Curriculum Resource with CD-ROM*. Not only are her exercises creative examples of learning by doing, Tammy understands that not all students learn the same way, and she has integrated a unique identification classification so that no matter how a student learns there is something available in this *Study Guide* to help them master the material. She has also written some beautiful PowerPoint slides, and helpful instructor tools that will make planning interesting and motivating classroom presentations easier for instructors. Tammy's educational background, like that of Tricia and Debby, is evident throughout both of these supplements, and I'm pleased to see they are some of the best I've seen on the market.

In my lifetime it is also wonderful to witness two new exciting supplements that have been added to the package that reflect the technical revolution that is happening in America's learning institutions. The EVOLVE learning management system now gives instructors and students a new platform for communication with one another, one that simulates a means of communicating that will dominate the medical assistant's professional career, as email and the digital age are so prevalent in the medical office. And the online courses for both Administrative and Clinical Medical Assisting now provide students with a convenient, anytime/anywhere opportunity to become confident in mastering the key concepts and skills they need to know, in order to prove competence when they reach the practice lab. This new learning platform reaches out to the many medical assisting students who would otherwise not be able to find the time to attend class, and it brings learning to life as only the Internet and its three-dimensional format can.

My heartfelt congratulations are extended to both Tricia Young and Debby Kennedy on the publication of their first textbook, and to Tammy Morton on the publication of the supplements. I also congratulate their advocates behind the scenes at WB Saunders/Elsevier who believe, as John Dusseau believed over 42 years ago, that success in life starts with the power of knowledge, and that that power comes in creating the right combination of training materials that together can turn a novice student into a highly qualified professional medical assistant ready to meet the challenges of today's busy and complicated medical office practice.

Mary E. Kinn, CPS, CMA-A
San Clemente, California
February 2003

Preface to the Fifth Edition

Medical assisting as a profession has changed dramatically since *The Administrative Medical Assistant* was first published in 1982. This new fifth edition continues to represent a long-standing commitment to quality medical assisting education, with its engaging, straightforward writing style and demonstrated positive outcomes. Hundreds of instructors in classrooms all across the country have used this text to teach thousands of students over the years. Many of these students have gone on to teach students of their own with this very same trusted resource. To continue the use and growth of this textbook and its features, the fifth edition has undergone a massive revision in an effort to offer you the most comprehensive, up-to-date, and innovative approach to teaching this subject today. I appreciate the opportunity to explore the existing field of administrative medical assisting with you!

DISTINCTIVE FEATURES OF OUR APPROACH

This textbook has endured throughout the years because it has been able to keep pace with an ever-changing profession while producing students who are well trained and qualified to enter medical practices across the country. This dependability is why the market continues to rely on this text, edition after edition. Underlying this dependability is a foundation of pedagogical features that has stood the test of time and that has been expanded and improved upon yet again in this new edition. Such pedagogical features include the following:

- An easy-to-read, highly interactive writing style that engages students through practical applications of administrative medical assistant competencies.
- An emphasis on skill development with procedural steps outlining each skill, supported by rationales that provide meaning to each step.
- A pedagogical framework based on the use of learning objectives, vocabulary terms, and supportive student supplements.
- A package of supportive materials to accommodate a wide variety of student learning types and instructor teaching styles.

NEW FEATURES IN THIS EDITION

The medical field is an ever-changing one, with constant advances in diagnostic procedures and treatment protocols. The influence of current risk management practices and the potential of electronic technology as a resource for student and patient education have both complicated and expanded the opportunities available to medical assistant professionals.

To build on the long-established strengths of the Kinn textbook, the fifth edition expands and supplements the techniques used so successfully in past editions. A combination of many talented individuals on the editorial and production staffs working with a new author and contributor team has resulted in a text that adheres to the Kinn tradition while meeting the needs of a new generation of administrative medical assistant educators and students. The result is an innovative text that comprehensively meets the educational and accreditation needs of all types of administrative medical assistant programs while effectively training tomorrow's front office medical assisting professionals.

The new edition of *Kinn's The Administrative Medical Assistant* incorporates a unique approach that is reflected in the new subtitle that has been added to the book for this edition: *An Applied Learning Approach.* It is believed that learning takes place only when students are engaged and when the learning requires something from them in response to information that is being imparted to them. I have therefore attempted to provide meaningful thought in the form of realistic scenarios that put information in context and provide a way for students to directly apply concepts they're learning by challenging them to consider how they would behave in certain situations.

This "applied" theme is set upfront in the first chapter, which introduces students to the concepts of critical thinking and the impact of individual learning styles on student success. This in turn transitions into time management and problem-solving skills, as well as effective study skills and test-taking strategies. The text develops from there true to the original Kinn textbook, and is rounded out by the last chapter, which helps students focus on preparing for and nurturing their career as an administrative medical assistant.

This pedagogical theme and other new enhancements can be found throughout the book and its supplements in the following features:

- Each chapter opens with a scenario related to the chapter's focus that introduces students to a medical assistant and a situation, or situations, that the medical assistant must approach.

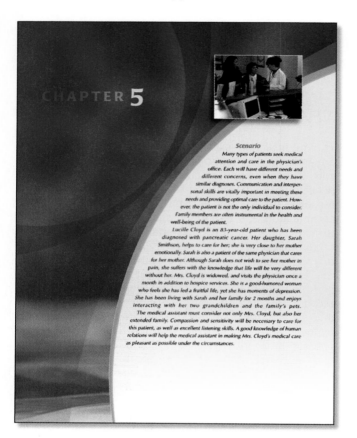

CHAPTER 5

Scenario

Many types of patients seek medical attention and care in the physician's office. Each will have different needs and different concerns, even when they have similar diagnoses. Communication and interpersonal skills are vitally important in meeting these needs and providing optimal care to the patient. However, the patient is not the only individual to consider. Family members are often instrumental in the health and well-being of the patient.

Lucille Cloyd is an 83-year-old patient who has been diagnosed with pancreatic cancer. Her daughter, Sarah Smithson, helps to care for her; she is very close to her mother emotionally. Sarah is also a patient of the same physician that cares for her mother. Although Sarah does not wish to see her mother in pain, she suffers with the knowledge that life will be very different without her. Mrs. Cloyd is widowed, and visits the physician once a month in addition to hospice services. She is a good-humored woman who feels she has led a fruitful life, yet she has moments of depression. She has been living with Sarah and her family for 2 months and enjoys interacting with her two grandchildren and the family's pets. The medical assistant must consider not only Mrs. Cloyd, but also her extended family. Compassion and sensitivity will be necessary to care for this patient, as well as excellent listening skills. A good knowledge of human relations will help the medical assistant in making Mrs. Cloyd's medical care as pleasant as possible under the circumstances.

- Throughout the chapter, Critical Thinking Applications are designed to allow the student to use a concept that has just been learned in the context of the overall chapter scenario. These exercises help students look at the big picture and consider various angles, or approaches, to the challenges in which they will eventually find themselves in the medical office. These exercises provide a wonderful opportunity for discussion and further reflection.

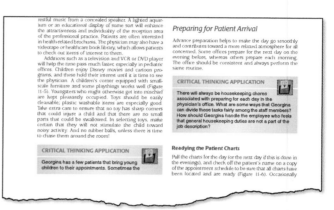

restful music from a concealed speaker. A lighted aquarium or an educational display of some sort will enhance the attractiveness and individuality of the reception area of the professional practice. Patients are often interested in health-related brochures. The physician may also have a videotape or healthcare book library, which allows patients to check out items of interest to them.

Additions such as a television and VCR or DVD player will help the time pass much faster especially in pediatric offices. Children enjoy Disney movies and cartoon programs, and these hold their interest until it is time to see the physician. A children's corner equipped with small-scale furniture and some playthings works well (Figure 11-5). Youngsters who might otherwise get into mischief are kept pleasantly occupied. Toys should be easily cleanable; plastic washable items are especially good. Take extra care to ensure that no toy has sharp corners that could injure a child and that there are no small parts that could be swallowed. In selecting toys, make certain that they will not stimulate the child toward noisy activity. And no rubber balls, unless there is time to chase them around the room!

CRITICAL THINKING APPLICATION

Georgina has a few patients that bring young children to their appointments. Sometimes the

Preparing for Patient Arrival

Advance preparation helps to make the day go smoothly and contributes toward a more relaxed atmosphere for all concerned. Some offices prepare for the next day in the evening before, whereas others prepare each morning. The office should be consistent and always perform the same routine.

CRITICAL THINKING APPLICATION

There will always be housekeeping chores associated with preparing for each day in the physician's office. What are some ways that Georgina can divide these tasks fairly among the staff members? How should Georgina handle the employee who feels that general housekeeping duties are not a part of the job description?

Readying the Patient Charts

Pull the charts for the day for the next day if this is done in the evenings), and check off the patient's name on a copy of the appointment schedule to be sure that all charts have been located and are ready (Figure 11-6). Occasionally

- Chapters end with a Summary of Scenario that identifies concepts for student focus, as well as a discussion, where relevant, of patient education as it relates to the chapter focus and concepts within the chapter.

SUMMARY OF SCENARIO

Susan looks forward to attending her medical assisting classes each day and works diligently to perform to the best of her ability in the classroom. She strives to do well on each procedure check-off and each examination that she completes. Her instructors provide excellent feedback and appreciate her contributions to the classroom experience.

Susan has the attitude that everything she is allowed to do in the medical office is a learning tool. She regularly asks for additional responsibilities and is always ready to assist a co-worker. Dr. Thomas has recognized that she has the desire to learn, and he gives her many opportunities to glean more knowledge through the everyday

experiences with their friends and relatives and may be an excellent source of referrals if they are treated with dignity and courtesy. If they have had a good experience, they will tell several people. If they have a poor experience, they tend to tell everyone they know! Be sure to have a part in each patient feeling a sense of satisfaction as they leave the office. All patients should feel that their time and money were well spent.

the medical profession, Susan logically. She knows the rules patient confidentiality and is information she provides to is never hesitant about asking guidance if she is unsure about

Patient Education

Offering a patient education center in the reception area is an effective way to provide up-to-date information about healthcare issues to patients. Brochures and information sheets can be displayed, and if the office is equipped with a VCR in the reception area, videotapes that deal with health topics can be available for viewing while the patient is waiting to see the physician.

Both the physician and the medical assistants caring for patients should ask if the patient has any questions during his or her visit to the office. Patients often complain that they did not have a chance to speak to the physician long enough to have their questions answered sufficiently. Be sure that this is not the case, and prompt the patient to ask about anything he or she is unclear on while the physician is still in the examination room.

- Improved integration of concepts that transcend chapter topics, such as legal and ethical issues, communications, professionalism, and office management.

- The artwork throughout has been updated and modernized, providing a more attractive textbook for student use. Many new photographs better support the revised content and are more relevant to the actual medical office. Many old photos were replaced with new photos that show more updated equipment and better illustrate key procedural steps.

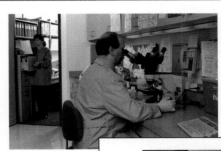

FIGURE 4-2   The physician [...] medical assistant to be at wor[...] Absent or tardy employees ca[...] greatly inconvenience the pati[...]

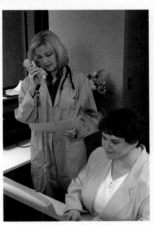

FIGURE 4-1   The professional medical assistant is an asset to the physician's office.

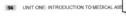

can be frustrating for patients when they must list their address and phone numbers on each of several forms. Review and revise the forms used in the office often so that they are user-friendly for the office and patient alike.

Patients may need reassurance that each staff member in the physician's office is committed to complete patient confidentiality. Always be open to answering questions regarding the patient medical record.

Legal and Ethical Issues

The authority to release information from the medical record lies solely with the patient unless required by law by subpoena. Ownership of the record is often a subject of controversy. The record belongs to the physician; the information belongs to the patient.

When a medical record is used as evidence in a court case, the person who entered information in the chart must be able to read it, no matter how much time has lapsed since the entry was created. When a chart is corrected, the proper method must be followed and the record should never be obliterated.

Be sure to understand the laws concerning records retention. Records should be kept through the period of the statute of limitations, and possibly longer in certain situations. Take care with the medical chart, as it is the lifetime of patient care in the medical facility.

56   UNIT ONE: INTRODUCTION TO MEDICAL ASS[...]

Credibility

Credibility is the perceived **competence** or character of a person. It leads to the belief that the person can be trusted. Since trust is a vital component of the physician-patient relationship, the credibility of the physician and those who assist in the office should be strong. The information provided to patients must be accurate. Patients expect that the physician and medical assistant will instruct them in a manner that will enhance their health and provide positive results. One must take care in giving any advice to patients, because they view the medical assistant as an agent of the physician. Patients may not distinguish between the medical assistant's advice and the physician's orders. To avoid charges of practicing medicine without a license, a medical assistant must be sure to suggest only what the physician has authorized.

Confidentiality

The importance of confidentiality cannot be stressed enough in the medical environment. Patients are entitled to privacy where their health is concerned, and they should be confident that medical professionals use information only to care for them. One must never reveal any information about any patient to anyone without specific permission to do so. If in doubt, be conservative and verify that the person seeking information has the right to see it. Casual conversations in hallways, elevators, and break rooms between staff can be overheard by a family member or friend of the patient.

The rules regarding confidentiality extend beyond the medical office. While at home, medical assistants should not discuss details about patients with their families and friends. Those outside the medical profession do not [...]understand how vital it is to keep information confidential[...] pass along damaging facts to others. Medical [...] it a rule never to discuss a patient [...] must be shared for

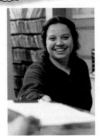

FIGURE 4-4   A good attitude goes a long way in patient and staff relationships.

and it can be hard to maintain a professional attitude in these cases. Some of the obstructions to professional behavior are discussed in this section.

Personal Problems and "Baggage"

Everyone has a life outside of the workplace, and sometimes we face challenges and difficult times that are hard to put aside. During working hours our thoughts should be on the job at hand, especially when we are dealing with patients. However, there may be situations in our lives that are so critical or important that we find ourselves [...]*baggage*, as it

- Well-developed learning objectives emphasize the cognitive and performance objectives addressed in the chapter, and are summarized at the end of each chapter for student review of learning.

Patient Reception and Processing

Learning Objectives

- Define and spell the terms listed in the vocabulary.
- Explain the purpose of the office mission statement.
- List several patient amenities and why these are important additions to the medical office.
- Describe how to prepare for patient arrivals.
- Explain why it is important to use the patient's name as often as possible.
- Discuss how the medical assistant may help the patient prepare for an examination.
- List and explain two methods of chart placement.
- Discuss how the medical assistant might deal with talkative patients.
- Explain how the medical assistant can recall closing duties.
- Discuss ways to make the patient feel at ease and comfortable in the medical office.
- Correctly prepare charts for registered patients who are scheduled.
- Demonstrate the correct way to register a new patient.

SUMMARY OF LEARNING OBJECTIVES

■ The office mission statement is the philosophy of why the office exists. Often physicians develop the mission statement themselves, which outlines their vision and reasons for entering medical practice. Some physicians allow the office staff to assist in its development. All employees should become familiar with the mission statement and promote its ideas to all patients and visitors.

■ Patient amenities include such things as a VCR, television, computer, telephone, and a desk where patients can sit and balance a checkbook or review work while away from the office. These features turn the time spent in the physician's office into productive minutes instead of wasteful ones.

■ Some offices prepare for patient arrivals the evening before, and some in the morning. Patient charts must be pulled and should be reviewed, checking for completed laboratory tests, posting of results, and to ensure that there are ample progress notes for this visit. Rooms should be checked and inventoried to make certain there are enough supplies on hand and that they present a clean, neat appearance.

■ People like hearing their own names; a better relationship is built between the staff and patients when the names are used often. Patients feel that the office staff care enough about them to acknowledge them, and this custom adds a personal touch.

■ The medical assistant should escort the patient to the examination rooms and other areas of the office. Always tell the patient when to disrobe and exactly what should be removed. Offer to assist with disrobing if the patient needs extra help. Take care that the patient's purse or wallet is in a secure [...] that doors do not open and expose [...] Instruct the patient as to [...] or should wait after

- Chapter 5 now includes an expanded and much more comprehensive discussion of interpersonal skills and human relations. This chapter provides information about the communication process, listening and observation skills, defense mechanisms, dealing with conflict, and perception. There is an emphasis on communication during difficult times, as well as a discussion about health self-esteem, self-improvement, and comfort zones.
- Chapter 8 on computers has been revised and thoroughly updated to include timely information to reflect the more sophisticated computer systems found in today's busy medical practice. It provides easy-to-understand details about subjects such as the elements of microprocessors, an "inside-the-computer" section, file formats, internet connectivity, networking basics, computer security, and ergonomics. The medical records management and health information chapters also include an in-depth discussion of computer-based medical records.
- More than any previous edition, customer service is stressed throughout the chapters. As patients become more involved in their healthcare, medical assistants must realize that the healthcare field is a service industry, and patients should be treated more like customers. Chapter 21 is devoted to practice marketing and customer service, and several sections stress the need for concern for the patient's time and working efficiently.
- New compliance regulations in medical billing and coding have lent a far greater emphasis on reimbursement than ever before. Both billing and coding have been expanded, and three new coding chapters have been added: Basics of Diagnostic Coding (Chapter 15), Basics of Procedural Coding (Chapter 16), and The Health Insurance Claim Form (Chapter 17).
- Major Internet sites relating to each chapter are provided for students to expand their understanding of chapter concepts and stay current on medical news and industry developments through research on the World Wide Web.

NEW INTERNET RESOURCE

Stay current with trends, developments, and news in the medical field, as well as access additional chapter supplemental features, advice on your externship, interviewing techniques, and more, through EVOLVE, the website that is provided complimentary to this textbook. This exciting website is your gateway to the World Wide Web. It is an interactive learning environment that adds an incredibly powerful set of instructional resources to your classroom experience. EVOLVE works in coordination with *Kinn's The Administrative Medical Assistant: An Applied Learning Approach, Fifth Edition* by providing Internet-based course content and Internet web links to reinforce and expand your learning experience.

The EVOLVE Course Management System (CMS) is also available to instructors who adopt this textbook. In addition to the Evolve Learning Resources available to students, there is an entire suite of tools available to instructors that allow for communication between instructors and students, including discussion boards, e-mail, chat rooms, and more.

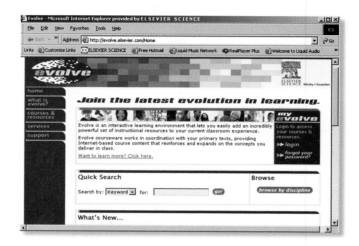

To access this comprehensive online resource, simply go to the EVOLVE Home Page at http://evolve.elsevier.com and enter your user name and password provided to you from your instructor. If your instructor has not set up a Course Management System, you can still access all the learning resources available free with this textbook by going to http://evolve.elsevier.com/Kinn/Admin/.

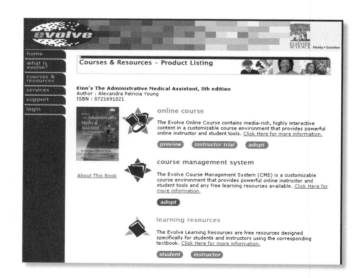

EXTENSIVE SUPPLEMENTAL RESOURCES

The diversity of students, instructors, programs, institutions, and teaching environments using this textbook required the development of an integrated, comprehensive, and flexible package of supplements to support *Kinn's The Administrative Medical Assistant: An Applied Learning Approach, Fifth Edition.* Each of these innovative supplements is designed to enhance the teaching and learning experience with the outcome of producing students well equipped to pass any certification examination, and who will go on to experience successful professional careers in medical assisting. These supplements and their unique features include:

Student Software Program

The free CD-ROM that comes with your textbook includes two programs designed for you to apply the key content and skills you've learned in the textbook. *The Virtual Medical Office Challenge* provides four realistic administrative scenarios, with you making the decisions and getting feedback on each decision you make, plus a skill-building section that lets you practice targeted administrative competencies. All forms used throughout are included for reference in a format suitable for printing. *Lytec Medical 2001,* a real medical office software program, lets you practice front office skills on the computer. A user's manual for the *Lytec* program is included in a format suitable for printing.

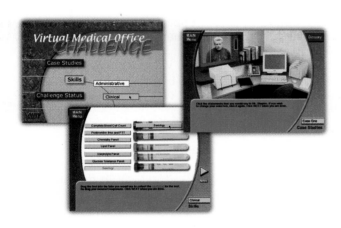

Student Study Guide
Tammy B. Morton, MS, RN, CS, CMA

This practical tool takes the "applied learning approach" to a whole new level, giving you the opportunity to apply the knowledge and skills you're learning in the textbook. Some of the outstanding features of this study guide include:

- Learning style icons that identify the targeted learning style of each exercise. Find out which learning style works best for you!
- Procedure checklists that serve as a valuable tool for checking your competency, as well as a tool for your

instructor to gauge your skill level and proficiency for each skill in the textbook.
- A multitude of exercises to reinforce key content throughout the textbook, including vocabulary exercises that help you recall and apply medical terms.
- Coding applications, documentation scenarios, and telephone screening examples provide you with the opportunity to apply administrative concepts to realistic situations.
- Chapter quizzes at the end of each chapter exercise set allow you to further test your knowledge.
- Study tips for all medical assisting students, as well as a section on study tips specifically designed for ESL (English-as-a-Second-Language) students, written by an ESL consultant.
- A glossary of English-Spanish terms, based on the text glossary, gives students an excellent resource for working with patients who speak English as a second language. This glossary is likewise extremely helpful for those medical assisting students who themselves speak English as a second language.

Instructor's Curriculum Resource
Tammy B. Morton, MS, RN, CS, CMA

This complete instructor teaching tool includes extensive curriculum materials in both print and electronic formats. Beginning and veteran instructors alike will be able to easily prepare their lectures, presentations, labs, and assessments with an extensive course syllabus, multiple course outlines, individual chapter lesson plans, chapter Internet addresses, and ready-made tests for each chapter. Answer keys for all text and Student Study Guide questions are also included. In addition, special tips for instructors with ESL (English-as-a-Second-Language) students have been provided, written by an ESL consultant. All of the printed materials from the Instructor's Curriculum Resource are also available in Word format on the free CD-ROM, making them fully customizable for use in any classroom.

Test Bank
Tammy B. Morton, MS, RN, CS, CMA

The test bank provides an accurate and exhaustive source of test items for a wide variety of examination styles. It contains more than 1,000 questions, and is available in both printed and electronic format so you can easily prepare your quizzes and exams, tailored to your classroom format.

PowerPoint Presentation Slides
Tammy B. Morton, MS, RN, CS, CMA

The instructor CD-ROM includes a PowerPoint viewer and a set of over 600 PowerPoint slides. The slides include a summary of key chapter material, and can easily be customized to support your lectures and enhance your classroom presentation. All slides have been formatted to reflect the text design, and include many images from the text. These slides can also be easily formatted within the PowerPoint program for student note taking or as overhead transparencies.

KINN'S ADMINISTRATIVE MEDICAL ASSISTING ONLINE
Available Summer 2003

Today's educational environment has the potential to be more interactive than ever before. The more resources available to facilitate learning, and the more varied those resources are, the greater the chances are for material to be comprehended and retained.

Kinn's Administrative Medical Assisting Online has been developed with this creative approach to education in mind. Offering a multidimensional experience that is not possible in a traditional classroom setting, these unique and innovative new products are complete courses that simulate the externship experience by creating a virtual medical practice where students have an opportunity to learn by doing.

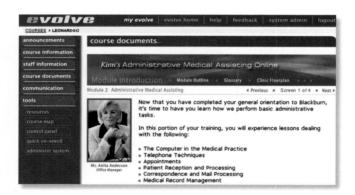

Designed to be used together with *Kinn's The Administrative Medical Assistant: An Applied Learning Approach, Fifth Edition,* course lessons draw upon the text for reading assignments, then provide an opportunity for you to apply text content by entering the simulated environment of "Blackburn Primary Care Associates," complete with an office manager who acts as your supervisor/mentor through the courses, other office personnel, physicians, and realistic patient cases. This environment is an exciting way for you to discover what it is like to work in the field of medical assisting before you ever enter your administrative externship.

A wide range of visual, auditory, and interactive elements create this exciting environment and work together to amplify key learning objectives from the textbook, giving you the opportunity to practice key skills first by being guided through a practice of each skill, then by trying to perform that skill in a realistic application exercise. This combination of guided practice and application of skills gives you the *confidence* to perform these skills with *competence* in your classroom or on the job.

Providing a myriad of learning opportunities, *Kinn's*

Administrative Medical Assisting Online accommodates diverse learning styles and circumstances through the use of a sophisticated learning management system that lets your instructor tailor the program's content either to support a traditional classroom learning experience or as a true distance education course. You log on through the Evolve portal to complete lessons, take quizzes and exams online, participate in threaded discussions, post assignments to your instructor, or chat with your instructor or fellow classmates, all from any location that has Internet connectivity.

DEVELOPMENT OF THIS EDITION

To ensure continuous improvement and accuracy of the material presented throughout this textbook, an extensive review and development process was used for all past editions. Building on that history, the fifth edition developmental process included several phases of evaluation by a variety of administrative medical assisting instructors. The first phase of the review process asked instructors who both used and did not use the text to suggest improvements to the organization of the text, to the text material, to the figures and tables throughout, and to the supplements. The second phase encompassed a more detailed review of each chapter as material was being prepared.

I am deeply grateful to the numerous people who have shared their comments and suggestions on this edition. Reviewing a book or supplement takes an incredible amount of energy and attention, and I am glad so many of my colleagues were able to take time out of their busy schedule to help ensure the validity and appropriateness of content in this edition. The reviewers provided many additional viewpoints and opinions that combined to make this text an incredible learning tool.

I wish to thank the following editorial reviewing team:

Kim Anthony Aaronson, BS, DC
Adjunct Instructor
Anatomy and Physiology and Medical Terminology
Truman College;
Adjunct Instructor
Pacific College of Oriental Medicine
Chicago, Illinois

Jannie Adams, PhD, RN, BSN, MSHA
Director/Assistant Professor
Medical Assisting
Clayton College and State University
Morrow, Georgia

Laura Baumgardner, CPC, CPC-H, CCS-P, CCS
Instructor, Health Careers Division
Harrisburg Area Community College
Harrisburg, Pennsylvania

Deborah Bedford, CMA, AAS
Program Coordinator and Instructor
Medical Assisting Program
North Seattle Community College
Seattle, Washington

Crystal Dawn Bennett, CMA, AAS
Instructor, Medical Assisting
Hocking College
Nelsonville, Ohio

Kathy Bonewit-West, BS, MEd, CMAC
Professor
Medical Assistant Technology
Hocking College
Nelsonville, Ohio

Carol J. Buck, MS, CPC
Program Director (Ret.)
Medical Secretary Programs
Northwest Technical College
East Grand Forks, Minnesota

Wendy Campbell, ADN
Medical Assistant Program Director
Concorde Career Institute
Portland, Oregon

Diana L. Carroll, CMA, CPC
Assistant Professor
Salt Lake City Community College
Salt Lake City, Utah

Janet Haggerty Davis, BSN, MS, MBA, PhD, RN
Dean, School of Health Studies
Robert Morris College
Chicago, Illinois

Judy Ehninger, RN, BS, CMA
Coordinator and Assistant Professor
Medical Assisting Program
Lehigh Carbon Community College
Schnecksville, Pennsylvania

Eugenia M. Fulcher, RN, BSN, MEd, EdD
Program Director, Medical Assisting
Swainsboro Technical College
Swainsboro, Georgia

Jesse Green, JD
General Counsel
Parker College of Chiropractic
Dallas, Texas

Helen Houser, RN, MSHA
Program Director
Medical Assisting Program
Phoenix College
Phoenix, Arizona

Carol Lee Jarrell, MLT, OPT
Instructor
Commonwealth Business College
Merrillville, Indiana

Karen D. Lockyer, BA, RHIT, CPC
Instructor
Montgomery College
Takoma Park, Maryland;
Administrative Assistant
National Institutes of Health
Bethesda, Maryland

Joseph E. McCann, BA, LVN, CMA
Medical Assisting Program Coordinator
San Antonio College
San Antonio, Texas

Catherine McCartney, MA, RN, CMA
Program Director/Instructor
Medical Assistant Program
Henry Ford Community College
Health Careers Division
Dearborn, Michigan

Shirley Jordan Oktay, BA, CMA, POLT(AAB)
Instructional Specialist III, Health Professions
Richland College
Dallas, Texas

Lauren Perlstein, RN, MSN
Coordinator of Medical Assistant Program
Norwalk Community Technical College
Norwalk, Connecticut

Janet Sesser, RMA(AMT), CMA, BSEd Admin
Director of Education for Allied Health
High-Tech Institute, Inc.
Phoenix, Arizona

Jane A. Shingler
Allied Health Department Chair
Allentown Business School
Allentown, Pennsylvania

Nina Thierer, CMA, BS, CPC-A
Associate Professor and Instructor
Medical Assisting Program
Ivy Tech State College—Fort Wayne
Fort Wayne, Indiana

Jana W. Tucker, CMA, LPRT
Medical Assistant Program Coordinator
Assistant Professor
Salt Lake City Community College
Salt Lake City, Utah

CONTRIBUTORS TO THIS EDITION

The preceding section demonstrates the amount of feedback and developmental input that went into shaping the fifth edition of this textbook. Because the medical assisting curriculum is so broad in scope, no individual can be an expert in all areas. I therefore extend a special acknowledgment to the following people who brought their expertise to bear by contributing one or more chapters to this edition:

Janet Beik, MEd
Administrative Instructor
Medical Assistant Program
Southeastern Community College
West Burlington, Iowa

Brenda K. Burton
President
Medextend, Inc
Cazenovia, New York

Carol A. Turiello, RN, RDMS, CPC
Administrator
Cardiology Division
Department of Medicine
State University of New York
Upstate Medical University
Syracuse, New York

Author Acknowledgments

It takes a dedicated group of individuals to produce an outstanding textbook such as this. I am thankful for the Elsevier team for the tireless work that was put into *Kinn's The Administrative Medical Assistant: An Applied Learning Approach, Fifth Edition.* Adrianne Cochran, Executive Editor for Vocational Publishing, provided encouragement, ideas, and a healthy dose of confidence as we undertook the project and throughout its development. I will be forever grateful for her belief in my ability as a writer. Beth LoGiudice, Associate Developmental Editor, was a tremendous asset to the project as we progressed from chapter to chapter. Her enthusiasm, sense of humor, and support were unending and greatly appreciated. It seemed that she was never frazzled, no matter what the challenge was before us. David Stein, Project Manager, was courteous and helpful throughout the production process. The photographer, Jack Foley of Jack Foley Photography, his team, and the Elsevier design team of Bill Donnelly and Mark Oberkrom all did a superb job in turning this book into a beautiful work of art. Finally, thanks also to Anne Rowe for introducing me to Adrianne Cochran and jump-starting my writing career. I could not have asked for a better team. Thanks to you all for your part in making this project become a reality.

Special thanks go to Debby Kennedy and Tammy Morton. I am privileged to know such talented individuals. You both did a wonderful job on this text and its supplements. Thanks also to Brenda Burton, Carol Turiello, and Janet Beik for writing the contributed chapters. They are truly fantastic.

I would like to thank my dad, Jim Crumley, attorney-at-law, for giving me a sense for law and ethics, and for allowing me to interrupt his black-and-white TV shows with my questions for the book. Without my mom, Patricia Crumley, I would have never made it through school and learned to spell and pronounce medical terms like "otorhinolaryngologist." Thanks to my sisters, Alisha and Karry, for their encouragement. I would also like to thank the physicians that I have worked with in the past, especially Dr. Brad Burns, Dr. Robert Wray, and my brother, Dr. Terry Watson, for their willingness to share and teach so that I might have a greater understanding of the healthcare industry. I would never have entered the medical field were it not for the foresight of Harry and Zylphia Dickerson, who founded the school where I obtained my medical assistant training. Without their dream of educating medical assistants, I would not have had the opportunities that have been placed before me over the years. It was with Carole Cannefax in mind that I pictured this book in use. She made my medical assistant courses intriguing, and without a great instructor, the textbook cannot take on life and reach the students.

Last, my family deserves so many thanks, because they allowed me to work on this text when they would rather have had me to themselves. My children—Jimmie, Jonathan, and Jessica—inspire me daily. Yes, Jonathan, the book is finished now. And to my precious husband, Jerry Homolka, thank you for your love and for encouraging me to do what I love the most in life—to write.

Alexandra Patricia Young, BBA, CMA, RMA
Dallas, Texas
February 2003

Contents

UNIT TWO
Administrative Medical Assisting

UNIT THREE
Financial Management

UNIT FOUR
Medical Practice and Health Information Management

UNIT FIVE
Assisting With Medical Specialties

UNIT SIX
Career Development

List of Procedures

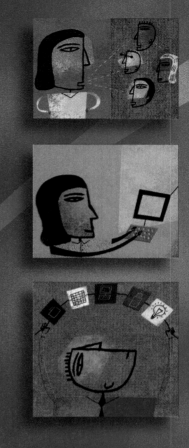

Introduction

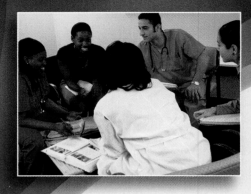

CHAPTER 1

Scenario

Shawna Long is a newly admitted student in a medical assistant program at your school. Shawna is anxious about starting classes and very concerned that she may not be a successful student. She had trouble with some of her classes in high school and must continue to work part-time while taking medical assistant classes. Based on what you discover about the learning process in this chapter, see if you can help Shawna take steps toward success.

Becoming a Successful Student

Deborah B. Kennedy

Learning Objectives

- Define and spell the terms listed in the vocabulary.
- Assess the importance of developing professional behaviors as a member of the allied health team.
- Evaluate the concept of critical thinking and how it affects your actions.
- Examine your learning preferences.
- Interpret how your learning style impacts your success as a student.
- Apply time management strategies to make the most of your learning opportunities.
- Utilize problem-solving techniques to manage conflict and barriers to your success.
- Integrate effective study skills into your daily activities.
- Design test-taking strategies that help you take charge of your success.
- Incorporate critical thinking and reflection to make mental connections as material is learned.

Vocabulary

critical thinking The constant practice of considering all aspects of a situation when deciding what to believe or what to do.

empathy Sensitivity to the individual needs and reactions of patients.

learning style The way that an individual perceives and processes information to learn new material.

perceiving How an individual looks at information and sees it as real.

processing How an individual internalizes new information and makes it his or her own.

professional behaviors Those actions that identify the medical assistant as a member of a healthcare profession including dependability, respectful patient care, initiative, positive attitude, and teamwork.

reflection The process of considering new information and internalizing it to create new ways of examining information.

You have taken the first step to becoming a successful student by choosing your profession and field of study. The medical assistant profession is both challenging and rewarding. Becoming a medical assistant opens the doors to a wide variety of opportunities in both administrative and clinical practice at ambulatory or institutional healthcare settings. Medical assistants are important members of the healthcare team, and as a healthcare professional you will be expected to practice certain **professional behaviors** (Figure 1-1). These professional behaviors, which are discussed in depth in Chapter 4, include dependability, respectful patient care, **empathy**, initiative, positive attitude, and teamwork. In order to become a successful medical assistant you must first become a successful student. This chapter helps you to discover the way that you learn best and provides multiple strategies to assist you in your journey toward success.

CRITICAL THINKING APPLICATION

Consider your history as a student. What do you think helped you to succeed? What do you think needs improvement? Create a plan for improvement that includes two or three ways you can become a more successful student.

Who You Are As a Learner: How Do You Learn Best?

Think about what you do when you are faced with something new to learn. How do you go about understanding and learning the new material? Over time you have developed a method for **perceiving** and **processing** information. This pattern of behavior is called your **learning style.** There are many different ways of examining learning styles, but most professionals agree that the success of students depends more on whether they can "make sense" of the information rather than on whether or not they are "smart." Education that is based on attention to individual learning styles is sensitive to the different ways that students learn and approaches new material with a wide variety of methods so that all students have the opportunity to learn. Determining your individual learning style and understanding how it applies to your ability to learn new material are the first steps to becoming a successful student (Figure 1-2).

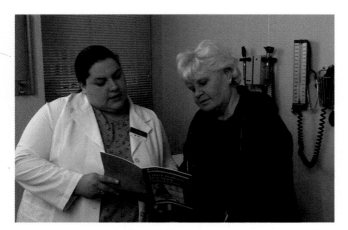

FIGURE 1-1 Professional interaction with patient.

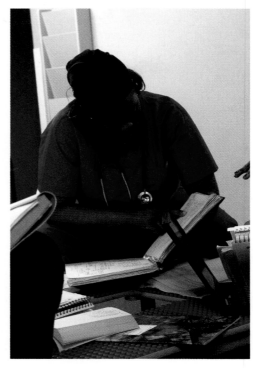

FIGURE 1-2 Student learning.

Learning Style Inventory

For you to learn new material, two things must happen. First you must perceive the information. This is the method you have developed over time that helps you examine the material and recognize it as real. Then you must process the information. Processing the information is how you internalize it and make it your own. By investigating various learning styles, you can figure out how to combine different methods of perceiving and processing information. In his book *Becoming a Master Student*, David Ellis discusses these different methods of information perception, processing, and learning.*

Information perception involves how you go about examining new material and making it real. There are two ways learners perceive new material. Some people are concrete perceivers who learn information through direct experience by doing, acting, sensing, or feeling. *Concrete* learners prefer to learn things that have a personal meaning or things that they feel are relevant. Other learners are *abstract* perceivers who take in information through analysis, observation, and **reflection.** Abstract learners like to think things through. They analyze the new material and build theories to help understand it. They prefer structured learning situations and use a step-by-step approach to problem solving.

Information processing is how you internalize the new information and make it your own. There are also two different methods for processing material. *Active* processors prefer to jump in and start doing things immediately. They make sense of the new material by immediately using it. They look for practical ways to apply the new material and typically do not mind taking risks to get the desired results. They learn best with practice and hands-on activities. *Reflective* processors, however, have to think about the information before they can internalize it. They prefer to observe and consider what is going on. The only way they can make sense of new material is to spend time thinking and learning a great deal about it before acting.

CRITICAL THINKING APPLICATION

- Consider the two ways to perceive new material. Are you a concrete perceiver who ties the information to a personal experience or do you prefer abstract perception in which you like to analyze or reflect on the meaning of the material? Choose which one you think most accurately describes your method of investigating new information.
- Then think about the way you process learning. Are you an active processor who is always looking for the practical application of what you learn or are you a reflective processor who has to think about new material before internalizing it?
- After completing this activity write down the combination of your perceiving/processing learning style and share it with your instructor.

---

*Ellis D: *Becoming a master student*, ed 10. Boston, 2002, Houghton Mifflin.

Using Your Learning Profile to be a Successful Student: Where Do I Go from Here?

No one falls completely into one or the other of these categories. However, by being aware of how we generally prefer to first perceive information and then process it, we can be more sensitive to our learning style and can approach new learning situations with a plan for learning the material in a way that best suits our learning preferences. Your preferred perceiving/processing learning profile will fall into one of the following stages in the Learning Style Inventory created by David Kolb of Case Western Reserve University.

Learners in *Stage 1* have a concrete/reflective style. These students want to know the purpose of the information and have a personal connection to the content. They like to consider a situation from many different points of view, observe others, and plan before taking action. Their strengths are in understanding people, brainstorming, and recognizing and creatively solving problems. If you fall into this stage, you enjoy small group activities and learn well in study groups.

Stage 2 learners have an abstract/reflective style. These students are eager to learn just for the sheer pleasure of learning rather than because the material relates to their personal lives. They like to learn lots of facts and arrange new material in a logical and clear manner. Stage 2 learners plan studying and like to create ways of thinking about the material but do not always make the connection with the practical application of the material. If you are a Stage 2 learner, you prefer organized, logical presentations of material and therefore enjoy lectures and generally dislike group work. You also need time to process and think about the new material before applying it.

Learners in *Stage 3* have an abstract/active style. Learners with this combination of learning style want to experiment and test the information that they are learning. If you are a Stage 3 learner, you want to know how techniques or ideas work and you also want to practice what you are learning. Your strengths are in problem solving and decision making, but you may lack focus and be hasty when making decisions. You learn best with hands-on practice by doing experiments, projects, and lab activities. You also enjoy working alone or in small groups (Figure 1-3).

Stage 4 is made up of concrete/active learners. These students are concerned about how they can use what they learn to make a difference in their lives. If you fall into this stage, you like to relate new material to other areas of your life. You have leadership capabilities, can create on your feet, and are usually vocal in a group, but you may have difficulty completing your work on time. Stage 4 learners enjoy teaching others and working in groups and learn best when they can apply the new information to real-world problems (Figure 1-4).

To get the most out of knowing your learning profile, you need to apply this knowledge to how you approach learning. There are pluses and minuses to each of the learning stages. When faced with a learning situation that does not match your learning preference, see how you can adapt your individual learning to make the best of the information. For example, if you are bored by lectures, look for an opportunity to apply the information being

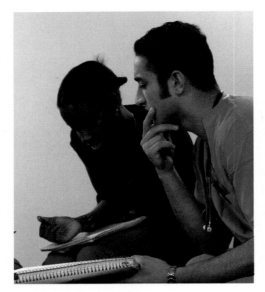

FIGURE 1-3 Learning in a small group.

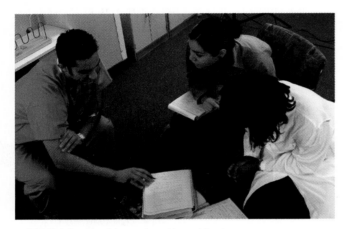

FIGURE 1-4 Teaching and working with others.

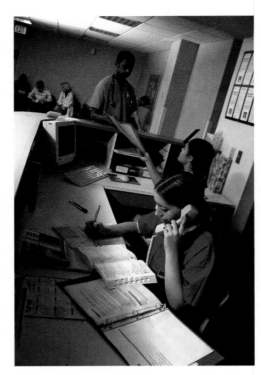

FIGURE 1-5 Time management in a busy medical practice.

presented to a real problem you are facing in the classroom or at home. If you are an abstract perceiver, take time outside of class to think about new information so that you are ready to process it into your learning system. If you benefit from learning in a group, make the effort to organize review sessions and study groups. If you learn best by teaching others, offer to assist your peers with their learning. By taking the time now to investigate your preferred method of learning, you will perceive and process information more effectively throughout your school career.

CRITICAL THINKING APPLICATION

Take a few minutes to reflect on a time when you really enjoyed learning about something new. How was the material presented and what did you do to "make it your own"? What do you need to do to become a more effective learner?

Time Management: Putting Time on Your Side

One of the most complicated tasks for a professional medical assistant is to effectively manage time. No other workplace can compete with the distractions and demands of a busy healthcare setting. Do you think that you practice effective time management skills? Do you believe that you are in control of your time or do you think that other people or situations control it? How frequently do you say that you just do not have enough time to do what you are supposed to do, let alone those things you would like to do? Time management gives you the opportunity to spend time in the way you choose. Effective time management is also crucial to your success as a student and as a future healthcare professional (Figure 1-5).

How to Put Time on Your Side

The following time management skills are designed to help you effectively deal with the demands on your time. Highlight the ones that you think will be most useful in helping you deal with your situation.

1. *Determine your purpose.* What do you want to accomplish this semester, in this course, or in this unit of study? What do you want to achieve as a student? What is one thing you can do to help achieve your goals?
2. *Identify your main concern.* Besides school, what other demands do you have on your time? Based on the learning goals you have established, what do you need to do to accomplish your goals?

- Plan time: Schedule projects in advance with notes to yourself on deadlines.
- Use down time: Take your work with you everywhere you go. Do small bits at every opportunity.
- Guard time: Avoid distractions (e.g., television, music) that will interfere with your concentration. Notice how others abuse your time. Learn to say no to outside demands on your time.
- Discover time: Steal time from other activities in your schedule.
- Assign time: Ask for help when you need it from friends and family.

3. *Be organized.* What materials (e.g., books, research, supplies) do you need to have an effective study session? What preparation is needed to make the most of your time?
   - Record time: Use a day planner or calendar to write down due dates for assignments and tests.
   - Optimal time: Take advantage of the time of day when you study and learn the best.

4. *Stop procrastinating.* If you avoid working on your goals, you may not achieve them. Examine the following suggestions as ways to break the procrastination cycle.
   - Make the work meaningful: What is important about the work you are putting off and what are the benefits of getting it done?
   - Plan work deadlines: Break assignments into achievable sections that can be completed in the time slots available.
   - Ask for help: Let your support system know you have work to get done. Ask them for encouragement to stay on track.
   - Prioritize: If you keep avoiding a certain task, re-evaluate its priority. If it is really worth worrying about, get started now not later.
   - Reward yourself: Create a reward that is meaningful and something you will work for. If you want to spend time with your family or friends on the weekend, develop a plan and stick to it so you can share that special time as a reward.

5. *Remember you.* It is very easy to become overwhelmed with responsibilities both in school and at home. Part of successful time management includes setting aside time to do things you enjoy. You have chosen a profession that can be very demanding. Now is the time to remember that you have to take care of yourself as well as meet your professional and personal responsibilities. So remember to plan some time for yourself as well (Figure 1-6).

CRITICAL THINKING APPLICATION

How do you spend your time? Over 3 days this week write down the amount of time you spend on each activity. How much TV do you watch? How much time do you talk on the phone? How about driving time, visiting time, work time, time for family and friends, and so on? At the end of the 3-day period, add up the various categories of time. Do you

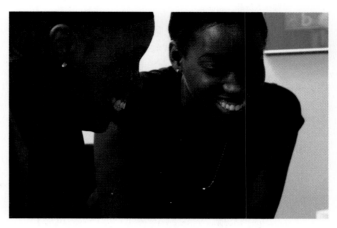

FIGURE 1-6   Making time for you.

recognize any time you might be wasting? Can you implement any of the suggested time management strategies to make more time available?

Problem Solving and Conflict Management

As a future member of the healthcare team, you will frequently face problems and conflict. Although we usually look at these situations as negative factors in our lives, problem solving and conflict management actually give us the opportunity to positively impact a potentially negative situation. Learning how to manage problems can be very useful for your practice as a medical assistant, as well as for your success as a student.

The first step in reaching an equitable solution to a problem or conflict situation is to identify the central issue. How many times have you known that you were upset about something but were not really sure why? You cannot solve a problem or a negative situation unless you are sure what is at the root of your feelings. You need to understand the problem and gather as much information about the situation as possible before you decide to act. One way of doing this is to ask yourself these questions:

- When does the situation occur and under what circumstances?
- Is there someone else involved?
- What interferes with making a decision or solving the conflict?

Once you understand the situation and how you feel about it, you need to decide if it is worth the effort to solve it. Prioritize your involvement. Sometimes there are situations and problems that you are unable to solve or ones that you decide are not important enough for you to act on.

After you have gathered the details about the problem or conflict, and you have decided to act, it is time to determine possible solutions. One way to do this is to ask for advice or brainstorm ideas with individuals you respect. Sometimes another person can give you special insight into the problem that you were unable to see on your own. After brainstorming for possible solutions, get feedback regarding the workability of the suggested solutions. Another way of approaching the problem is to list the pros and cons of possible solutions. Simply looking at a list of the positive and negative aspects of the solution may clarify how you should solve the problem. Before deciding on a solution, critically analyze the consequences of each proposed solution: Which one best meets your needs and has the potential of providing an outcome you can live with?

Finally you are ready to implement the chosen solution. However, your work is not over yet. You need to evaluate the outcome of your decision and see if it truly did meet your needs. If not, it may be time to review possible solutions and try another approach.

Conflict management requires some additional consideration. If you are in conflict with a peer, instructor, or co-worker, it is important to follow certain guidelines. You should attempt to solve the conflict in a private place at a prescheduled time. This ensures that the person will meet with you and that neither one has to worry about others overhearing the conversation. At the meeting clearly state your feelings about the conflict and how you would like it solved. Then try to come to an agreeable solution. The best way to deal with conflict situations is through open, honest, assertive communication. However, just as with problem solving, it is important to follow up on the decided course of action to see if it effectively dealt with the source of the conflict (Figure 1-7).

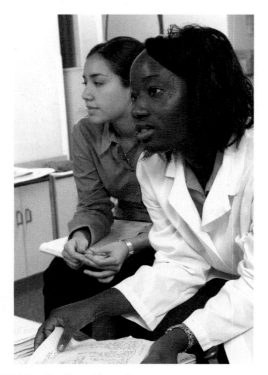

FIGURE 1-7 Dealing with conflict.

CRITICAL THINKING APPLICATION

Think about a serious problem you are currently facing. Utilize the brainstorming and/or pros-and-cons method for creating solutions to the problem. Implement your chosen solution and follow up on its effectiveness. Did the problem-solving process help you manage the situation more effectively?

Study Skills: Tricks to Becoming a Successful Student

So far in this chapter we have looked at the influence of individual learning styles and time management on learning success. Now we will investigate some ideas that are useful in learning new material. These study skills include memory techniques, active learning, brain tricks, reading methods, and note-taking strategies.

There are several techniques you can utilize to help you store and remember information. The first of these involves organizing information into recognizable groups so the brain can easily find it. You can organize information by getting the big picture first before trying to learn the details. One way to implement this strategy is to skim a reading assignment before actually reading and taking notes on the material, thus getting a general impression of what you need to learn before tackling the details. Depending on your learning style, it may also help to find a way of making the new information meaningful. Think about your educational goals and how the new material will help you achieve those goals. Another way of remembering material is to create an association with something you already know. By grouping new material with already stored material, your brain will remember it much easier.

A useful study skill for some learners is to be physically active while learning. Some students learn best if they walk or talk out loud while studying. Besides encouraging learning, moving and talking while studying relieve boredom and keep you awake. Another way to be actively involved in learning is to use pictures or diagrams to represent the material you are studying. Some people are visual learners, and creating pictures of the material is the easiest method for them to retain the information. Other students find that rewriting notes or making lists of information helps them retain the material. Writing also helps those students who need to "do" something in order to learn.

Studying will go much smoother if you work with your brain rather than against it. If you tend to get anxious and worried while studying, you may act as your own worst enemy. One way of dealing with a topic that you find anxiety producing is to overlearn it. If material is overlearned, you are much less likely to experience test anxiety. Another method for remembering material is to quickly review it after class. This mini-review will help the new information become part of your long-term memory system. Many students find creating songs, dances, or word associations an effective way to learn and remember new material. Putting details into a familiar song and moving to it can help trick the brain into remembering the information. This is especially helpful when trying to learn anatomy and physiology. Another excellent way of learning information is to actually teach it to someone else. Teaching requires you to have a good understanding of the material as well as the ability to describe it for others. It can be an effective reinforcer of complicated material (Figure 1-8).

A great deal of the learning process is expected to take place from assigned readings. There are methods that you can use to make reading assignments more meaningful. If you find a reading assignment challenging or difficult to understand, the first step is to take the time to read it again. Sometimes the first time through the material is not enough to gain understanding. As you read, highlight important words or thoughts and stop periodically to summarize the material. If you get bored while reading, use your body—walk or talk your way through the assignment. Take the time to look up words or terms you do not understand or ask your instructor or tutor for help. Outlining the material can help you create a brief overview of what you need to learn. And finally, the best way to determine if you learned anything from your reading is to try to explain it to someone else. If that is effective, you know you acquired the knowledge needed from the reading assignment.

Many students find effective note taking a challenge. The big question is, "How much of what the instructor says do I actually need to write down?" The first step in effective note taking is to come to class prepared. The more familiar you are with the material, the easier it will be to determine the important parts of the instructor's lecture. Pay attention to the instructor and look for clues about what he or she thinks is important. Ask questions about the material if you do not understand it rather than writing down information that makes no sense to you. Think critically about what you hear before you write it down so you can start to build relationships between what you want or need to know.

When it comes to actual note taking, there are some strategies that can make the process of recording notes an active learning tool. Organize the information as much as possible while you are writing in either an outline or paragraph format. Use only one side of the paper for easier reading and leave blank spaces where needed to fill in details later. Use key words to help you remember the material and create pictures or diagrams to help visualize it. If permitted, use tape recorders when appropriate and make sure you have either handouts or notes that cover material written on the board, in an overhead, or in a PowerPoint presentation. Another helpful tool is to develop your own system of abbreviations to help simplify the writing load.

The most effective way to use your notes is to review them shortly after class. This is the time to add details, clarify information, or make notes about asking the instructor for explanations during the next class. You could even exchange notes with students you trust to compare information (Figure 1-9). Some students find it beneficial to type or rewrite their notes. This can give you an opportunity to learn the material as you are transcribing it. As you are reviewing your notes you can also draw mind maps of the information or diagram outlines to help you better understand and remember the material.

Creating mind maps is a way of representing the main idea of the topic and supporting important details with a figure or picture. Healthcare textbooks are made up of complicated concepts with multiple main ideas, each with its own important details. Mind maps are a way of consolidating complex details and organizing them into a format that is easier to remember. The Spider map example in Figure 1-10 presents a method for including several main ideas with details in one study guide. The Fishbone map in Figure 1-11 can be used to learn complicated causes of disease. The Chain of Events map in

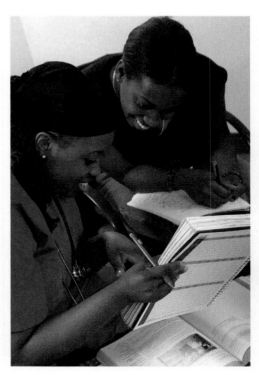

FIGURE 1-9   Sharing notes.

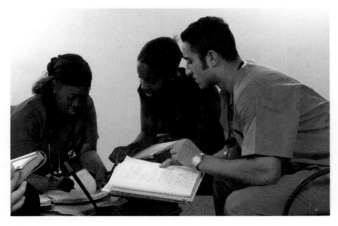

FIGURE 1-8   Effective study skills.

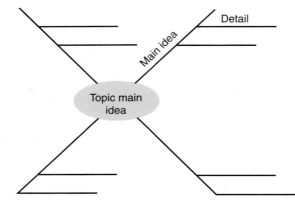

FIGURE 1-10 Spider map displays multiple main ideas with supporting details.

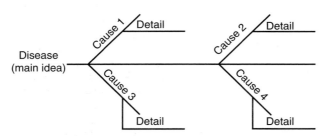

FIGURE 1-11 Fishbone map used to describe causes of disease.

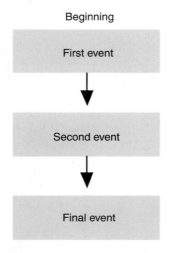

FIGURE 1-12 Chain of events map displays the cause and effect of events.

Figure 1-12 displays the cause and effect of events such as infection control or the history of medicine. The Cycle map in Figure 1-13 shows the connection between factors such as with the chain of infection. Creating your own mind maps is a way of making the information more meaningful and easier for you to understand.

Although there are many techniques you can use to help you study, perhaps the most important one is your attitude toward learning. Some students fall into the "I can't possibly learn this material" trap. That type of attitude only leads to self-defeat. The way to solve barriers is to first recognize that they exist. Once you know your weak spots, use the suggested study skills to improve in those areas. Do not be afraid to ask questions or to seek

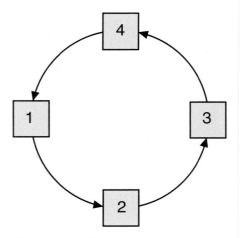

FIGURE 1-13 Cycle map shows how one action leads to another.

out help if you do not understand the material. Employ as many different strategies as necessary to become a successful student.

CRITICAL THINKING APPLICATION

Write down at least two barriers to your learning. Review the study skill suggestions above and choose four you want to try out. Use them over the next week to help you when learning new material. Reflect on whether the chosen study skills helped you learn the material better.

Test-Taking Strategies: Taking Charge of Your Success

What happens when you do not know the answer to the first question on a test? What if you do not know the next one? Are you able to go on without panicking? Many people find taking tests the most challenging part of being successful students. There are multiple approaches that you can employ to take charge of your success and improve your ability to take tests. These include such strategies as adequate preparation, controlling negative thoughts during test time, and understanding how to manage various types of questions.

The first step is to go into a test adequately prepared. Use the time management skills already outlined in this chapter to get prepared for the big day. Recognize and employ your preferred learning style to overlearn the material and increase your confidence. Use memory tools like flash cards, checklists, and mind maps to help visualize the material. Form a study group if you are the type of learner who benefits from studying in groups (Figure 1-14). Schedule and plan study time and reward yourself for your hard work. It is also important to go into the test rested and relaxed, so eat, exercise to relieve stress, and sleep before the test so that you are as alert as possible.

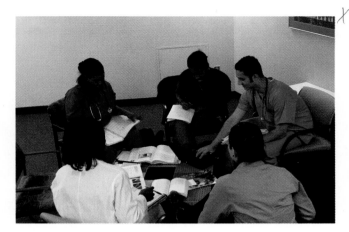

FIGURE 1-14 Study group.

Before you start the test make sure you read directions carefully and, if possible, begin with the easiest or shortest questions to build your confidence. Be aware of the amount of time allotted for the examination and pace yourself accordingly. As you go through the test, look for clues to answers in other questions. During test time remember to use positive self-talk at the first indication of panic. Repeatedly remind yourself that you are well prepared, relax, and think about the material before you get worried. You need to stop negative thoughts as soon as they arise, and instead visualize yourself being successful. Use slow deep breathing to relax and, if helpful, close your eyes for a minute and visualize a relaxing place before you go on with the test. You may find it helpful to wear a thick rubber band on your wrist and snap it as soon as you start to think negatively. This will provide a physical reaction to interfere with the power of your negative thoughts and serve as a reminder of what you should be concentrating on.

There are some strategies that you can employ when answering certain types of questions. With multiple choice questions, try to identify key words or clues in each question. Read the question carefully and answer it in your head before you review the provided answers. If you are not absolutely sure of the answer, make an educated guess or follow your instincts in choosing an answer. "True/false" questions give you a "50/50" chance of being correct. Remember that if any part of the question is not true, then the statement is false. Again, check the statements for key words that will help indicate the direction of the answer. Look for qualifying terms (e.g., "always," "never," "sometimes") that are key to understanding the meaning of the true/false statement.

CRITICAL THINKING APPLICATION

Think about a time you experienced test anxiety. Write down the details about the situation and how you felt. Choose four test-taking strategies that you think would be beneficial in handling similar situations in the future.

Becoming a Critical Thinker: Making Mental Connections

The ability to process information and arrive at reasonable conclusions is crucial to all healthcare workers. The process of **critical thinking** involves sorting out conflicting information, weighing the knowledge you possess about that information, ignoring or letting go of personal biases, and deciding on a reasonable belief or action. Critical thinking is actually an active search for the truth. Critical thinking could be described as thorough thinking because it requires learners to be open-minded to all possibilities. Successful students are thorough thinkers because they must determine the facts about the topic being learned and come to logical conclusions about the material. Critical thinkers are also inquisitive learners who are constantly in the process of analyzing and sorting out conflicting information to reach conclusions. A crucial step in critical thinking is evaluating the results of your learning. Reflection is key to critical thinking. "How did I learn what I learned" and "What does it mean in my life" are questions that must be consistently asked in order to continue to learn. Becoming a successful student and, ultimately, a successful member of the allied health team requires the possession of critical thinking skills. Both the material presented in this chapter and the critical thinking application exercises are designed to encourage you along this life-long learning path of critical thinking.

SUMMARY OF SCENARIO

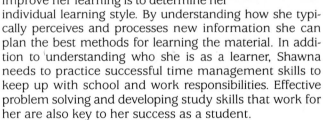

One of the things Shawna can do to improve her learning is to determine her individual learning style. By understanding how she typically perceives and processes new information she can plan the best methods for learning the material. In addition to understanding who she is as a learner, Shawna needs to practice successful time management skills to keep up with school and work responsibilities. Effective problem solving and developing study skills that work for her are also key to her success as a student.

SUMMARY OF LEARNING OBJECTIVES

- Medical assistants play a vital role in the healthcare team and are expected to display such professional behaviors as dependability, respectful patient care, empathy, initiative, positive attitude, and teamwork.
- Critical thinkers can evaluate conflicting information and make a decision to act based on their knowledge and willingness to be open-minded to all possibilities.
- Learning preferences are the ways that you like to learn and have proven successful in the past.
- Learning styles are determined by your individual method of perceiving or examining new material and the way that you process it or make it

your own. People are either concrete or abstract perceivers and either active or reflective processors.

■ Effective time management strategies such as setting goals, prioritizing, getting organized, and avoiding procrastination will make you a more successful student as well as an effective medical assistant.

■ Problem-solving and conflict-management techniques are key to your success. First, identify the central issue and how you feel about it; then consider possible solutions and their potential results, implement the chosen solution, and analyze the results.

■ Study skills such as memory techniques, active learning, brain tricks, effective reading methods, note-taking strategies, and mind maps all help students to be more successful.

■ Test-taking strategies include preparing adequately for the examination, controlling negative thoughts during the examination, and understanding how to deal with different types of questions.

■ Critical thinking can be described as thorough thinking because it considers all sides of the information without bias. Reflection is the process of thinking about or reviewing information before acting.

INTERNET CONNECTIONS

LEARNING STYLES

- AT&T Learning Network. What is Your Learning Style? A Self Quiz.
  www.att.com/learningnetwork/virtualacademy/success4.html
- Coastline Community College. Online Study Skill Module.
  http://pelican.ccc.cccd.edu/ ~ module/
- Fastrack Consulting. Online Learning Styles.
  www.fastrak-consulting.co.uk
- Funderstanding. About Learning Theories.
  www.funderstanding.com

TIME MANAGEMENT

- Learning Skills Program
  www.yorku.ca/cdc/lsp/lsphome.html

- Time Management Resources
  www.learningcommons.uoguelph.ca/learning/tmres-bhtm#links

STUDY SKILLS

- Memory Improvement
  www.memoryweb.freeuk.com/index.hts
- Strategies for Success
  www.mtsu.edu/ ~ studskl/

TEST-TAKING STRATEGIES

- Academic Success-CAPS
  www.unc.edu/depts/unv_caps/TestTake.html
- Study Guides and Test-taking Strategies
  www.eop.mu.edu/study/index.html
- Test Taking Strategies
  www.shsu.edu/ ~ counseltest_taking.html

CHAPTER 2

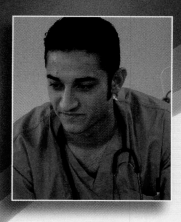

Scenario

Carlos Santos, CMA, is a medical assisting instructor with 10 years' experience in the clinical area. He has worked for a group of family practitioners and for an allergist during his career as a medical assistant. Mr. Santos believes that it is very important to give his students an overview of the healthcare industry early in their training. He feels that it is exciting to show them the history and progress of medicine and introduce them to the current types of facilities available for patient care on both a national and local level. This helps the student to understand where he or she fits in the whole picture as a medical assistant. Often Mr. Santos assigns the students a short report on one person who contributed to the growth of medicine. He finds that this is a good way to encourage the students to use the Internet right from the start of their training. It also offers the student a chance to grow more comfortable in speaking in front of a group. The knowledge that the students will learn about the different areas of patient care will be very useful once they graduate and begin working in a physician's office. They will frequently be required to provide patients with information about health and community resources. All of these skills will make Mr. Santos' students more versatile and valuable to their eventual employer.

The Healthcare Industry

National Curriculum Competencies

TRANSDISCIPLINARY COMPETENCIES

3e. Identify community resources

Vocabulary

accreditation The process through which an organization is recognized for adherence to a group of standards that meet or exceed expectations of the accrediting agency.

advent A coming into being or use.

allopathy A word coined by Samuel Christian Hahnemann to contrast homeopathic medicine with mainstream medicine; medicine supposedly characterized by an effort to counteract the symptoms of a disease by administration of treatments that produce an opposite effect from the symptoms.

ambulatory Able to walk about and not be bedridden.

amenities Something that contributes to comfort, enjoyment, or convenience.

cardiac arrhythmias Irregular heartbeat resulting from a malfunction of the electrical system of the heart.

case management The process of assessing and planning patient care, including referral and follow-up to ensure continuity of care and quality management.

chiropractic A medical discipline in which chiropractic physicians focus on the nervous system and painlessly, manually adjust the vertebral column to affect the nervous system, resulting in healthier patients.

cited Quoted by way of example, authority, or proof or mentioned formally in commendation or praise.

contamination A process by which something is made impure, unclean, or unfit for use by the introduction of unwholesome or undesirable elements.

credentialing The act of extending professional or medical privileges to an individual; the process of verifying and evaluating that person's credentials.

dissection Separation into pieces and exposure of parts for scientific examination.

encounter Any contact between a healthcare provider and a patient that results in treatment or evaluation of the patient's condition; not limited to in-person contact.

fermentation An enzymatically controlled transformation of an organic compound.

holistic Related to or concerned with all of the systems of the body, rather than breaking it down into parts.

indicators An important point or group of statistical values that, when evaluated, indicate the quality of care provided in a healthcare institution.

indicted Charged with a crime by the finding or presentment of a jury with due process of law.

indigent Totally lacking in something of need.

innate Existing in, belonging to, or determined by factors present in an individual since birth.

mysticism The experience of seeming to have direct communication with God or ultimate reality.

naturopathy An alternative to conventional medicine in which holistic methods are used, as well as herbs and natural supplements, with the belief that the body will heal itself. Naturopathic physicians can currently be licensed in 12 states.

osteopathy A medical discipline based primarily on the manual diagnosis and holistic treatment of impaired function resulting from loss of movement of all kinds of tissues.

pandemic Affecting the majority of the people in a country or a number of countries.

peer review organizations A group of medical reviewers contracted by the Centers for Medicare and Medicaid Services (CMS) (formerly HCFA) to ensure quality control and medical necessity of services provided by a facility.

philanthropist An individual who makes an active effort to promote human welfare.

putrefaction Decomposition of animal matter that results in a foul smell.

robotics Technology dealing with the design, construction, and operation of robots in automation.

staff privileges Allowance of a healthcare professional to practice within a specific facility.

standards Item or indicator used as a measure of quality or compliance with a statutory or accrediting body's policies and regulations.

subluxations Slight misalignments of the vertebrae or a partial dislocation.

telemedicine The use of telecommunications in the practice of medicine, in which great distances can exist between healthcare professionals, colleagues, patients, and students.

teleradiology The use of telecommunications devices to enhance and improve the results of radiological procedures.

treatises Systematic expositions or arguments in writing including a methodical discussion of the facts and principles involved and the conclusions reached.

triage The sorting of and allocation of treatment to patients according to a system of priorities designed to maximize the number of survivors and treat the sickest patients first.

In the first decade of the new millennium, the growth of the healthcare industry seems unstoppable. Thanks to modern technological advances, medicine speeds forward faster than ever in its quest to improve the health of humankind. **Telemedicine** is experiencing a significant growth spurt, and the images produced with **teleradiology** have vastly improved in their resolution. **Robotics** is assisting healthcare professionals in surgery and even delivers drugs to hospital floors using laser sensors. Education in medicine has grown exponentially: computers, the Internet, and video have enabled an instructor in New York to communicate with a student in Los Angeles. The key to this technology lies within the development and widespread use of elaborate information systems that have revolutionized the way that medicine is practiced today. The rate at which technology is advancing is clearly far ahead of the pace of 20 years ago, and we can barely imagine the benefits to healthcare of the future. This chapter looks back at the history of medicine, gazes at its present, and glances toward its future.

The History of Medicine

Medical Language and Mythology

Today's medicine uses words whose origins stem from the romance and fantasy of classical and ancient languages. In particular, the study of anatomy reaches back to the dawn of recorded history, and today's modern terms are almost unchanged from their original version. Some terms are inaccurate when translated literally, because the ancients did not fully understand body functions. For example, *artery*, which comes from the Greek word *arteria*, literally means "a windpipe." The Greeks believed that the arteries carried air, not blood. Greek and Roman mythology has contributed a major portion of our medical terminology, but we have also borrowed liberally from Arabic, Anglo-Saxon, and German sources. Several terms originate from the Bible.

The human head rests on the first cervical vertebra, which is called the *atlas*. Atlas was the famous Greek titan who was condemned by Zeus to bear the heavens on his shoulders. Achilles was held by the heel by his mother and dipped into the river Styx so that he would become invulnerable. However, his heel was not immersed, and he later died from a wound in that area. Thus a common expression used today to show a point of weakness is "Achilles heel." Aphrodite, the Greek goddess of love and beauty, is the source of the name for drugs used to enhance sexual arousal, called *aphrodisiacs*. The equivalent Roman goddess of love, Venus, is associated with lustful desires. A portion of the female anatomy, the mons veneris (mons pubis), as well as venereal diseases, was named after her. Venus carried quite a legacy into future centuries!

Aesculapius, the son of Apollo, was revered as the god of medicine. The early Greeks worshiped the healing powers of Aesculapius and built temples in his honor, where patients were treated by trained priests. His daughters were Hygeia, goddess of health, and Panacea, goddess of all healing and restorer of health. Our modern word "*hygiene*" has its origin in Hygeia, and the modern meaning for *panacea* is "a remedy for all ills and difficulties." A common medical icon is the staff of Aesculapius. It depicts a serpent encircling a staff and signifies the art of healing. The staff of Aesculapius has been adopted by the American Medical Association as the symbol of medicine. The mythological staff belonging to Apollo, the caduceus, which is a staff encircled by two serpents, is the medical insignia of the U.S. Army Medical Corps and is often misused as a symbol of the medical profession (Figure 2-1).

Medicine in Ancient Times

Although religious and mythological beliefs were the basis of care for the sick in ancient times, there is evidence of the use of drugs, surgery, and other treatments based on theories about the body from as early as 5000 BC. In the well-developed societies of the Egyptians, Babylonians, and Assyrians, certain men acted as physicians and used the little knowledge they had to try to treat illness and injury.

Moses presented rules of health to the Hebrews about 1205 BC. He was thus the first advocate of preventive medicine and is considered the first "public health officer." Moses knew that some animal diseases could be passed to humans and that **contamination** existed, so a religious law was developed forbidding humans to eat or drink from dirty dishes. The people of that era believed that doing so would defile their bodies, and they would lose their souls.

Hippocrates, known as the Father of Medicine, is the most famous of the ancient Greek physicians (Figure 2-2). He was born in 450 BC on the island of Cos in Greece. He is best remembered for the Hippocratic Oath, which his pupils repeated. This oath has been administered to physicians for more than 2000 years. Hippocrates is

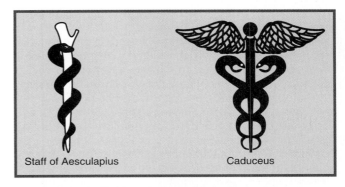

Staff of Aesculapius   Caduceus

FIGURE 2-1   Staff of Aesculapius and the caduceus.

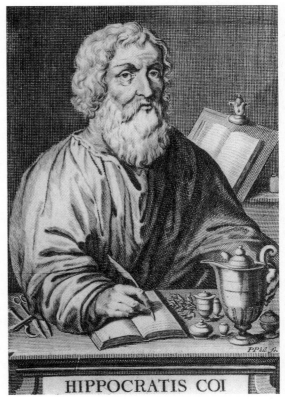

HIPPOCRATIS COI

FIGURE 2-2   Hippocrates is known as the Father of Medicine. (Courtesy the National Library of Medicine.)

credited with taking medicine from **mysticism** and giving it a scientific basis. During this period of history, most believed that illness was caused by demon possession, and to cure the illness, the demon must be removed from the body. Hippocrates' clinical descriptions of diseases and his volumes on epidemics, fevers, epilepsy, fractures, and instruments were studied for centuries. He believed that the body had the capacity to heal itself and that the physician's role was to help nature. Very little was known about anatomy, physiology, and pathology, and there was no knowledge of chemistry. Despite these limitations, many of the classifications of diseases and descriptions of symptoms that Hippocrates developed are still being used today.

Galen was a Greek physician who migrated to Rome in 162 AD and became known as the Prince of Physicians. He is said to have written more than 500 **treatises** on medicine. He wrote an excellent summary on anatomy as it was known at the time, but his work was faulty and inaccurate, because it was largely based on the **dissection** of apes and swine. He is considered the Father of Experimental Physiology and the first experimental neurologist. He was the first to describe the cranial nerves and the sympathetic nervous system, and he performed the first experimental section of the spinal cord, producing hemiplegia. Galen also produced aphonia by cutting the recurrent laryngeal nerve, and he gave the first valid explanation of the mechanism of respiration. Galen was also a champion of medical ethics: he felt that physicians "must learn to despise money," and that if a physician was interested in profit, he was not serious in his devotion to the art of medicine. His thoughts parallel those of many modern leaders in the healthcare industry. Although much of what he believed about the body was incorrect, his teachings remained intact until human dissections began, when physicians were able to visualize exactly what was inside the human body.

Because both Hippocrates and Galen were highly respected, the authority of their observations went unquestioned, and this had a negative effect on the progress of science throughout the Dark Ages and well into the sixteenth century. Their theories and descriptions were considered immutable principles, so few physicians were innovative and curious enough to challenge them. Those who did experiment in medicine were scorned by their colleagues, and physicians continued to use methods that were at best ineffectual or innocuous and at worst harmful to the patient. However, the establishment of universities led to a study of theories of disease rather than observation of the sick.

Early Development of Medical Education

Medical knowledge developed slowly, and distribution of such knowledge was poor. Before the printing press was invented in the mid-fifteenth century, there was very little exchange of scientific knowledge and ideas, and scientists were not well informed about the investigations of others. The printing press allowed books to be distributed faster and over a widespread area. Another development important to science occurred in the seventeenth century, when European academies or societies were established, consisting of small groups of men who met to discuss subjects of mutual interest. The academies provided freedom of expression that, with the stimulus of exchanging ideas, contributed significantly to the development of scientific thought.

One of the earliest of the academies was the Royal Society of London, formed in 1662. A significant aspect of this organization was their publications, such as *Philosophical Transactions*. The development of communications during this era was important.

Society became more complex over the centuries, which prompted a greater need for regulation. The passage of the Medical Act of 1858 in Great Britain was considered one of the most important events in British medicine. It established a statutory body, the General Medical Council, which controlled admission to the medical register and had great power over medical education and examinations.

In the United States, medical education was greatly influenced by the Johns Hopkins University Medical School in Baltimore, Maryland. The school admitted only college graduates with a year's training in the natural sciences. Its clinical work was superior because the school partnered with Johns Hopkins Hospital, which had been created expressly for teaching and research by members of the medical faculty. The first four professors at Johns Hopkins were Sir William Osler (Professor of Medicine), William H. Welch (Chief of Pathology), Howard A. Kelley (Chief of Gynecology and Obstetrics), and William D. Halsted (Chief of Surgery). Together these four men transformed the organization and curriculum of clinical teaching and made Johns Hopkins the most famous medical school in the world. The earliest medical school **accreditation** resulted from a report published by Abraham Flexner. He received a grant from the Carnegie Foundation Commission to study the quality of medical colleges in the United States and Canada. His report, called the Flexner Report, resulted in the closure of many low-ranking schools and the upgrading of others. These events legitimized medical education and opened new doors for many individuals to the world of medicine.

CRITICAL THINKING APPLICATION

- Mr. Santos asks his class to identify which of the individuals involved in early medicine have had the most impact on modern healthcare. Which would you choose and why?
- The students point out that early research was often viewed in a negative manner. How does research affect us now and how is it viewed by the public?

Early Medical Pioneers

Andreas Vesalius (1514 to 1564) was a Belgian anatomist known as the Father of Modern Anatomy (Figure 2-3). At the age of 29 he published his great *De Corporis Humani Fabrica*, in which he described the structure of the human body. This work marked a turning point by

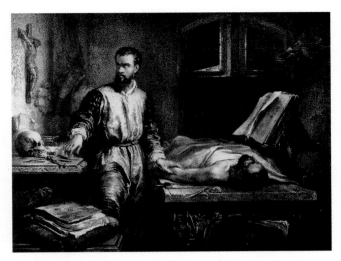

FIGURE 2-3   Andreas Vesalius is known as the Father of Modern Anatomy. (Courtesy National Library of Medicine.)

breaking with past traditional beliefs in Galen's theories. Vesalius introduced many new anatomical terms, but because of his radical approach, he was subjected to some persecution from his colleagues, teachers, and pupils. Despite his great contributions to the science of anatomy, his name is not used to identify any important anatomic structures.

Other important advances and discoveries took place throughout the world. Gabriele Fallopius (1523 to 1562), an Italian student of Vesalius, was also an accurate dissector. He described and named many parts of the human anatomy. He named the oviducts, or fallopian tubes, after himself, and also named the vagina and placenta. In 1628 William Harvey (1578 to1657) announced his discovery that the heart acts as a muscular pump, forcing and propelling the blood throughout the body. He revealed that the blood's motion is a continuous cycle, basing his conclusion on his experimental vivisection, ligation, and perfusion as well as brilliant reasoning. Harvey's writings were recognized in Germany before the English permitted their publication at home. Modern England now considers Harvey to be its medical Shakespeare.

There were few great advances in medicine for a century or more, but the unseen world of microorganisms was first revealed by Anton van Leeuwenhoek (1632 to 1723), a Dutch linen draper and haberdasher. Haberdashers made their living dealing in men's clothing and accessories, but Leeuwenhoek's hobby of grinding lenses eventually led to his discovery of the magnification process. He ground more than 400 lenses during his lifetime, some of which were no larger than a pinhead. In the grinding process, Leeuwenhoek learned how to use a simple biconvex lens to magnify the minute world of organisms and structures, which had never been seen before. Leeuwenhoek was the first to ever observe bacteria and protozoa through a lens, and his accurate interpretations of what he saw led to the sciences of bacteriology and protozoology.

Marcello Malpighi (1628 to 1694) was born near Bologna, Italy and attended the University of Bologna, where he earned a doctorate in both medicine and philosophy. He pioneered the use of the microscope in the study of plants and animals, after which microscopic anatomy became a prerequisite for advances in physiology, embryology, and practical medicine. In 1661 he described the pulmonary and capillary network connecting the smallest arteries with the smallest veins. This was one of the most important discoveries in the history of science, and it validated Harvey's work. Malpighi is commonly regarded as the first histologist.

Scientific Advances in the Eighteenth and Nineteenth Centuries

English scientist John Hunter (1728 to 1793) is known as the Founder of Scientific Surgery. An army surgeon, he became an expert on gunshot wounds and experimented with tissue transfer. His surgical procedures were soundly based on pathological evidence. He was the first to classify teeth in a scientific manner and introduced artificial feeding by means of a flexible tube passed into the stomach. He provided a classic description of the syphilitic chancre, which is sometimes called a *hunterian* chancre. During his studies of venereal diseases, he inoculated himself with what he thought was gonorrhea, but instead he acquired syphilis. His results in this study actually caused confusion in the medical community, because he mistakenly thought that gonorrhea was a symptom of syphilis. This confusion was not corrected until the beginning of the twentieth century. His collection of anatomic and animal specimens formed the basis for the museum of the Royal College of Surgeons. After Hunter's death he was buried in St. Martin. His remains were later moved, however, to Westminster Abbey as a gesture of honor, and a tablet was placed over his grave by the Royal College of Surgeons to "record their admiration of his genius as a gifted interpreter of the Divine Power and Wisdom at work in the laws of Organic Life and their grateful veneration for his services to mankind as the Founder of Scientific Surgery." Today in Australia, the John Hunter Hospital serves more than 570 inpatients and 980 outpatients per day.

Edward Jenner (1749 to 1823) was a student of John Hunter and a country physician from Dorsetshire, England. He is considered one of the immortals of preventive medicine for his development of the smallpox vaccine. While Jenner was serving as an apprentice, he assisted in treating a dairymaid. Smallpox was mentioned and she commented, "I cannot take that disease, for I have had cowpox." Smallpox at that time was a deadly **pandemic**. Jenner observed that those who had contracted cowpox never contracted smallpox. Later, as a practicing physician, Jenner continued investigating the relationship between cowpox and smallpox almost obsessively, and the medical society members grew bored with his obsession and threatened to expel him from their ranks. On May 14, 1796 Dr. Jenner took purulent matter from a pustule on the hand of Sarah Nelmes, a dairymaid, and inserted it through two small superficial incisions into the arm of James Phipps, a healthy 8-year-old boy. This was the first vaccination. On July 1 a virulent dose of smallpox matter was given to the boy in the same arm. Phipps' vaccination kept him safe from the dreaded disease, and Jenner's method of vaccination spread throughout the world. The results of his experiments were published in 1798. He called this method of protection *vaccination*, from the Latin word *vacca*, which means "cow," and at that time, cowpox was called *vaccinia*. Today smallpox has been eradicated throughout the world as a result of a planned program of world vaccination.

Austrian physician Leopold Auenbrugger (1722 to 1809) developed the use of percussion in diagnosis. He became physician-in-chief to the Hospital of the Holy Trinity at Vienna in 1751, and there he tested his discovery. Although scorned and ignored by his contemporaries, his techniques later made him famous and are still used today during physical examinations. René Laennec (1781 to 1826) was a French physician who developed the stethoscope in 1819. At first, he used only a cylinder of rolled paper in his hands, then a wooden device was used for its sound-conducting properties. With today's sophisticated stethoscopes physicians are able to hear sounds in the body, including a fetus inside the mother. Laennec's book, *Treatise on Mediate Auscultation and Diseases of the Chest*, was readily accepted and translated into many languages. It is said to be the most important treatise on diseases of the thoracic organs ever written.

Several men of the early 1800s are remembered for their fight against puerperal fever and their concern for women's health. Puerperal fever, an infectious disease that can be contracted during childbirth, was also called *puerperal sepsis* or *childbed fever*. The term *puerperal*, denoting a woman in childbed, originates from the Latin *puer*, "a child," and *pario*, "to bring forth." The word *puerperium* now designates the period from delivery to the time the uterus returns to normal size (about 42 days after childbirth).

The best known of these men was the Hungarian physician Ignaz Philipp Semmelweis (1818 to 1865); history has called him the Savior of Mothers. His fight against puerperal fever is a sad story of hardships. His theories were resisted by many professionals, including his instructors. Semmelweis noted that the fever often attacked women who were delivered by medical students coming straight from the autopsy or dissecting rooms. Semmelweis directed that in his wards, the students were to wash and disinfect their hands before going to examine the women and deliver the children. This process brought about a marked reduction of cases of puerperal fever on his ward, but he still faced unrelenting opposition. As his theories were proved correct, Semmelweis felt an incredible guilt that the doctors themselves had caused so many deaths. He died at the age of 47—ironically, from the very infection he had fought. He was infected with puerperal fever from a cut on his finger during an autopsy. His grave had hardly been closed when scientists began to understand the causes of this disease, largely as a result of the investigations of two great scientists, Louis Pasteur and Joseph Lister.

Pasteur (1822 to 1895) was a Frenchman who did brilliant work as a chemist, but it was his studies in bacteriology that made him one of the most famous men in medical history (Figure 2-4). He was bestowed the title of Father of Bacteriology and has also been honored as

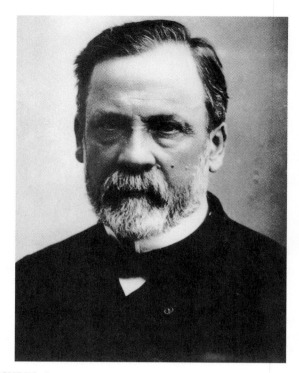

FIGURE 2-4 Louis Pasteur was a brilliant chemist who made numerous contributions to medicine. (Courtesy National Library of Medicine.)

the Father of Preventive Medicine. He gave unselfishly of his time outside his profession to help others solve problems. Pasteur's adventures included studying the difficulties in the **fermentation** of wine. He averted disaster in the most important industry of France at that time, winemaking, by a process he developed, now called *pasteurization*; this achievement alone would have made him an immortal among the French. Through a process of supplying enough heat to destroy microorganisms, wine was prevented from turning to vinegar. The French people called on Pasteur again to help the ailing silkworm industry. He devoted 5 years to the conquest of diseases that infected the silkworm. His efforts were impeded when he was stricken with hemiplegia, but after a long, difficult recovery, he was able to continue with a stiff hand and a limp.

Convinced that the infinite world of bacteria held the key to the secrets of contagious diseases, Pasteur left chemistry again to continue studying his theory. Many renowned scientists denied the germ theory of disease and devoted themselves to degrading Pasteur's theories and experiments. In the midst of this controversy, he became involved in the prevention of anthrax, which threatened the health of cattle and sheep. Pasteur was eventually honored for his work on many other diseases, such as rabies, chicken cholera, and swine erysipelas. He devoted the last 7 years of his life to the Pasteur Institute, which was founded as a clinic for rabies treatment, a research center for infectious disease, and a teaching center. The Pasteur Institute still exists today. He died in 1895, with his family at his bedside. It is said that his last words were, "There is still a great deal to do."

Joseph Lister (1827 to 1912) revolutionized surgery through the application of Pasteur's discoveries. He understood the similarity between infections in postsurgical wounds and the processes of **putrefaction**. Pasteur had proved that these processes were caused by microorganisms. Before this time surgeons had accepted that infections in surgical wounds were inevitable. Lister reasoned that microorganisms must be the cause of infection and should be kept out of wounds. His colleagues were indifferent to his theories, because most believed infections were God-given and natural. Lister disagreed, and he developed antiseptic methods by using carbolic acid for sterilization. By spraying the rooms with a fine mist of the acid, soaking the instruments in carbolic solutions, and washing his hands in a similar solution, he was able to prove his theories. He is honored as the Father of Sterile Surgery. Pasteur and Lister met after years of great mutual admiration. The meeting was filled with emotion, and it was written in *Pathfinders in Medicine* that "a new star should have appeared in the heavens to commemorate the event." Medicine truly owes a deep gratitude to these two pioneers for the knowledge they imparted to the art.

Robert Koch (1843 to 1910) is a familiar name to all bacteriologists, because of his famous Koch's Postulates. These are his theory of rules that must be followed before an organism can be accepted as the causative agent in a given disease. Koch was a German physician who earned great honors in bacteriology and public health. He introduced many of the tools used in the laboratory, such as the culture-plate method for isolation of bacteria. He discovered the cause of cholera and demonstrated its transmission by food and water. This discovery completely transformed health departments and proved the importance of bacteriology in everyday life. Koch's greatest disappointment was his failure to find a cure for tuberculosis, but in his attempt he isolated tuberculin, the substance produced by tubercle bacteria. Its use as a diagnostic aid was of immense value to medicine. In 1885 the University of Berlin created the Chair of Hygiene and Bacteriology in honor of Robert Koch. He became the Nobel Laureate in 1905.

One of Koch's students was a German physician named Paul Ehrlich (1854 to 1915). He pioneered the fields of bacteriology, immunology, and especially chemotherapy, which was a new science. He was only 28 when he wrote his first paper on typhoid, but his greatest gift to humanity was called his "magic bullet," or formula 606, which was designed to fight syphilis. With the organism identified by scientists Bordet and Wasserman, Ehrlich set out to find a chemical that would destroy the organism but not harm the host, specifically, the human body. The six hundred-sixth drug that Ehrlich tried finally brought about healing. He called it *salvarsan* because he believed that it offered mankind salvation from the disease. This endeavor also marked the beginning of the practice of injecting chemicals into the body to destroy a specific organism. In 1908 Ehrlich shared the Nobel Prize with Eli Metchnikoff, who is remembered for his theory of phagocytosis and immunology.

Crawford Williamson Long (1815 to 1878) was the first to employ ether as an anesthetic agent. Early in 1842 a group of students would have a social gathering after chemistry lectures and inhale ether, a chemical commonly found in chemistry labs, as a form of amusement. Ether, a similar intoxicant to nitrous oxide, functions as a soporific, or sleep-inducing agent. However, at one of these "ether frolics," as they were called, Dr. Long also observed that people under the influence of ether did not seem to feel pain. After considerable thought, he decided to use ether for a surgical operation. In March 1842 he removed a tumor from the neck of James M. Venable after placing him under the influence of ether. Dr. Horace Wells was a dentist who reported using nitrous oxide as an anesthetic in 1844. Another dentist, Dr. William T.G. Morton, reported using ether in 1846 when he extracted a tooth from a patient, and he also used the gas at Massachusetts General Hospital for a surgical procedure.

Surgeons are grateful to Wilhelm Konrad Roentgen (1845 to 1922), a professor of physics at the University of Wurzburg, Germany. Roentgen discovered the x-ray in 1895 while experimenting with electrical currents passed through sealed glass tubes. He was awarded the Nobel Prize in Physics in 1901. Although he called it an *x-ray*, history has honored him by calling it the *roentgen ray*. Marie and Pierre Curie discovered radium in 1898, and they were awarded the 1902 Nobel Prize in Physics for their work on radioactivity. Unfortunately, Pierre was killed 3 years later while crossing a street in a rainstorm. Marie was awarded his teaching position at the Sorbonne, a medical university in France, where no woman had taught in its 650-year history. In 1911 she was awarded the Nobel Prize for her discoveries of radium and polonium, the first person to receive the award twice. She died in 1934 from pernicious anemia, which was believed to have been caused by her overexposure to radiation and years of overwork.

Nineteenth Century Women in Medicine

Many other women made great contributions to medicine in the early nineteenth century. Florence Nightingale (1820 to 1910) is known as the founder of nursing and fondly called the Lady With the Lamp (Figure 2-5). She was of noble birth, and somewhat late in life she sought nurse's training in both England and Europe. By the dawn of the Crimean War in 1854, she had established a fine reputation for her work in hospital organization. She was invited by the British Secretary of War to visit the Crimea to help correct the terrible conditions that existed in caring for the wounded. She created the Women's Nursing Service in Scutari and Balaklava. The physicians treated her and the other 38 nurses poorly, until a crisis brought thousands of wounded and sick soldiers to the army hospitals. The bravery and competence of the nurses helped the doctors realize their value to the medical profession. In 1860 she founded the Nightingale School and Home for Nurses in London, which marked the beginning of professional nursing education.

Clara Barton (1821 to 1912), an American, began her nursing career early in life. When she was 11 years of age her brother fell from the roof of their barn, and

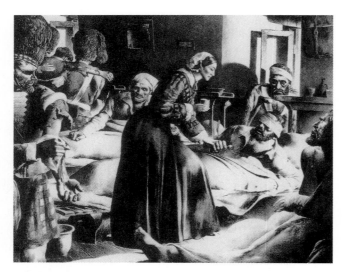

FIGURE 2-5 Considered the founder of nursing, Florence Nightingale is also known as the Lady With the Lamp. (Courtesy National Library of Medicine.)

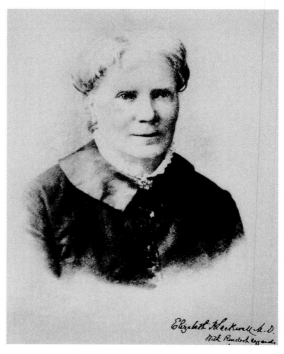

FIGURE 2-6 Elizabeth Blackwell was the first female to receive a degree as a medical doctor in the United States. (Courtesy National Library of Medicine.)

Clara nursed him back to health over a 2-year period. She later was a battlefield nurse and **philanthropist** whose work during the Civil War led her to recognize that very poor records were kept in Washington to aid in the search for missing men who were wounded or killed in combat. Her efforts to remedy this led to the formation of the Bureau of Records. Her organization and recruitment of supplies for the wounded led to her eventual involvement with the Red Cross in the Franco-Prussian War. In 1881 she organized a Red Cross Committee in Washington, forming the American Red Cross. She served as its first president from 1881 to 1904. Her retirement came at the age of 82, just after personally leading dangerous expeditions to help victims of fires, hurricanes, and floods.

Elizabeth Blackwell (1821 to 1910) was the first woman in the United States to receive the Doctor of Medicine degree from a medical school (Figure 2-6). Blackwell's family immigrated to New York from England in 1832. She began her medical education by reading medical books and later obtained private instruction. Medical schools in New York and Pennsylvania initially refused her applications for formal study, but finally in 1847 she was accepted at the Geneva Medical College in New York. Ten years later, as she was practicing medicine, she established the New York Infirmary for Indigent Women and Children, the first hospital staffed entirely by women. In 1869 Blackwell returned to her native England and became a professor of gynecology at the London School of Medicine for Women, of which she was a founder.

Lillian Wald (1867 to 1940), a social worker and nurse, made great contributions to medical care when she founded the Henry Street Settlement in New York City. Wald operated a visiting nurse service from this establishment. When one of her nurses was assigned to the city's public schools in 1902, the New York City Municipal Board of Health established the world's first public school nursing system.

Margaret Sanger (1883 to 1966) was born in Corning, New York and trained as a nurse at the White Plains Hospital. She became the American leader of the birth control movement. While working among the poor in New York City, she came to understand the public's need for information about contraception. She left nursing to devote herself to that objective. In 1873 the federal Comstock law declared it illegal to import or distribute any device, medicine, or information designed to prevent conception or induce abortion, or to mention in print the names of sexually transmitted diseases. Nurses and physicians were legally prohibited from providing this information to their patients. In 1914 Sanger was **indicted** for circulating the magazine *The Woman Rebel*, in which she attacked the legislative restrictions of the Comstock law. The case was dismissed 2 years later. In the same year she established the first American birth control clinic; this led to her arrest, conviction, and time in the county jail. She continued her work, and after World War II, she successfully advocated research into hormonal contraception, because of the newfound concern about population growth. This research ultimately led to development of the birth control pill. When the Planned Parenthood Federation of America was formed in 1941, she was named honorary chairperson.

CRITICAL THINKING APPLICATION

- Mr. Santos asks his students to tell him which of these early pioneers they would most like to have worked with. Which would you choose and why?

Twentieth Century Medicine

In recognition of the achievements of scientists of the past, it has been said of our ability to discover and innovate, "We stood on the shoulders of giants." Great strides in medicine accompanied the twentieth century, and technology began to advance rapidly. Medical leaders continued their contributions, and knowledge, treatment, and research grew by leaps and bounds. Walter Reed was a U.S. Army pathologist and bacteriologist who proved that yellow fever was transmitted by the bite of a mosquito. Persons with diabetes should be grateful to Sir Frederick Grant Banting, a Canadian physician who isolated insulin for treatment, along with Charles Herbert Best, a Canadian physiologist. In 1928 Sir Alexander Fleming discovered penicillin accidentally while researching influenza and working with staphylococcal bacteria. He found a substance in mold that prevented growth of bacteria even when the substance was diluted 800 times. Children born with cyanosis resulting from a malformed heart benefit from the work of cardiologist Helen Taussig of Baltimore, who developed a lifesaving operation for "blue babies" while working with surgeon Alfred Blalock. This became known as the Blalock-Taussig procedure, first performed at Johns Hopkins University. Jonas Edward Salk and Albert Sabin almost eradicated poliomyelitis, once the killer and crippler of thousands in the United States. Salk's injectable vaccine was developed in 1952, and following wide-scale testing in 1954, it was distributed nationally, greatly reducing the incidence of the disease. Sabin's live-virus vaccine, in a form that could be swallowed, became available less than a decade later. Werner Forssmann, a German surgeon, originated a cardiac technique called *catheterization* that is used in the diagnosis and treatment of heart disease. Christiaan Barnard, a South African surgeon, performed the first human-heart transplant in 1967. Dr. Elisabeth Kübler-Ross, a Swiss-born psychiatrist, was shocked at the treatment of terminally ill patients at her hospital in New York. She wrote the best-selling book *On Death and Dying*, which helped professionals and laypersons alike to understand the stages of grief.

Leaders of the Millennium

Dr. David Ho. Dr. David Ho (Figure 2-7) is considered by many to be one of the most brilliant minds today helping to piece together the puzzle of the human immunodeficiency virus (HIV). Ho is the scientific director and chief executive officer (CEO) of the Aaron Diamond AIDS Research Center in New York City and is also a professor at Rockefeller University. He was born in Taiwan in 1952, and his family immigrated to the United States when he was 12 years of age. He eventually entered college to study physics—medicine was actually his second choice—but once he discovered molecular biology and the concept of gene splicing, he decided to become a researcher. He still does calculations in Chinese. Ho was named *Time* magazine's "Man of the Year" in 1996 for his work in the battle against HIV and acquired immunodeficiency syndrome (AIDS).

Dr. Eve Slater. Dr. Eve Slater serves as the Assistant Secretary for Health at the U.S. Department of Health

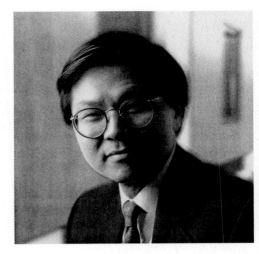

FIGURE 2-7   David Ho. (Courtesy David Ho, MD.)

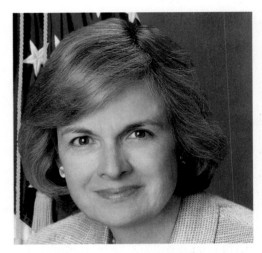

FIGURE 2-8   Eve Slater (Courtesy Eve Slater, MD.)

and Human Services (DHHS). She assumed this position in February 2002. Dr. Slater serves as Secretary Tommy G. Thompson's primary advisor on matters regarding issues concerning the nation's public health and oversees DHHS's U.S. Public Health Service (PHS). Before she joined DHHS, Dr. Slater served as a senior vice president of Merck Research Laboratories' external policy, and also as Vice President of Corporate Public Affairs. Dr. Slater was the first woman to hold this rank. During her time with Merck, she spearheaded the approval of major medicines used to treat the HIV infection, osteoporosis, cardiovascular disease, arthritis, chickenpox, and many others. In 1976, Dr. Slater became the first woman appointed chief resident in medicine at Massachusetts General Hospital. She served as an assistant professor at Harvard Medical School and directed laboratory research funded by the National Institutes of Health (NIH) and the American Heart Association.

Dr. C. Everett Koop. Dr. Koop (Figure 2-9) was graduated from Cornell University as a medical doctor in 1941 and spent most of his career as a pediatric surgeon. During his terms as the U.S. Surgeon General, he became a proponent of tobacco awareness, insisting that tobacco

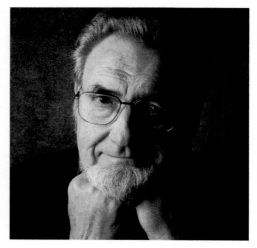

FIGURE 2-9   C. Everett Koop. (Courtesy C. Everett Koop, MD.)

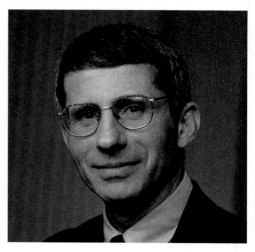

FIGURE 2-11   Anthony Fauci. (Courtesy Anthony Fauci, MD.)

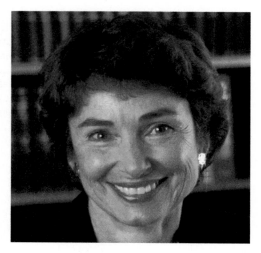

FIGURE 2-10   Marcia Angell. (Courtesy Marcia Angell, MD.)

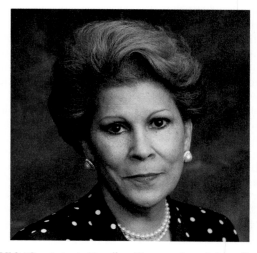

FIGURE 2-12   Antonia Novello. (Courtesy Antonia Novello, MD.)

advertisements must be less attractive to the youth of today. Dr. Koop is a professor at Dartmouth Medical School. He founded the Koop Institute, an organization whose mission is to "promote the health and well-being of all people." Dr. Koop has been honored with many awards, including 41 honorary doctorates.

Dr. Marcia Angell. Dr. Marcia Angell (Figure 2-10) is the former editor-in-chief of the *New England Journal of Medicine* (NEJM), one of the most prestigious medical publications in the United States. Her career with NEJM began in 1979, and her excellent articles spanned a variety of subjects, from the pharmaceutical companies' profit margins to the effects of socioeconomic status on Americans seeking healthcare services. Angell was named one of the 25 most influential Americans in 1997 by *Time* magazine. She has written and contributed to several books, including *Science on Trial: the Clash of Medical Evidence and the Law in the Breast Implant Case*. Angell is a board-certified pathologist and currently serves as senior lecturer in the Department of Social Medicine at Harvard Medical School.

Dr. Anthony S. Fauci. As the director of the National Institute of Allergy and Infectious Diseases at the NIH, Dr. Anthony Fauci leads research efforts on immune–medicated disorders. His scientific leadership has resulted in major advances in several diseases, such as polyarteritis nodosa and Wegener's granulomatosis. Many of his studies now relate to HIV and the body's response to the AIDS virus, and ways to improve HIV treatment and prevention, including HIV vaccine development. Out of more than one million scientists who published during the period between 1981 and 1994, Dr. Fauci was the fifth most cited. He received his MD from Cornell University Medical College, and his career with the NIH has spanned more than 30 years.

Dr. Antonia Novello. Dr. Antonia Novello (Figure 2-12) was the first woman, and the first Hispanic, to be honored with the post of Surgeon General. She served at the NIH and was the honorary chairperson of the National Youth Summit for Mothers Against Drunk Driving (MADD). Novello played a key role in writing the warning labels on cigarette packages. She supported and promoted the National Organ Transplant Act of 1984 and has contributed to the efforts of the United Nations Children's Fund (UNICEF). Novello was a clinical professor at Georgetown University Hospital and in 1994 was inducted into the National Women's Hall of Fame. She currently serves as New York State's health commissioner.

CRITICAL THINKING APPLICATION

- During class discussion, Mr. Santos points out that these Leaders of the Millennium had specific goals for their career and achieved worldwide recognition for their contributions. What other individuals not listed have made contributions to medicine in recent years?
- How can the individual medical assistant make a contribution to medicine?

The National View of Healthcare

World Health Organization

The World Health Organization (WHO), founded in 1948, is a specialized agency of the United Nations. The organization promotes cooperation between nations in their efforts to control and eliminate diseases worldwide. The purposes of WHO are to give worldwide guidance in the field of health; set global standards for health; cooperate with governments in strengthening national health programs; and develop and transfer appropriate health technology, information, and standards. One of the greatest accomplishments of this agency was the eradication of smallpox. Other diseases, such as polio and leprosy, are on the verge of eradication. WHO is committed to research and delivery of needed drugs and medical supplies to various areas of the world. In addition, WHO promotes the sharing of health information, and WHO officials meet with the leaders of the worldwide health industry to discuss various ethical and moral implications that face today's healthcare professionals.

Department of Health and Human Services

DHHS is the principal U.S. agency for providing essential human services and protecting the health of all Americans, especially those who are unable to help themselves. DHHS is made up of more than 300 programs that comprise medical and social science research, immunization services, financial assistance for low-income families, child support enforcement services, improvement of infant and maternal health, child and elder abuse prevention services, and various programs for elderly Americans. DHHS also oversees the Medicare and Medicaid programs. Medicare is the nation's largest health insurer, and DHHS processes more than 900 million claims every year. It is the largest grant-making agency in the federal government, providing approximately 60,000 grants annually. With a budget of more than $429 billion and more than 63,000 employees, DHHS works side by side with local and state governments in its effort to serve the healthcare needs of the public.

U.S. Army Medical Research Institute of Infectious Diseases

The primary focus of the U.S. Army Medical Research Institute of Infectious Diseases (USAMRIID) is protecting military service members, but the Institute conducts key research programs in national defense and infectious diseases that benefit everyone. USAMRIID, located at Ft. Detrick in Maryland, works extensively with the Centers for Disease Control and the World Health Organization (Figure 2-13). USAMRIID also controls an internationally known reference laboratory with state-of-the-art facilities. This laboratory is instrumental in identifying biological threats and the diseases those threats produce. USAMRIID is the only laboratory facility operated by the Department of Defense that is equipped to study Biosafety Level IV viruses and pathogens.

There are four Biosafety Levels commonly accepted among laboratory professionals. Biosafety Level I consists of well-known agents that have a minimal or low biohazard potential to laboratory personnel and to the environment as a whole. At this level, the laboratory is not necessarily separated from the regular areas of the facility. Examples of Level I pathogens include *Pneumococcus* and *Salmonella*. In the Biosafety Level II section of the laboratory, substances with a moderate biohazard potential are studied. At Levels I and II, laboratory personnel have specific training in handling pathogens, and specialized equipment is used to avoid splashes and splatters. Pathogens classified as Biosafety Level II are hepatitis, the Lyme disease virus, and influenza virus.

Personnel working in Biosafety Level III have very specific training in working with the potentially deadly pathogens found at this level. All procedures performed on Level III have a high biohazard risk and are done inside protective safety cabinets. Laboratory personnel are required to wear heavy personal protective equipment. Special regulations concerning exhaust air and ventilation are strictly followed, and there is limited access to the laboratory when work is in progress. HIV, anthrax, and typhus are some of the pathogens classified as Biosafety

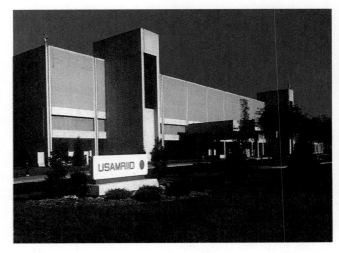

FIGURE 2-13 U.S. Army Medical Research Institute of Infectious Diseases in Fort Detrick, Maryland.

Level III. Biosafety Level IV contains the most deadly pathogens, which often produce incurable diseases. There is an extreme biohazard risk of transmission of these agents, including the risk of airborne transmission. Laboratory personnel are highly trained in the manipulation and handling of these dangerous pathogens. Laboratory access is strictly controlled in this section. Some of the pathogens studied at Biosafety Level IV include *Ebola*, *Lassa*, and the *Hantavirus*.

Centers for Disease Control and Prevention

The headquarters for the Centers for Disease Control and Prevention (CDC) are located in Atlanta, Georgia (Figure 2-14). The CDC is the principal U.S. federal agency concerned with the health and safety of people throughout the world. It is a clearinghouse for information and statistics associated with healthcare. There are 12 divisions within the CDC that focus on specific health-related issues, such as the National Center for HIV, STD, and TB Prevention; the Public Health Practice Program Office; the National Center on Birth Defects and Developmental Disabilities; and the National Center for Health Statistics. Branch offices are located throughout the United States and in several foreign countries. The CDC has approximately 8600 employees who are dedicated to public health. Extensive publications and information services provide healthcare professionals all over the world with the information needed to care for patients.

The agency conducts research into the origin and occurrence of diseases and develops methods for their control and prevention. Additionally, it develops immunization services and aids in the training of healthcare workers. In recent years the CDC has been intricately involved in the battle against HIV, the human immunodeficiency virus, which in its advanced form is called AIDS. The agency has developed guidelines emphasizing that universal blood and body fluid precautions be used in all situations where the risk of contamination by body

fluids exists. These recommended precautions are the basis for the laws enforced by the Occupational Safety and Health Administration (OSHA) regarding bloodborne pathogens.

National Institutes of Health

The National Institutes of Health (NIH) began as a one-room laboratory in the marine hospital on New York's Staten Island in 1887. Its first major contribution to medicine was the isolation of the bacterium that causes cholera. Tuberculosis was the number one cause of death at that time. There were few drugs that could alleviate or cure diseases, and there were no vaccines, except for smallpox vaccine. There were no antibiotics, and even aspirin was not yet available. Doctors could diagnose some conditions but fell short on treatments. In 1891 the laboratory moved from Staten Island to Washington, DC. In 1930 this laboratory became the National Institutes of Health, an agency of the U.S. Department of Health and Human Services. The mission of the NIH is to uncover new knowledge that will lead to better health for everyone. As a part of the public health service, it seeks to improve the health of the American people, supports and conducts biomedical research into the causes and prevention of diseases, and uses a modern communications system to furnish biomedical information to the healthcare professions.

The NIH moved from Washington, DC to Bethesda, Maryland in 1938 and today occupies more than 60 buildings covering 30 acres. It consists of 13 research institutes, four divisions, and the National Library of Medicine. Thousands of research projects are under way in NIH laboratories and clinics at any given time. The NIH also provides support to other research projects conducted at universities, medical schools, and hospitals.

Health Industry Councils

Health industry councils are organizations that seek to organize and unify all of the entities providing healthcare in a certain region or community. These organizations keep statistical records about the medical trends in the area and are an important factor in drawing new businesses related to the medical field to the area that they represent. These councils are designed to function as a developmental group that promotes the industry in their area and works together for the good of all those involved in healthcare. The organizations represented within the council may fiercely compete in the area market, but they work together to promote the healthcare industry in the region in which they are located. The councils usually are made up of task forces and committees that study communications concepts, home health, managed care, membership and development, new business promotion, and design and construction. They also are an excellent source of medical information and trends in medicine locally, statewide, and nationally. These councils are valuable assets to any region that wishes to remain on the cutting edge of healthcare.

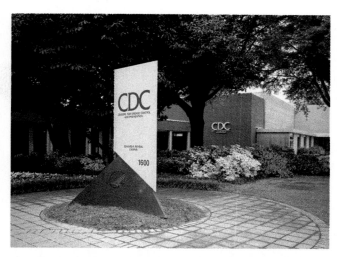

FIGURE 2-14 The headquarters of the Centers for Disease Control and Prevention (CDC) are located in Atlanta, Georgia. (Courtesy Centers for Disease Control and Prevention, Atlanta, GA.)

Types of Healthcare Facilities

Hospitals

There are several different types of hospitals. They are classified according to the type of care and services that they provide to patients. Acute care hospitals offer intensive care units and emergency or trauma departments and are equipped to handle the most severely ill or injured patients. Subacute hospitals offer patient care for those who do not require extensive services but still need hospital supervision and treatment. Specialty hospitals offer specific services, such as a psychiatric hospital. Teaching hospitals provide a learning environment and often have research departments as well. These hospitals are usually affiliated with medical schools, and interns provide care supervised by licensed physician instructors. Community hospitals provide care in rural areas or in specific areas within a metropolis. Regional hospitals are usually acute care facilities and serve a large area that may not offer intensive care in its local communities.

Private hospitals are run by a corporation or other organization and are usually designed to produce a profit for the owners or stockholders. Nonprofit hospitals exist to serve the community in which they are located and are normally run by a board of directors. The term *nonprofit* is sometimes misleading, because there is a difference in "profit" and "making money." A nonprofit hospital or organization may make money in a campaign or fund-raiser, but all of the money is returned to the organization. Nonprofit hospitals and organizations must follow strict guidelines in the area of finance and must account to the government how much money is brought in and for what purposes it is used. Sometimes the term *county hospital* is used to designate the hospital to which **indigent** patients are taken. These are hospitals that will provide emergency care to those who cannot pay for medical expenses. Today, however, many people without insurance go to the emergency department for routine illnesses. This is one reason that emergency departments are busy and full. If patients have no other options, the emergency department physicians become the primary care providers, and this is a major cause of the long waiting times experienced in hospital emergency departments. Managed care has eased this problem somewhat by refusing to cover visits to the ER that are not true emergencies. **Triage** procedures are used to determine which patients have the most severe conditions and should be seen first.

Hospitals have various departments that are organized to provide efficient patient care. The admissions department gathers information and enters it into a computer for use by the rest of the hospital staff. Nursing service supervises all of the nursing care given to the patients and is involved in **case management**. The laboratory provides diagnostic testing on blood, body fluids, and tissues, while the radiology or nuclear medicine department offers diagnostic imaging and x-ray services. Respiratory services offers a broad spectrum of diagnostic tests and various treatments. Most hospitals also have a physical medicine and rehabilitation department, which offers both physical and occupational therapy. The dietary department employs professionals who carefully plan menus to meet the needs of each patient served. Most modern hospitals have a surgery department, and many offer day surgery services, which allow patients to have a procedure performed and go home the same day, if they recover as expected. The medical records department is responsible for the patient records related to every **encounter** that takes place in the facility. Social services works with patients to ensure continuity of care, patient education, and social intervention to assist the patient with emotional, economic, and social concerns.

The hospital administrators manage the hospital on a day-to-day basis, and human resources is usually a part of the administration department. Almost every hospital has a board of directors to assist the administrators in governing the hospital, and there is usually a medical staff committee, led by the hospital's chief of staff, who assist in the management of the facility and the **credentialing** process for the physicians that have **staff privileges** there. Credentialing involves determining whether a practitioner should be allowed to practice medicine in a facility, based on his or her education, license, past performance, and other qualifications.

The National Practitioner Data Bank also gathers information that helps healthcare facilities identify physicians who are incompetent. It provides information about physicians who have had licensure problems, made malpractice payments, had clinical privileges revoked or restricted, or had action taken against them by a professional society. This is an incredibly important process, because if an incompetent physician is allowed to have staff privileges at a hospital, patients could be harmed, and the facility could easily be held liable for the physician's actions and named as a codefendant in medical professional liability cases. Physicians' backgrounds should be carefully scrutinized by the credentialing committee and staff to avoid this threat of liability. Various types of **peer review organizations (PROs)** are also critical to good healthcare facility management.

Accreditation is considered the highest form of recognition for the quality of care that a facility or organization provides. Not only does it indicate to the public that the facility is concerned with offering quality care, it also provides professional liability insurance benefits and plays a role in regulatory agency relicensure and certification efforts. Hospitals and other healthcare facilities are often accredited by the Joint Commission on Accreditation of Healthcare Organizations (JCAHO), an organization that is concerned with the quality of care given in healthcare facilities. **Standards** or **indicators** have been developed that help to determine when patients are receiving quality care. There is much more to the term *quality* than whether the patient liked the food served or had to wait to have a procedure or test performed. Categories of compliance include such areas as the assessment and care of patients; use of medication; plant, technology, and safety management; orientation, education, and training of staff; medical staff qualifications; and patient rights. Ratings from 1 to 5 are given to the facility on their performance in specific areas. A "1" rating means that the facility is in full compliance with that standard, and the other ratings indicate different levels of non-compliance. DHHS also regulates healthcare facilities, as does the Occupational Safety and Health Administration (OSHA).

CRITICAL THINKING APPLICATION

- Mr. Santos has assigned his students to groups and asked them to investigate local hospitals. What types of hospitals are found in your local area?
- How might Mr. Santos' students find out whether a physician has staff privileges at a certain hospital?

Ambulatory Care

There are many other types of healthcare facilities that operate in the industry today. **Ambulatory** care centers includes a wide range of facilities that offer healthcare services to patients who are able to walk around and are not bedridden. Physician's offices, group practices, and multispecialty group practices are a common type of ambulatory care facility. Group practices may be of a single specialty, such as pediatrics, or may be multispecialty. A multispecialty practice might consist of an internal medicine specialist, an oncologist, a family practitioner, and an endocrinologist. Usually the physicians within the practice refer to each other, where indicated. This is not only more convenient for the patients, but also more profitable for the physicians.

Occupational health centers are concerned with helping the patient return to work and productive activity. Often physical therapy is used in conjunction with rehabilitation services that assist the patient in regaining as much of their previous ability as possible. There are also freestanding rehabilitation centers that assist patients with a wide range of services. Pain management centers help patients deal with the pain associated with their condition. Sleep centers diagnose and treat people who have sleep problems. Difficulty in sleeping is a symptom, like pain, and the cause of the disturbance must be found so that proper treatment can be provided. Freestanding urgent or emergency care centers provide patients with an alternative to hospital emergency departments. They are less expensive, have a shorter waiting time, and are conveniently located in many areas. Most have flexible hours, often are open well into the evening hours, and walk-in appointments are usually accepted.

Surgery has become easier and more convenient because of the number of ambulatory surgical centers that exist today. Day surgery performed in hospitals has continued to provide patients with better alternatives than overnight hospital care after surgery. Many insurance companies now prefer day surgery, because it is more cost effective. Not many years ago, however, the only alternative to inpatient surgery was that hospital's day surgery department. Today there are an ever-increasing number of freestanding surgical centers. Patients can be treated with laser surgery, radial keratotomy, and cataract removal during the day and recover at home that same evening. Plastic surgeons are becoming very innovative in the physical structure of their offices and the types of surgery they offer on an outpatient basis. Many plastic

surgeons offer breast augmentation and reduction and even abdominoplasty (tummy tuck) and liposuction in the office setting. It was not long ago that a tummy tuck surgical procedure meant several days in the hospital. This new trend is becoming more accepted partially as a result of the new "office-based surgery" accreditation offered by the Ambulatory Care Accreditation Program of the JCAHO.

Dialysis centers offer services to patients with severe kidney disorders, and many of the larger cities across the country offer cancer centers for patients who need treatment by oncologists. There are many other types of ambulatory care facilities, including centers that provide magnetic resonance imaging (MRI), student health clinics, dental clinics, endoscopy centers, community health centers, mobile health services, podiatric care centers, and women's health centers.

Geriatric and long-term patients have more options today for ambulatory care than ever before. In the past, nursing homes were the only alternative to keeping an elderly patient in their own home. These nursing homes provided care for residents that needed more than just assistance with day-to-day activities. Now there are many attractive options to traditional nursing homes, or skilled nursing facilities. One of the most popular is assisted living. Most assisted living facilities provide 24-hour supervision of their residents, all meals, and a broad range of services, from the very basic, such as transportation to physician office visits, to the extravagant, such as shopping trips taken by limousine. Most also provide exercise programs, social services, laundry and linen services, and housekeeping. The cost ranges from approximately $1000 to $3000 per month, depending on the location and the **amenities** desired by the resident. There are many new assisted-living facilities specifically designed for Alzheimer's or other memory-care patients.

Independent retirement communities offer residents the opportunity to come and go as they please. Many have a resortlike design, catering to the desire of retirees to enjoy their golden years. Usually the communities consist of apartments or duplex units, and some even offer small cottages. Activities are planned to enhance the social life of the residents, and some offer libraries with computer access, restaurant-style dining, beauty salons, and even gardens to grow food. Keeping safety in mind, the units usually have special emergency call bells and other protective devices.

Other Healthcare Facilities

Several other types of healthcare facilities deserve attention in the broad overview of the healthcare industry. Diagnostic laboratories offer testing services for patients referred by their physician. Since the enactment of the Clinical Laboratory Improvement Act (CLIA) in 1967 and its amendment in 1988, many physician offices stopped providing laboratory tests that were performed inside their offices. These types of labs are called physician office laboratories (POLs). The regulations set forth by both OSHA and CLIA rules made it more cost-effective to have the patient go to an outside laboratory to have tests done. It should be noted that OSHA is an organization and division of the U.S. Department of Labor. CLIA is a law, not an agency. However, both influence workplace safety and quality testing.

Home health agencies were tremendously successful in the late 1980s to the mid-1990s, but cuts in Medicare funding have caused them to suffer severe losses in recent years. This concept of care is very popular, but the influx of too many agencies and the subsequent drop in payments made to them have resulted in fewer home healthcare providers today. In addition, many hospitals began offering home healthcare, which added to the already heavy competition that smaller firms faced. Home healthcare offers its patients home care, therapy services, administration and assistance with medications, and other services so that the patient can remain at home yet still obtain the care that is needed.

Medical suppliers are retail operations that offer all types of medical devices and products. Diabetic patients can purchase glucose monitoring machines. Special hospital beds can be ordered for those who need them. All types of aids, such as bedpans, crutches, bathing assistance devices, wheelchairs, and walkers, are available, often without a physician's prescription. Most medical suppliers serve both the public and the profession.

Medical Practices

Three general types of business structure exist in medical practices today: the sole proprietorship, the partnership, and the corporation. Sole proprietorships dominated medical practice until the last quarter of the twentieth century. These practices are on the decline as a result of the **advent** of managed care and its favor of the multispecialty group practice.

The Sole Proprietorship

A sole proprietor is an individual who holds exclusive right and title to all aspects of the medical practice. The sole proprietor may employ other physicians to participate in the practice. The employed physician is entitled to employee benefits, but by contrast, the owner is not considered an employee, and is not so entitled. Additionally, the owner would be potentially liable for all of the acts of his or her professional employees and staff members. Although there are many advantages to practicing alone, including flexibility and independence, there are also heavy disadvantages. The drawbacks include having total responsibility for the practice 24 hours a day, 7 days a week. In an unincorporated solo practice, the business dies when the owner leaves it, unless it is sold to someone else. Many modern physicians do not see the sole proprietorship as an avenue for a decent income as a doctor, because so many of the managed care companies have selectively chosen to offer participation to group practices over the single-practice physician. Some doctors organize associate practices. In this case, physicians share office space, and often equipment and employees, but they operate their practices as sole proprietorships. Agreements such as these should always be in writing to avoid misunderstandings and legal concerns.

The Partnership

When two or more physicians elect to associate in the practice of medicine, they may enter into a partnership agreement. This agreement specifies all of the rights, obligations, and responsibilities of each partner. They have more potential for profit as a partnership than they would in practice as sole proprietors. Each of the physicians has more freedom, because the doctors rotate an "on-call" schedule so that there is some time away from the office and patients. However, one disadvantage of the partnership is the liability of each for the actions and conduct of all the others. In a partnership arrangement, the partners often pool employees, equipment, insurance, facilities, and even profits, and these resources are divided according to the specifications of the partnership agreement or contract.

A group practice is a body of at least three licensed physicians who engage in full-time practice in a formally organized and legally recognized entity. A group practice may take the form of a partnership, or it may be formed as a corporation. The group may share income and expenses, equipment, records, and personnel, and may combine patient care and business management. The group practice may be an association of the same specialty or be a multispecialty organization. Usually, a group practice will take the form of a partnership or a corporation.

The Corporation

A corporation may be defined as an artificial entity having a legal and business status that is independent of its shareholders or employees. Corporations are regulated by statutes of the state in which the incorporation takes place. In most cases, the physician shareholders are employees of the corporation. Even one physician in a solo practice can incorporate the practice. All employees of the corporation receive income and tax advantages. Corporations are usually able to offer better benefit packages, which may include pension and profit-sharing plans, medical expense reimbursement, life insurance, disability income insurance, and many other benefits. Some offer *cafeteria plans*, which the employees can customize to their specific needs, including benefits such as child care reimbursement and tuition reimbursement. Most benefits are tax deductible to both the employer and employee, and some plans offer pretax benefit packages as well. Professional employees of a corporation are liable only for their own acts, although it is always a good idea for any professional in the medical field to carry their own malpractice insurance. Another advantage of the corporate entity is the continuous life of the corporation. It does not dissolve with a change in shareholders.

Healthcare Professionals

See Tables 2-1 to 2-3.

The Title of "Doctor"

Doctors of Medicine. Medical doctors, or MDs, are considered to be **allopathic** physicians and are the most

TABLE 2-1	Types of Medical Specialties	
Specialty	**Title of Practitioner**	**Description of Specialty**
Allergy and immunology	Allergist/immunologist	An allergist/immunologist is trained to evaluate disorders and diseases of the immune system. This includes such conditions as adverse reactions to drugs and foods, anaphylaxis, problems related to autoimmune diseases, asthma, and insect stings.
Anesthesiology	Anesthesiologist	An anesthesiologist provides pain relief and management during surgical procedures and for patients with long-standing conditions accompanied by pain, such as cancer patients. Anesthesiologists also provide critical care and resuscitation for patients during cardiac or respiratory emergencies.
Colorectal surgery	Colorectal surgeon	This type of surgeon diagnoses and treats conditions affecting the intestines, rectum, and anal area, as well as organs that can cause intestinal disease. They often treat cancers that appear in these areas, as well as disorders such as hemorrhoids and fissures.
Dermatology	Dermatologist	The dermatologist works with adult and pediatric patients in treating disorders and diseases of the skin, hair, nails, and related tissues. Dermatologists are specially trained to manage conditions such as skin cancers, cosmetic disorders of the skin, scars, allergies, and other disorders, both malignant and benign.
Emergency medicine	Emergency physician	An emergency physician is an expert in triage and treating a patient to prevent the patient's death or serious disability. This physician gives immediate care to stabilize the patient and then refers the patient to the appropriate professional for further care. These physicians are usually found in hospital emergency rooms or freestanding emergency centers.
Family practice	Family practitioner	The family practitioner offers care to the whole family, from newborns to elderly adults, and is familiar with a wide range of disorders and diseases. Preventive care is of primary concern. This is one of the more common specialties that physicians choose.
General surgery	Surgeon	Surgery is the correction of deformities, defects, diseases, or injured parts of the body by means of operative treatment. A surgeon must be familiar with the various specialties to effectively treat patients. General surgery includes all of the aspects of surgery other than those separated into a subgroup specialty.
Internal medicine	Internist	Internists are concerned with comprehensive care, often diagnosing and treating those with chronic, long-term conditions. They also offer treatment for common illnesses and preventive care. Internists must have a broad understanding of the body and its ailments to diagnose and provide treatment to the patient.
Medical genetics	Geneticist	A geneticist is a physician trained to diagnose and treat patients who have conditions related to genetically linked diseases and may provide special genetic counseling when indicated. Often associated with research projects, this physician may participate in screening programs for defects and abnormalities, sometimes prior to birth of an infant.
Neurological surgery	Neurological surgeon	The neurological surgeon offers nonoperative and operative care for patients with conditions of the central, autonomic, and peripheral nervous systems. This includes the supporting structures and vascular supplies of related organs.
Neurology	Neurologist	The neurologist diagnoses and treats disorders of the brain, spinal cord, nerves, and the blood vessels that support those organs. Generally, the neurologist manages infectious, metabolic, degenerative, and systemic involvement of the nervous system.
Nuclear medicine	Nuclear medicine specialist	This specialist uses radioactive substances for the diagnosis and treatment of disease. Radiation and imaging devices are used to detect diseases, often before the organ is seen as abnormal by other methods. The nuclear medicine specialist is aware of the effects of radiation on various structures, as well as the fundamentals of the principles of radiation and physics.
Obstetrics and gynecology	Obstetrician/ gynecologist (OB/Gyn)	Obstetricians provide care to women of child-bearing age and monitor the progress of the developing child. They deliver the baby, and care for the mother for approximately 6 weeks after birth. Gynecologists are concerned with the diagnosis and treatment of the female reproductive system.

TABLE 2-1	Types of Medical Specialties—cont'd	
Specialty	**Title of Practitioner**	**Description of Specialty**
Ophthalmology	Ophthalmologist	Ophthalmologists diagnose, treat, and provide comprehensive care to the eye and its supporting structures. These physicians also offer vision services, including corrective lenses. Screening tests are promoted as a measure of preventive care.
Otolaryngology	Otolaryngologist	These physicians treat diseases and conditions that affect the ear, nose, throat, and structures related to the head and neck. Problems that affect the voice and hearing are also referred to this specialist.
Pathology	Pathologist	Pathologists study the causes of diseases that affect the body, and determine what may have caused the death of a patient. These physicians study tissues and cells, body fluids, and actual organs to assist in diagnosing the patient's ailments. Pathologists often perform autopsies.
Pediatrics	Pediatrician	Pediatricians promote preventive medicine and treat diseases that affect children and adolescents. They monitor the child's growth and development, and provide a wide range of health services to keep their patients healthy.
Physical medicine and rehabilitation	Physiatrist	This specialty assists patients who have physical disabilities. This may include those with musculoskeletal disorders, or who are suffering from pain as a result of injury or trauma. Their primary goal is to restore the patient to his or her state of health prior to the injury or trauma as nearly as possible through rehabilitation.
Plastic surgery	Plastic surgeon	The plastic surgeon works with patients who have had some type of injury or condition that has left them with a physical defect. The surgeon performs reconstructive procedures, using grafts, flaps, and tissue transfer and replanting. These surgeons also provide cosmetic enhancements and procedures that are elective in nature.
Preventive medicine	Preventive medicine specialist	Preventive medicine is concerned with preventing the occurrence of both mental and physical illness and disability. Analysis of present health services and planning for future medical needs are part of this specialty. Preventive medicine consists of several components, including biostatistics, environmental studies, occupational studies, and clinical preventive medicine activities.
Psychiatry	Psychiatrist	A psychiatrist is a physician whose specialty is the diagnosis and treatment of persons with mental, emotional, or behavioral disorders. The psychiatrist is qualified to conduct psychotherapy and to prescribe medications when necessary.
Radiology	Radiologist	Radiology is a specialty in which x-rays are used for diagnosis and treatment of disease. A diagnostic radiologist specializes in using x-rays, ultrasound, nuclear medicine, computed tomography, and magnetic resonance imaging for detection of abnormalities throughout the body.
Thoracic surgery	Thoracic surgeon	This surgical specialty is concerned with the operative treatment of the chest and chest wall, lungs, and respiratory passages. Specialists in this field are involved with heart surgery, including both valvular and coronary heart surgery.
Urology	Urologist	Urology is a medical specialty concerned with the treatment of diseases and disorders of the urinary tract. Urologists diagnose and manage problems with the genitourinary system and practice endoscopic and percutaneous procedures related to these structures.

widely recognized type of physician. They diagnose illness and disease and prescribe treatment for their patients. MDs are allowed to write prescriptions and perform surgeries. They offer advice on nutrition and preventative medicine. To become a medical doctor, 4 years of undergraduate training (premed) usually precede 4 years of medical school. Some extraordinary students are allowed entry after 3 years of undergraduate studies, but competition for entry to medical school is intense, so grades and other experience in healthcare is strongly considered. Premed students study biology, physics, organic and inorganic chemistry, mathematics, English, humanities,

and social sciences. There are approximately 125 allopathic medical schools in the United States. After medical school the student faces 3 to 8 years of internship and residency programs. An intern is a medical student still in training at medical school, but treating patients under the supervision of licensed doctors. A residency is a graduate medical education program, often in a specialty, and is usually a paid "on-the-job training" hospital position. Often MDs specialize in a certain field, such as cardiology or pediatrics. These doctors usually invest 3 to 6 years of training in the specialty after medical school and can obtain board certification in one or more of 24 different specialty areas recognized by the American Board of Medical Specialties (see Table 2-1). An MD must have a state license to practice, and continuing education is required to maintain the license. Graduates of foreign medical schools can usually obtain a license in the United States after passing an examination and completing a residency program in this country.

Doctors of Osteopathy. Osteopathic physicians, or DOs, complete similar requirements as medical doctors to graduate and practice medicine. Osteopaths use medicine and surgery, as well as osteopathic manipulative therapy (OMT), in treating their patients. Andrew Taylor Still is considered the originator of osteopathic medicine, which he began in 1874. He believed in a more **holistic** approach to medicine, and although he was an MD, he founded the American School of Osteopathy in Kirksville, Missouri. The school was originally chartered to offer an MD degree but later focused more on the osteopathic approach. DOs stress preventive medicine and holistic patient care, as well as a special focus on the musculoskeletal system and OMT. Osteopathic medicine also promotes the **innate** ability of the body to heal itself, and many osteopaths tend to take a more conservative approach to using medications and surgical procedures than allopathic physicians. Premed students moving toward osteopathic medicine also study biology, physics, organic and inorganic chemistry, mathematics, English, humanities, and social sciences. They also usually attend 4 years of undergraduate studies and then begin 4 years of medical studies at a school for osteopathic medicine. Most DOs participate in a 12-month rotating internship in the various specialty areas before entering a residency program lasting from 2 to 6 years, and they are eligible for board certification through either the American Board of Medical Specialists or the American Osteopathic Association. Approximately one in 20 physicians in the United States is an osteopathic physician. DOs participate in continuing education programs to renew their licenses annually.

Doctors of Chiropractic. Chiropractors, or DCs, are typically thought of as "bone doctors," but actually focus on the nervous system to help patients live healthier lives. The nervous system is the master system of the body, controlling and coordinating all the other systems. Information from the environment, both internal and external, moves through the spinal cord to get to the brain, and in the same manner, information from the brain moves through the spinal cord to reach the body in a two-way flow of communication. The intention of the **chiropractic** adjustment is to remove any disruptions or distortions of this energy flow that may be caused by slight misalignments called **subluxations**. Chiropractors are trained to locate these subluxations and remove them, using touch as well as x-ray films, thereby restoring the normal flow of nerve energy so that the entire body functions in an optimal fashion. They believe that the same innate inner intelligence that grows the body from a single cell into a complex human being can also heal the body if it is free of disturbance to the nervous system. The philosophy is that health, not merely absence of symptoms, comes from within the body, not from the outside. Chiropractic

colleges require undergraduate studies in biology, organic and inorganic chemistry, physics, English, and the humanities, and then 3 years are spent studying chiropractic. Each state offers licensing, and some devote their practices to a specific specialty, but more often practice general chiropractic. Continuing education is required for relicensure.

CRITICAL THINKING APPLICATION

- Mr. Santos challenges his new medical assisting students to interview several types of doctors at some point during their studies. The class discusses the different philosophies of medicine among allopathic, osteopathic, and chiropractic physicians. Discuss with your class the similarities and differences of these three aspects of medicine.
- Most of Mr. Santos' students have visited one or more of these types of doctors. What experiences have you had with MDs, DOs, or chiropractors?

Dentists. There are two basic types of dentists in the United States: Doctors of Dental Medicine (DMD) and Doctors of Dental Surgery (DDS). Dentists treat and prevent problems dealing with the teeth, gums, and tissue surrounding them. They can perform oral surgery and write prescriptions for antibiotics and analgesics. Some specialist dentists perform straightening, called *orthodontics*, and some perform root canal therapy, called *endodontics*. Dental school usually lasts 4 years after completion of undergraduate studies, and state licensing is required.

Optometrists. The optometrist (OD) is trained and licensed to examine the eyes to test visual acuity and to treat vision defects by prescribing correctional lenses and other optical aids. A program of exercise may be planned for the patient's eyes. Optometrists study at accredited schools for optometry for 4 years after completing undergraduate studies in the sciences, mathematics, and English. They must be licensed in the state in which they practice. Optometrists should not be confused with ophthalmologists, who are licensed MDs.

Podiatrists. Podiatrists, or Doctors of Podiatric Medicine (DPM), are educated in caring for the feet, including surgical treatment. Normal persons spend an extraordinary amount of time on their feet, resulting in wear and tear and chronic pain. Podiatrists are trained to find pressure points and weight distribution problems. These doctors train for 4 years at accredited colleges after undergraduate studies in the sciences.

Other Doctorates. Other individuals may be called "doctor" based on the degree they have earned in their field. For instance, a person with a PhD has a doctoral degree in philosophy, may be addressed as "doctor," and might work as a professor at a university or in a field related to his or her discipline. A PsyD is a doctor of psychology, and an EdD is a doctor of educational psychology. Doctors who practice **naturopathy** use only natural means to help the body to heal. These medical professionals are licensed in several states.

TABLE 2-2	Healthcare Occupations Accredited by the Commission on Accreditation of Allied Health Education Programs (CAAHEP)	
Occupation	**Credential**	**Brief Job Description**
Anesthesiologist assistant	AA	Functions under the direction of a licensed and qualified anesthesiologist. Assists in developing and implementing the anesthesia care plan.
Athletic trainer	AT	Functions under supervision of attending and/or consulting physician. Provides a variety of services, including injury prevention, recognition, immediate care, treatment, and rehabilitation after physical trauma.
Cardiovascular technologist	CVT	Performs diagnostic examinations at the request or direction of a physician in one or more of three areas: (1) invasive cardiology, (2) noninvasive cardiology, and (3) noninvasive peripheral vascular study.
Cytotechnologist	CT	Works with pathologist. Prepares cellular samples for study under the microscope and assists in the diagnosis of disease by examining the samples.
Diagnostic medical sonographer	DMS	Provides patient services using medical ultrasound under the supervision of a physician. Assists in gathering sonographic data necessary to diagnose a variety of conditions and diseases.
Electrodiagnostic technologist	EEG-T	Works in collaboration with the electroencephalographer. Possesses the knowledge, attributes, and skills to obtain interpretable recordings of patients' nervous system function.
Emergency medical technician–paramedic	EMT-P	Works under the direction of a physician—often through radio communication—and is able to recognize, assess, and manage medical emergencies of acutely ill or injured patients in prehospital care settings.
Health information administrator	RRA	Manages health information systems consistent with the medical, administrative, ethical, and legal requirements of the healthcare delivery system. Works with medical and hospital administrative staff involving medical records.
Health information technician	ART	Maintains components of health information systems in all types of facilities including hospitals and ambulatory healthcare centers. Processes, maintains, compiles, and reports patient data.
Medical assistant	CMA	Multiskilled practitioner who works primarily in ambulatory settings such as physicians' offices and clinics, performing both administrative and clinical procedures.
Medical illustrator	MI	Working with many different media, medical illustrators create visual material designed to facilitate the recording and dissemination of medical, biological, and related knowledge.
Ophthalmic medical technician/technologist	OMT	Renders supportive services to the ophthalmologist. Administers diagnostic tests, takes ocular measurements, tests ocular functions, and performs other tasks assigned by the ophthalmologist.
Orthotist/prosthetist	OP	Both the orthotist and the prosthetist work directly with the physician in the rehabilitation of the physically challenged. The orthotist designs and fits orthoses to provide care to patients who have disabling conditions of the limbs and spine. The prosthetist designs and fits devices for patients who have partial or total absence of limb.
Perfusionist	PERF	A perfusionist operates extracorporeal circulation equipment during any medical situation in which it is necessary to support or temporarily replace the patient's circulatory or respiratory function (e.g., cardiopulmonary bypass).
Physician assistant	PA	The physician assistant is academically and clinically prepared to practice medicine with the supervision of a licensed doctor of medicine or osteopathy. The functions of the physician assistant include performing diagnostic, therapeutic, preventive, and health maintenance services.
Respiratory therapist	RRT	The respiratory therapist working under the supervision of a physician evaluates all data to determine the appropriateness of the prescribed respiratory care and participates in the development of the respiratory care plan.
Respiratory therapy technician	CRTT	The respiratory therapy technician works under the supervision of the respiratory therapist and a physician in administering general respiratory care.

Continued.

TABLE 2-2	Healthcare Occupations Accredited by the Commission on Accreditation of Allied Health Education Programs (CAAHEP)—cont'd	
Occupation	**Credential**	**Brief Job Description**
Specialist in blood bank technology	SBB	Specialists in blood bank technology perform both routine and specialized tests in blood bank immunohematology in technical areas of the modern blood bank and perform transfusion services.
Surgical technologist	ST/CST	Works in the surgical suite with surgeons, anesthesiologists, registered nurses, and other surgical personnel.

From *Allied Health and Rehabilitation Professions Education Directory*, ed 24. American Medical Association, Chicago, IL, 1996-1997.

TABLE 2-3	Healthcare Occupations Accredited by Agencies Other Than CAAHEP Under the AMA Umbrella
Occupational therapist	
Occupational therapy assistant	
Dietetic technician	
Dietitian/nutritionist	
Dental assistant	
Dental hygienist	
Dental laboratory technician	
Audiologist	
Speech-language pathologist	
Radiation therapist	
Radiographer	
Nuclear medicine technologist	
Clinical laboratory technician/medical laboratory technician—associate degree	
Clinical laboratory technician/medical laboratory technician—certificate	
Clinical laboratory scientist/medical technologist	
Histologic technician/technologist	
Pathologist's assistant	

From *Allied Health and Rehabilitation Professions Education Directory*, ed 24, Chicago, 1996-1997.

Licensed or Certified Professionals

There are numerous categories of licensed or certified professionals who assist the physician in diagnosing and treating the patient. Some of the professionals that the medical assistant will commonly encounter are listed in this section.

Physician Assistants. Physician assistants (PAs) provide direct patient care services under the supervision of licensed physicians. They are trained to diagnose and treat patients as directed by the physician, and in 46 states and the District of Columbia, they are allowed to write prescriptions. These professionals take patient histories, order and interpret tests, perform physical examinations, and even make diagnosis decisions. They can be found in physician offices, hospitals, military bases, and other healthcare facilities.

Nurse Practitioners. Nurse practitioners (NPs) provide basic patient care services, including diagnosis and prescribing for common illnesses. These professionals must have advanced academic training beyond the RN degree and also have vast clinical experience. Usually the focus of nurse practitioners is on preventive care and disease prevention, and an NP is allowed to practice independently or as a part of a team of healthcare professionals.

Nurse Anesthetists. Nurse anesthetists are registered nurses who administer anesthetics to patients during care by surgeons, physicians, dentists, or other qualified health professionals. They practice in many different settings, including offices, traditional hospitals, labor and delivery units, ophthalmology offices, plastic surgery offices, and many others. This practice is quite advanced, and they are compensated well for their skills. Nurse anesthetists can be found in metropolitan and rural communities alike.

Registered Nurses. The registered nurse (RN) has many career options available. Many nurses work in an administrative capacity within hospitals or other types of healthcare facilities as managers. They also provide direct patient care, where they are vital in assessing the patient and providing a care plan. Usually nurses find a specialty area that they enjoy and practice within that area, although they may also "float" to different departments within the hospital. Some function as home health nurses, visiting the patients and providing home care. Some work in nursing homes or in public health, and others serve in physicians' offices.

Licensed Practical/Vocational Nurses. Licensed practical/vocational nurses (LVNs/LPNs) offer bedside care, assisting with the actual day-to-day personal care required by inpatients. They assess patients, chart their progress, and administer medications and intravenous fluids where allowed by law. They often work in hospitals or skilled nursing facilities and are also found in physicians' offices. They sometimes supervise nursing assistants and may also provide patient education services.

Medical Technologists. Medical technologists (MTs) perform diagnostic testing on blood, body fluids, and other types of specimens to assist the physician in obtaining a diagnosis. These professionals work with bacteria and viruses and use their technical skills combined with their knowledge of disease to perform their duties. They can make quality control decisions and can act independently within their profession. Hospitals, teaching universities, research organizations, and laboratories employ most of the medical technologists. Usually they have a bachelor of science (BS) degree in addition to their certification or license.

Medical Laboratory Technicians. Medical laboratory technicians (MLTs) perform most of the same test procedures that the medical technologist performs; the difference between the two is that they do not work independently. They are usually supervised by an MT and have at least an associates degree and a certification or license. MLTs work in the same types of facilities as MTs.

Physical Therapists. Physical therapists (PTs) assist patients in regaining their mobility and improving their strength and range of motion, which may have been impaired by an accident or injury, or as a result of disease. After assessing the patient, the physical therapist devises a treatment plan in conjunction with the patient's physician. The goal of the physical therapist is to improve how the patient functions at work and at home.

Respiratory Therapists. Most respiratory therapists (RTs) work in the hospital environment. All types of patients receive respiratory care, including newborns and geriatric patients. RTs commonly use oxygen therapy to assist with breathing, and they also perform diagnostic tests that measure lung capacity.

Occupational Therapists. Occupational therapists (OTs) work with patients who have developed conditions that disable them developmentally, emotionally, mentally, or physically. They assist in helping the individual to compensate for loss of function. The goal of OTs is to bring their patients to a level of living healthy, productive lives.

Diagnostic Cardiac Sonographers. Diagnostic cardiac sonographers (DCSs) assist in the diagnosis and treatment of cardiac and vascular diseases and disorders. They perform noninvasive tests, including echocardiographs and electrocardiographs. Often ultrasonography is used by the cardiovascular technician to assist the physician in discovering the malfunction of the heart and its structures.

Diagnostic Medical Sonographers. Diagnostic medical sonographers (DMS) assist physicians in the diagnosis of various disorders by means of ultrasound waves, which produce images of the internal structures of the body. These professionals are often called *sonographers*. Ultrasonography is used to assist the physician in many ways, including the monitoring of fetal development.

Radiology Technicians. Radiology technicians (RTs) use various machines to help the physician diagnose and treat certain diseases. These machines may include x-ray equipment, ultrasonographic machines, and magnetic resonance (MR) scanners. RTs explain procedures to patients and know correct positioning techniques, so that the images recorded are accurate and helpful for the diagnosing physician.

Paramedics. Paramedics are specially trained to provide emergency care to patients in life-threatening situations. Paramedics are highly efficient and well versed in the functions of the body. They perform advanced skills and, with more experience, are able to supervise or direct the operations of an emergency care ambulance facility.

Emergency Medical Technicians. Emergency medical technicians (EMTs) progress through several levels of training, each providing more advanced skills. Their medical education encompasses managing respiratory, cardiac, and trauma cases, and often emergency childbirth. There are also specialties within the EMT field

in certain states, such as EMT Cardiac, which includes training in **cardiac arrhythmias**, and EMT Shock Trauma, which includes starting intravenous fluids and administration of medication.

Registered Dietitians. Registered dietitians (RDs) have thorough training in nutrition and the different types of diets that patients are placed on to improve or maintain their condition. They use the advice of the physician and information about the patient to design healthy diets during hospital stays and even help to plan menus for home use. They also provide education for the patient about the diet and alternatives that will help in choosing attractive foods.

Closing Comments

The healthcare industry is certainly one of the most exciting career fields to enter in today's world. The constant change and development of new technology and theories make medicine an attractive option for career choices. The needs of medicine extend far beyond the boundaries of the United States, and collaborative efforts between countries promote a faster move forward with new discoveries and hope for those affected by disease. New headlines grace the papers and computer screens daily, and stories of human cloning, designer babies, genetic discoveries, and computer capabilities amaze us all. Medications are being developed that bring us to the brink of eliminating certain diseases. The mapping of the human genome may lead to incredible breakthroughs in the study of colon cancer, breast and ovarian cancer, cystic fibrosis, neurological degeneration, sickle cell anemia, and countless other conditions. There has never been a more thrilling time to become a part of the world of medicine and make a contribution as a healthcare professional.

Patient Education

The medical assistant must be able to help patients find community resources to improve their quality of life and provide needed services. The office should keep a current listing of all of the local resources as well as state and national resources. Service agencies such as the American Heart Association, American Red Cross, American Cancer Society, and others provide assistance and literature, often at no charge. Remember that not all of the patients seen in the office will be Internet savvy. Phone numbers and literature will be helpful, as well as Internet addresses.

Information about these agencies can be found in the phone book, library, newspaper, local Chambers of Commerce, and Internet sites. The medical assistant can provide information to patients with written leaflets and correspondence, as well as in-person discussions and over the phone. It is critical that the office conducts follow-up to be sure that the patient acted on the suggestions of the physician. When a referral to an outside agency is made, documentation of such should be made in the patient's chart.

Legal and Ethical Issues

The medical assistant should have a good understanding of the history of medicine so that there is an appreciation of those who paved the way and pushed to achieve today's level of medical care. These pioneers of medicine and patient care should be respected for their efforts to expand and improve healthcare, because many of them sacrificed their reputations and even their lives to prove the theories in which they believed. Their historical legacy, often taken for granted, represents enormous endeavors by these discoverers of new principles and treatments.

The ethical medical assistant will always strive above and beyond the call of duty to assist patients. Having information on hand to use in referring patients to various agencies is a way to ensure the patient's health and well-being outside the physician's office.

SUMMARY OF SCENARIO

Mr. Santos is an effective instructor, and one who is concerned about providing interesting material for his students. He wishes to instill a strong respect in the students for the people who played a role in early medical advances. His classroom discussions will help the students to think about what it was like to present new ideas to the public and often be ridiculed.

While teaching them about the history of medicine and the state of healthcare today, he also provides opportunities for the students to work together in discussion groups and present information to the class. He also encourages Internet research, a valuable skill that will help the medical assisting student in many areas of their training. In allowing the students to speak in front of the classroom while giving reports on the medical forefathers, Mr. Santos teaches them to be more at ease when speaking in public and when articulating instructions and details to patients and co-workers. All of these skills make a well-rounded medical assistant who will become a great asset to the facility in which he or she is employed.

SUMMARY OF LEARNING OBJECTIVES

- Greek and Roman mythology contributed the major portion of the medical terms we use today. Terms have also been borrowed from Anglo-Saxon, German, Arabic, and other sources, including the Bible.
- The American Medical Association adopted the staff of Aesculapius as the symbol of medicine. It is a staff encircled by a serpent. The caduceus is often mistakenly used to represent medicine, but is actually the medical insignia of the U.S. Army Medical Corps. This is a staff encircled by two serpents, bearing wings at the top.
- The Oath of Hippocrates is still administered to new medical graduates of many medical schools. It was written by Hippocrates, and contained ethical guidelines for the art of medicine. Clearly, medicine was to be considered a highly respected profession and honor was of the utmost importance. The Oath of Hippocrates can be found in more detail in Chapter 6 of this text.
- Johns Hopkins University Medical School has been recognized as a leader in healthcare education for over a century and was one of the first institutions to partner with a hospital for training purposes. It contained a research department as well, where faculty members investigated new methods and treatments for patients. Today Johns Hopkins is a $2.25 billion organization, containing three acute care hospitals and other entities of an integrated healthcare system.
- Numerous early pioneers made tremendous contributions to the medical field. Constant growth and research have pressed the medical profession forward, and with the assistance of technology, the growth speeds along today, faster than ever.
- World healthcare organizations provide information, medication, and personnel to attempt to eradicate disease and treat those diseases for which there is no cure. Many of these organizations operate with restricted funding and rely often on volunteer donations and volunteer workers to operate. WHO and the CDC often work together in an effort to effectively solve problems of epidemics and learn more about diseases. These organizations are a vital part of the medical industry today.
- Physicians' offices, group practices, and multispecialty group practices are a few types of ambulatory care. This division of medicine also includes occupational health centers, dialysis centers, rehabilitation clinics, and sleep centers. Patients who are ambulatory are able to move from place to place, usually on their own or with the assistance of a wheelchair or walker.
- There are three main provider portals of entry into the healthcare system today, which include medical doctors, osteopathic physicians, and chiropractic physicians. These different disciplines have some similar training, but osteopathic physicians usually use a holistic approach, and chiropractors concentrate many of their efforts on the alignment of the spine in an effort to promote a healing of the body.

INTERNET CONNECTIONS

- American Cancer Society
  www.cancer.org
- American Chiropractic Association
  www.amerchiro.org
- American Heart Association
  www.americanheart.org

- American Medical Association
  www.ama-assn.org
- American Osteopathic Association
  www.aoa-net.org
- American Public Health Association
  www.apha.org
- American Red Cross
  www.redcross.org
- Centers for Disease Control and Prevention
  www.cdc.gov
- Department of Health and Human Services
  www.os.dhhs.gov

- Hospice Foundation of America
  www.hospicefoundation.org
- National Council on Aging
  www.ncoa.org
- National Institutes of Health
  www.nih.gov
- U.S. Army Medical Institute of Infectious Diseases
  www.usamriid.army.mil
- United Way of America
  www.unitedway.org
- World Health Organization
  www.who.int

UNIT one

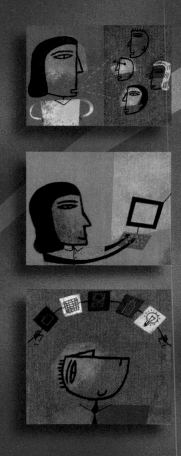

Introduction to Medical Assisting

CHAPTER 3

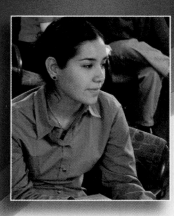

Scenario

Sandra Rameriz is a single mother who has decided on medical assisting as a career. She has always been interested in the medical field and wants a job that will allow her to spend evenings and weekends with her 3-year-old son, Roberto. The idea of working in a physician's office appeals to her, and she has applied to a school that is close to her apartment and day care provider. She plans to attend day classes and work part-time after school until it is time to pick up her son. Sandra is very excited about her new career and has set several goals for her training. First, she hopes to attain perfect attendance, and second, she would like to graduate with honors. She has budgeted her study time and plans to ask her instructors during the first 2 weeks of school for suggestions about how she can better prepare for classes and examinations. Sandra will find medical assisting to be a rewarding career and respected profession.

The Medical Assisting Profession

Learning Objectives

- Define and spell the terms listed in the vocabulary.
- Briefly discuss the history of medical assisting as a profession.
- Differentiate between administrative and clinical medical assisting duties.
- Discuss the versatility of a career in medical assisting.
- Explain the reasons that "bargain help" is often the most expensive.
- Identify several considerations when choosing a position as a medical assistant other than financial compensation.
- Discuss the aspects of the medical assistant's performance on a successful externship.
- List three unacceptable behaviors on the externship site.
- Explain why continuing education is so important to the medical assistant.
- Discuss the difference between a CMA and RMA.

Vocabulary

allied health fields Occupational disciplines in which professionals involved with the delivery of health-care or related services assist physicians with the diagnosis, treatment, and care of patients in many different specialty areas.

benefits Services or payments provided under a health plan, employee plan, or some other agreement, including programs such as health insurance, pensions, retirement planning, and many other options that may be offered to employees of a company or organization.

certification To attest as being true, as represented, or as meeting a standard; to have been tested, usually by a third party, and awarded a certificate based on proven knowledge.

continuing education units (CEUs) Credits for courses, classes, or seminars related to an individual's profession, designed to promote education and to keep the professional up-to-date on current procedures and trends in their field; often required for licensing.

cross-training Training in more than one area, so that a multitude of duties may be performed by one person, or so that substitutions of personnel may be made when necessary or in emergencies.

externship/internship A training program that is part of a course of study of an educational institution and is taken in the actual business setting in that field of study; these terms are often interchanged in reference to medical assisting.

intangibles Incapable of being perceived, especially by touch; incapable of being precisely identified or realized by the mind.

invasive Involving entry into the living body, as by incision or insertion of an instrument.

mandatory Containing or constituting a command.

perks Extra advantages or benefits from working in a specific job that may or may not be commonplace in that particular profession; a shortened form of *perquisites*.

phlebotomy The invasive procedure used to obtain a blood specimen for testing, experimentation, or diagnosis of disease.

profit sharing Offer of a part of the company's profits to employees or other designated individuals or groups.

stock option Offer of stocks for purchase to a certain group of individuals or certain groups, such as employees of a for-profit hospital.

versatile Embracing a variety of subjects, fields or skills; having a wide range of abilities.

According to the U.S. Department of Labor's *Occupational Outlook Handbook*, medical assisting is expected to be one of the ten fastest growing occupations through the year 2008. This exciting field is considered one of the most **versatile** of the healthcare professions. A career as a medical assistant is challenging and offers job satisfaction, opportunities for service, financial reward, and possibilities of advancement. Both men and women can be equally successful as medical assistants. Individuals considering the medical assisting discipline must be dedicated, committed, and have a strong desire to become *caregivers*. Caregivers are people who have the ability to put the needs of the patient first and have a sincere concern for those who are not at their best. A caregiver must feel an obligation to assist the patient in whatever way possible and have patience with those who, at times, are more difficult. This strong inner desire is one of the most important qualities of the successful, professional medical assistant. By developing this "caregiving" mentality, many personal rewards will follow, as will a long and beneficial career.

The History of Medical Assisting

The first medical assistant was probably a neighbor of a physician who was called on to help when an extra pair of hands was needed. As time passed and the practice of medicine became more organized and more complicated, some physicians hired registered nurses to help in their office practices. Gradually, record keeping, data reporting, and an increasing number of business details became important to physicians, and they realized a need for an assistant with both administrative and clinical training. Nurses were likely to have training only in clinical skills, so many physicians began training them or other individuals to assist with all of the office duties. Community and junior colleges began offering training programs that focused on both administrative and clinical skills in the late 1940s. Medical assistant organizations at the local and state level began developing around 1950, and soon after, certifying examinations were available. Today, medical assisting is one of the most respected **allied health fields** in the industry, and training is readily available through community colleges, junior colleges, and private educational institutions throughout the United States.

The Scope of Practice of a Medical Assistant

Versatile is an excellent descriptive term for today's medical assistant. The duties that medical assistants perform vary not only from office to office, but even within the same clinic. They perform routine duties within the offices of many types of health professionals, including physicians, chiropractors, podiatrists, and others. Individuals with medical assisting training can accomplish many jobs in the hospital environment, and some are employed by freestanding emergency centers or surgery centers. There are growing opportunities for medical assistants because of the constant change within the medical profession and the surge of **cross-training**, which means that one individual is trained to do a variety of duties. Medical assistants work under the direct supervision of a physician in the office and perform tasks delegated by the doctor or supervisor.

The American Association of Medical Assistants defines the scope of practice as the performance of delegated clinical and administrative duties within the supervising physician's scope of practice consistent with the medical assistant's education, training, and experience. The duties performed by the medical assistant do not constitute the practice of medicine.

There are two major categories of duties that medical assistants perform—administrative and clinical (Figure 3-1). On the administrative end of the spectrum, medical assistants greet patients who arrive in the office or clinic and obtain basic registration information from them. They may enter information into a computer and construct the patient's chart. They are trained to do office accounting, which may be done electronically or manually. The medical assistant is trained in filing procedures and in proper techniques for adding information to the patient's chart. A basic knowledge of procedure and diagnosis coding is important to today's medical assisting professional, and some medical assistants concentrate strictly on the billing and coding career option. The medical assistant is able to complete insurance claim forms and determine insurance coverage and limitations for the patient. Medical assistants answer telephones, schedule appointments, update medical records, and handle all types of correspondence. Often the medical assistant schedules outpatient procedures and hospital admissions, and may coordinate consultations with other physicians. Medical assistants who enjoy the administrative side of the profession often enter into office management positions.

The clinical duties that medical assistants perform are just as broad as the administrative duties. These professionals assist the physician with patient examinations and prepare the patient and the equipment needed before the examination. They assist with or perform basic testing procedures and are usually proficient in **phlebotomy**. Medical assistants are trained in first aid skills and cardiopulmonary resuscitation. They collect and prepare laboratory specimens and know how to adhere to OSHA and CLIA regulations. Often medical assistants working in the clinical area are responsible for inventorying and ordering supplies. If directed by a physician, they may administer various types of medications in most states. Medical assistants also perform electrocardiograms and prepare patients for x-ray evaluations. They assist in minor surgical procedures, prepare sterile trays, and perform autoclave sterilization procedures for instruments. Another clinical duty involves taking medical histories from patients, patient teaching, and obtaining and recording vital signs.

Medical assistants who enjoy the clinical side of the profession may also become office managers or may supervise other medical assistants. Duties and restrictions related to medical assisting vary from state to state, but in most of the United States, the medical assistant performs as an agent of the physician and is under the physician's supervision.

CRITICAL THINKING APPLICATION

- Sandra is not sure whether she will enjoy administrative or clinical assisting more. How can she begin to explore both avenues during her classroom training? During her externship/internship?
- How could Sandra explore the medical specialties and determine what areas might be of interest to her as a potential job site?

A Career in Medical Assisting

A trained medical assistant is equipped with a flexible, adaptable career (Figure 3-2). The skills acquired by the medical assistant are valuable, and employment is readily available anywhere in the world that medicine is practiced. Individuals working in the medical assisting field do not have a **mandatory** retirement age. Many medical assistants pursue their careers far beyond the usual retirement age, because physicians realize the value of the experienced, mature employee. This career attracts the nontraditional student who may be older than the average postsecondary student by a decade or more. Although many older students feel intimidated by the classroom, they normally have excellent experiences in school and become top in their class. Medical assisting is more than suitable for the student just exiting high school, who may plan on continuing his or her education and plans to use medical assisting as a viable income during further studies.

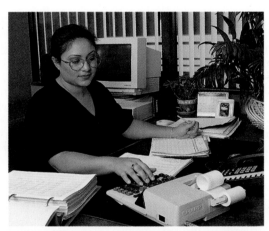

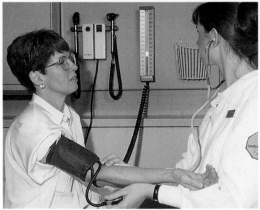

FIGURE 3-1 The responsibilities of a medical assistant include both administrative and clinical duties. (Bottom photo from Chester GA: *Modern medical assisting*, Philadelphia, 1998, WB Saunders.)

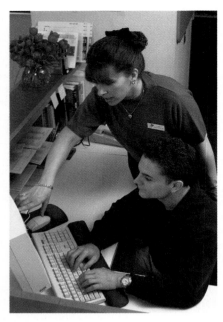

FIGURE 3-2 Medical assisting is a career with many benefits and perks, not to mention the internal rewards of assisting patients in need.

The practice of medicine has changed dramatically in the past several decades. Increasing costs have created a trend away from hospital-based treatment and moved toward the delivery of care in physicians' offices and in outpatient ambulatory clinics. Although physicians have employed medical assistants in their practices for many years, computerization and technologic advances have created more opportunities for formally trained medical assistants and their responsibilities have similarly increased. Clearly defined educational requirements have been determined by the nation's two certification organizations. These requirements have resulted in improvement of the quality and accessibility of medical assistant training, and have produced a healthy respect for medical assistants, who are considered a part of the allied health field.

Employment for medical assistants is abundant. There were 329,000 jobs held by medical assistants in the United States in 2000, and 60% of those were in physicians' offices. Career opportunities abound in public health facilities, hospitals, laboratories, medical schools, research centers, voluntary health agencies, and medical firms of all kinds. Jobs may also be available with federal agencies such as the Department of Veterans Affairs, the U.S. Public Health Service, and armed forces clinics or hospitals.

Most medical assistants derive a high degree of satisfaction from their work. Job turnover among medical assistants is surprisingly low; some medical assistants begin working with a physician when the practice is opened and stay until the physician's retirement. Most physicians have learned that "bargain help" is often the most expensive.

Medical assistants are compensated in various ways, some hourly and some by salary. The earnings vary from place to place. Overall, medical assistants can expect a healthy return on their investment in training, experience,

and skills. Most physicians realize that a good medical assistant is worth a higher-than-average wage, and a medical assistant with formal training often is compensated on a higher scale than one with no training. The *Occupational Outlook Handbook*, a Department of Labor publication, keeps statistics on the average salaries for many different career fields, including medical assisting. This information can be accessed at http://stats.bls.gov/ocohome.htm. More information on salaries may be obtained by monitoring the local help-wanted advertisements and by checking online job offer information on sites such as Yahoo! Careers. It is important to determine a realistic entering salary. Often graduates in many fields expect to make a much higher salary than is reasonable right after graduation.

The medical field often offers very good **benefits** to employees. Usually, the larger the organization, the better the benefits and **perks**. Most employers offer a health insurance plan or managed care plan to their employees. Often a moderate life insurance program is included, and dental insurance is always a valuable benefit. There are companies that have **profit sharing** plans and **stock options**. Some organizations give their employees access to credit unions, and many have discount options to local businesses, such as at a uniform shop. Remember that benefits and perks should be included when considering a certain job. Many medical assistants may choose to work for less money if the benefits and the opportunities for advancement are good. One should also consider driving time, holidays, paid parking, sick days, vacation days, and facilities when choosing a job. Do the co-workers seem to enjoy each other and get along? Is the physician friendly or more "stand-offish" and cold? All of these should be weighed carefully before making the final decision as to which position to accept. It is a truism that "money is a by-product of services rendered." Nowhere is this more accurate than in the medical field. When the patients are served well, the medical assistant becomes more and more valuable to the employer and is compensated accordingly.

CRITICAL THINKING APPLICATION

- Sandra knows that she needs certain benefits as a single mother. What might she need to look for in a potential job after her graduation?
- What are some ways that Sandra can compare positions and opportunities?
- What types of websites might help Sandra in learning about opportunities in her geographic location?

Education and Training

Ideally, a medical assistant should have both administrative and clinical skills, although he or she may have a personal preference for one or the other. The physician's staff must be able to handle all responsibilities of the office except those requiring the services of the physician or another licensed professional. Where there are several assistants, each should be able and willing to substitute in an emergency for any of the others and should be cross-trained on the basics of each other's duties. Teamwork is a very important part of any occupation, and even more so in the medical environment.

Certain knowledge and skills are expected of a trained medical assistant. The skills listed here are not all inclusive but suggest what may be expected on entry to employment as a professional medical assistant.

Classroom Training

Formal training is essential for today's medical assistant. Many community colleges, junior colleges, and private career institutions offer courses in medical assisting (Figure 3-3). After satisfactory completion of the program, the student receives a certificate or diploma. Students who attend community and junior colleges to study medical assisting may complete additional educational requirements to obtain an associate degree. Courses at the community college level usually take 1 to 2 years to complete, and offer enrollment two or three times per year. Private career institutions offer training that usually takes 7 to 10 months to complete, and offer enrollment as often as monthly.

Currently the trend is toward offering the medical assisting program in modules, so that the student receives some clinical training, some administrative training, and some theory in each module taken. Some classes are taught in traditional classrooms, and the clinical aspect is usually taught in a laboratory at the school. Much of the equipment that the medical assistant will use in practice is found in the laboratory, such as an autoclave, medical instruments and trays, and specimen collection equipment.

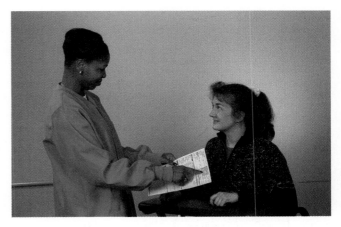

FIGURE 3-3   Get to know instructors and ask their advice on study habits and test preparation. Instructors are valuable references when the medical assistant begins the job search.

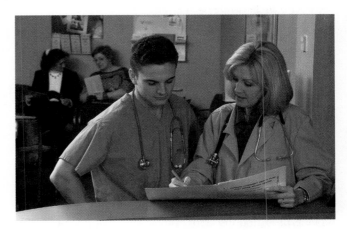

FIGURE 3-4   The externship/internship provides practical experience in the skills learned in the classroom. It is usually listed first on the resume once the medical assistant graduate prepares a resume, so it is vital to perform well and make a good impression.

CRITICAL THINKING APPLICATION

- How can Sandra develop a positive, nurturing relationship with her instructors?
- What should she do if she has difficulty in the classroom or if her grades begin to fall?
- How can Sandra study effectively and prepare for examinations?

Externships/Internships

Most medical assisting training programs require an **externship** or **internship** before the student graduates. For the purposes of this text, the terms are interchangeable and have the same meaning. This is a type of on-the-job training that allows students to put the skills they have learned in the classroom setting to use with real patients and staff members. The physician, probably more than any other employer, expects employees to carry out their duties independently, with little or no direct supervision. Someone at the externship site will be designated as the

student's supervisor. The medical assisting student should consult frequently with the externship supervisor to determine what is expected of the student and what progress is being made (Figure 3-4).

The student must be open to constructive criticism and be a willing learner. Techniques may be learned on the externship that were not included in the classroom training, or optional methods may be taught for various procedures. The medical assistant should never argue with the staff at the clinical site that a method taught by the school is the only correct way. Often there are several methods available to obtain the same result. The medical assisting student should treat the externship experience as if it were a probationary period on an actual job. Remember, the externship is often the first medical reference that the student will be able to list on the resume.

There are several general rules to remember while on the externship site. First, the medical assistant will have to gain the trust of the employees there. This is done by willingly performing the duties assigned in a timely manner and performing those duties to the best of the student's ability. If there are any questions at any time, the student should ask the externship supervisor instead of assuming or performing the duties the wrong way.

It is often helpful to read the job description of the medical assistant so that the student will understand what is expected of him or her. The student medical assistant must show responsibility and dependability. There should never be a time that the student is not busy while at the externship site. If all assigned duties are completed, the extern should offer to assist others in their duties or ask for additional responsibilities. There is always a counter that can be cleaned or filing to be done. The student who does these duties without being told shows initiative and a strong work ethic.

There are a few other unwritten rules for externs to know. A medical assisting student must never attempt to form a romantic relationship with patients or co-workers on the externship site. Patient confidentiality must be respected at all times, and anything that the student discovers about a patient must not be revealed or discussed under any circumstances. The student must not use any of the drug samples at the office unless specifically given permission by the physician. The student should never go to the drug storage area alone without permission or unless directed by the supervisor or physician. Externs should be extremely careful if asked to handle petty cash in the office. No student wants to be accused of any impropriety while performing their externship hours. Students must never ask the physician to treat them or any members of their family or friends. If the physician offers this as a benefit, it is acceptable, but one must not assume the physician is available for and willing to give free treatment. An extern must not ask the physician to provide prescriptions; most physicians will not prescribe medications for people who are not their patients for liability reasons.

CRITICAL THINKING APPLICATION

- If Sandra has any difficulty on her externship, whom should she contact?
- What should Sandra do when she has completed her normal duties for the day at the externship, and it is not yet time to leave the clinic?
- How can Sandra glean more knowledge from her co-workers on the externship?

BENEFITS FROM AN EXTERNSHIP

- The school has a line of communication to the community and is better able to assess the needs and expectations of the public for which it is training prospective employees.
- The externship agency benefits from the new ideas and methods that the trainee may introduce. If the facility is looking for additional help, this is an ideal way to evaluate the performance of a trainee without involvement in the hiring process.
- The trainee benefits most of all by exposure to practical experience in a variety of settings. This experience in the real world removes a great deal of the anxiety that might otherwise be present in a first employment situation.

The externing student should bring many **intangibles** to the physician's office not found in any job description. Courtesy toward others and a capacity for teamwork, a positive attitude, enthusiasm, initiative, and dedication are important personal attributes for the professional medical assistant. After becoming comfortably acquainted with what is expected on the externship, the student should concentrate on developing his or her skills and learning as much as possible during this short period. An extern becomes a valuable team player by assisting others and being reliable. By performing at peak level, the student gains the respect and trust of those on the externship site, and these people can become an excellent reference to use in beginning the search for that first paid position. Remember, the professional services of a medical assistant are extremely personal. Therefore the manner in which these services are performed can affect the health and welfare of a patient in either a positive or a negative way. When medical assisting students do their best to be sure that all contact with patients is positive in nature, they win the praise of patients, supervisors, and co-workers alike.

Continuing Education

Education does not end with the completion of formal training. The amount of medical knowledge gained is said to double every 5 years. The practicing medical assistant must keep current with the rapid changes within the profession. Most physicians appreciate the medical assistant who asks questions about unfamiliar conditions and procedures and are willing teachers about the function of the body and treatments that benefit the patient. Much can be learned by reading or reviewing the medical literature that arrives in the daily mail or articles that appear in newspapers, magazines, and medically related newsletters.

Continuing education classes are available to enhance the knowledge of the professional medical assistant. **Continuing education units (CEUs)** may be required to maintain the medical assistant's certification. These credits can be obtained through many sources, including the American Association of Medical Assistants, the American Medical Technologists, and various other agencies and educational institutions. Professional seminars and workshops often offer CEUs. Notices of continuing education classes are sent in bulk to medical facilities and physicians' offices, so the staff should watch for courses that pertain to their particular job duties and take advantage of them as available.

Professional Appearance

A well-groomed medical assistant in appropriate attire has a positive psychological effect on patients. The essentials of a professional appearance are good health, good grooming, and suitable dress.

Good health requires getting adequate sleep, eating balanced meals, and exercising enough to keep fit. Medical assistants can set a good example by following a sensible and healthful lifestyle that includes regular checkups of their own physical condition, both medical and dental. A radiantly healthy office staff promotes the best possible public relations image for the physician.

Good grooming is little more than attention to the details of personal appearance. Personal cleanliness, which includes taking a daily bath or shower, using deodorant, and practicing good oral hygiene, is vital. The use of perfume or aftershave cologne should be avoided or limited, because patients and co-workers may be allergic to some scents. A female medical assistant's makeup should be conservative and moderately applied. Heavy or exaggerated makeup is out of place in the professional office; subtle eye and lip makeup is best for the physician's office. Clear or muted shades of nail polish are best, and long nails are not only inappropriate, but can be dangerous to the patient and the medical assistant. Nails must be kept clean and at a conservative length. Both male and female assistants should be sure that the hair is shiny clean, neatly styled, and off the collar.

The medical assistant usually wears a uniform or lab coat, which not only presents a professional appearance, but also identifies the assistant as a member of the health-care team (Figure 3-5). Fashionable styling makes it possible for the medical assistant's uniform to be both practical and attractive. Women may choose to wear pantsuits, which are available in white or a variety of colors; a two-piece dress uniform in white or a color; an attractively styled traditional white uniform; or a scrub set. Scrubs have become increasingly popular and much more attractive over the past decade. They are now often made of pretty fabrics in rich colors and patterns and are much better suited for the professional office than the old green or blue scrubs worn in the surgical suites of hospitals. Men may also wear the newer scrubs or may choose white

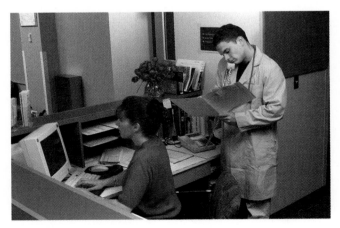

FIGURE 3-5   Medical assistants must have a professional appearance and demeanor in the medical office environment.

slacks with a white or colored shirt, jacket, or pullover top. If it is acceptable in the facility, a lab coat worn over street clothes may be worn, but it is important that the lab coat be buttoned when performing **invasive** procedures. Uniforms should be laundered daily, since medical assistants are exposed to ill patients throughout their workday. Shoes should be appropriate for a uniform and be spotless and comfortable. White shoes must be kept white by daily cleansing. Remember that if laced shoes are worn, the laces also need cleaning.

In some facilities, the physician prefers that the staff not wear uniforms. Some psychiatrists and some pediatricians, for example, believe that the clinical appearance of a uniform may affect patients adversely. However, today's uniforms reflect so many styles and patterns that the right one for the particular office should be readily available. Some of the fabrics depict cartoon characters or drawings that will appeal to children and still function as a durable uniform. A medical assistant who does not wear a uniform should follow the dictates of good taste and propriety in choosing a professional wardrobe.

The garments worn while on duty must be comfortable, allow easy movement, and still look fresh at the end of a busy day. Whatever uniform style the assistant chooses, it should be personally becoming and worn over appropriate undergarments. The lines, colors, and ornamentation of the undergarments should not be seen through the uniform; therefore it is best to wear a neutral color without a pattern. When wearing a uniform, jewelry should be limited to an engagement ring, wedding band, and professional pin. No more than two earrings per ear lobe should be worn, and the clothing or hairstyle should cover tattoos. A name badge worn on the right shoulder will help patients identify each staff person by name.

Be sure that there is a clear understanding of the dress code that is required in the office setting. Then adhere to that code as a demonstration of responsibility and the willingness to cooperate with office rules.

Professional Organizations

By joining a professional organization and taking part in the activities it affords, a medical assistant can grow personally and professionally, keeping abreast of current trends. Participation in a recognized professional organization shows that the employee takes the career seriously and wants to be an asset to the employer. There are national organizations, state chapters of these organizations, and local groups that meet to promote the profession of medical assisting. The organizations offer many benefits to members. Some offer health, disability, and malpractice insurance programs. Some offer VISA or MasterCard options and discount programs that are exclusive to their membership. All extend an opportunity for continuing education and learning beyond the classroom.

CRITICAL THINKING APPLICATION

- When should Sandra get involved with professional organizations for medical assistants?

CRITICAL THINKING APPLICATION—Cont'd

- How can she contribute to professional organizations in her area once she has graduated and secured a position as a medical assistant?
- Is it important that Sandra participate in volunteer organizations?

American Association of Medical Assistants and Certified Medical Assistants

The AAMA was formally organized in 1956 as a federation of several state associations that had been functioning independently. Today the AAMA has 43 state societies and more than 350 local chapters. The organization, whose national headquarters are located in Chicago, Illinois, has been a driving force behind establishing a national certification program for medical assistants. It has also been instrumental in the accreditation of medical assisting training programs in community colleges and private career institutes and in setting the minimum standards for entry-level medical assistants. Meetings are held on a national, state, and local level, where medical assistants can participate in workshops, learn about all types of advancement in the field, hear prominent speakers, and network with other medical assistants from other parts of the country. AAMA publishes a bimonthly journal called the *Professional Medical Assistant* (PMA), which includes articles with tests that may be submitted for CEU credit.

Since 1963 the AAMA has administered the CMA examination. Those who pass the examination are awarded the certified medical assistant (CMA) credential (Figure 3-6). Examinations are given in January and June of each year at more than 280 centers throughout the United States. **Certification** is available to graduates of medical assisting programs accredited by the Commission on Accreditation of Allied Health Education Programs (CAAHEP) or by the Accrediting Bureau of Health Education Schools (ABHES). Recertification is required every 5 years and can be accomplished through CEUs or reexamination. More information is available at www.aama-ntl.org.

American Medical Technologists and Registered Medical Assistants

In the early 1970s the American Medical Technologists (AMT), a national certifying body for laboratory professionals, began offering a certifying examination for medical assistants. This led to the formation of the registered medical assistant (RMA) program within the AMT organization in 1976. AMT offers this national certification to medical assistants who meet established standards and pass the examination (Figure 3-7). There are several other certification examinations offered by AMT that may be of interest to medical assistants. The certified office laboratory technician (COLT) examination is available to those who have completed certain educational and work experience requirements. Most medical assistants who work in the clinical area and have at least 6 months' experience qualify to take the examination. Medical assistants may also qualify to take the phlebotomy technician certi-

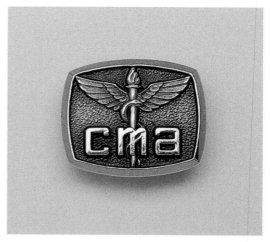

FIGURE 3-6   This pin is worn by the certified medical assistant. (Courtesy American Association of Medical Assistants, Chicago, Illinois.)

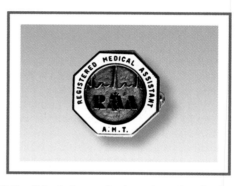

FIGURE 3-7   This pin is worn by the registered medical assistant. (Courtesy RMA/American Medical Technologists, Park Ridge, Illinois.)

fication examination (RPT) offered by AMT after meeting specific work-related requirements. AMT also provides societal benefits, including publications such as *AMT Events*, a quarterly magazine with useful information and articles relating to the professions served by the organization. AMT also offers national, state, and local meetings to enhance the knowledge and networking opportunities of its members. CEU credits are available to assist in increasing a medical assistant's level of competence.

The RMA examination can be scheduled nearly every day of the year other than Sundays and holidays at Prometric Testing Centers, with more than 300 locations throughout the United States. To find the nearest testing center, go to the Prometric website, which is www.2test.com. Applicants for the RMA examination must be graduates of a medical assisting course accredited by the Accrediting Bureau of Health Education Schools (ABHES) or by the Commission on Accreditation of Allied Health Education Programs (CAAHEP). The national headquarters for AMT are located in Park Ridge, Illinois, and more information about the RMA examination is available on their website, which is www.amt1.com.

The Difference Between CMAs and RMAs

Both of the certifying examinations are national credentials. The CMA credential is offered by the American

Association of Medical Assistants, and the RMA credential is offered by the American Medical Technologists. Since medical assistants are not required to be licensed, both of these examinations are voluntary. A medical assistant may practice in the United States without either certification, but most employers today require at least one certification. Both organizations have committees that develop the examinations, and they are both based on the roles that medical assistants fulfill in the workplace. Graduates from CAAHEP- or ABHES-accredited schools are immediately eligible to take the CMA or RMA examination. Both organizations publish a list of the programs they have approved for accreditation.

The major difference between these two credentials and organizations is the cost. The CMA examination fee for the 2002 testing year is $80 for CAAHEP graduates, but ABHES graduates must be members of the AAMA to obtain the $80 fee. The membership fees vary from state to state and will be substantially less expensive if joined while one is still a student. Student membership costs range from $20 to approximately $32 but must be applied for before graduating. Nonmembers must pay $155 to take the CMA examination. Annual dues thereafter are between $67 and $92, depending on the state association joined. The RMA examination cost is $85, which includes the first year's dues. Annual dues thereafter are currently $48.

CRITICAL THINKING APPLICATION

- Why is it important for Sandra to obtain one of the medical assisting certifications after graduation?
- How might certification help her career as a medical assistant?
- When can the tests be taken in your area?

MEDICAL ASSISTANT'S CREED

I believe in the principles and purposes of the profession of medical assisting.
I endeavor to be more effective.
I aspire to render greater service.
I protect the confidence entrusted to me.
I am dedicated to the care and well-being of all patients.
I am loyal to my physician-employer.
I am true to the ethics of my profession.
I am strengthened by compassion, courage, and faith.

Closing Comments

This chapter has presented the advantages of becoming a trained medical assistant and some of the many career opportunities available. The necessary skills that must be developed and the general knowledge that must be acquired to function effectively have been presented. However, skills and knowledge alone do not ensure success. Personality traits and professional appearance are also

critical. Professional societies and continuing education are vital to the professional medical assistant. The individual who accepts this career must be willing to accept the responsibilities inherent in its standards. Whatever the career goals of the medical assistant, the ideas expressed in this chapter will be useful to all.

Patient Education

The medical assistant may find it necessary to educate the patient about the definition of what a medical assistant is and does. Often, patients assume that those assisting in the offices are nurses, but medical assistants should never represent themselves in this manner. When making introductions with the patient, one should state: "I am Sandra Rameriz, Dr. Patrick's medical assistant." These words accurately portray the duties performed and help the patient to know who is who in the physician's office.

Medical assisting has grown into one of the most respected professions in the allied health field. When asked about the field, one should share the role a medical assistant plays in the office and the training involved. Others may be interested in a career change or have a desire to enter the medical field. A medical assistant should always be a good ambassador for the profession.

Legal and Ethical Issues

In the course of a medical assistant's daily work, a vast amount of personal and intimate knowledge will surface about the patients who entrust their care to the physician and the practice. Such information must be held in strict confidence and never be discussed or relayed to others, including professional associates, unless the lack of knowledge will affect the patient's care in a negative way.

On an externship, a medical assisting student should expect to observe all the office protocols of regular attendance, being on time, and in appropriate attire. The extern should hold the rules and regulations of the office in high regard and not expect special treatment. One should never expect or ask for payment for serving as an extern, because this is usually a part of the school curriculum.

During the externship practice, medical assisting externs should restrict practice to areas in which they have been trained. If the state has a scope of practice for medical assistants, know the boundaries within which they are expected to perform and do not exceed them. Some medical assistants carry their own personal malpractice or medical liability insurance policies, and externing students may be covered under a blanket policy held by their school. Remember, if ever in doubt about what is acceptable during the externship, or even in actual practice as a medical assistant, ask the physician or supervisor.

SUMMARY OF SCENARIO

Sandra has chosen to embark on an exciting career and will find her work very rewarding. She knows that she will be proud of her efforts and looks forward to becoming a respected member of the healthcare team in a physician's office. She has set goals for her class work and attendance, and is determined to meet them.

There are many opportunities for the medical assistant in both administrative and clinical positions, and as Sandra progresses through her training, she will find areas that appeal to her more than others. All are vitally important so that she will be a versatile medical assistant, able to perform front and back office duties. More exposure to various duties will be provided during the externship, and these experiences will help her to determine where she might enjoy working once she graduates. It is important that Sandra glean as much experience and knowledge as possible while in school so that she will have more options after her training.

Sandra should develop a good relationship with her instructors and go to them when she has questions or concerns. These professionals are anxious to share their knowledge and experiences with students to best prepare them for the work environment. If there is ever a situation in which her grades drop or she is struggling, Sandra should seek the advice of the instructor to improve her performance. The externship is also critically important, because it is usually the first medical reference a new graduate will have. Any difficulties at the externship site should be brought to the attention of the externship supervisor or an instructor at her school.

There are many benefits to working in the medical field, and Sandra will need to carefully weigh what she needs for herself and her son before taking any position. She should look at all of her options and choose the best one after careful evaluation. This will result in her satisfaction with her job and new career.

SUMMARY OF LEARNING OBJECTIVES

■ The first medical assistants were probably neighbors and friends of the physician. The field has grown into one of the most respected and versatile professions in allied health.

■ Administrative duties are those that involve running the office, such as scheduling appointments and filing insurance. Administrative medical assistants usually spend most of their day in the front office of the facility. Clinical duties include more patient contact and assisting the physician in the back office. Often new graduates move toward one or the other divisions but should always be ready and willing to adapt to new duties or fill in other areas when necessary.

■ Medical assistants are versatile enough to work in many different settings. Most often they are found in physician offices, but also work in hospitals, insurance companies, clinics, laboratories, and many other facilities. The combination of administrative and clinical training makes the medical assistant quite valuable to the employer.

■ Medical assistants who have been formally trained certainly deserve a fair wage, comparable to the national average for a person in whatever position they hold. When a supervisor or employer attempts to find "bargain help" at a cheaper rate, often they do not hire the quality employee that is so necessary in the physician's office. Since medical assistants help care for the patient, they should be compensated well so that the retention of the office staff will be continuous and stable. This can only help the physician care for patients in a more effective manner and gives the patients a sense of familiarity and security as well.

■ The medical assistant should consider many other factors than the salary when choosing a position. Location, perks, benefits, and the atmosphere of the office are all important. Many assistants are interested in growth within the organization and welcome those opportunities. Working for a friendly, caring physician and/or supervisor is invaluable. Sometimes, taking a lesser position in a well-known and reputable facility is temporarily worth a lower wage, because of future opportunities. Consider all aspects of a position before saying "Yes" to a job offer.

■ The medical assisting externship offers the student an opportunity to put the skills learned in the classroom to good use. If completed successfully, this is an excellent reference for the resume. The student should perform at the optimal level and never hesitate to complete duties assigned. Offer to go above and beyond to secure the support of the externship site as the job search begins.

■ An externing medical assistant should never attempt to form relationships with patients outside the office or view the chart for personal information. Do not ask the physician to treat family members or take medications without explicit permission from the physician or supervisor. Be very careful when handling cash and drugs in the office. The student should make every effort to never be late or tardy to the externship site, unless there is a severe emergency.

■ Continuing education is important to medical assistants so that the latest trends and information are readily available and accessible. Take advantage of local seminars and continuing education classes. Often the employer will agree to pay for classes or seminars that the medical assistant takes if they relate to his or her employment at the facility. Some will provide tuition reimbursement for college expenses, often even if the college courses are not related to the position the employee holds at the facility.

■ The main difference between the CMA and RMA credentials is the agency that provides each certification. The CMA credential is awarded by the American Association of Medical Assistants, and the RMA is awarded by the American Medical Technologists. Both are nationally recognized certifications.

INTERNET CONNECTIONS

- American Association of Medical Assistants
  http://www.aama-ntl.org/
- American Medical Technologists
  http://www.amt1.com/

CHAPTER 4

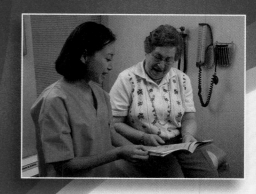

Scenario

Karen Yon has wanted to work in the medical field for most of her adult life. She volunteered in a local hospital during high school, and then after working for 3 years in the restaurant business, she enrolled in medical assistant classes. She studied very hard in school and graduated with honors. After her externship, she was asked to continue as a regular employee at a family practice in her area.

Karen strives to do all of her duties well in the physician's office. She wants to project a professional image to the patients and her co-workers. However, these are aspects of her job that are sometimes difficult to learn in the classroom setting. Since this is her first experience in the medical field, she wants to make a good impression on her employer and be a team player.

Professional Behavior in the Workplace

Learning Objectives

- Define and spell the terms listed in the vocabulary.
- Explain the meaning of the word *professionalism*.
- Discuss several of the characteristics of professionalism.
- Explain why confidentiality is so important in the medical profession.
- Discuss the role of the medical assistant's attitude in caring for patients.
- List some examples of office politics.
- Identify specific ways that teamwork can be promoted in the physician's office.
- Discuss the meaning of insubordination and why it is grounds for dismissal.
- Identify several categories of prioritizing tasks and their meaning.
- Talk about goal setting and how this helps in achieving career success.

National Curriculum Competencies

TRANSDISCIPLINARY COMPETENCIES

2a. Identify and respond to issues of confidentiality
2b. Perform within legal and ethical boundaries
2d. Document appropriately

Vocabulary

characteristics Distinguishing traits, qualities, or properties.

commensurate Corresponding in size, amount, extent, or degree; equal in measure.

competence The quality or state of being competent; having adequate or requisite capabilities.

connotation An implication; something suggested by a word or thing.

credibility The quality or power of inspiring belief.

demeanor Behavior toward others; outward manner.

detrimental Obviously harmful or damaging.

discretion The quality of being discrete; having or showing good judgment or conduct, especially in speech.

disseminated To disburse; to spread around.

initiative To cause or facilitate the beginning of; to initiate something into happening.

insubordination Disobedience to authority.

morale The mental and emotional condition, enthusiasm, loyalty, or confidence of an individual or group with regard to the function or tasks at hand.

persona An individual's social facade or front that reflects the role in life the individual is playing; the personality that a person projects in public.

procrastination Intentionally putting off doing something that should be done.

professionalism The conduct or qualities characterized by or conforming to the technical or ethical standards of a profession; exhibiting a courteous, conscientious, and generally businesslike manner in the workplace.

reproach An expression of rebuke or disapproval; a cause or occasion of blame, discredit, or disgrace.

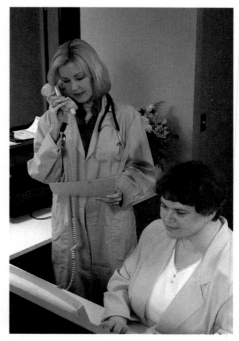

FIGURE 4-1   The professional medical assistant is an asset to the physician's office.

The word *professional* comes to mind when we think of physicians and those employed in their offices. What is professional behavior? We tend to hold medical personnel to a higher standard of **professionalism** than those in most other career fields. The medical assistant who works to improve his or her professional approach in the workplace will become quite valuable to the employer and will be promoted to positions of more responsibility more quickly within the healthcare industry.

The Meaning of Professionalism

Professionalism is defined as exhibiting a courteous, conscientious, and generally businesslike manner in the workplace. It is characterized by or conforms to the technical or ethical standards of a certain profession. Conducting oneself in a professional manner is essential for successful medical assistants. The attitude of those in the medical profession is generally more conservative than in other career fields. Patients expect professional behavior and will base much of their trust and confidence in those that exhibit this type of **demeanor** in the physician's office (Figure 4-1).

Characteristics of Professionalism

There are many **characteristics** that make up the professional posture required of medical assistants. It is critically important that a student medical assistant begin developing these characteristics while in school, because these qualities will not magically appear when the student begins working with actual patients. Although we might think that we would always behave appropriately during an externship or in a job setting, the habits developed in school will carry over into these experiences. If the behavior is unacceptable, it will be **detrimental** to the medical assistant's professional career. If the medical assistant wishes to advance and receive wage increases, promotions, and the trust of the employer, the following characteristics must be a part of his or her **persona**.

CRITICAL THINKING APPLICATION

- How can students practice professional behavior while still in the classroom experience?
- When students are practicing clinical skills, how can they incorporate professional behavior proficiency?

Loyalty

Loyalty is a faithfulness or allegiance to a cause, ideal, custom, institution, or product. Loyalty to an employer means that the employee is appreciative of the opportunity provided through the job and supports the company by giving the best effort possible. There are many

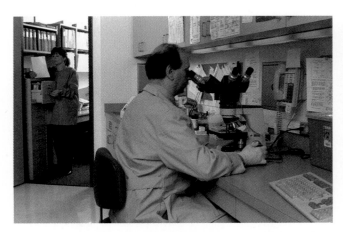

FIGURE 4-2 The physician will count on the dependability of the medical assistant to be at work on time and on each scheduled day. Absent or tardy employees cause scheduling difficulties and can greatly inconvenience the patients and remaining staff.

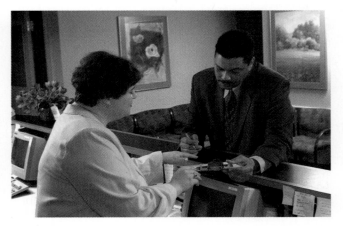

FIGURE 4-3 Taking a few moments to explain forms and bills to a patient is a courteous way to avoid misunderstandings and promote goodwill.

individuals today who are interested only in what the employer can provide them. However, this is an immature approach to take toward a job. When a person is employed by a company, there is an exchange of skills for different types of compensation. Each party benefits the other. Often we forget that experience alone is a great benefit from working. Loyalty to the employer is important, and the employee should feel a sense of loyalty from the company as well.

CRITICAL THINKING APPLICATION

- How can Karen demonstrate loyalty to her employer?
- What are some ways that her employer can reciprocate Karen's loyalty?

Dependability

One of the most valuable traits of a successful medical assistant is dependability. One should always be on time and make every attempt to be at work every day. When staff members arrive late, the entire day's schedule can be delayed (Figure 4-2). A medical assistant must follow through when the physician or supervisor gives an order. That person will count on the medical assistant to remember and complete all assigned duties. Supervisors should be confident that once given a task to do, the medical assistant will carry it out accurately and in a timely manner.

Courtesy

There is no excuse for not showing courtesy to the patients and co-workers in the physician's office. Kind words and compassion go far in building trust between the medical assistant and patients (Figure 4-3). It is essential that all visitors and staff members in the office be shown kindness and consideration. The fact that a medical assistant is having a bad day is no excuse for inflicting his or her

anger or irritation on patients. Always demonstrate a good attitude and offer patients and visitors a sincere smile.

Initiative

One of the more common complaints from supervisors is an employee's lack of **initiative**. Taking initiative means that the medical assistant looks for the opportunity to be of help, assisting others as the workload demands. Instead of waiting to be told to perform a task, look for jobs that need to be completed; never remain idle. There is always something that can be done in the medical office. There is never a lack of filing to be done. Inventories, supply ordering, or restocking can be performed when there is extra time in the medical facility. The medical assistant should also keep an eye on the reception area, since it may need to be tidied up several times during the day.

CRITICAL THINKING APPLICATION

- How can Karen show her initiative on the job?
- What types of duties can she perform when she has finished her workload for the day and there is still time left before leaving the office?

Flexibility

A medical assistant must be able to adapt to a wide variety of situations. An emergency could occur in the office, and the staff must be flexible enough to adjust the schedule and care for all of the patients. Being flexible also means that there is a willingness among staff members to assist each other in the performance of their duties. No one in the physician's office should say, "That's not my job." The patients must come first, and every staff member must be willing to lend a hand where needed. Some medical assistants trade or rotate their duties. If there is a task that one assistant does not particularly enjoy doing, perhaps another assistant would be willing to trade tasks. This way, both are more satisfied with their jobs. Being able to adapt quickly and cheerfully will make the medical assistant a valuable asset to the office.

Credibility

Credibility is the perceived **competence** or character of a person. It leads to the belief that the person can be trusted. Since trust is a vital component of the physician-patient relationship, the credibility of the physician and those who assist in the office should be strong. The information provided to patients must be accurate. Patients expect that the physician and medical assistant will instruct them in a manner that will enhance their health and provide positive results. One must take care in giving any advice to patients, because they view the medical assistant as an agent of the physician. Patients may not distinguish between the medical assistant's advice and the physician's orders. To avoid charges of practicing medicine without a license, a medical assistant must be sure to suggest only what the physician has authorized.

Confidentiality

The importance of confidentiality cannot be stressed enough in the medical environment. Patients are entitled to privacy where their health is concerned, and they should be confident that medical professionals use information only to care for them. One must never reveal any information about any patient to anyone without specific permission to do so. If in doubt, be conservative and verify that the person seeking information has the right to see it. Casual conversations in hallways, elevators, and break rooms between staff can be overheard by a family member or friend of the patient.

The rules regarding confidentiality extend beyond the medical office. While at home, medical assistants should not discuss details about patients with their families and friends. Those outside the medical profession do not understand how vital it is to keep information confidential and may pass along damaging facts to others. Medical assistants must make it a rule never to discuss a patient with anyone unless information must be shared for patient care and treatment.

Attitude

Possibly the most important asset a medical assistant brings to the office is a good attitude. This trait alone can influence promotions, terminations, and the entire atmosphere of the office (Figure 4-4). We are able to control our attitude, with practice. It takes skill to react calmly to people who are very upset, rather than to respond in kind, especially if we are being harassed or accused. If you speak in an even tone and perhaps a little softer than normal, the listener will have to lower his or her voice to hear yours. Offer to help resolve the problem and attempt to move to a private room out of the hearing range of other patients to talk.

Obstructions to Professionalism

It is not always easy to be a professional. Sometimes patients, co-workers, and supervisors try our patience,

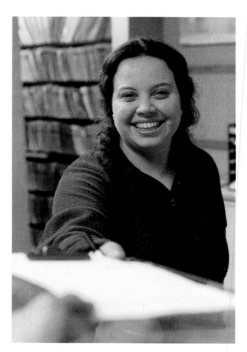

FIGURE 4-4   A good attitude goes a long way in patient and staff relationships.

and it can be hard to maintain a professional attitude in these cases. Some of the obstructions to professional behavior are discussed in this section.

Personal Problems and "Baggage"

Everyone has a life outside of the workplace, and sometimes we face challenges and difficult times that are hard to put aside. During working hours our thoughts should be on the job at hand, especially when we are dealing with patients. However, there may be situations in our lives that are so critical or important that we find ourselves thinking of them constantly. This personal *baggage*, as it is called, can interfere with our ability to properly perform job duties.

When there is a situation intruding on your thoughts at work, it is often best to take the time to talk with your supervisor. It is not necessary to share the intimate details, but a quick explanation that some difficulties are occurring outside of work will help the supervisor to understand any changes in your habit or attitude. However, there are some supervisors who are uncaring and are only concerned with satisfactory job performance. The medical assistant will have to use some **discretion** when discussing private affairs with the supervisor.

CRITICAL THINKING APPLICATION

- It is often hard to keep from thinking about a problem while you are working. How can Karen do this if she is concerned about a grandmother who is critically ill?

Rumors and the "Grapevine"

A rumor by definition is talk or widely **disseminated** opinion with no discernible source, or a statement that is not known to be true. The definition alone suggests that a rumor should be avoided. Most people enjoy working in an environment in which employees cooperate and get along with each other, but rumors can cause problems with employee **morale** and are often great exaggerations or manipulations of the truth. By promoting the grapevine, rumors are passed along and become more and more outrageous with each retelling. A medical assistant should refuse to participate in the office rumor-mill and attempt to be cordial and friendly to everyone at work (Figure 4-5). Supervisors regard those who spread or participate in rumors as unprofessional and untrustworthy.

Personal Phone Calls and Business

It is wise to avoid receiving unnecessary phone calls to the office from friends and family. The office phone should be considered a business line and must be used as such, except in emergencies. Visitors should not frequent the office, especially not in the area where the medical assistant is working. If someone must come to the office, always offer the reception area as a waiting room.

Checking personal email should also be avoided in the workplace. Any type of personal business, such as studying, looking up information on the Internet for personal use, or balancing a personal checkbook, should be done at home, not in the office setting. All of these distract the medical assistant from the job at hand; the focus should be on serving the patients in the office at all times.

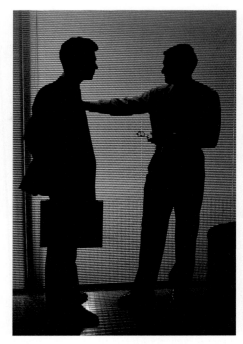

FIGURE 4-5   Gossip and rumors have no place in the medical profession. Avoid employees who participate in this type of activity.

productive workers, accept responsibility, be dependable, and always conduct themselves in a professional manner.

Procrastination

Procrastination is often a symptom of the fear of failure. Some people procrastinate because this gives them an excuse for failure. Others procrastinate because they are perfectionists and feel that only they can complete a project the right way. Procrastination is the surest way to see that goals remain unfulfilled. The best way to stop this habit is to DO something. Divide projects into small steps and complete one at a time. When a project is divided into small segments, it is much less overwhelming. The stronger the motivation, the easier it is to fight the urge to procrastinate.

CRITICAL THINKING APPLICATION

- Karen has a friend who works in a video store close to her office. Her friend has begun the habit of stopping in daily during her lunch hour to chat with Karen. How can Karen politely discourage her friend from doing this?
- Karen feels the need to check on her grandmother's condition as often as possible during the days she is ill. How might she accomplish this in a professional way?

Professional Attributes

Teamwork

If managers were asked what the most important attributes would be for medical professionals, teamwork would be high on the list (Figure 4-6). Staff members must work together for the good of the patients they care for. They must be willing to perform duties outside their formal job description if they are needed in other areas of the office. Many supervisors frown on employees who state, "That's not in my job description." Any order that is given by a supervisor becomes mandatory, and an individual who refuses to perform such a task can have his or her employment terminated for **insubordination**. A medical assistant should perform the duty and later discuss with

Office Politics

Most people associate office politics with some underhanded scheme or plans to move upward in the company in whatever way possible, whether the methods used are ethical or not. The tendency is to give the word *politics* a negative **connotation**. Politics can be defined as the art or science of influencing and guiding government or some other organization. The same can be applied to medical office politics. When an individual wishes to move upward in an organization, a certain strategy should be used. Many people develop a specific plan as to how they will advance, and in what time period they will accomplish this. Medical assistants who wish to advance should be

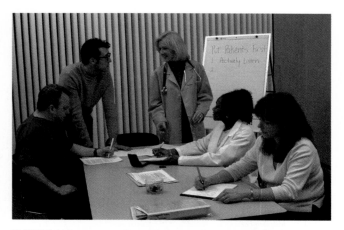

FIGURE 4-6 Teamwork is a vital part of the medical profession. All staff members must work together to care for the patient and perform required duties in the physician's office.

the supervisor any valid reasons that it should have been assigned to someone else.

Although we would all enjoy working in an office in which everyone gets along and likes every other employee, this does not always happen. Personal feelings must be set aside at work, and all employees must cooperate with others to get the job done efficiently. If a medical assistant has an issue with another employee, the first move would be to discuss it privately with the other person. Then, if the situation does not improve, perhaps a supervisor should be involved for further discussions.

Time Management

We have often heard the expression "work smart." This means that we are to use our time efficiently and concentrate on the duties that are most important first. To do this we must first prioritize our duties and arrange our schedule to ensure that these duties can be performed (see the next section). The first way to improve time management is to plan the tasks that need to be done that day. Taking 10 minutes to write down the day's tasks will help to ensure that they are done. Then it is important to stay on schedule throughout the day, unless emergencies disrupt the schedule. Even then, when office days are well planned, allowances can be made for emergencies, even if they happen often, and the majority of the tasks can still be completed. The key to managing time is prioritizing.

Prioritizing

Prioritizing is simply deciding which tasks are most important. Many people make a "to do" list for the day's activities, but the secret to success is prioritizing those activities into categories that give order to the tasks.

Most tasks can be prioritized into three general categories. There are activities that *must* be done that day, some that *should* be done that day, and those that *could* be done if there is time. Once you have a general list of tasks, review the list and further prioritize it, using a code such as *M* for must, *S* for should, and *C* for could (or this might be further simplified by using the letters

A, *B*, and *C*). Once the tasks are divided into these categories, they can be further classified within each section. For instance, if there are six A category duties, meaning they *must* be done today, these six can be numbered in the order they should be performed. The same process is completed with the B and C categories, and then as the tasks are completed, they are checked off for that day. Other categories can be added to customize the list. For example, an *H* category can be used for duties to perform at home, *P* could represent phone calls that need to be made, and *E* could represent errands to run. Customizing the categories will make the list more user-friendly.

Goal-Setting

Those who succeed in life are planners and goal-setters. The first step in becoming a proficient goal-setter is to take the time to really think about what is to be accomplished throughout one's lifetime. These goals must be written down and reviewed often. Goals should be set for all areas in a person's life, including personal growth, career, home life, family, spiritual needs, and any others that apply to the individual. The goals should not be unreasonable. They should be measurable and specific, with written steps detailing how they will be reached. Determination and persistence in reaching the goals will help to make them happen, along with a healthy dose of hard work. The goals should be reviewed often and progress evaluated; then goals can be reset as necessary.

Remember to celebrate the accomplishments and move past any goals that are missed, evaluating and restating the goals if necessary. Charles Kettering, an inventor who is most well-known for his invention of the automobile self-starter, once said, "The only time you can't afford to fail is the last time you try." Never quit trying to improve and experience personal growth.

CRITICAL THINKING APPLICATION

- What are some goals that Karen might set related to her behavior on the job?
- List several goals for the new medical assistant to work toward during his or her first year in the field.

Knowing the Facility and its Employees

A much-circulated story tells of a college professor who used to end a critical test with the question, "What is the name of the woman who cleans our wing of the building?" This would perplex most students, but the question makes a good point. A professional medical assistant should attempt to get to know the people who work in the facility and should have a good idea of who handles which duties (Figure 4-7). When patients have specific problems with which they need help, they can be referred to the person

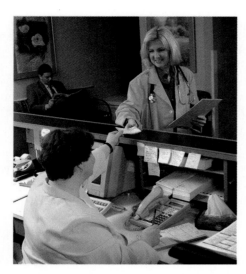

FIGURE 4-7 Knowing which employee to call when help is needed promotes goodwill among employees and often gets a task done more efficiently.

who knows the most about that particular issue. It is wise to express appreciation to others whenever possible. Say "thank you" often or "I appreciate your help" when working with others. This will make co-workers more likely to assist at other times when their help is needed.

Documentation

From the standpoint of professional behavior, documentation skills are vital to medical assistants. Charting accurately with legible, neat handwriting can make a difference in the perception of professionalism in the medical office. Be complete in any narrative regarding patients. Be sure to state facts, not opinions, and never use sarcastic remarks when charting. Phone messages must be documented carefully as well, and handled in a professional manner. Never use sarcasm when reporting messages to the physician or anyone else in the office. Use conservative speech and proper wording in all situations in the medical facility.

Note-Taking

Whenever office meetings or seminars are held, be prepared by having a pad and pencil ready for note-taking. A medical assistant should never be without paper and pen so that accurate information from the meeting can be jotted down for future reference. It is wise to keep a notebook or file on office meetings to refer to in case clarification of an order or a point is needed. Another good idea is to keep a small spiral notebook in a pocket with a pen, so that if an order is given in passing by the physician, the medical assistant will have a place to jot it down until he or she has access to the patient's chart. This avoids giving incorrect dosages of medication or forgetting to order a laboratory test, as well as many other errors that could be made by relying on memory.

Work Ethics

Work ethics can involve a whole range of activities, from individual acts to the philosophy of the entire facility. A person who has good work ethics is one who arrives on time, is rarely absent, and whose work output is **commensurate** with the pay received. Work ethics also involves other situations. If another employee is seen taking drugs from the supply cabinet or money from the cash box, the act should certainly be reported. However, if the guilty employee is also a close friend of the person who witnesses the act, an ethical dilemma is present. Ways to solve ethical problems will be discussed in Chapter 6. A medical assistant must always act in such a way that his or her actions are above **reproach**.

Communication

Communication skills are paramount in working with patients and other health professionals. A medical assistant should work hard to perfect his or her communication techniques. Often the success of a business is directly related to its ability to communicate effectively. Communication skills will be discussed in detail in Chapter 5.

Closing Comments

Patients expect and deserve professional behavior from those who work in medical facilities. Always show compassion, caring, and consideration for a person who comes to the office, whether a patient, visitor, or co-worker. By displaying these traits, the medical assistant will earn the respect of co-workers and become indispensable to the physician-employer.

Patient Education

When speaking to patients and providing them with information, remember that most do not have any medical background and do not understand many of the phrases used by the medical community. A medical assistant must be patient and explain in a courteous manner any aspect of the instructions or details that the patient does not understand. When educating the patient, the medical assistant should have a professional attitude of concern and helpfulness. Assure the patient that medical assistants and the rest of the staff in the facility are bound by rules of patient confidentiality if the patient seems concerned about revealing pertinent information.

Never transfer personal problems and baggage to the patient. A professional medical assistant does not share personal information with anyone at the medical facility. It is forbidden to pass along rumors of any type to patients or their families. The workday should be centered around patient care, so never allow personal business to impinge on time that should be spent assisting patients and the physician.

Legal and Ethical Issues

Behaving in a professional manner in the medical office will help to gain the patient's trust. Trust is one of the most important factors in avoiding cases of medical professional liability. Treating patients with care and not subjecting them to poor attitudes and unnecessary information will keep the patient-physician relationship a strong one, conducive to the health and recovery of the patient.

SUMMARY OF SCENARIO

Karen is happy to be employed in a family practice in which providing quality patient care is paramount. She is learning to be careful of what she says and to remain focused on the patient instead of any difficulties she may be having. She made an appointment to speak with her supervisor and explained the situation with her grandmother. The supervisor was very sympathetic and encouraged Karen to call and check on her grandmother whenever she felt she needed to, even offering the use of her phone and office. Karen was happy to find support in this area, and she has not taken advantage of the time she has been given to provide support to her own family.

Karen knows that it is her responsibility to be a team player and to assist the other staff members as much as possible. She maintains a good attitude, even when personal issues could distract her from her duties. Karen gets a strong sense of pride in being a part of the medical profession. She insists on a neat appearance and arriving on time for each scheduled workday. She always asks others if they need help when she has any extra time throughout the day. Karen looks forward to a long relationship with her employer. The rewards she feels as a member of the health team are second to none.

SUMMARY OF LEARNING OBJECTIVES

- Professionalism is the characteristic of being or conforming to the technical or ethical standards of a profession. It involves exhibiting courtesy, being conscientious, and conducting oneself in a business-like manner at the workplace. Professionalism is vitally important in the medical profession.

- Some of the characteristics of professionalism include loyalty, dependability, courtesy, initiative, flexibility, credibility, confidentiality, and a good attitude.

- Confidentiality is vitally important in the medical profession. Patients depend on medical personnel to keep their health information confidential and private. Breach of patient confidentiality is one reason that an employee could be immediately terminated from his or her position and can result in litigation between the patient and the physician-employer.

- Because most patients are not at their best when visiting the physician's office, the attitude of the staff plays an important role in patients' attitude while in the office. Medical assistants need patience when working with those who are ill. A smile or a reassuring pat on the back will go a long way and be encouraging.

- Office politics can be negative or positive. A person who uses others to be promoted through the company or takes credit for a team effort may be using office politics in a negative way; a person who strategically plans advancement by outstanding performance, dependability, and teamwork uses office politics in a positive manner. Knowing when to speak and when to listen will help the medical assistant to play the game of politics well in the medical facility.

- Teamwork makes any job easier to complete. By helping those who may be overwhelmed with duties, the medical assistant may find willing co-workers who will help when the situation is reversed in the future. If two assistants both have duties they dislike, they might trade the duties and both be satisfied.

- Insubordination can be used as grounds for immediate dismissal. Insubordination is being disobedient to any type of authority figure, usually the supervisor. When given a task to complete, the medical assistant should carry out the order unless it is unlawful or unethical. If the medical assistant feels that the duty should have been performed by someone else or there was some reason it should not have been performed, the supervisor should be consulted. Discuss the issue and attempt to reach an agreement about the appropriateness of performing the task in the future.

- Prioritizing tasks can help the medical assistant to accomplish more tasks. Prioritizing can be used for work, home, and extracurricular activities. Tasks can be identified as those that must, should, or could be done today. Then within each of these categories, the tasks can be numbered in the order they should be completed.

■ Goals should be written down and reviewed often to check progress. Taking small steps toward goals will help ensure that they are eventually reached. Individuals should set goals in each area of their lives, breaking the tasks down into manageable parts. Goals should not be unreasonable or unattainable, but should provide the opportunity for small successes along the way to reaching the ultimate goal.

CHAPTER 5

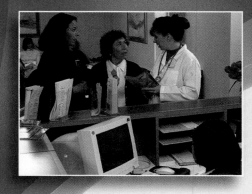

Scenario

Many types of patients seek medical attention and care in the physician's office. Each will have different needs and different concerns, even when they have similar diagnoses. Communication and interpersonal skills are vitally important in meeting these needs and providing optimal care to the patient. However, the patient is not the only individual to consider. Family members are often instrumental in the health and well-being of the patient.

Lucille Cloyd is an 83-year-old patient who has been diagnosed with pancreatic cancer. Her daughter, Sarah Smithson, helps to care for her; she is very close to her mother emotionally. Sarah is also a patient of the same physician that cares for her mother. Although Sarah does not wish to see her mother in pain, she suffers with the knowledge that life will be very different without her. Mrs. Cloyd is widowed, and visits the physician once a month in addition to hospice services. She is a good-humored woman who feels she has led a fruitful life, yet she has moments of depression. She has been living with Sarah and her family for 2 months and enjoys interacting with her two grandchildren and the family's pets.

The medical assistant must consider not only Mrs. Cloyd, but also her extended family. Compassion and sensitivity will be necessary to care for this patient, as well as excellent listening skills. A good knowledge of human relations will help the medical assistant in making Mrs. Cloyd's medical care as pleasant as possible under the circumstances.

Interpersonal Skills and Human Behavior

National Curriculum Competencies

TRANSDISCIPLINARY COMPETENCIES

1b. Recognize and respond to verbal communication

1c. Recognize and respond to nonverbal communication

Vocabulary

adage A saying, often in metaphorical form, that embodies a common observation.

aggression A forceful action or procedure intended to dominate; hostile, injurious, or destructive behavior, especially when caused by frustration.

ambiguous Capable of being understood in two or more possible senses or ways; unclear.

animate Full of life; to give spirit and support to expressions.

battery An offensive touching or use of force on a person without his or her consent.

caustic A remark or phrase marked by sarcasm.

channels Means of communication or expression; courses or directions of thought.

comfort zone A place in the mind where an individual feels safe and confident.

congruent Being in agreement, harmony, or correspondence; conforming to the circumstances or requirements of a situation.

decode To convert, as in a message, into intelligible form; to recognize and interpret.

defense mechanisms Psychological methods of dealing with stressful situations that are encountered in day-to-day living.

encode To convert from one system of communication to another; to convert a message into code.

encroachments That which advances beyond the usual or proper limits.

enunciate To utter articulate sounds; the act of being very distinct in speech.

external noise Sounds or factors outside the brain that interfere with the communication process.

externalization To attribute an event or occurrence to causes outside the self.

feedback The transmission of evaluative or corrective information to the original or controlling source about an action, event, or process.

grief An unfortunate outcome; a deep distress caused by bereavement.

internal noise Factors inside the brain that interfere with the communication process.

language barrier Any type of interference that inhibits the communication process that is related to languages spoken by the people attempting to communicate.

litigious Prone to engage in lawsuits.

malediction To speak evil of or curse.

media Term applied to agencies of mass communication, such as newspapers, magazines, and telecommunications.

paraphrasing To express an idea in different wording in an effort to enhance communication and clarify meaning.

perception Capacity for comprehension; an awareness of the elements of the environment.

physiological noise Physiological interferences with the communication process.

pitch Highness or lowness of a sound; the relative level, intensity, or extent of some quality or state.

proxemics The study of the nature, degree, and effect of the spatial separation individuals naturally maintain.

sarcasm A sharp and often satirical response or ironic utterance designed to cut or give pain.

stereotype Something conforming to a fixed or general pattern; a standardized mental picture that is held in common by many and represents an oversimplified opinion, prejudiced attitude, or uncritical judgment.

stressors Stimulus that causes stress.

subtle Difficult to understand or perceive; having or marked by keen insight and ability to penetrate deeply and thoroughly.

thanatology The description of the study of the phenomena of death and of psychological methods of coping with death.

vehemently Marked by forceful energy; intensely emotional.

volatile Easily aroused; tending to erupt in violence.

The interpersonal skills developed by the medical assistant help to set the tone of a medical office. Human relations can be defined as the study of the problems that arise from organizational and interpersonal contact. The two entities intersect each other, and a successful medical assistant will work to enhance these attributes on a continual basis. Patients who visit the healthcare facility may not be at their best, and the way in which the medical assistant reacts and interacts with them can make an incredible difference in their perception of the office, the physician, and the medical staff.

First Impressions

Our elders have stressed all of our lives that first impressions are lasting ones, and this old **adage** is still true! The opinions formed in the early moments of meeting someone remain in our thoughts long after the first words are spoken. The first impression is much more than just physical appearance or dress; it includes attitude and compassion, and the all-important smile (Figure 5-1)!

One of the primary objectives of the professional medical assistant is to care for and about the people that are being served. Patients are the reason for the existence of the facility, and they should be offered the best customer service available. They must be warmly welcomed, and it is important to call patients by their names. People enjoy hearing their name, and it gives the patient confidence that the medical staff knows whom they are caring for.

Although you may function comfortably in your facility, try to put yourself in the place of the new patient, who is entering unknown territory. As a staff member of the facility, you are in familiar surroundings and already have some information about the new patient. However, the patient knows nothing about you or the other staff members. One way to break that barrier is to have all staff members wear name badges, with letters large enough to be read at a distance of 3 feet. Include the staff position

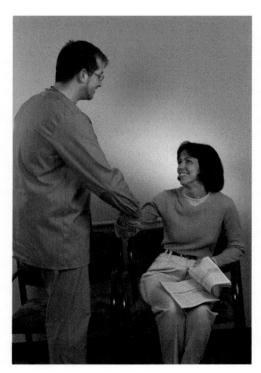

FIGURE 5-1   First impressions are critical in gaining the patient's trust.

if there are several divisions of responsibility; for instance, "medical assistant," "insurance biller," and "office manager." When the patient approaches, even though you are wearing a name badge, introduce yourself and smile. Let your smile show both facially and in your voice and eyes and genuinely welcome the patient to the office. This small effort will help to put the patient at ease in your environment.

Many physicians make brief notes in the chart about the personal lives of the patient. Then, when the patient arrives for the appointment, the physician can ask about his or her recent trip abroad or new grandchild. This tells the patient that the doctor and the office staff see him or her as more than just an illness or a chart number. It gives the impression that they truly care, and that impression should be an accurate one. Once an impression is formed in the patient's mind, it is very difficult to change, so make the first impressions of your office positive ones.

Communication Paths

Verbal Communication

Messages are conveyed by the use of language, which may be written, spoken, or communicated in another way. Verbal communication depends on words and sounds. The **pitch** of the voice is a part of verbal communication. The voice lifts at the end of a question. It drops at the end of a statement. Usually, when a speaker intends to continue a statement, the voice will hold the same pitch, the head will remain straight, and the eyes and hands will be unchanged. This is not an appropriate time to

interrupt. If the message is interrupted, the train of thought may not be completed. Tone of voice and choice of words also affect messages.

The medical assistant should speak clearly and **enunciate** words properly. Speak loudly enough that the patients are able to hear clearly and pay particular attention to those who wear some type of hearing assistance device. It is wise to note this information on the patient's chart to jog the memory when a patient with a hearing problem visits the office. Never assume that just because a patient is elderly, he or she has a hearing problem. When talking with patients, be sure to use the volume of speech to an advantage. Always speak at a clearly audible level, but at times it will be necessary to increase or decrease the volume of speech. When a patient is upset, for instance, it often helps to lower the volume of speech, because the patient tends to get quieter to hear the person speaking.

Eye contact is critical. Look at the person being spoken to, and do not forget a genuine smile. Many people feel that a person who speaks and cannot look another in the eyes is being deceptive. It can also mean that the speaker is very shy and has little self-confidence. Use gestures where appropriate to liven speech and **animate** the conversation.

Medical assistants must become aware of how they express themselves and how they affect the feelings of others. The tone of voice is vitally important. There is no place for **sarcasm** or **caustic** remarks. For example, saying "I hope you can manage to be on time for your next appointment" to a patient is needless and rude. The medical assistant must be conservative when speaking and not be too familiar. The patient expects professionalism and has the right to demand this in the healthcare setting. Never make an inappropriate remark and follow with "I was just kidding." This has no place in a medical facility. Take special care not to hurt anyone's feelings with words and phrases. Be very careful about what is said, especially to patients.

Remember that patients are in the facility to be treated or cared for by the physician and staff. They are usually concerned about their illness and may have great apprehensions and fears about the future. It is completely out of place for the medical assistant to talk about his or her personal life and challenges with the patients. Allow the patient to speak, and listen, instead of offering personal information. Often patients will casually mention things to the medical assistant that might influence their care. The saying that we are given "one mouth and two ears" stresses which should get more use!

Nonverbal Communication

Both verbal and nonverbal communications are important in the art of expression, and both are needed to succeed in the communication exchange. Nonverbal communications are messages conveyed without the use of words. They are transmitted by body language, gestures, and mannerisms that may or may not be in agreement with the words a person speaks. Body language is partly instinctive, partly taught, and partly imitative. It involves eye contact, facial expression, hand gestures, grooming, dress, space, tone of voice, posture, touch, and much more. We are often unaware of our own nonverbal signals and consciously recognize only a small number of the signals sent by others. Our ability to help others increases as we hone our own skills in interpreting nonverbal communication.

Appearance is an integral part of nonverbal communication. It influences the way others view us, and can present a conflicting message, or even a totally incorrect message. When we see someone who dresses or grooms in a way that is very different from our own style, we tend to assume that the personalities are opposite. This is not always true. Although we should not judge people by the way they dress, it is difficult not to form opinions based on what is seen. Visible piercings and tattoos are often looked on unfavorably in the medical profession, as are brightly painted long nails. Although these do not signify that the wearer is not professional, many patients, especially older patients, look on these trends unfavorably. For this reason alone, the medical assistant who is less conservative may be diminishing the chance for certain jobs and advancements. It is healthy to express oneself, yet in the medical profession, professional appearance is mandatory to avoid blocks in communications.

The successful medical assistant expresses self-esteem and confidence by stance, vocabulary, facial expression, and a caring attitude. The experience of speaking to someone who does not make eye contact helps one to realize the importance of greeting the patient with the eyes as well as the voice and body language. Facial expressions often convey our true feelings and are not masked by the words we use. Our eyes often tell the truth when our words are misleading or false. It is important to have an open body stance when dealing with patients. Crossed arms and legs hint that one is "closed" to the person being spoken to, and this may be construed as disinterest or disbelief. Nonverbal and verbal communications are dependent on one another (Figure 5-2). They must be in harmony to convey an accurate message, easily interpreted by the receiver. If the two are not **congruent**, the nonverbal is usually dominant and expresses the true message.

Our need for personal space is demonstrated by how patients in the reception area will choose a seat. **Proxemics** is defined as the study of the nature, degree, and effect of the spatial separation individuals naturally maintain and how this separation relates to cultural and environmental factors. Seldom will a person sit in an adjoining seating space with a stranger, if there is another option. Although the need for space varies with the individual culture, some might even remain standing to satisfy the need for personal space. Public space is usually accepted as a distance of 12 to 25 feet, and social space is usually considered to be 4 to 12 feet. Personal space ranges from 1.5 to 4 feet, and intimate contact includes physical touching to about 1.5 feet. The medical assistant can often tell when he or she has invaded someone's personal space, because the person will tend to back up a step or two. If this happens, take a small step back and respect the boundaries that are being set. The more familiar and comfortable patients are with the medical assistant, the closer the space they will allow.

Touch is a powerful communicator. The soft acceptance of someone's hand in yours, to the good-natured pat on the back, to the harsh slap on the face, all relay different messages that need no words to accurately express. In the medical profession, as in any business, touch can be comforting or can promote a sexual harassment suit. Unfortunately, one must be extremely careful when using this effective communication tool. In today's **litigious** atmosphere, any nonconsensual touching may be considered **battery**, and touch should be used with great discretion and cautious care.

The medical assistant should not, however, be afraid to touch the patient appropriately, such as a pat on the back or a squeeze of the hand (Figure 5-3). Some patients are receptive to a brief sideways hug, whereas others would take this as an intrusion into their personal space. Certainly patients with serious illnesses appreciate touch as an expression of empathy. Never be afraid to touch sick patients, especially those with diseases such as AIDS, as long as proper precautions are followed where indicated. These individuals need to feel acceptance, and the attitude of the medical staff members they encounter will directly influence their adherence to keeping their appointments with the physician. If they do not feel accepted and cared for, they will not return to the physician's office. A gentle touch and a smile do wonders for showing that you care.

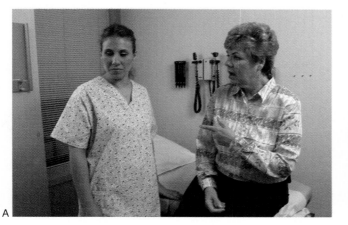
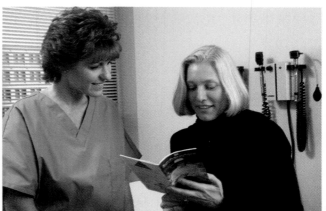

A   B

FIGURE 5-2   **A,** Pointing is often an accusatory gesture and causes discomfort. **B,** A bright smile helps to put the patient at ease and relax.

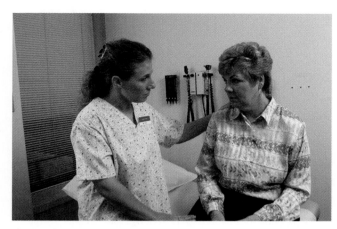

FIGURE 5-3   Touching the patient communicates care and compassion.

CRITICAL THINKING APPLICATION

- How might touch be an important communication tool with Mrs. Cloyd?
- How can Sarah be affected by using touch?
- Could laughter affect either of these women as they deal with death?

Posture can signal depression, excitement, anger, or even an appeal for help. When the physician sits at the front of the chair and leans forward, he or she is giving the message of caring and interest. Positioning is important as well. Sitting behind a desk promotes an air of authority. Standing or sitting across a room may convey a negative message of denying involvement or reluctance to talk. The medical assistant should practice good postural techniques as a part of projecting a positive image and for personal health reasons.

The Process of Communication

Anyone who works within the realm of public service should develop good communication skills. It is critically important to be able to interact with others and put them at ease, so that their comfort level increases and they develop trust. To communicate well, we must first have a general understanding of the process of communication. Once a message is sent, it cannot be retrieved and restated or expressed in a different way. Especially in the medical profession, communication must be clear and concise, and the message we intend to send must match what the receiver understands.

Although there are many different scientific models of communication, the one that best fits most types of communication is the *transactional communication model*. Before understanding how this model works, one must understand the elements we use to communicate.

Usually, when two people interact, both people act as a sender and as a receiver. The sender is the person who sends a message through a variety of different **channels**. Channels can be spoken words, written messages, and body language. The sender **encodes** the message, which simply means that he or she chooses a specific way of expression using words and other channels. The receiver **decodes** the message according to his or her understanding of what is being communicated. However, there are times that the receiver understands the message incorrectly. This is often because of noise, which is anything that interferes with the message being sent. It can be literal noise, such as a radio or a jackhammer on the street outside. This is called **external noise**. Or, it could be **internal noise**, which would include the receiver's own thoughts or prejudices and opinions. **Physiological noise** interferes with communication as well. This includes any biological factor that would preclude the communicator from sending or receiving accurate messages, such as not feeling well or being overly tired. **Feedback** can be verbal expressions or body language, such as a simple nod of understanding. The **perception** of the receiver is very important, and will be discussed later in this chapter.

The transactional communication model (Figure 5-4) depicts "communicators" instead of one sender and one receiver. If two people are communicating, both are sending and receiving messages and both are encoding and decoding what is being offered. Even when two people are speaking one at a time, messages are continually sent with words, body language, facial expressions, and gestures. Various channels of communication are used, and both communicators offer feedback, even if it is done subconsciously. Noise may or may not be present, but even the best communicators experience some type of noise, even if that is only thinking of what to say next.

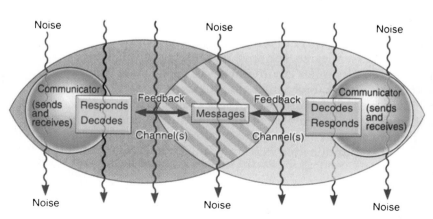

FIGURE 5-4   The transactional communication model. (From Adler RB, Towne N: *Looking out, looking in: interpersonal communication*, San Antonio, 1996, Harcourt Brace.)

Listening

Listening is just as important to good communication as the spoken word. People need to know that they are being heard. This is true in all interpersonal relationships, including husband/wife, parent/child, supervisor/employee, and doctor/patient interactions. When listening to someone who is attempting to communicate, the first rule is to look at the speaker and pay attention. Sometimes it is important not to respond immediately, but to remain silent and offer an understanding and reassuring nod.

There are times when it is hard to listen. We may not be able to listen effectively because we are distracted by our own thoughts. Perhaps the situations occurring in our own lives make the conversation we are hearing seem meaningless and unimportant. Or, there may be so many messages attacking at once that we are unable to focus on any specific one to hear what is being communicated. At other times, such as in anger, we are so rapidly preparing our response that we cannot hear what is being said. We may simply be too tired to listen or may have prejudged the speaker and decided that there is no need to listen. However, while working with patients, the medical assistant must be diligent in not only hearing the words being spoken, but also listening to them and what the patient is attempting to communicate.

Active listening is the skill whereby **paraphrasing** and clarifying what the speaker has said take place. Paraphrasing is listening to what the sender is communicating, analyzing the words, and then restating them to confirm that the receiver has understood the message as the sender intended it. This process clarifies the speaker's thoughts and helps to indicate that there is a common understanding of the message between both people. When communicating in this way, the receiver should reword what the sender has said and then ask a clarifying question. Consider the example below:

Patient: I have not been feeling well lately.
MA: You say you have not been feeling well. What exactly is the trouble?

This type of communicating may seem awkward at first, because most of us believe that listening involves lack of speech. Active listening means that the speaker's words are heard and there is a restatement that is used to verify that the message was understood correctly. This statement gives the speaker the opportunity to correct any misconceptions or misunderstandings. Consider the following example:

Patient: My back hurts.
MA: Where does it hurt?
Patient: In the middle.
MA: Can you point to exactly where it hurts?
Patient: Yes, right here (points).
MA: Is it a sharp or dull pain?
Patient: Very sharp.
MA: How often does it occur?
Patient: Several times a day.
MA: Can you tell me on an average day how many times it bothers you?
Patient: About six times.
MA: How long does it last?
Patient: About 10 or 15 minutes.
MA: How long has this been a concern?
Patient: For about 2 weeks.
MA: So you have had a sharp pain in this part of your back, about six times a day lasting for up to 15 minutes for 2 weeks? Is that correct?
Patient: Yes.

It would have been easier for the patient to have said, "I have had a sharp pain in my back that lasts up to 15 minutes, and it happens about six times a day," but this example shows how the medical assistant can continue clarifying until the answer is specific enough. This is critical when obtaining information from the patient.

It is also helpful to ask "open" questions, as opposed to "closed" questions. An open question requires more than a "yes" or "no" answer. It forces the patient to provide more detail and expand on his or her thoughts. A closed question can be answered with "yes" or "no" and compel the medical assistant to spend more time obtaining the answers needed to accurately document the patient's needs.

Often when a person or patient is talking with the medical assistant, he or she is looking for a specific type of response. Some patients want advice, some want sympathy, and others are looking for reassurance. Many patients will open up to the medical assistant faster and more completely than to the physician. Since it is important to build good rapport with patients, this can be a very positive aspect of the relationship the medical assistant has with the patient. However, the medical assistant should never agree to withhold information from the physician under any circumstances. If the patient asks that the assistant not reveal something to the physician, the medical assistant should politely explain that there is an ethical obligation to report any and all pertinent information to the physician, especially if it affects medical care. For example, if the patient asks the medical assistant not to tell the physician that the patient has been smoking against medical advice, the assistant could be jeopardizing the patient's care if the information is not reported.

This does not mean that specific details must always be aired. If the patient reveals that stress levels have been high because they have filed a sexual harassment suit against their boss, the medical assistant could report to the physician that the patient is having some legal problems, which have resulted in additional stress at work.

Never agree to lie to the physician! The patient must understand that if the physician questions any information given by the patient, it must be revealed so that the physician is assured that the care being provided is the right care. It is also critical to note that the physician may have worked with the patient for a long period and have a better understanding of the patient's needs than the medical assistant does. One patient may be able to handle a high degree of stress, and another may crumble at the first sign of stress. A good physician knows his or her patients and keeps accurate, complete records that will help with decision-making in these situations.

If ever in doubt about telling the physician something a patient has said, the best solution is to tell. Remember, medical professionals are legally bound to confidentiality, and the patient may need to be reminded of this. Encourage him or her to talk to the physician and communicate all of his or her concerns, no matter how insignificant they may seem. Never display a judgmental attitude or express negativity about the patient's activities, thoughts, or behavior. Offer to be with the patient, if he or she desires, as the patient discusses difficult issues with the physician, or to make arrangements for a special counseling session with the physician if this is indicated. Some patients are hesitant to initiate conversation with the physician because they feel they are taking too much time. The medical assistant can help to ensure that critical issues receive the doctor's attention.

Advising a Patient

The medical assistant must be extremely careful when giving advice to a patient in order to avoid legal accusations of practicing medicine without a license. Often a patient will ask for an opinion as to which course of action to take. Strict laws in most states prohibit anyone other than a licensed physician from giving medical advice. Even if the patient asks what the medical assistant would do if presented with the same options, the assistant cannot encourage the patient to choose one option over another. The assistant can offer a listening ear though, and help the patient process his or her own thoughts. This can be done in much the same way as using active listening techniques (Figure 5-5). When a patient expresses a concern, the medical assistant should restate the concern and then ask a clarifying question. For example:

> Patient: I don't know if I should take the chemotherapy treatments the doctor suggested.
> MA: You seem worried about the treatments. What are you concerned about specifically?

Patients must come to their own decisions about treatments and options that they have when faced with a medical decision. The medical assistant is often looked on not only as an authority figure, but also as an extension of the physician. Patients may mistakenly think that the medical assistant reflects the same opinion as the physician. Always attempt to get the patient to openly discuss all of his or her concerns and fears with the physician.

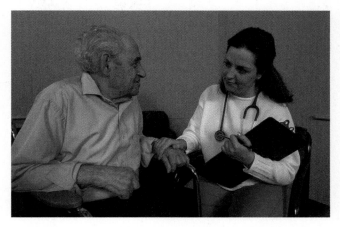

FIGURE 5-5 Careful listening and asking questions will help the patient express thoughts and feelings.

CRITICAL THINKING APPLICATION

- How should the medical assistant handle Sarah's questions about her mother's refusal to accept further chemotherapy treatments?
- How does this decision affect Sarah's ability to communicate with medical professionals? What barriers to communication might be present?

Observing Carefully

In the fast-paced world of medicine, there are times that nonverbal signals sent by patients are missed, which play a critical role in their care. Hesitancy while the patient is speaking may indicate that there is more to say. As mentioned previously, the inability to look a person directly in the eyes sometimes, but not always, indicates deception. The medical assistant must play close attention to what is seen as well as what is heard when communicating with the patient. Look in the eyes, and watch intently for signs of trouble.

When a patient cries, the medical assistant should always question what is causing the tears. Some patients may refuse to discuss the issue or insist that nothing is wrong, but tears are always a symptom of some emotion, whether it is anger, frustration, fear, pain, or some other concern. It is unwise to allow patients that are obviously emotionally upset to leave the office without reasonable assurance that they are going to be safe. The medical assistant might wish to suggest that a friend come to the office and escort the patient home. On rare occasions, it is better to be firm with the patient and insist on help getting home than later to find that the patient hurt herself or himself or someone else because of his or her **volatile** state. Careful observation of the patient as a whole is worth the time investment and may even save the patient's life.

Defense Mechanisms

Anxiety or stress causes the human body to react in many different ways. Some people handle **stressors** more easily than others. Most people use **defense mechanisms** during times in which they feel pressured or attacked in some way. These are often subconscious reactions designed for emotional protection; they help us to deal with whatever difficult event has triggered such a response. Often people may not even realize that they are using these mechanisms, and may even **vehemently** deny that they do so. There are many types of defense mechanisms, and the medical assistant should be familiar with them to better communicate with patients and others they come into contact with in the course of their duties.

Verbal Aggression

When a person verbally attacks another without addressing the original complaint, or disregards it, he or she is being verbally **aggressive** (Figure 5-6). Some individuals get very angry at any suggestion of wrongdoing; their response is to change the subject. They lash out, usually quite loudly, and attack back quickly in hopes of diminishing their role in any wrongdoing.

> "When are you going to clean the garage?"
> "Who are you to ask me that? You are late paying the rent again!"

Sarcasm

This word has its origin in the Greek *sarkasmos*, which means "to tear flesh" or "to bite the lips in rage." This is quite an accurate definition of the nature of sarcasm. It is a biting edge added to words that a person states with the intent to cause pain or anger. Sarcasm is hostile and cruel in most cases, and there are some individuals who use it constantly, thinking that it is quite witty. On the contrary, it often makes bitter enemies of its victims.

> "Of course it's a nice dress, if you like tents."

Rationalization

Rationalizing is attributing actions to rational and credible motives without analyzing underlying methods. When

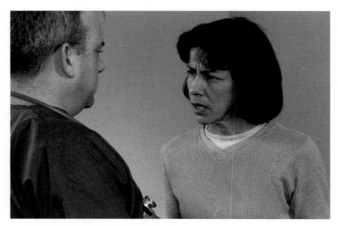

FIGURE 5-6 Remain calm even if a patient becomes verbally aggressive and attempt to calm him or her by listening and expressing empathy whenever possible.

people rationalize their behavior, they are offering excuses for what has been done or said and trying to convince others that the behavior was completely justified.

> "He only hits me because he is stressed at work."

Compensation

A person who compensates makes up for one behavior by stressing another. Compensation is a psychological mechanism through which feelings of inferiority, frustration, or failure in one area are counterbalanced by achievement in another. Compensation is not always a negative response, but it is often used as an excuse for not accomplishing what should be accomplished.

> "I know I gained 5 pounds, Dr. George, but I exercised three times last week."

Regression

Regression is the reversion to an earlier mental or behavioral level. Some people regress to a childlike state or period or exhibit qualities inherent to an earlier time in life. This can include making excuses for not doing a certain thing, saying that it cannot be done, instead of the truth, which is that the person does not want to do it. Replacing the word "can't" with "won't" is a good gauge of using regression.

> "I'd like to get better grades, but I can't find time to study."

Repression

The process whereby unwanted desires or impulses are excluded from the consciousness and left to operate in the unconscious is called *repression*. Blocking a problem out of the mind, or changing the subject when it is mentioned, are both types of repression. The repressed urges or desires may seethe beneath the surface, absorbing energy, and force the continual repression of the desires, which takes more and more concentration to do successfully.

> "I should phone my brother since our fight, but I just can't deal with that now."

Apathy

Apathy is a lack of feeling, emotion, interest, or concern. It is an indifference to what is happening or a pretense of not caring about a situation. Usually, apathy is not a true reflection of the inner feeling. It is a defense mechanism that is similar to repression, but with a more flippant attitude.

> "I don't care what grade I made on the test, because I am not going to pass the class anyway."

Displacement

Displacement is defined as the redirection of an emotion or impulse from its original object, such as an idea or person, to another object. When challenged or attacked by one person or event, displacement is used to channel negative feelings to some other area, which gives a false sense of control over issues that may not be controllable. The venting of hostile feelings is directed somewhere other than where it should be directed, but usually this is a result of a lack of confidence in addressing the true issues at hand.

> "I have enough problems at work and don't need to come home to a nagging wife!"

Denial

Denial is a psychological defense mechanism in which confrontation with a personal problem or with reality is avoided by denying the existence of the problem or reality. This is where the common expression, "He's in denial" originates. For whatever reason, the individual is unable to cope with the stress of a situation and completely pushes it or any person or thing representing it away.

> "My husband can't have cancer. He is completely healthy."

Physical Avoidance

Some events are so painful for people that they completely avoid any representation of the event. This could be a person, a place, an object, or just about anything that serves as a reminder of the event that induces the negative feelings. If the problem is a person, that person may be avoided for the rest of their life. If it is a place, such as a home that a couple lived in before one of them died, the other person may physically move. In some cases, such as physical abuse, the avoidance may be necessary, but it can also be quite unhealthy and may need to be explored further through therapy.

> "I will never go to that restaurant again, because that is where my ex-husband proposed to me."

Projection

Projection as a defense mechanism is defined as the attribution of one's own ideas, feelings, or attitudes to other people or to objects. This especially includes the **externalization** of blame, guilt, or responsibility as a defense against anxiety. Some people project their feelings about a certain thing onto others, who may not be affected by the negative connotations the first person feels. Projection is a way to avoid dealing with the root issues of a problem.

> "Everyone else is always late, so why am I getting written up for it?"

Dealing with Conflict

Conflict is defined as the struggle resulting from incompatible or opposing needs, drives, wishes, or external or internal demands. We deal with conflict in our lives in some capacity almost daily. Knowing how to recognize the traits of conflict and what patterns people use to deal with conflict will be of great benefit to the medical assistant. This will enable the professional to be understanding and empathetic to patients, co-workers, supervisors, and others in the day-to-day work environment.

Conflict is not always negative; sometimes it is beneficial to relationships. It can be constructive and allow people to learn more about each other. This may promote a stronger understanding and deeper levels of intimacy. Unless both parties are aware that a problem exists between them, there is no conflict. The conflict begins when both realize there is a problem that needs resolution. People handle conflict in different ways. Some avoid it at all costs, and on the other end of the spectrum, some seem to thrive on it.

It is helpful to define some of the many types of conflict to understand the thought processes of others and how best to respond to them, as well as discerning how others respond. Of itself, assertion is not conflict; assertion is stating or declaring positively, often forcefully or aggressively. Being assertive or aggressive can be very productive. Assertive people often receive job promotions and reach the goals they set for their lives. Too much aggression can make a person seem pushy, so it should be controlled and used at the appropriate times. Remember, there is a difference between assertion and aggression, which will be discussed in the following paragraphs.

Nonassertion is the inability to express needs and thoughts or the refusal to express them. Some avoid conflict and some accommodate by putting others before their own desires. There are times that nonassertion is justifiable. Anyone who has been involved in a long-term relationship realizes that there will be occasions when the other person's needs must come first. Many have learned the truth of the old saying, "Choose your battles wisely."

CRITICAL THINKING APPLICATION

- Why might Mrs. Cloyd and Sarah experience conflict at this stage in their lives?
- How might each deal better with disagreements, especially regarding Mrs. Cloyd's decisions about her medical care?

Aggression is defined in several ways. It can be a hostile, injurious, or destructive behavior or outlook, especially when caused by frustration. It is also the practice of making attacks or **encroachments**, especially if the acts are unprovoked. In the realm of psychological studies, there are different types of aggression. Direct aggression occurs when a person directly attacks another, whether by criticism, **malediction**, ridiculing, or other methods. This behavior causes the victim to feel embarrassment, shame, anger, or a range of other emotions. *Passive aggression* is a familiar term, but most may not know its definition. A passive-aggressive person expresses himself or herself in an obscure, **ambiguous** way. People who experience passive aggression may have feelings or rage, inadequacy, or resentment that they cannot articulate in a direct manner. Unfortunately, this behavior usually will not provide the results that are needed or expected.

The Crazymakers: Passive-Aggressive Communications

In the book *Looking Out, Looking In: Interpersonal Communication* by Ronald B. Adler and Neil Towne, the concept of "Crazymakers" is discussed and credited to George Bach. Bach was a psychologist who developed the theory of creative aggression; he nicknamed this passive-aggressive behavior *crazymaking*. He said that there are two types of aggression—clean fighting and dirty fighting. Crazymaking was his name for dirty fighting, which is a detrimental behavior for all involved. The term *partner* is loosely used to indicate the opposite side or victim of the crazymaker.

Following are brief descriptions of the characteristic types of passive-aggressive persons described by Bach.*

The Avoider. Avoiders refuse to fight. When a conflict arises, they leave, fall asleep, pretend to be busy at work, or keep from facing the problem in some other way. This behavior makes it difficult for the partner to express feelings of anger and hurt, because the avoider will not fight back.

The Pseudoaccommodator. Pseudoaccommodators refuse to face up to a conflict either by giving in or pretending there is nothing wrong. This drives the partner crazy, who definitely feels there is a problem and causes feelings of guilt and resentment toward the accommodator for bringing up the situation in the first place.

The Guiltmaker. Instead of saying straight out that they don't want or approve of something, guiltmakers try to make their partners feel responsible for causing pain. A guiltmaker's favorite line is, "It's OK, don't worry about me…" followed by a long sigh.

The Subject Changer. Really an avoider, the subject changer escapes facing up to aggression by shifting the conversation whenever it approaches an area of conflict. Because of their tactics, subject changers and their partners never have the chance to explore their problems and do something about them.

The Distracter. Rather than come out and express their feelings about the object of their dissatisfaction, distracters attack other parts of their partner's life. Thus they never have to share what is really on their minds and can avoid dealing with painful parts of their relationships.

The Mind Reader. Instead of allowing their partners to express feelings honestly, mind readers go into character analysis, explaining what the other person really means or what is wrong with the other person. By behaving this way, mind readers refuse to handle their own feelings and leave no room for their partners to express themselves.

The Trapper. Trappers play an especially dirty trick by setting up a desired behavior for their partners and then when it's met, attacking the very thing they requested. An example of this technique is for the trapper to say, "Let's be totally honest with each other," and then attack the partner's words of honesty.

The Crisis Tickler. Crisis ticklers almost bring what is bothering them to the surface, but never quite come out and express it. Instead of admitting concern about the finances, they innocently ask, "Gee, how much did that cost?" dropping a rather obvious hint, but never really dealing with the crisis.

The Gunnysacker. Gunnysackers do not respond immediately when angry. Instead, they put their resentment into a gunnysack, which after a while begins to bulge with both large and small gripes. Then, when the sack is about to burst, the gunnysacker pours out all the pent-up aggressions on the overwhelmed and unsuspecting partner.

The Trivial Tyrannizer. Instead of honestly sharing their resentments, trivial tyrannizers do things they know will get their partner's goat—leaving dirty dishes in the sink, clipping fingernails in bed, belching out loud, turning up the television too loud, and so on.

The Beltliner. Everyone has a psychological "beltline," and below it are subjects too sensitive to be approached without damaging the relationship. Beltlines may have to do with physical characteristics, intelligence, past behavior, or deeply ingrained personality traits a person is trying to overcome. In an attempt to "get even" or hurt their partners, beltliners will use intimate knowledge to hit below the belt, where they know it will hurt.

The Joker. Because they are afraid to face conflicts squarely, jokers kid around when their partners want to be serious, thus blocking the expression of important feelings.

The Blamer. Blamers are more interested in finding fault than in solving a conflict. Needless to say, they usually do not blame themselves. Blaming behavior almost never solves a conflict and is an almost sure-fire way to make receivers defensive.

The Contract Tyrannizer. Contract tyrannizers will not allow their relationships to change from the way they once were. Whatever the agreements the partners had for roles and responsibilities at one time, they will remain unchanged.

The Kitchen Sink Fighter. Kitchen sink fighters are so named because in an argument they bring up things that are totally off the subject—as in everything including the kitchen sink. It may be the way the other person behaved last New Year's Eve, or bad breath, the unbalanced checkbook, any past imperfection is fair game.

The Withholder. Instead of expressing their anger honestly and directly, withholders punish their partners by keeping back something—courtesy, affection, good cooking, humor, sex. This is likely to build up even greater resentments in the relationship.

The Benedict Arnold. Benedict Arnolds get back at their partners by sabotage, by failing to defend them from attackers, and even by encouraging ridicule or disregard from outside the relationship.

Barriers to Communication

Physical Impairment

Patients may have physical troubles that impair their ability to communicate effectively. This could be a vision

---

*Modified from Adler RB, Towne N: *Looking out, looking in: interpersonal communication*, San Antonio, 1996, Harcourt Brace College.

or hearing problem, or one of many other conditions that makes communicating a bit more difficult than usual. The medical assistant should use more descriptive language when speaking with the patient who has a visual disturbance. This helps the patient to "see" what is being discussed in his or her thoughts. The person with diminished hearing may be very sensitive and in denial of the condition. Be certain that you have his or her attention and that you are face to face with the person while speaking. People who are hearing impaired are often very dependent on lip-reading for comprehension. Being elderly is not an impairment at all. Many older patients will be physically fit and mentally sharp and do not expect special treatment. Never increase the volume of your speech in an assumption that an older patient is hard of hearing.

CRITICAL THINKING APPLICATION

- What must be considered when communicating verbally with Mrs. Cloyd? With Sarah?
- How can the medical assistant show compassion to a terminally ill patient during her appointment when the office is extremely busy?

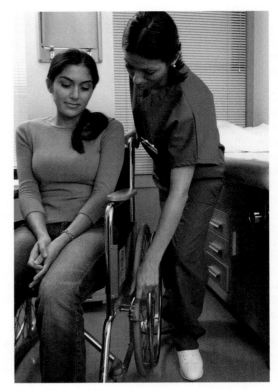

FIGURE 5-7 Bilingual staff members are valuable in ensuring accurate communications with patients who speak a different language.

Language

With non–English-speaking patients, the medical assistant may need to use gestures and more body language to convey messages. In such cases, be alert to the possibility of misunderstandings. Confirm that the message being sent is the message that the listener received by asking for feedback. Ask the listener to repeat the message, and if family members are present, be sure they have a good understanding of what is being communicated as well.

It is always helpful to have a bilingual staff member so that there is less chance of miscommunication with those who speak a different language (Figure 5-7). Many regions offer bilingual classes for medical professionals to assist them with basic communications with their patients. It would be well worth the time and financial investment to investigate such classes, because bilingual assistants are quite valuable to the physician and may be able to command a higher salary.

Prejudice

Personal and social bias, or prejudice, brings about discrimination. *Discrimination* is a word that is used to describe unfair treatment of a person because of race, gender, religious affiliation, handicap, or any other reason. Discrimination is unethical, morally and socially wrong, and in many situations, it is illegal. It also prevents us from communicating effectively.

Some discrimination is very **subtle**; it is not expressed openly or in a blatant manner. Subtle discrimination is based on a person's appearance, values, lifestyle, or some other personal factor. Examples include discrimination against those who are obese, divorced individuals, homo-

sexuals, welfare recipients, or those with sexually transmitted diseases. Sometimes we are not aware that our words or actions reflect subtle discrimination against others.

Personal prejudices must be recognized before one can change them. Medical professionals are exposed to a wide variety of persons who need excellent medical care. The professional cannot allow personal prejudice to affect the care of any individual. Everyone has the right to be honored as a human being and treated respectfully. This enforces the Golden Rule, treating others as you would wish to be treated. Realize the worth of each individual person and allow that attitude to reflect in all of the actions taken with a patient.

Stereotyping

Stereotyping is defined as a standardized mental picture that is held in common by members of a group and that represents an oversimplified opinion, prejudiced attitude, or uncritical judgment. It is unfair to **stereotype** anyone or categorize him or her based on preconceived, often incorrect, assumptions. Although sometimes there is a degree of truth to the assumption based on stereotypical categories, people should not be judged before there has been an opportunity to get to know them as individuals. The medical assistant should push preconceived notions aside and look at the individual when forming and building a relationship. In the medical profession, stereotypical categories should not be considered when caring for patients and developing good rapport with them.

Perception

Perhaps one of the most important issues to consider when discussing barriers to communication is the concept of perception. *Perception* means the capacity for comprehension, or the discernment of what is being communicated, according to the message receiver's point of reference. When we discussed the transactional communication model earlier in the chapter, it was obvious that because of different types of noise and channels, there would be times that the message sent would be distorted; the receiver would not always get the message that the sender meant to send. The receiver's perceptions could completely alter the message, no matter how clearly it was sent. If the receiver believes that all attorneys are corrupt, he or she will probably be unable to get past this perception when speaking with a lawyer and therefore may not be able to trust.

Often our perceptions stem from some experience with a certain group of people from the past. This perception goes unresolved or has affected us so strongly that we group all people from that walk of life into a negative category. This is an unfair way to deal with people; everyone should be viewed as an individual, not as a part of a stereotypical group. Remember, perception is an individual's point of view, right or wrong. There is also the issue of interpretation and the determination of what is meant by a certain message. There must be an attempt to understand both points of view and be willing to discuss them calmly, even in the most heated of discussions. No one truly enjoys conflict, and we should have a healthy respect for others' opinions. The differences between individuals are part of what makes each of us unique.

Communication During Difficult Times

Communication is not an art that comes easily to everyone. It is often difficult to express feelings in an honest and open way. When a crisis occurs, it is much harder to communicate effectively and we sometimes say things that we do not mean. The medical assistant must develop communication skills that can be used in times of trouble. There must be an understanding of why a patient or co-worker is unable to communicate.

Patience is important, too, because people are not always at their best when they are concerned about their condition or that of a loved one. Always remain calm when dealing with a person who is experiencing a traumatic event or has any depressive condition. Remember that he or she may be reacting to many emotions—fear, anger, doubt, inadequacy, or many others. The key is to listen and determine the best way to help the patient out of any immediate danger, and help them establish some type of support system.

Anger

One of the most difficult times to communicate is when we are angry. Anger is a normal emotion that all of us feel at one time or another. Usually the expression of anger is a healthy thing. Some people bottle up their emotions and do not express what they truly feel inside. If this is done repeatedly, at some point the anger will erupt, possibly over a tiny event. Others explode over every little situation, and people who do this need anger management skills and training.

Anger, like most emotions, can cause physiological changes. When a person feels anger, the blood pressure rises and the heart rate increases. Many things can trigger anger, from a simple traffic backup to a real or perceived betrayal, the diagnosis of a disease, or the death of a close relative. Road rage is one example of anger out of control and is a serious problem on our public highways today. Unexpressed anger can cause or contribute to all types of health problems, including depression and hypertension.

The medical assistant can help to calm an angry patient by speaking calmly and refusing to return the emotion. If the volume is gradually lowered with every sentence spoken, the angry person will have to lower the volume as well to hear what the assistant is saying. Suggest that the person breathe deeply and stop talking for a few minutes. Remember that the anger that is being expressed is usually not directed intentionally toward the medical assistant. Be a good listener and allow the person to speak as long as it is not abusive speech. Using logic with the angry individual may also help. Some will use words such as "never" and "always"; for example, "My wife never balances the checkbook!" or "You always make me wait for my appointment!" These statements are broad generalizations and usually untrue. Using a logical approach and maintaining a calm attitude will help the angry individual.

It is very important to address the root of the problem and be willing to admit if the office has made a mistake or contributed to a problem. Do not be afraid to say, "I'm sorry, we made an error." Arguing will never solve the situation and will only increase the intensity of the patient's feelings. Four words that will often disarm an angry person are "Let me help you." There will be times while working in the medical profession that a patient, co-worker, or even the physician will lash out, even though the medical assistant is not the source of their anger. Realize that this is a part of being human, and be as caring and kind as possible. If the anger becomes abusive, either refer the situation to a supervisor, or if that is not possible, tell the patient that you can no longer discuss the situation and offer to schedule an appointment so that the matter can be discussed at a later time. By then, the patient will probably have calmed down and will be able to discuss the situation rationally.

Shock

When an event or a circumstance arises that is especially painful, we may experience emotional shock. A person who has just been told that a family member has been killed in an automobile accident may go into what we call *shock*. There are many different types of shock, but in this chapter, the emotional aspect will be discussed. Often the person cannot think or move, and other coping reactions may take place. One person may scream in agony, whereas another may calmly sit down and begin to talk about a completely unrelated subject. The person who appears calm is probably more at risk, because in addition to shock, there may be a denial process. We never really know in advance how we will react to events that are traumatic. Also, our reactions may differ from time to time. So much depends on what else is happening in a person's life as to how they will be able to cope with a traumatic event.

The first rule is to never leave a person in emotional shock alone. If the healthcare professional cannot stay close by, arrangements should be made for someone to stay near, especially during the early stages, if at all possible. Since the thought processes the person is experiencing may not be under control, he or she could be a danger to himself or herself or others. People who are in shock have a strong need to get away from the situation they have found themselves in. They may try to literally run away, or may speed off in a car, which compounds the situation. The event does not have to be a life-threatening one, but the patient may perceive it as such. For instance, a teenager who becomes pregnant may not be able to focus on anything except her perception that her life is ruined. As with anger, listening is a good disarming tool for dealing with a person in emotional shock.

There are several symptoms of emotional shock that the medical assistant should watch for, including hyperactivity, disruptions in breathing patterns, a blank staring, sudden hysterics, and shaking. Humans have an innate sense of threat or danger, and this sense may initiate what psychologists call the "fight or flight" syndrome. When a person feels a threat of some kind, the hormone adrenaline is released in the body quickly, and this hormone promotes an increased heart rate and blood pressure. The oxygen level in the body increases, which prepares the muscles to help the body flee. Awareness is increased, as is energy and performance. The individual either runs, avoiding the danger, which is the "flight" aspect, or stays to "fight," facing the stressors or threat. With either choice, the body must have this increased energy level and awareness to deal with the situation. When the immediate period of shock abates, the individual may feel a debilitating, drained sensation as the hormonal levels return to normal.

CRITICAL THINKING APPLICATION

- Is it possible that Sarah might experience shock months after her mother's death?
- How can the medical assistant help Sarah to deal with these emotions?

Death and Dying

Years ago patients who were considered terminally ill were placed in hospital wards and left to their demise. The medical community did not focus on understanding the fears and concerns of the dying, and very few measures that preserved their dignity were offered to them. However, in 1969 a ground-breaking book, *On Death and Dying*, was published by Dr. Elisabeth Kübler-Ross, who studied **thanatology**. Kübler-Ross (Figure 5-8), a Swiss psychiatrist, realized that terminally ill patients

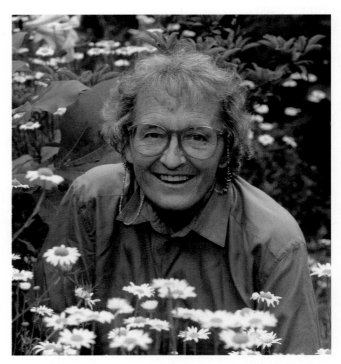

FIGURE 5-8 Dr. Elisabeth Kübler-Ross is the author of more than 20 books, many of which deal with the subject of death and dying, and is considered an international authority on the stages of grief. (Photograph copyright Ken Ross, 1985.)

were somewhat ignored, even by medical professionals, and she spent many hours interviewing these patients, discovering their fears and concerns. Kübler-Ross listened to them and realized that there were certain stages that patients passed through as they dealt with their impending death. She held seminars during which she interviewed dying patients as medical students listened. When the book was published, she was recognized internationally as an authority on the subject of death. She has written more than 20 books about the process of dying. Kübler-Ross's latest book is about the living. In *Life Lessons*, she shares many of the truths she has learned from the dying to encourage us to live.

Kübler-Ross states that there are five specific stages of the process of **grief**. These stages include denial, bargaining, anger, depression, and acceptance. She believes that all people go through each stage in the grieving process, but they may not go through the stages in the same order. A stage could take days to work through or several months. Although she relates these stages to dying patients, they are not exclusively limited to those who are dying. Anyone experiencing grief may progress through these five stages, and having a good understanding of them will help the medical assistant to better care for the patient.

Denial is the first stage, during which the patient or grieving person denies the issue that is causing the grief and thinks, "No, not me." The person is shocked and rejects the facts. The denial is a defense mechanism that helps the individual to deal with the news. The second stage is anger, when the dying patient begins to ask, "Why me?" The anger is often directed at others, and that may include the people in the family taking care of the patient, or may include healthcare workers who cannot present a cure. In the third stage, the patient begins to bargain in an attempt to postpone death or eliminate it altogether. This bargaining is usually with God, and the patient may pray to see a child marry or to witness some other upcoming event. The event is not the true hope of the patient, but life itself is. These patients say, "Yes, me, but…" in their attempt to postpone their death. The fourth stage is depression, and during this stage patients realize that they are going to die and may feel regret for the goals they did not accomplish or for not taking better care of themselves. These patients say, "Yes, it's me…." and they must be allowed this period of grieving. However, family and friends should watch the patient carefully for signs of deep depression. The final stage of grief is acceptance, during which the patient is able to say, "Yes, me, and I'm ready…." The reality of the impending death is accepted, and although the patient may continue to experience some depression, he or she is better equipped to deal with the arrangements that have to be made and may even demonstrate good humor during this time.

Patients who are dying must be treated with dignity and respect. This does not mean that they are unable to laugh and enjoy the life they are still living. Gentle touch and kind words will help patients to know the medical assistant cares for them. It is important to be careful with words and phrases around dying patients, but be natural in your conversations with them and do not be afraid to laugh. Never suggest to such patients that you "know how they feel." This phrase belittles their situation, and it is a fact that we will really never know how another person feels. Asking questions is a good method of communication when you are not sure what to say. Use questions such as, "How do you feel about that?" or "What does your family think about your plans to discontinue treatment?" Then listen to the patient and make eye contact with him or her as you listen. You may also ask, "How can I help you?" as opposed to "Is there anything I can do?" There will be a natural tendency for the patient to say "No" to the second question. However, if you ask specifically how to help, they may open up and allow you or the office staff to be of help. They may simply need suggestions about who could cut their grass or how to contact Meals on Wheels. Hospice services provide terminally ill patients and their families with care and support, often from the point of diagnosis to bereavement. Many have found hospice services invaluable in the process of coping with a loved one close to death. The medical office should have listings of community resources to assist in many types of situations.

CRITICAL THINKING APPLICATION

- How can the medical assistant help Sarah to deal with her mother's impending death?
- What stage of grief might Mrs. Cloyd currently be experiencing? What stage might Sarah be experiencing?

CRITICAL THINKING APPLICATION

- Often people put off writing a will. Could this be procrastination or a fear of death?
- When is it important to have a will?

Multicultural Issues

Cultural differences influence the way we deal with those from various parts of the world. We often become isolated in our thinking and incorrectly assume that people all over the world think and do things the same way that we do. However, there are vast differences in cultures from country to country, and even from areas within the same country. In the United States we see a difference between Northerners and Southerners. The speech of people in New York is significantly different from that of people in south Texas, and there is still another change in dialect from Texas to the West Coast. We picture Texans with cowboy boots and hats, but that is not how most Texans dress. Some of us still associate Alaska with Eskimos and igloos. Perhaps this stems from the books we read in elementary school, but cultures today are much more widely mixed in the United States, and since many others immigrate to our country for various reasons and opportunities, it is wise to learn a bit more about the cultures and the variety of people that inhabit the world.

We sometimes stereotype people of other cultures and think that we understand what they are like and how they live. Often, some type of **media** has influenced our thinking. There is much to learn from other cultures, and sharing is a way to gain an understanding of the experiences in other places. This helps us to be more well-rounded individuals and to enjoy and appreciate our own cultural differences. Remember that those people who have come to the United States from other countries have to deal with their ideas of both their own homeland and this country as well. There may be significant misconceptions, so in the medical facility, patience will be necessary as explanations are provided. Take extra time and care with patients of other cultures without assuming they know or understand this culture. Also understand that culture is something that is passed from generation to generation, so many of the ideas people hold dear have been handed down for centuries.

Some people who enter a new country go through a period of what is called "culture shock," a state of being in unfamiliar surroundings and being away from the things that were present in everyday life in the homeland. Street signs are different; in some cases, people drive on the opposite side of the street. There is a quick realization that the person's "normal" way of doing things no longer works, and there must be some type of adaptation to survive. This adaptation may mean changing the habits and customs of a lifetime. This can be a very exciting prospect for some, but a very frightening prospect for others. Simple processes, such as enrolling in school, become difficult tasks. Patience is a critical tool to help others adjust to the American way of life.

WHAT OTHER CULTURES THINK OF AMERICANS

We are not the only ones with stereotypical ideas of other cultures—here is what some other cultures think of Americans!

- Outgoing and friendly
- Informal
- Loud, rude, and boastful
- Immature
- Hard-working
- Extravagant
- Wasteful
- Sure they have all the answers
- Disrespectful of authority
- Racially prejudiced
- Ignorant of other countries
- Wealthy
- Generous
- Promiscuous
- Always in a hurry
- Careless with money

From *www.studyabroad.com*.

EXAMPLES OF VARIOUS CULTURAL TRADITIONS

- A husband speaks for his wife. The wife does not speak to the physician.
- The palm of the hand, facing down, is used to beckon someone. The hand motion signaling one to come or follow, performed with the back of the hand toward the patient, is used only when calling an animal. An open hand is used to point, rather than one finger.
- A female's clothing is not removed without the presence of another female family member.
- Emotional crying and sobbing denote femininity.
- Going to the doctor is a sign of weakness.
- The female medical assistant never touches the male patient.
- Acquaintances are not permitted to stand within 3 feet of the patient; only immediate family members are permitted to stand within this space.
- The Chinese do not like to be touched by people they do not know.
- The Laotian's "yes" response may not mean "yes," because it is considered rude to say "no" to others or to cause conflict.
- A native of Cambodia, as well as a Laotian, will not look into the eyes of the person being addressed because long eye contact means disrespect and is impolite.
- Cambodians do not like to have their blood drawn because they believe it will weaken them.
- Afghans and Mexicans have a concept of time that is less precise than in the United States.
- Vietnamese consider the head to be a sacred part of the body and are offended by being touched on the head or shoulders. Only the elderly may touch the head of a child without giving offense.

Communicating With People of Other Cultures

People from other cultures want to be treated just as you would like to be treated if you were visiting another country; they wish to be respected and treated fairly. There is so much to learn about the background of others, and much to share about the culture we know, too. Cultural differences are responsible for many misunderstandings. We must make an attempt to understand people of other walks of life.

When speaking with those from a foreign country, there may be a **language barrier**. Even if the person knows some English, there will be words and phrases that do not make sense in the way that we use them in America. A period of time must pass when the words are heard frequently before they will take on meaning to a person who is unfamiliar with them. It is important to speak a little slower than usual to a person whose primary language is not English. This is not to insinuate they are less intelligent, but it does give them a chance to absorb the words and mentally translate them into their own language, then prepare a response. There is no need to increase the volume of speech—people from other cultures are not hard of hearing. They merely need a little more time to process the words that are said.

Medical assistants should have an awareness of the nonverbal messages being sent by the persons that are interacting. In our society, a simple up-and-down nod of the head means "yes" and a side-to-side shake means "no." However, in Bulgaria and among the Eskimos, these signals have the opposite meaning. It is important to be sensitive to and aware of the beliefs of the many cultures that will be represented in the patient population. If you work in a practice that predominantly serves a distinct ethnic group, discuss possible cultural differences with the physician and with influential people within the cultural group. Learning to understand cultural differences helps you to gain the confidence and respect of patients.

Emotional and Physical Needs

As human beings, there are certain emotional and physical needs that must be met for us to live balanced lives and a healthy existence. Many of us take these needs for granted until they become an absolute necessity, and then our focus becomes directed toward meeting the need. Few in the United States have faced hunger as those in some Third World countries have, and when hunger is our need, it suddenly becomes our prime concern. This section will provide some insight into the needs we have as humans and their role in the total health of the body, mind, and spirit.

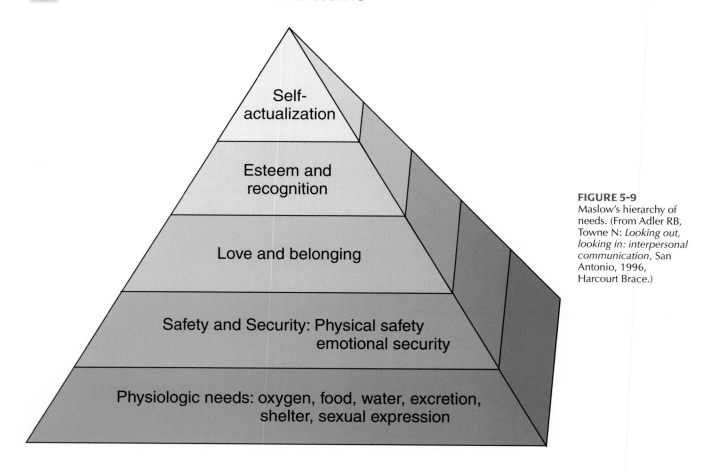

FIGURE 5-9
Maslow's hierarchy of needs. (From Adler RB, Towne N: *Looking out, looking in: interpersonal communication*, San Antonio, 1996, Harcourt Brace.)

Maslow's Hierarchy of Needs

Psychologist Abraham Maslow created what he called the *hierarchy of needs* (Figure 5-9). A hierarchy is defined as "things arranged in order, rank, or a graded series." Maslow believed that our human needs could be categorized into five levels and that the needs on each level had to be satisfied before moving to the next level. These levels are often depicted as a triangle, with the most basic needs at the bottom and the highest potential for growth as a human being at the top.

The needs we have as humans, at the most basic level, are those that involve our physical well-being. This includes food, rest, sleep, water, air, and sex. The second level includes issues related to our safety. We need to feel safe and secure in our homes and our environments, as well as the places where we work. The third level involves our social needs for love, a sense of belonging, and interaction with others. The fourth level relates to our self-esteem. We have an inner need to feel good about ourselves and to know that others view us in a positive manner. The last level is the self-actualization stage, in which we maximize our potential. In this level, we attempt to be at our best, and live our lives to the fullest extent possible.

Approval, Acceptance, and Achievement

There are three specific needs that we have, apart from Maslow's hierarchy of needs, that are critical to our happiness. These three needs include approval, acceptance, and achievement. Although most would agree that we do not need everyone's approval at all times, there are specific people whose approval we do seek. Children usually wish to please their parents, even when the child is an adult. We seek to please our supervisors, and even our own children. However, there is the danger of taking this need to please too far. There are books that address personalities called *pleasers*, who often place their own needs second to those they feel they must please.

We have a healthier self-esteem if we feel accepted by others. This is similar to the sense of belonging discussed earlier, but is a bit more extensive in nature. A feeling of acceptance includes the belief that our actions, words, dress, mannerisms, and other personality traits are acceptable to others we wish to impress.

Last, we have an inner need for achievement. Most humans want to do something great and contribute to their world in some way. A great thing to one person may be winning an Olympic race, but to another it may be reading to an elderly grandmother at a nursing home. We all enjoy praise for a job well done, or for losing weight, or for passing a difficult examination. It is beneficial to all when legitimate praise is shared freely and appreciated. This is especially true in our close relationships, but just as important in the workplace. It is much easier to work for a supervisor who praises for work well done than for one who never offers a pat on the back.

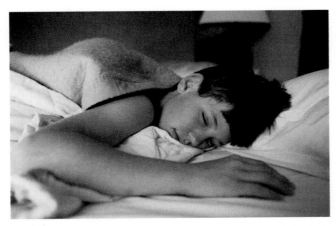

FIGURE 5-10 Sleep is a critically important physical need, the lack of which will eventually take a toll on the body, both physically and mentally.

A Good Night's Sleep

Many of us do not realize the value of our sleep time. Sleep is one of the most important physical needs that we have and is the one most often sacrificed during busy, stressful periods of life. This is called *sleep deprivation*. Human beings need about 8 hours of sleep each night, although many can function for a period of time with less sleep. Eventually this lack of sleep will take a physical and emotional toll on the body (Figure 5-10).

There are two main phases of sleep: nonrapid eye movement (NREM) and rapid eye movement (REM). During NREM sleep the eyes are fairly still and the body relaxes and slows down. There are four stages of NREM, which progress into a deeper sleep. After the body moves through the four stages of NREM, it enters REM sleep. During REM sleep the brain is highly active and the eyes move rapidly. Breathing is more irregular, and most people experience REM sleep in the last few hours of the sleep cycle. Dreaming occurs during REM sleep.

Many professionals who study and treat sleep disturbances agree that if an individual does not reach REM sleep, he or she will have provided physical rest for the body, but not mental rest. This rest is critical in stress management, and because it occurs at the end of most sleep cycles, or during its last hours, those who cut their sleep time short may not enter REM sleep often. Thus they do not get the mental rest that is needed to perform at optimal levels.

Healthy Nutrition

We have been taught since we were children that good nutrition is vital to healthy bodies. Our bodies are machines whose performance depends on good health. We care for the body with a balance of good nutrition, activity, and health care. A balanced diet is essential to ensure that the organs and systems within us function at optimal levels. When the body is not receiving the nutrients and vitamins that it needs, various parts may malfunction, and this can lead to conditions or diseases, or a worsening of the problems already present.

In today's diet-conscious society, some people attempt to lose weight by eating less food or cutting out meals altogether. This is a dangerous practice that prompts the body to hoard the fat stores it has built up, and there is no resulting weight loss. Losing weight quickly through fad diets and miracle supplements is usually a guarantee that the weight will eventually return.

One should always begin weight loss programs under the advice and care of a physician. Do not skip meals in an effort to lose weight and choose foods from the four basic food groups. Avoid unhealthy snacks and sodas, and drink at least 8 to 10 glasses of water every day. Exercise regularly and take walks to provide cardiovascular benefits to the body. By taking good care of your body, the chances are increased that it will function properly for a longer period of time, resulting in a longer, healthier lifetime to enjoy to the fullest.

CRITICAL THINKING APPLICATION

- Could Sarah's sleep and nutrition habits affect her ability to care for her mother?
- How might these affect Sarah's personal stress levels and how can she ensure that she is caring for herself, when her thoughts are primarily on her mother?

Positive Relationships

As mentioned earlier in this chapter, all of us need to feel approval, acceptance, and achievement. This is a vital component within our relationships as well. When we are involved in a relationship that is not going well, it will naturally reflect in our attitude, our opinions, and our sense of self-esteem. This can greatly influence the performance we offer at work. Often, because of infatuation, we find ourselves in a situation that might not be a positive one. Once the relationship is in progress, it is sometimes hard to end it and find a connection with a supportive, caring individual.

Many individuals really have not determined what they need from a relationship. It is helpful to make a list of what you are looking for in a partner and commit not to compromise the critical points on the list. The sparks and fireworks that appear in the beginning of a relationship may lose their intensity as time goes on, and there must be a firm foundational base after the newness wears off. Choose carefully and wisely, and the chances of becoming involved in healthy relationships greatly increase. Additionally, more and more individuals are choosing to remain single and enjoying life to the fullest. Certainly this choice is better than being a part of a destructive partnership.

Harmful relationships are not always just between partners. Often we experience stress and strain with relatives, friends, and co-workers. There are times when contact with the person causing the discontent cannot be avoided, at least for a period of time. In these cases, we must learn coping techniques for dealing with the difficult relationship. Open, honest communication is of paramount importance.

Healthy Self-Esteem

Self-esteem is a confidence and satisfaction in oneself. To have good self-esteem, an individual must also be self-aware, and that takes some honesty. It means taking a look at your strengths and your weaknesses, and knowing what you have to offer as a person. To feel well and accomplish goals in life, you must develop positive attitudes and positive responses to the pressures in life (Figure 5-11). It can sometimes be difficult to keep a positive attitude when others around us are being negative. Some people believe that if they inflict their bad feelings on others, they will feel better about themselves. It is important to remember, though, that no one can make you feel a certain way; it is a choice that you make. Blaming others for our situation in life or our negative emotions is self-defeating.

There are two things in life that we are able to control—our attitude and our actions. Even when faced with a potentially volatile situation, our attitude and reactions are decisions that we make. These decisions should be made with careful thought, even if the reaction must be a swift one. Think before speaking. Pause a moment if needed, before reacting. Take a time out. Choose your battles wisely. All of these suggestions will help you to

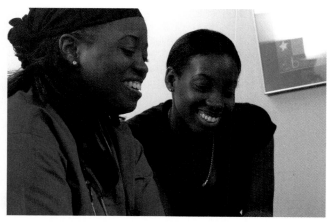

FIGURE 5-11 A healthy self-esteem will help the medical assistant keep a positive attitude and seek to improve performance. It will also encourage growth in the profession and personally.

react in a more positive, constructive way when faced with a difficult situation.

Improving Yourself

No matter how great the training or how many opportunities are placed in front of a person, fear and doubt can sabotage efforts to improve the self-image, confidence, and future potential of an individual. Almost every failure or mistake experienced can be traced to fear or doubt; either we are afraid to take a specific action or we doubt our own abilities. Blaming the circumstances around us is no excuse for a poor performance. It is also important to remember that it is the small, daily decisions that make a huge impact on our lives, sometimes even more so than what we consider critical life decisions. For example, a student decides not to study for 30 minutes daily for an upcoming major examination, and then fails it. This small decision to do something other than study results in failing an examination that may force course repetition and delay the graduation date.

Self-esteem will improve if a person is able to adapt to situations well. To be human is to be a changing, growing, imperfect, but amazing living creation. Adapting means being flexible and open to the actions of others. Although we should have empathy for others, we cannot allow others to ruin our day or lower our confidence level. Inventor-philanthropist Charles Kettering once said, "The only time you can't afford to fail is the last time you try." Our failures often teach us much more than our successes. The important thing is to get up, evaluate why the failure occurred, and then move forward armed with the new knowledge gained from mistakes.

Procrastination is often a symptom of the fear of failure and the fear of success. Many people procrastinate because they feel it will give them an excuse for their failure. They say, "There is no way I could pass that test—I only had 2 days to study!" Others are perfectionists and put off doing a job or delegating because they feel no one can do it as well as they can. The best way to stop procrastinating is to do something! Divide projects into small steps and complete one at a time. This makes tasks much less overwhelming.

The self-improvement process is ongoing. Periodically stop and evaluate where you stand in relation to the goals you have set for your life. Set goals for all of the areas of life—short- and long-term—including career, relationships, and personal growth. Write the goals down and make them specific and measurable. Be sure that the goals are reasonable. Start with smaller, short-term goals and work toward long-term goals. Be persistent and never give up. Post a list of them on the refrigerator and note progress. Do not count on having a whole lifetime to pursue goals; instead, move toward them consistently and enthusiastically.

Comfort Zones

We all have comfort zones. When faced with new ideas or changes, many of us tend to be a bit unsure of ourselves. Think back to the first day at school, the first day on a new job, the first time going to a fancy restaurant, a first date—

these events often make us feel a bit uncomfortable. New experiences may be outside of our **comfort zone**. Psychologists often speak about a comfort zone, which is a place in the mind where we feel safe and comfortable, where we can perform comfortably and confidently. Most goals, however, require movement outside the comfort zone to reach them. Striving to reach a goal means trying new things, and this can be quite stressful. Since we do not want to become so stressed that we give up on our goals, we should take slow, small steps that are challenging and then move to the next step. Procrastination is a failure concept, but can be overcome through dedication and consistent planning.

Remember, too, that patients are usually outside of their comfort zones while visiting the physician's office. Do everything possible to make them feel at home and comfortable.

Closing Comments

Interpersonal skills are critically important to the successful medical assistant. Communication will be a part of all interactions throughout the day, and the better developed these skills are, the better the medical assistant will be able to serve the patients in the facility. Every attempt should be made to enhance the interpersonal and human relations skills that the medical assistant currently has, and strive to better these skills continually. This will ensure that effective communication will be a part of the relationship with patients as well as others with whom the medical assistant interacts.

Patient Education

The medical assistant has the opportunity to provide an educational service to every patient who enters the medical facility. Patients will often have questions about their care or treatment, and the medical assistant with good communication skills will be able to assist the patient in understanding.

Patients must have clear knowledge of the role they play in their own care. The medical assistant can communicate information to the patient in many ways other than verbally. Leaflets and brochures can help patients to understand their illness better and will educate them, but the medical assistant should always explain each piece of literature given to a patient. Never just hand them out and expect them to be read. Have patients clarify instructions given by repeating them if there is a question of their understanding.

Often patients will need to be educated about the community resources available to them. It is wise to keep an ongoing list of local community services and agencies that can assist patients. Remember that physical care is not the only aspect of patient care; they have emotional needs as well. Often the very things we take for granted, such as food and shelter, are struggles for patients, and this stress can worsen their physical condition. Ask questions and be aware of what the patient is communicating to the staff. This will help the medical assistant to best serve the patient.

Legal and Ethical Issues

Patients see the medical assistant as an extension of the physician, so it is important that all communication with the patient be professional and accurate. Never give a patient advice that is not approved by the physician to avoid accusations of practicing medicine without a license. Always discuss issues with the physician that affect the patient's care in any way. Never agree to withhold any information from the physician, because even a small piece of information could completely change his or her plan of treatment. When giving instructions to patients, it is always best to have them in writing and keep a copy for the patient's chart so that there is a written record of what was communicated to the patient. Use excellent documentation technique when adding information to the patient's chart. Remember that all of the patients in the facility deserve to be treated with respect and compassion. Help the physician to establish trust with the patient. An open, trusting relationship with the patient will help to avoid legal issues in the future.

SUMMARY OF SCENARIO

Mrs. Cloyd and her daughter are facing a difficult time. Death is inevitable for everyone, but when a loved one is diagnosed with a terminal illness, it is particularly distressing. Both of these women need compassion and caring from the medical team. They will need to feel as if they are being heard and that their opinions are important. Some of their needs are similar, but they have differing needs as well. A gentle touch and laughter will brighten their day, and these expressions are critical to a person experiencing the stress of a devastating illness.

The medical assistant must ensure that Mrs. Cloyd understands her medications and treatments. The office should assist her and her daughter in finding community resources for which she might be eligible. Be sure to instruct Mrs. Cloyd primarily, and make certain that Sarah also understands any directions her mother should follow. Sarah will need compassion as she deals with her mother's illness and impending death. Since she is also a patient of the clinic, she should be given care and attention and may have emotional needs or periods of great stress also. Even on the busiest of days, these two women deserve warmth from the staff and should be made as comfortable as possible as they seek medical care.

SUMMARY OF LEARNING OBJECTIVES

- First impressions are critical in the medical profession. Dress, attitude, and appearance will all influence the credibility of the medical assistant. The medical assistant should always treat patients and visitors to the office as individuals who deserve the best in customer service.

- Verbal communication depends on words and sound, while nonverbal communication is messages that are conveyed to another without the use of words. Body language, eye contact, facial expressions, and hand gestures are some of the many ways we use body language. Sometimes our body language conflicts with verbal communication and sends mixed signals to the receiver. Often we are unaware of nonverbal signals and notice only a small number of the signals that other people send.

- Spatial separation can be defined as the space of comfort between individuals. Public space is usually considered to be 12 to 25 feet, whereas social space is about 4 to 12 feet. Personal space is the range of 1.5 to 4 feet, and intimate space would include touching up to about 1.5 feet.

- Touch is important in the process of communication because it projects an air of care and compassion to the receiver. The medical assistant should never be afraid to touch patients, as long as precautions are taken with those who are contagious. Touching the patient shows empathy and often can be more eloquent than the spoken word.

- The transactional communication model includes a sender and a receiver who both offer messages to each other using various channels. The sender encodes a message and then the receiver decodes it, to the best of his or her ability. Often some type of noise interferes as well, such as internal, external, and physiological noise. Perception is important when communicating because messages are sometimes easily misinterpreted.

- Some of the barriers to communication include physical impairment, language differences, prejudice, stereotyping, and perception. Barriers may also be present during difficult times, such as a crisis, when angry or in shock, or when a patient or family member is experiencing an impending death or serious accident or illness.

- Maslow's hierarchy of needs includes five levels, beginning with our most basic needs, such as food, rest, sleep, water, or anything that involves our physical well-being. The second level is related to safety issues, and the third, our social needs, such as love and interaction with others. The fourth level deals with our self-esteem, and the fifth is self-actualization, where our potential is maximized.

- Defense mechanisms are psychological methods of dealing with stressful situations, and include sarcasm, denial, repression, compensation, and several others. Often these mechanisms are our only way of dealing with circumstances that are difficult to cope with.

- Listening is one of the most important skills the medical assistant can possess. Listening involves not only silence, but active feedback as well. Open-ended questions help the medical assistant to restate what the patient is saying, to be sure that the patient is understood clearly.

- Everyone experiences conflict in daily living, so it is necessary to develop skills in dealing with conflict in as positive a way as possible. Conflict is not always negative and can be quite beneficial to relationships. Knowing the different types of conflict, as well as how people attempt to process conflict, will help the medical assistant to recognize patterns and respond appropriately.

- Elisabeth Kübler-Ross suggests that there are five stages to the process of grief, which include denial, bargaining, anger, depression, and acceptance. She believes that all stages are experienced while grieving, but not necessarily in the same order. The medical assistant can better care for the patient and the patient's loved ones when there is a good understanding of the grieving process.

■ Everyone needs physical and emotional rest to function throughout the day. A good night's sleep, consisting of at least 8 hours, regular exercise, and healthy nutrition will help to keep the medical assistant fit for duty.

INTERNET CONNECTIONS

- Elisabeth Kübler-Ross
  www.elisabethkublerross.com
- Hospice Foundation of America
  www.hospicefoundation.org
- Toastmasters International
  www.toastmasters.org

CHAPTER 6

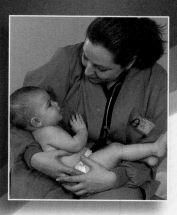

Scenario

Monica Johnson has been employed for 6 months as a medical assistant in a family practice. She works as the clinical medical assistant for Dr. Richard Wray. One of Dr. Wray's patients, Anna Walsh, recently adopted a baby after 8 years of trying to conceive a child. The baby, Delaney Gracelia, was born to a single mother, Susan, who participated in an open adoption in which she and the Walshes met and got to know each other during her pregnancy.

Dr. Wray performed some genetic testing on Delaney, and the adoptive parents were involved throughout the pregnancy, even meeting Delaney's birth mother for physician appointments from time to time. Monica observed both Susan and the Walshes and saw many benefits from the arrangement, noticing that everyone was primarily concerned with Delaney and her happiness and well-being. However, there were periods that were difficult as well for both sides. This prompted Monica to give some thought to her own feelings and ideas about many different ethical situations and issues and how she would react in the face of making ethical decisions.

Medicine and Ethics

National Curriculum Competencies

TRANSDISCIPLINARY COMPETENCIES

2a. Identify and respond to issue of confidentiality
2b. Perform within legal and ethical boundaries

Vocabulary

allocating Apportioning for a specific purpose or to particular persons or things.

advocate One who pleads the cause of another; one who defends or maintains a cause or proposal.

annotation A note added by way of comment or explanation.

beneficence The act of doing or producing good, especially performing acts of charity or kindness.

clinical trials Research studies that test how well new medical treatments or other interventions work in the subjects, usually human beings.

disposition The tendency of something or someone to act in a certain manner under given circumstances.

duty Obligatory tasks, conduct, service, or functions that arise from one's position, as in life or in a group.

euthanasia The act or practice of killing or permitting the death of hopelessly sick or injured individuals in a relatively painless way for reasons of mercy.

fidelity Faithfulness to something to which one is bound by pledge or duty.

gametes Mature male or female germ cells usually possessing a haploid chromosome set and capable of initiating formation of a new diploid individual.

genome The genetic material of an organism.

idealism The practice of forming ideas or living under the influence of ideas.

infertile Not fertile or productive; not capable of reproducing.

introspection An inward, reflective examination of one's own thoughts and feelings.

nonmaleficence Refraining from the act of harming or committing evil.

opinion A formal expression of judgment or advice by an expert; the formal expression of the legal reasons and principles on which a legal decision is based.

philosopher A person who seeks wisdom or enlightenment; an expounder of a theory in a certain area of experience.

postmortem Done, collected, or occurring after death.

public domain The realm embracing property rights that belong to the community at large, are unprotected by copyright or patent, and are subject to use or appropriation by anyone.

ramifications Consequences produced by a cause or following from a set of conditions.

reparations The act of making amends, offering atonement, or giving satisfaction from a wrong or injury.

sociological Oriented or directed toward social needs and problems.

surrogate A substitute; to put in place of another.

unique identifiers Codes used instead of names to protect the confidentiality of the patient in a method of anonymous HIV testing.

veracity A devotion to or conformity with the truth.

*E*thics is defined as the thoughts, judgments, and actions on issues that have implications of moral right and wrong. The concept of ethics concerns itself with the philosophies underlying ideal relationships between human beings, as well as the promotion of the highest good for humanity as a whole. There are various beliefs about what is and is not ethical in everyday life and in the medical profession. The decisions that people make based on ethical beliefs can quite possibly alter the course of human existence.

A medical assistant must not only have a strong knowledge base about ethical issues that might be faced throughout the profession, but must also come to terms with some of the deeply rooted value systems that have been a part of his or her life since youth. The trials and tribulations we have experienced, as well as the joys, will all influence our thought patterns when we are faced with an opportunity to make a good ethical decision.

History of Ethics in Medicine

From earliest recorded history, humans have pondered ethics—the judgment of right and wrong. Ethics should not be confused with etiquette. *Etiquette* refers to courtesy, customs, and manners, whereas ethics explores the moral right or wrong of an issue. It is not surprising that for centuries the field of medicine has set for itself a rigid standard of ethical conduct toward patients and professional colleagues.

The earliest written code of ethical conduct for medical practice was conceived about 2250 BC by the Babylonians and was called the Code of Hammurabi. It elaborated on the conduct expected of a physician and even set the fees that a physician could charge. The Code was quite lengthy and detailed, which is the probable reason it did not survive the ages. About 400 BC Hippocrates, the Greek physician known as the Father of Medicine, developed a brief statement of principles that remains an inspiration to the physicians of today. The Oath of Hippocrates has been administered to many medical graduates (Figure 6-1). The most significant contribution to medical ethics after the time of Hippocrates was that of Thomas Percival. Percival was a physician, **philosopher**, and writer from Manchester, England. In 1803 he published his Code of Medical Ethics. Percival was very interested in **sociological** matters and took a great interest in the study of ethical concepts as related to the medical profession.

In 1846, as the American Medical Association (AMA) was being organized in New York City, medical education and medical ethics were already considered important aspects of the profession. At the first annual AMA meeting in 1847, a Code of Ethics was formulated and adopted. It specifically acknowledged Percival's code as its foundation, and this document became a part of the fundamental standards of the AMA and its component parts. Even today there are sections of the AMA Code of Ethics that stem from Percival's writings.

Who Decides What is Ethical?

When we weigh the question of who decides what is ethical, the answer is evident: you do. Every day medical professionals face the task of making ethical decisions.

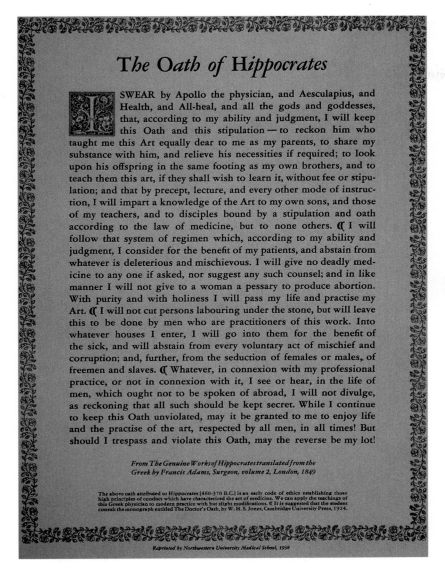

The Oath of Hippocrates

I SWEAR by Apollo the physician, and Aesculapius, and Health, and All-heal, and all the gods and goddesses, that, according to my ability and judgment, I will keep this Oath and this stipulation — to reckon him who taught me this Art equally dear to me as my parents, to share my substance with him, and relieve his necessities if required; to look upon his offspring in the same footing as my own brothers, and to teach them this art, if they shall wish to learn it, without fee or stipulation; and that by precept, lecture, and every other mode of instruction, I will impart a knowledge of the Art to my own sons, and those of my teachers, and to disciples bound by a stipulation and oath according to the law of medicine, but to none others. ¶ I will follow that system of regimen which, according to my ability and judgment, I consider for the benefit of my patients, and abstain from whatever is deleterious and mischievous. I will give no deadly medicine to any one if asked, nor suggest any such counsel; and in like manner I will not give to a woman a pessary to produce abortion. With purity and with holiness I will pass my life and practise my Art. ¶ I will not cut persons labouring under the stone, but will leave this to be done by men who are practitioners of this work. Into whatever houses I enter, I will go into them for the benefit of the sick, and will abstain from every voluntary act of mischief and corruption; and, further, from the seduction of females or males, of freemen and slaves. ¶ Whatever, in connexion with my professional practice, or not in connexion with it, I see or hear, in the life of men, which ought not to be spoken of abroad, I will not divulge, as reckoning that all such should be kept secret. While I continue to keep this Oath unviolated, may it be granted to me to enjoy life and the practise of the art, respected by all men, in all times! But should I trespass and violate this Oath, may the reverse be my lot!

From The Genuine Works of Hippocrates translated from the
Greek by Francis Adams, Surgeon, volume 2, London, 1849

The above oath attributed to Hippocrates [460-370 B.C.] is an early code of ethics establishing those high principles of conduct which have characterized the art of medicine. We can apply the teachings of this Greek physician to modern practice with but slight modifications. ¶ It is suggested that the student consult the monograph entitled The Doctor's Oath, by W. H. S. Jones, Cambridge University Press, 1924.

Reprinted by Northwestern University Medical School, 1938

FIGURE 6-1   The Oath of Hippocrates. (Courtesy National Library of Medicine.)

Although many different groups of people meet to discuss the ethics of a procedure or decision from the local level to national and worldwide levels, fundamentally, each individual decides what is ethical and what is not for him or her and the individuals these decisions will affect. As with any important choice, one must consider the short- and long-term effects and consequences. Although it is a completely acceptable practice to depend on groups and committees to guide ethical decisions, the responsibility for making these decisions ultimately rests with the individual (Figure 6-2).

Organizations that study ethical dilemmas may decide that a concept such as abortion is an ethical medical practice. But if an individual does not find abortion to be an acceptable practice for religious or other reasons, abortion is not ethical for that individual. A great freedom that Americans often take for granted is that we can exercise free will in decisions related to individual conscience in this country, that we can choose from a variety of options—but we must exercise this responsibility carefully.

CRITICAL THINKING APPLICATION

- Monica knows that she has deep-rooted thoughts and ideas about many ethical matters. However, she has never really thought about where she formed her ideas. Where do we get most of our opinions on ethical or moral issues?
- What is the difference between an opinion's being "our own" and being someone else's?

The Role of the AMA and CEJA Regarding Ethics

The AMA serves physicians as a national organization providing various types of information and support. One of the most important facets of the AMA is its Council on Ethical and Judicial Affairs (CEJA). The CEJA consists of

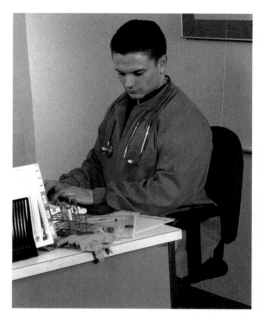

FIGURE 6-2 Medical assistants may find themselves making ethical decisions on a daily basis.

nine active members of the AMA, including one resident physician member and one medical student member, and is responsible for interpreting the Principles of Medical Ethics as adopted by the House of Delegates of the AMA. The AMA's Code of Ethics has four components:

- Principles of medical ethics
- The fundamental elements of the patient-physician relationship
- Current opinions of the CEJA with **annotations**
- Reports of the CEJA

The *Code of Medical Ethics: Current Opinions with Annotations* is a publication that contains the first three components, with discussion of more than 135 ethical issues encountered in medicine. A separate publication, *Reports of the Council on Ethical and Judicial Affairs*, discusses the rationale of the Council's **opinions** (Figure 6-3).

The AMA Principles of Medical Ethics has been revised several times to follow current trends in medicine, but there has never been a change in the moral intent or overall **idealism** of the statements. In 1957 the AMA Principles of Medical Ethics was condensed to a preamble and ten sections. In 1980 the principles were reduced to seven sections to clarify and update the language, eliminate ref-

---

FUNDAMENTAL ELEMENTS OF THE PATIENT-PHYSICIAN RELATIONSHIP

From ancient times, physicians have recognized that the health and well-being of patients depend on a collaborative effort between physician and patient. Patients share with physicians the responsibility for their own healthcare. The patient-physician relationship is of greatest benefit to patients when they bring medical problems to the attention of their physicians in a timely fashion, provide information about their medical condition to the best of their ability, and work with their physicians in a mutually respectful alliance. Physicians can best contribute to this alliance by serving as their patients' advocates and by fostering these rights:

1. The patient has the right to receive information from physicians and to discuss the benefits, risks, and costs of appropriate treatment alternatives. Patients should receive guidance from their physicians as to the optimal course of action. Patients are also entitled to obtain copies or summaries of their medical records, to have their questions answered, to be advised of potential conflicts of interest that their physicians might have, and to receive independent professional opinions.
2. The patient has the right to make decisions regarding the healthcare that is recommended by his or her physician. Accordingly, patients may accept or refuse any recommended medical treatment.
3. The patient has the right to courtesy, respect, dignity, responsiveness, and timely attention to his or her needs.
4. The patient has the right to confidentiality. The physician should not reveal confidential communications or information without the consent of the patient, unless provided for by law or by the need to protect the welfare of the individual or the public interest.
5. The patient has the right to continuity of healthcare. The physician has an obligation to cooperate in the coordination of medically indicated care with other healthcare providers treating the patient. The physician may not discontinue treatment of a patient as long as further treatment is medically indicated, without giving the patient reasonable assistance and sufficient opportunity to make alternative arrangements for care.
6. The patient has a basic right to have available adequate healthcare. Physicians, along with the rest of society, should continue to work toward this goal. Fulfillment of this right is dependent on society providing resources so that no patient is deprived of necessary care because of an inability to pay for the care. Physicians should continue their traditional assumption of a part of the responsibility for the medical care of those who cannot afford essential healthcare. Physicians should advocate for patients in dealing with third parties when appropriate.

FIGURE 6-3 Fundamental elements of the patient-physician relationship. (From *Report of the Council on Ethical and Judicial Affairs of the American Medical Association*. Originally adopted June 1990; last updated August 2001. http://www.ama-assn.org/ama/pub/category/5425.html Report #26 1990.)

erence to gender, and seek a proper and reasonable balance between professional standards and contemporary legal standards in our changing society. The most recently adopted changes, presented at the 2001 Annual Meeting of the AMA House of Delegates, reflect wording consistent with today's privacy issues and stress the importance of informed consent in DNA database information in genomic research. Several opinions were issued at the 2001 Interim meeting involving filming patients in healthcare settings, performing procedures on newly deceased persons for training purposes, and confidentiality of health information **postmortem**.

Making Ethical Decisions

Before discussing the opinions of AMA's Council on Ethical and Judicial Affairs, it is best to understand a few of the elements of ethics, the different types of ethical problems, and how a good ethical decision is made. Then, as some of the opinions are presented in this text, students can begin to evaluate their own positions regarding each issue. This section will enable the medical assistant to recognize the type of ethical problem that might present in the physician's office and provide a pattern to follow when making an ethical decision.

Elements of Ethics

Ruth Purtilo, in her book, *Ethical Dimensions in the Health Professions*, presents three general elements of ethics: duties, rights, and character traits. A **duty** is an obligation that a person has or perceives himself or herself to have. A daughter may feel the obligation to care for her elderly parents, or a husband who has hurt his spouse may feel an obligation to somehow make up for his act.

There are several types of duties that Purtilo mentions that relate to the medical profession. **Nonmaleficence** refers to refraining from harming the self or another person. **Beneficence** refers to bringing about good. **Fidelity** is the concept of promise-keeping, and **veracity** refers to the duty of telling the truth. Justice, in relation to medical ethics, deals with the fair distribution of benefits and burdens among individuals or groups in society having legitimate claims on those benefits. When a person has wronged another, he or she has a duty to make **reparations**, or right the wrong. Last, a person should feel grateful after being the beneficiary of someone else's goodness. This is also a type of duty.

Rights are defined as claims that a person or group makes on society, a group, or an individual. The Bill of Rights appended to the U.S. Constitution guarantees certain liberties that we enjoy as American citizens. However, some individuals think that they have rights that are really privileges. For instance, Americans do not have the "right" to healthcare services. There are some countries that provide medical care to all its citizens, but the United States is not one of those countries. A right applies to all people within a group, without prejudice. One of the most intense ethical arguments faced today is the right-to-life concept. If our Constitution states that we all have the right to life, liberty, and the pursuit of happiness, how can abortion be considered ethical? Or if an individual is trying to end his or her suffering from a terminal illness, could the "pursuit of happiness" be interpreted to include seeking a physician's help in committing suicide? These are the types of ethical questions that arise in the healthcare field.

Character traits are defined in Purtilo's book as a **disposition** to act in a certain way. A person who feels honesty is an important character trait can usually be trusted to speak the truth. One who feels that it is acceptable to take small items from work for use at home may not be able to resist an opportunity to take something more valuable. Character traits will certainly not always provide an indication of how a person will react in all situations. No human being is perfect, and we are sometimes unpredictable. Stress can also interfere with our normal reactions, and there are other factors, such as depression or anger, that will influence how we act as well. The phrase that someone is acting "out of character" usually means that he or she is deviating from his or her normal behavior patterns.

With an understanding of these basic elements of ethics, we have a good foundation that will help us to look more objectively at ethical problems and then solve them to the best of our ability.

Types of Ethical Problems

Purtilo presents four basic types of ethical problems (Figure 6-4). They are:
* Ethical distress
* Ethical dilemmas
* Dilemmas of justice
* Locus of authority issues

Ethical distress is the type of problem faced when a certain course of action is indicated, but there is some type of hindrance or barrier preventing that action. A professional knows the right thing to do, but for whatever reason, cannot do it.

An ethical dilemma is a situation in which an individual is faced with two or more choices that are acceptable and correct, but doing one precludes doing another. A choice must be made, and there may be a loss of something of value if a second choice is eliminated. This could be viewed as the proverbial "being caught between a rock and a hard place," whereby a choice must be made that has more of an affect than what may be seen on the surface.

The third type of ethical problem is the dilemma of justice. This problem focuses on the fair distribution of benefits to those who are entitled to them. Choices must be made as to who receives these benefits and in what portion. A few examples of the dilemma of justice would include organ donations and distribution of scarce or pricey medications.

In locus of authority issues, there are two or more authority figures with their own ideas about how a situation should be handled, but only one of those authorities will prevail. If one physician feels a patient should have surgery and another does not, how does the patient decide (Figure 6-5)?

Recognizing the type of ethical problem is not always easy. Sometimes a medical professional is faced with an issue that is a mixture of one or more types of ethical problems. When possible, it is wise to take some time in weighing the right course of action to take before making

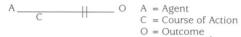

WHAT SHOULD BE DONE?

1. **Ethical Distress**
   I know which course of action I (the "agent") should take for the patient's benefit, but there is a structural barrier to my being able to do it.

   $$A \underset{C}{\rule{4cm}{0.4pt}} \| \quad O \qquad \begin{aligned} A &= \text{Agent} \\ C &= \text{Course of Action} \\ O &= \text{Outcome} \end{aligned}$$

2. **Ethical Dilemma**
   There are two (or more) courses of action, each of which is right (or wrong). No matter which one I (the "agent") choose, something of value will be compromised.

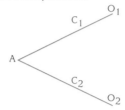

3. **Distributive Justice**
   There are benefits to be distributed among several potential beneficiaries. Not everyone can receive a full measure of the benefit. On what basis should the distribution be made?

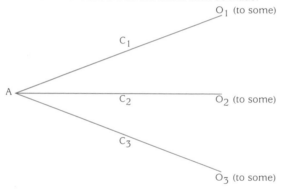

WHO SHOULD DO IT?

4. **Locus of Authority**
   There are 2 (or more) agents or "authorities" in this situation. Each believes he or she knows what outcome will benefit the patient the most, but only one authority will prevail.

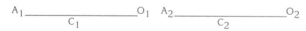

FIGURE 6-4 Summary of types of ethical problems. (From Purtilo R: *Ethical dimensions in the health professions*, ed 3, Philadelphia, 1999, WB Saunders.)

an important decision. Unfortunately, this is not always possible in the fast pace of the medical profession. Some decisions must be made in a split second, so it is wise to have a thorough grasp of ethical decision-making before the need arises.

The Ethical Decision-Making Process

Purtilo presents a five-step process for ethical decision-making in her book. The steps include:

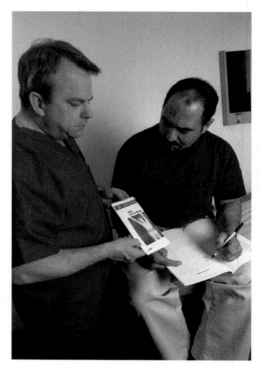

FIGURE 6-5 One of the duties of a medical assistant is to ensure that the patient understands the instructions given.

- Gathering relevant information
- Identifying the type of ethical problem
- Determining the ethics approach to use
- Exploring the practical alternatives
- Completing the action

While gathering information, a medical professional should ask questions, review charts, talk to the patient and other professionals, and search for other data so that the full view of the situation is available for scrutiny. Once the information is gathered, the medical professional must decide which ethical problem or problems are being presented. In determining the ethical approach to use, we must consider duties, rights, and character traits of all the individuals involved with this issue, paying close attention to the **ramifications** of all possible decisions. All of the alternatives must be considered and evaluated, and then an action should be taken.

CRITICAL THINKING APPLICATION

- What are the ramifications of an open adoption such as Delaney's? What problems might occur during the first year of her life?
- How might these problems be avoided?
- What are the positive aspects of the adoption?

Although it is best to have a space of time to give these areas some thought, this may not always be possible. It is a good practice for those entering the medical profession to take stock of what their core beliefs are. Scan the news-

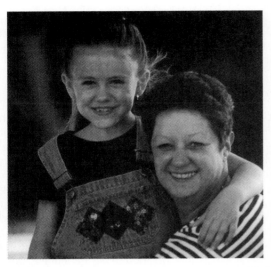

FIGURE 6-6   Norma McCorvey was "Jane Roe" in *Roe v. Wade*, the Supreme Court decision that legalized abortion. More than 20 years later, she became one of the pro-life movement's biggest advocates.

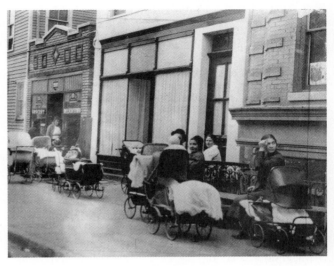

FIGURE 6-7   Margaret Sanger and her associates opened America's first birth control clinic on October 16, 1916, and women lined up on the street before the doors opened. The police closed the clinic on its tenth day, after providing advice and counseling to just 488 women. (Photo from Margaret Sanger Papers, Sophia Smith Collections, Smith College.)

papers and search professional journals for ethical situations, think about the facts, and then decide how you would react to each one. This is excellent preparation for the day that you will be faced with making a quick ethical decision.

Current Opinions of the CEJA and Medicine's Ethical Issues

Now, armed with a basic knowledge about the types of ethical problems and the process used to solve them, we will take a look at some of the Council opinions. Remember, physicians and other medical professionals are not bound to abide by the CEJA opinions. They have the freedom to make their own decisions, but many of the medical professionals in our country tend to agree with the decisions made by the committee.

Abortion

In 1973 the U.S. Supreme Court heard the case of *Roe v. Wade*. Since that ruling, abortion has been one of the most volatile issues with which the CEJA deals. According to the Principles of Medical Ethics, the AMA does not prohibit a physician from performing an abortion in accordance with good medical practice and under circumstances that do not violate the law (Figure 6-6). In recent years laws have been passed in some states requiring mandatory parental notification of a minor's intent to have an abortion. In some cases this means that the minor must have parental consent, and in others, parents must only be notified of their daughter's intent to have an abortion. Some states also require a 24-hour or more waiting period after the notification has been made.

The AMA strongly encourages physicians to persuade the minor toward seeking counseling with someone she trusts, such as a school counselor, teacher, or relative, if the minor's parent is not to be involved in the abortion decision. However, the AMA agrees that the physician should not feel compelled to require minors to involve the parent in the decision. Medical professionals must be aware of the laws in their respective states that deal with the mandatory notification requirements and should contact the medical societies in their region to determine what constitutes proper notification.

In early 2002 the Bush administration proposed a change in the regulations of the Department of Health and Human Services (DHHS) that would give states the right to classify a fetus as an unborn child eligible for some government-paid health assistance, including prenatal care. This move enraged abortion supporters, who felt that the prenatal care definition could have been extended to pregnant women instead of the unborn child, which they felt sets the stage for anti-choice legislation. The change would alter the definition so that states would be able to provide coverage for children from *conception* to age 19, instead of the current wording, which defines a child as an individual under the age of 19. The issue of abortion continues to spark disagreement in the United States and abroad (Figure 6-7).

Case to Discuss: Should a woman who has been raped and become pregnant seek an abortion?

Abuse

The AMA requires that a physician be familiar with the signs of physical, psychological, and sexual abuse of spouses, children, mentally incompetent persons, and the elderly. Discovery of abuse creates a difficult situation for a medical professional. The patient may be the object of abuse but deny its existence because of fear of further attacks. The law requires that abuse be reported, and if the physician does not report abuse, ethical standards have also been breached. In addition, the abuse may continue. Any medical assistant who suspects abuse must report this information to the physician first, who must determine whether the incident is reportable by law and take action. If action is not taken, the medical assistant is responsible for making a report.

Case to Discuss: What harm can come to a patient's family if the medical professionals are incorrect about their assessment of abuse?

Allocation of Health Resources

Sometimes society must decide who will receive care when serving all who need care is not possible. Decisions must be made fairly and should be weighed carefully. The criteria to consider when **allocating** health resources include urgency of need, likelihood of benefit, duration of benefit, amount of resources required for successful treatment, and potential for change in quality of life. Nonmedical criteria should not be considered, such as ability to pay, social worth of the individual, age, obstacles to treatment, or the patient's contribution to the illness. The physician who is treating the patient must remain the **advocate** of the patient and should not be involved in making allocation decisions for that patient. Procedures for such allocations are determined in an objective manner by the institutions involved in the patient care.

Case to Discuss: If the CEO of American Airlines, the winner of last year's Academy Award for Best Actor, and a drug-abusing mother of three all were equally ill and needed a liver transplant, which should receive the organ, and on what would you base the decision?

Artificial Insemination

Any individual or couple considering artificial insemination must be thoroughly counseled and endure a lengthy group of screening procedures for infections, such as HIV, and genetic diseases and disorders that the donor and/or recipient may have. Informed consent must be provided, and there are further regulations based on the marital status of the people involved. If the recipient is married to the donor, the resultant child will have all of the rights of a child naturally conceived. If the donor is anonymous, the husband must sign consent if he is to become the legal father of the resultant child. If the donor and recipient are not married, the recipient is considered the sole parent, unless both parties agree to recognize a right to paternity.

There is much discussion on the use of extra embryos that are harvested for reproductive purposes. The control and use of these **gametes** should logically be left to the man and woman who produced them, but the AMA agrees that both must give their consent as to how they are used. In vitro fertilization is considered an ethical procedure, but there are new discussions as to stem cell research, which is done using human embryos. Many organizations feel that using human embryos for stem cell research destroys the most vulnerable of beings, and laws are designed to protect them. Others want to explore the possibility of developing cures from this research for diseases such as Alzheimer's disease, diabetes, Parkinson's disease, and heart disease.

Case to Discuss: If a man dies who fertilized eggs that were frozen for later use, but he made no provision for the use of those eggs before his death, should the wife be able to use those eggs after her marriage to a second man?

Surrogate Motherhood

Surrogate motherhood introduces many different ethical, legal, and social problems to the individuals involved. However, this could be the only opportunity for **infertile** couples to have a child. The risks of **surrogacy** must be heavily weighed against the possible problems that might arise. The AMA feels that the birth mother must be given a period of time during which she can reverse her decision to give up the child she has delivered and void the contract. However, in cases of gestational surrogacy, the legality and ethical implications are more complicated. In gestational surrogacy, the child is not genetically linked to the birth mother. Usually the couple engaging the surrogate mother would be the genetic parents of the resultant child. One must also consider what would happen if the child is born with a deformity or handicap. This is a contract that should never be entered into without strong forethought and counseling.

Case to Discuss: What is a fair length of time to give a surrogate mother to petition to void a surrogacy contract?

Human Cloning

The AMA agrees that physicians should not at this time participate in human cloning, or *somatic cell nuclear transfer*, because of the numerous legal and moral issues that must be explored. Most agree that our current ethical and moral standards would interpret that a "cloned human" be granted the same rights as "normal humans," much in the same way as an adopted child is accepted legally and socially as part of a family. The AMA does not feel there has been nearly enough research into the long-term effects of cloning and therefore does not advocate the practice today.

Case to Discuss: If a couple loses a child through death but it were possible to clone the child, what concerns would be present for the family?

Genetic Counseling

Genetic counseling is also an area in which the AMA recommends caution. Through genetic counseling, parents of tomorrow may be able to choose eye color, talents, and intellect levels for their children (Figure 6-8). There are already humans who were conceived as "designer babies" in the world today. In 1980 the Repository for Germinal Choice (more commonly known as the "Genius Sperm Bank") was founded. Although it was not established to create a perfect "master race," it did attempt to produce leaders and creators. As with cloning, the AMA recommends that much more research be done before instituting genetic counseling on a global scale.

Case to Discuss: What could happen if parents "designed" a baby, but it arrived flawed in some way or did not meet their expectations?

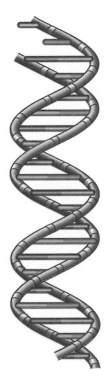

FIGURE 6-8   DNA, known as the "blueprint of the body," contains all the genes and chromosomes that make each human a unique creation, unlike any other human. (From Chester GA: *Modern medical assisting*, Philadelphia, 1998, WB Saunders.)

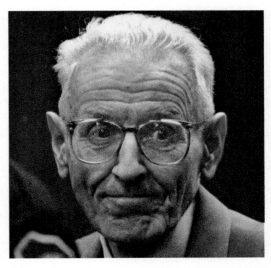

FIGURE 6-9   Dr. Jack Kevorkian, after being acquitted for numerous assisted suicides, was convicted in 1999 of second-degree murder and delivery of a controlled substance in the death of Thomas Youk, 52, who had amyotrophic lateral sclerosis (ALS or Lou Gehrig's disease). He will be eligible for parole in 6 years. (©AFB/CORBIS.)

CRITICAL THINKING APPLICATION

- How might the genetic testing done in Delaney's case have caused an ethical dilemma?
- Discuss whether genetic testing can be counted on to predict disease.
- How many in your class would have genetic testing done on their own child before birth?

Physician-Assisted Suicide

The AMA believes that physician-assisted suicide interferes with the fundamental purpose of being a physician—being a healer. The CEJA advocates that physicians aggressively provide care and alternatives in treatment for those who are near the end of life, but not promote or provide the means with which the patient could end his or her own life. This includes not only assisting the patient to inject chemicals that will induce death, but also prescribing drugs and information about lethal doses, or administering a lethal dose of a drug to a patient to promote death (Figure 6-9). This is sometimes called **euthanasia**, or mercy-killing.

Case to Discuss: If a parent mentioned in passing that he or she would want the right to commit suicide in the event of a terminal illness, would you support that decision if the situation did in fact arise?

Withholding or Withdrawing Life-Prolonging Treatment

A physician is committed to saving life and relieving suffering. Sometimes these two goals are incompatible, and a choice between them must be made. If possible, the patient should decide what treatment is given. Often the patient makes his or her wishes known to a responsible relative or other representative, in case the patient becomes incapacitated. Some patients wish to have a "do not resuscitate" (DNR) or "no code" order added to their charts. Usually such an order is desired so that no heroic measures are taken in a situation in which a patient would be unable or incompetent to make a decision. Advance directives are oral and/or written instructions for healthcare and usually are in the form of a living will or a durable power of attorney. Advance directives are strongly recommended by the AMA.

Patients of today are urged to create a living will. This is a document that states the wishes of the patient in case of terminal illness or an accident after which the patient cannot express his or her wishes. A durable power of attorney is a legal document that allows the patient to appoint someone who is trusted to make medical decisions for the patient in the event that the patient cannot make those decisions. This person is sometimes called a *healthcare proxy*. Federal law requires that patients be given information about advance directives by all facilities that participate in the Medicare and Medicaid programs.

Case to Discuss: How would a medical assistant handle the family of a patient who asks for advice about withdrawing life-prolonging treatment?

Quality of Life

Physicians must sometimes participate in or advise on decisions affecting the fate of a person whose prognosis is poor, such as a deformed newborn or a person of advanced age with many physical problems. The first thought may be the burden that the patient will be to the family or society in caring for this person. However, the AMA insists that the physician's primary consideration be what is best for the patient.

Case to Discuss: If a child is born deaf and has a severe liver disorder to a mentally ill single mother who is institutionalized, should the child continue to be fed by the hospital staff?

Clinical Trials and Investigation

Without **clinical trials** and investigation, no new drugs or procedures would be developed. However, all such investigation must follow a competently designed systematic program with due concern for the welfare, safety, and comfort of patients. The physician-patient relationship does exist in clinical investigation, and when treatment of the patient is involved, voluntary written consent must be obtained from the patient or the patient's legally authorized representative. Additional restrictions apply to minors or mentally incompetent adults. Physicians must show the same concern for the welfare and safety of the person involved in the clinical trials as they would if the person were a private patient.

Case to Discuss: If your brother were homosexual and wanted to participate in clinical trials for a vaccination against HIV, would you support his decision?

Cost of Healthcare Services

Concern for the quality of patient care should be the physician's first consideration. However, the physician should be conscious of costs and not provide or prescribe unnecessary services. Access to an adequate level of healthcare for all members of our society is now a moral expectation, but certainly not a right. Cost must be considered when providing these services, as well as the degree of benefit to the patient, the duration of the benefit, and the number of people who will benefit.

Case to Discuss: Should an 87-year-old patient with cardiovascular disease and stomach cancer have an expensive breast reconstruction surgery?

Organ Donation

Organ donation is not only considered ethical by the AMA but is encouraged when appropriate. However, it is considered unethical to participate in proceedings in which the donor receives payment, except reimbursement of expenses directly incurred in the removal of the donated organ. The rights of both the patient and the donor must be equally protected. In cases in which the donor has lost his or her life, the death must be certified by a physician other than the recipient's physician.

The most common organ transplantation is a blood transfusion. Some religions do not believe in transfusing blood, and cases in which such beliefs come to bear must be dealt with carefully. If the patient is a minor and the parents refuse the child a blood transfusion, some states would hold the parents liable for danger to or abuse of a child. However, the court system is reluctant to fight the parents over their religious beliefs and would intervene only in extreme circumstances.

Case to Discuss: A woman dies with a living will that states that she wishes her organs to be donated. Her mother, still living, disagrees with the decision and does not want her daughter's organs donated. What should health professionals do in this situation?

CRITICAL THINKING APPLICATION

- Monica has often thought about being an organ donor. She is very much in favor of organ donation because of her interest in the medical field. Her parents are very opposed to this because of their religious beliefs. How can Monica deal with this conflict within her family?
- If Monica dies before her parents do, how can she ensure that her wishes are carried out?

Capital Punishment

The CEJA does not consider participation in the act of capital punishment by a physician to be ethical. The physician may certify the death of the person but should not administer a lethal injection or induce death in any way. This conflicts with the physician's role as a healer, much in the same manner as physician-assisted suicide.

Case to Discuss: A very emotional patient, the parent of a child who was raped and killed, has been given the opportunity to attend the execution of the murderer. She expresses concerns about being able to cope with the memory of her daughter during the execution and asks you if you would attend in the same situation. What advice do you give the patient?

Ethical Issues Surrounding HIV

Being HIV positive creates a whole new world of ethical concerns for patients as well as those who support and care for them. When the HIV crisis first came to public attention, so many variables about the virus were unknown, and this created a wealth of misinformation. Those infected with the virus were often forced to leave their homes, were shunned in society, and faced rejection seemingly everywhere they turned, all because of fear of the illness (Figure 6-10).

Today clinical trials are underway for vaccinations against HIV, but clinical trials need volunteers for testing. Because vaccinations are often made of an attenuated or weakened strain of a virus, there are serious concerns as to who will receive the vaccination. Researchers have considered testing the vaccination in several Third World countries that have a high number of prostitutes and a thriving sex industry. These people, with no intentions of changing their lifestyle no matter the risks, may see vaccination trials as their chance of not contracting HIV. However, there is a question of the ethics of not submitting our own citizens to testing instead of those from disadvantaged countries.

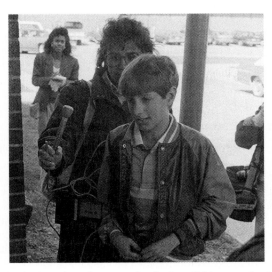

FIGURE 6-10   After a long court battle, Ryan White won the right to attend public school, despite his HIV status. (© Bettmann/CORBIS.)

Because of the discrimination practiced even today against people who are infected with HIV, there are problems with testing in some states that report the names of HIV-positive patients to various health departments and agencies. Although the stated intention is to ensure that these patients receive care, the accompanying effect is the risk of discriminatory practices. Some states use code systems called **unique identifiers** to assist in helping maintain the confidentiality of those getting tested for HIV. However, other states insist by statute that the names be reported. Some states require mandatory HIV testing for prisoners and those who have committed sex crimes. Insurance is a difficult issue when a person is infected with HIV, and some policies can be cancelled if HIV infection is discovered. This may prompt providers who want to treat patients infected with HIV to delay reporting the infection as long as possible, using other diagnoses regarding symptoms as opposed to the underlying cause of the patient's problems. All of these ethical issues are difficult to resolve, especially since currently there is no cure for HIV infection.

Ethics and the Human Genome

The mapping of the human **genome** has been in the news for several years. The genome project formally began in 1990 with the primary goal of identifying all of the approximately 30,000 genes present in the human body. Access to genetic information prompts many concerns and presents ethical, legal, and moral questions. Most of the major healthcare agencies and organizations in the United States and worldwide will be involved in the decisions made about this type of information, including the Centers for Disease Control and Prevention (CDC), National Institutes of Health (NIH), DHHS, Food and Drug Administration (FDA), Centers for Medicare and Medicaid Services (formerly HCFA), and many others. Experts will be needed to educate Congress, federal agencies, and state and local governments, because laws must be passed regarding the use of genetic information. The rapid pace of science surpasses the ability of lawmakers to keep up, so the challenge ahead with regulation of the use of genetic information is a mammoth one.

The mapping of the human genome and the information provided have raised concerns about privacy and confidentiality issues: Who actually owns genetic information, and who will be allowed to control it? Logically, it would seem that the patient owns his or her own genetic information, but if that is so, then the patient should be able to control access to it. Also, decisions must be made on the fair use of genetic information. Employers, schools, courts, insurance companies, adoption agencies, and the military are just a few examples of organizations that could potentially misuse genetic information and discriminate against those whom they may wish to target for inclusion or exclusion. There are reproductive issues as well, and questions about the reliability of genetic testing.

Patients will have to be counseled thoroughly on the risks and limitations of genetic technology. The answers to many questions are uncertain. Should a parent be allowed to test a minor child for adult-onset diseases? Should testing be performed for diseases that have no cure? All of these issues need resolution before the widespread use of genetic information.

Other Ethical Issues

Interprofessional Relationships

If a medical assistant recognizes or suspects an error in a physician's orders, there is an ethical obligation to report this to the physician. Questioning a possible error is necessary, even if it means risking the displeasure of the physician or supervisor. It could save a life or prevent a lawsuit if there is an error.

Physicians often refer a patient to another physician for diagnosis and treatment when it is necessary. A physician should make these referrals only when confident that the patient will receive competent treatment.

Unless there are legal restrictions in the state, a physician in private practice is free to choose whom he or she will treat. Although private practitioners may refuse certain patients, they must treat those who have already been accepted in the practice, or face possible charges of neglect. This does not include referring a patient to another physician for a condition that is not within the scope of the original physician's practice.

A sports medicine physician must keep in mind that the professional responsibility at a sporting event is to protect the health and safety of the participants, with personal judgments being governed only by medical considerations.

In years past it was considered unethical for a physician to have any type of romantic relationship with nurses or assistants in the office or hospital. Although this is not as stringent a rule today, it is very wise to not fraternize with co-workers, especially subordinates, at the workplace.

Confidentiality

Confidentiality is one of the cardinal rules of the medical profession. It is completely unethical and unacceptable to divulge any information about a patient to any other person not directly related to the patient's care. The easiest places to breach confidentiality are in an elevator, break room, or lunch room. One never knows whose relative is behind the medical assistant, listening to conversations that are inappropriate. Breach of patient confidentiality is grounds for immediate termination from a healthcare facility or physician's office.

When minors request confidential services, physicians should encourage them to include their parents. However, if the minor does not wish to involve them and the law does not require otherwise, physicians should allow competent minors to consent to medical care and should not notify the parents without the minor patient's consent.

Confidentiality restrictions apply to information in patient records and charts, as well as what the medical assistant is told by the patient or patient's family (Figure 6-11). Never investigate a patient record strictly for curiosity. All information in the record must be kept in the strictest confidence. If records are computer based, accessing records for patients that do not fall directly under the medical assistant's realm of duty is also considered unethical. Never share information on patients with anyone outside the medical facility or office, including your own immediate family.

CRITICAL THINKING APPLICATION

- Susan, Delaney's birth mother, comes to the office for a check-up 6 weeks after the baby is born. Susan looks a little sad, and when Monica questions her, she asks how Delaney is doing. What should Monica tell her?
- How can the office protect itself from issues about confidentiality in this unusual adoption scenario?

Advertising

The only restrictions on advertising by physicians are those that specifically protect the public from deceptive practices. Standards regarding advertising and publicity have been liberalized over the years, but any advertise-

ment or publicity must be true and not misleading. Testimonials of patients, for instance, should not be used in advertising, because they are difficult to verify or measure by objective standards. Statements regarding the quality of medial services are highly subjective and difficult to verify.

Communications with the Media

Although information regarding some patients such as celebrities and politicians may be considered news, the physician cannot discuss any patient's condition with the press without authorization from the patient or the patient's legal representative. The physician may release only authorized information or that which is public knowledge. Certain kinds of news are a part of public records. This is known as news in the **public domain** and includes births, deaths, accidents, and police cases.

A medical assistant must be aware that only the physician is authorized to release information, and under no circumstances should the medical assistant violate the confidential nature of the physician-patient relationship. It is unethical even to certify or verify that the patient is under the physician's care without the patient's permission.

Computers

The expanding uses of computer technology permit the accumulation of an unlimited amount of medical information. With the use of computers in the physician's office and the employment of computer service organizations, confidentiality becomes even more difficult to maintain. In general, all information must only be entered and accessed by authorized personnel, and a tracking system should be used to identify which employees access information. Breaches in computer policies should be considered a breach of patient confidentiality, and the consequences should be stringent enough to deter employees from accessing information to which they are not entitled (Figure 6-12). Information from the computer should only be disseminated to those who have a legitimate reason for needing the information.

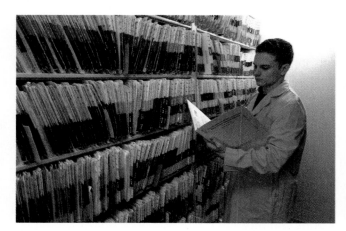

FIGURE 6-11 Confidentiality issues apply to all information about the patient, including what is charted and what is spoken between the patient and the medical assistant.

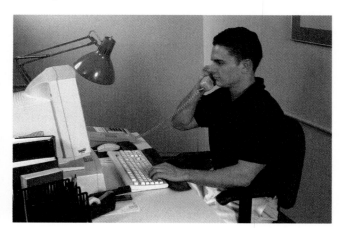

FIGURE 6-12 With the advent of advanced computer technology, a medical assistant must be particularly careful about using information about patients on the computer.

Fees and Charges

Charging or collecting an illegal or excessive fee is unethical. The medical assistant is responsible for keeping informed about current billing regulations and to see that they are conscientiously followed.

Requesting that payment be made at the time of treatment is entirely appropriate, and very common in today's medical offices. Often managed care patients are asked to remit their co-payment before seeing the physician on the day of their visit. If the patient is notified in advance, adding interest or other reasonable charges to delinquent accounts is also considered ethical. Most offices use a patient information booklet that provides a written reference of all policies and that is given to new patients on their first visit. A reasonable charge may be made for the cost of duplicating patient records.

Fee Splitting and Contingent Fees

If a physician accepts payment from another physician solely for the referral of a patient, both are guilty of an unethical practice called *fee splitting*. This practice, whether with another physician, a clinic, a laboratory, or a drug company, is unethical.

Although attorneys often accept a case on a contingent fee basis, it is unethical for a physician to engage in this practice. The fee in this case is contingent on a successful outcome, but a physician should never set his or her fee on the successful outcome of medical treatment. A physician's fee must always be based on the value of service provided to the patient.

Insurance Forms

Although physicians' offices in times past would willingly file the claim on all insurance policies for their patients, some have changed their policies to a payment up-front system and give patients the information needed to file the claim themselves. Many offices will still file at least one insurance claim for established patients but may charge for multiple or complex insurance filing. This practice is entirely ethical if in conformity with local custom.

Waiver of Insurance Co-payments

Physicians may opt to write off or waive co-payments to facilitate patient access to medical care. If access to care is directly threatened because the patient cannot make the co-payment, the physician may forgive the payment. However, routine waiver of the co-payments may violate the policies of some insurers, both public and private. Physicians should ensure that their policies on co-payments are consistent with applicable law and within legal boundaries of their contracts with insurers.

Professional Courtesy

Professional courtesy is defined as the provision of medical care to physician colleagues or their families and staff free of charge or at a reduced fee. This is a long-standing tradition, but certainly not an ethical requirement. Physicians make the decision as to who will receive professional courtesy in their offices, and this should be written into the office policy manual.

Appointment Charges

It is ethical for a physician to charge for a missed appointment or one that was not cancelled within a stated time if the patient has been fully advised in advance that such a charge may be made. Discretion should be used in applying such charges, however, since the patient may have encountered an emergency. Often adding a missed appointment charge to the bill of a patient who never cancels in advance will prompt a call in the future when the appointment cannot be kept.

Prescribing Drugs and Devices

The physician should not be influenced in the prescribing of drugs, devices, or appliances by a direct or indirect financial interest in the supplier. A physician may own or operate a pharmacy but generally may not ethically refer his or her patients to that pharmacy. Patients should enjoy the same freedom of choice in deciding who will fill their prescriptions as they do in choosing a physician.

Health Facility Ownership by a Physician

A physician may ethically own or have a financial interest in a for-profit or other health care facility, such as a free-standing clinic or health club. However, before admitting or referring a patient to that facility, the physician has an ethical obligation to reveal such ownership to the patient. In general, physicians should not refer patients to a health facility that is outside their office practice and at which they do not directly provide care or services.

Ghost Surgery

The substitution of another surgeon without the patient's consent is called *ghost surgery*. The patient has a right to choose his or her own physician or surgeon. To make a substitution without consulting the patient is deceitful and unethical.

Discipline Within Medicine

A physician should expose incompetent, corrupt, dishonest, or unethical conduct on the part of members of the profession, without fear of loss of favor. A physician may be subject to civil or criminal liability for violation of government laws. Expulsion from membership is the maximum penalty that may be imposed by a medical society for violation of ethical standards.

Physicians and Infectious Disease

A physician who knows that he or she has an infectious disease should not engage in any activity that creates an identified risk of transmission to the patient. Simple colds and other minor illnesses will arise occasionally, but illnesses that would cause a significant risk to the patient should not be given a chance to cause infection.

Substance Abuse

It is unethical for a physician to practice medicine while under the influence of a controlled substance, alcohol, or other chemical agents that could impair the ability to properly care for the patient or perform procedures.

Closing Comments

The study of ethics requires much thought and honest appraisal of what the medical assistant believes. Sometimes **introspection** of this type is difficult. Often our beliefs are a result of our environment, upbringing, and other factors that have influenced our thinking and actions from the time we were small children to our current age. It is important that our belief system be one that we have created personally, not just a set of beliefs accepted from another source. Medical assistants should take a serious look at the thoughts and concepts that make up their own concepts of ethics. It is important to approach ethical decisions calmly, logically, and without haste.

Patient Education

Patients may not always understand the ethical standards that physicians and medical assistants adhere to. They may ask a medical assistant questions about their own health or the health of a fellow patient. Medical assistants must educate patients regarding the issues of confidentiality in such a way that the patient does not take offense, explaining that all patients deserve to have their medical and personal information kept private. Now more than ever, there are ethical obligations to privacy as well as legal ones. A medical assistant must be certain that all patients understand that they are entitled to confidential treatment of their records and that the facility is dedicated to that principle.

Legal and Ethical Issues

The prime objective of the medical profession is to render service to humanity, and this must be a medical assistant's first concern as well. The importance of respecting the confidentiality of information learned from or about patients in the course of employment cannot be overemphasized. It is unethical to reveal patient confidences to anyone, and this includes family, spouse, best friends, and other medical assistants. A medical assistant must never mention the names of patients outside the place of employment, because sometimes the doctor's specialty reveals the patient's reason for consultation.

Never discuss one patient's case with another patient. If curious patients ask questions about others, simply explain that medical assistants are obligated to keep all patient information confidential. This can be done in a tactful and kind manner. Patients who ask questions of a medical nature about his or her own case should be referred to the physician for information and instructions, unless the physician has authorized the medical assistant to provide this information. A medical assistant must

avoid giving advice of a personal or professional nature to the patient, because they tend to identify remarks made by any of the assistants as reflecting the advice of the physician. By avoiding these situations, medical assistants protect themselves, the physician, and the patient. Confidential papers, case histories, and even the appointment book should be kept out of sight of curious eyes.

Medical assistants have an ethical obligation to keep abreast of current developments that affect the practice of medicine and care of the patients. Membership in a professional organization provides access to continuing education for maintaining knowledge and skills pertaining to the performance of medical assisting.

In rare instances a medical assistant is faced with a situation in which the physician-employer's conduct appears to violate established ethical standards. Before making any judgments, the medical assistant must be absolutely sure of all the information and circumstances. If unethical conduct occurs, the medical assistant must then make his or her own decision about continued employment in the facility: Would it be wise to remain in the office under the circumstances? Would it be better to seek other employment? Would remaining adversely affect future opportunities for employment with another physician?

These decisions are difficult, especially if the relationship and employment conditions have been favorable and congenial. An ethical medical assistant will not wish to participate in known substandard or unlawful practices, especially those that might be harmful to patients.

SUMMARY OF SCENARIO

Pregnancy is usually a joyous time, but Monica has learned that even such an anticipated event can bring ethical issues to light. She has realized that there are two or more sides to every situation and that she must be open and willing to look at all sides when making an ethical decision.

Medical assisting is a rewarding career, but sometimes the decisions that the medical professional is faced with making are quite difficult. Monica must learn to be nonjudgmental and not to inflict her opinions on her patients. They must make their own decisions regarding their health and emotional well-being, and the medical assistant should not influence their thinking unfairly.

Monica will continue to evaluate her own ideas and beliefs throughout her career as a medical assistant. Periodic self-evaluation is good for everyone, and she will grow emotionally from the experiences that patients bring about where ethical issues are concerned.

SUMMARY OF LEARNING OBJECTIVES

■ Ethics are judgments of right and wrong or actions on issues that have implications of a moral right and wrong. Etiquette deals with courtesy, customs, and manners. Rights are claims that are made by a person or group on society, a group, or an individual.

Although these terms have different definitions, the concepts are interrelated, and often all are involved in ethical questions.

■ Ethical distress is a problem to which there is an obvious solution, but some type of barrier hinders the action that needs to be taken. An ethical dilemma is a situation in which there are two or more solutions, but in choosing one, something of value is lost in not choosing the other. A dilemma of justice involves allocation of benefits and how they are to be fairly distributed. Two or more authority figures, each with his or her idea of how to handle a certain situation, are the center of the locus of authority ethical problem. Only one of the authority figures can prevail. Often an ethical problem has several aspects and more than one type of problem is presented.

■ Making an ethical decision is easier when approached logically and considered using a five-step process. First, one gathers relevant information; then identifies the type of problem. After determining the ethical approach to use, one should explore alternatives. Finally, all that is left is to complete the action and make the decision.

■ Although healthcare professionals do not have to abide by the opinions of the CEJA, the Council's opinions are highly regarded, and many professionals practice in accordance with these opinions. Often providers will abide by the opinions to avoid controversy, but there are still many who openly oppose the decisions of the CEJA.

■ Unique identifiers maintain the confidentiality of patients who are tested for HIV. Some individuals might hesitate to be tested if they were concerned that their name would be reported to various agencies. Using the unique identifiers, patients may have much more confidence that the chances of discrimination resulting from their HIV status are lessened.

■ There are many ethical concerns regarding genetic testing. Many patients are concerned about how the information gained will be used and who will have access to the information. Questions arise regarding the ownership of the information. When negative information is found, other ethical problems arise that will need to be addressed. Knowledge of a person's genetic blueprint could lead to discrimination. There are countless issues that must be examined before the use of genetic information becomes widespread.

■ Confidentiality is of major importance in the medical profession. The patient's privacy should be of prime concern to a medical assistant. It is a serious enough issue that a breach of patient confidentiality is sufficient reason for immediate termination of an employee. Because it is such a critical aspect of patient care, it is considered highly unethical to reveal any information about a patient to anyone else. All medical assistants are required and expected to uphold the confidentiality of the information with which they come into contact.

INTERNET CONNECTIONS

- American Medical Association Council on Ethical and Judicial Affairs
  http://www.ama-assn.org/ama/pub/category/2498.html

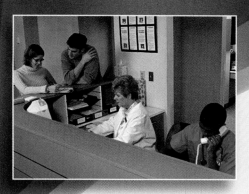

CHAPTER 7

Scenario

Barbara Johnson is the new office manager for two neurologists in an urban area. Recently she was subpoenaed to appear in court with medical records to testify about a patient who was referred to one of the physicians for whom she works. Dr. Rebecca Patrick saw the patient several years ago; this patient has brought a medical professional liability case against a surgeon in another city. Barbara is considered the custodian of records and will take the records to court and answer questions about the information in the patient's chart.

One of Barbara's first priorities is to make certain that the office is operating in compliance with the legal regulations that affect the facility. She is knowledgeable about OSHA requirements, and because her father was an attorney, she is very familiar with legal issues.

Two of the employees Barbara supervises, Samantha and Lynda, are newly graduated from medical assisting school and are anxious to learn more about the statutes and laws that affect the physicians' office. Barbara is more than happy to share what she has learned with them. She is excited about her new job and eager to be a great success.

Medicine and Law

National Curriculum Competencies

TRANSDISCIPLINARY COMPETENCIES

2a. Identify and respond to issues of confidentiality
2b. Perform within legal and ethical boundaries

Vocabulary

act The formal action of a legislative body; a decision or determination of a sovereign state, a legislative council, or a court of justice.

allegation A statement by a party to a legal action of what the party undertakes to prove, an assertion made without proof.

appeal A legal proceeding by which a case is brought before a higher court for review of the decision of a lower court.

appellate Having the power to review the judgment of another tribunal or body of jurisdiction, such as an appellate court.

arbitration The hearing and determination of a cause in controversy by a person or persons either chosen by the parties involved or appointed under statutory authority.

arbitrator A neutral person chosen to settle differences between two parties in a controversy.

assault An intentional, unlawful attempt of bodily injury to another by force.

assent To agree to something, especially after thoughtful consideration.

bailiff An officer of some U.S. courts usually serving as a messenger or usher, who keeps order at the request of the judge.

battery A willful and unlawful use of force or violence on the person of another.

Code of Federal Regulations (CFR) A coded delineation of the rules and regulations published in the Federal Register by the various departments and agencies of the federal government. The CFR is divided into 50 titles that represent broad subject areas, and then chapters that provide specific detail.

concurrently Occurring at the same time.

contributory negligence Statutes in some states that may prevent a party from recovering damages if he or she contributed in any way to the injury or condition.

damages Loss or harm resulting from injury to person, property, or reputation; compensation in money imposed by law for losses or injuries.

decedent A legal term for a deceased person.

docket A formal record of judicial proceedings; a list of legal causes to be tried.

due process A fundamental constitutional guarantee that all legal proceedings will be fair; that one will be given notice of the proceedings and given an opportunity to be heard before the government acts to take away life, liberty, or property; a constitutional guarantee that a law will not be unreasonable or arbitrary.

emancipated minor A person under legal age who is self-supporting and living apart from parents or guardian; a mature minor considered to possess a sufficient understanding of self-care and responsibility.

expert witness A person who provides testimony to a court as an expert in a certain field or subject to verify facts presented by one or both sides in a lawsuit, often compensated and used to refute or disprove the claims of one party.

felony A major crime, such as murder, rape, or burglary; punishable by a more stringent sentence than that given for a misdemeanor.

fine A sum imposed as punishment for an offense; a forfeiture or penalty paid to an injured party or the government in a civil or criminal action.

guardian ad litem Legal representative for a minor.

implied consent Presumed consent, such as when a patient offers an arm for a phlebotomy procedure.

informed consent A consent in which there is understanding of what treatment is to be undertaken and of the risks involved, why it should be done, and alternative methods of treatment available (including no treatment) and their attendant risks.

infraction Breaking the law; a minor offense of the rules.

judicial Of or relating to a judgment, the function of judging, the administration of justice, or the judiciary.

jurisdiction A power constitutionally conferred on a judge or magistrate to decide cases according to law and to carry sentence into execution; jurisdiction is original when it is conferred on the court in the first instance, called original jurisdiction; or it is appellate, which is when an appeal is given from the judgment of another court.

jurisprudence The science or philosophy of law; a system or body of law or the course of court decisions.

law A binding custom or practice of a community; a rule of conduct or action prescribed or formally recognized as binding or enforceable by a controlling authority.

liable Obligated according to law or equity; responsible for an act or circumstance.

libel A written defamatory statement or representation that conveys an unjustly unfavorable impression.

litigious Prone to engage in lawsuits.

manifestation Something that is easily understood or recognized by the mind.

misdemeanor A minor crime, as opposed to a felony, punishable by fine or imprisonment in a city or county jail rather than in a penitentiary.

municipal A court that sits in some cities and larger towns and that usually has civil and criminal jurisdiction over cases arising within the municipality.

negligence Failure to exercise the care that a prudent person usually exercises; implies inattention to one's duty or business; implies want of due or necessary diligence or care.

ordinance An authoritative decree or direction; a law set forth by a governmental authority, specifically a municipal regulation.

other potentially infectious material (OPIM) Substances or material other than blood that has the potential to carry infectious pathogens, such as body fluid, urine, semen, and others.

paraphrased A restatement of a text, passage, or work giving the meaning in another form.

perjured testimony The voluntary violation of an oath or vow either by swearing to what is untrue or by omission to do what has been promised under oath; false testimony.

precedence To surpass in rank, dignity, or importance; to be, go, or come ahead or in front of.

precedents A person or thing that serves as a model; something done or said that may serve as an example or rule to authorize or justify a subsequent act of the same kind.

preponderance of the evidence Evidence that is of greater weight or more convincing than the evidence offered in opposition to it; evidence that as a whole shows that the fact sought to be proven is more probable than not.

physician office laboratories (POLs) Laboratories owned by a private physician or corporation, such as the lab inside a physician's office or a free-standing laboratory.

prudent Marked by wisdom or judiciousness; shrewd in the management of practical affairs.

quackery The pretense of curing disease.

reasonable doubt Doubt based on reason and arising from evidence or lack of evidence; it is not doubt that is imagined or conjured up, but doubt that would cause reasonable persons to hesitate before acting.

relevant Having significant and demonstrable bearing on the matter at hand.

statute A law enacted by the legislative branch of a government.

stipulate To specify as a condition or requirement of an agreement or offer; to make an agreement or covenant to do or forbear something.

subpoena A writ or document commanding a person to appear in court under a penalty for failure to appear.

testimony A solemn declaration usually made orally by a witness under oath in response to interrogation by a lawyer or authorized public official.

Uniform Commercial Code (UCC) A unified set of rules covering many business transactions; it has been adopted in all 50 states, the District of Columbia, and most U.S. territories.

verdict The finding or decision of a jury on a matter submitted to it in trial.

Law is a fascinating subject. When law is applied to medicine, it can provoke interesting case studies and complex decisions. In today's **litigious** society, medical assistants, as well as physicians and other staff members, must take steps to protect themselves from lawsuits. Legal issues underlie many aspects of the provision of healthcare in a physician's office. Although the wording of statutes and regulations is often long and complicated, medical assistants must stay abreast of the rules governing medical facilities and do everything possible to remain in compliance with the standards and regulations for all organizations that oversee the medical industry.

Jurisprudence and the Classifications of Law

Jurisprudence, the science and philosophy of law, comes from the Latin words *juris*, which means "law, right, equity, or justice," and *prudentia*, which means "skill or good judgment."

Law is a custom or practice of a community. It is a rule of conduct or action prescribed or formally recognized as binding or enforceable by a controlling authority. Law is the system by which society gives order to our lives. The U.S. Constitution is the supreme law of the land, which takes **precedence** over federal statutes, court opinions, and state constitutions. However, within the states, the state constitution is the supreme law within the boundaries of that state, unless it conflicts with the U.S. Constitution. States cannot pass laws that conflict with the U.S. Constitution, nor can local governments pass laws that conflict with the state constitution.

A law enacted at the federal level, which must be passed by Congress, is called an **act. Statutes** are laws that have been enacted by state legislatures. Local governments create and enact **ordinances**. Much of our law is based on previous **judicial** and jury decisions, which are called **precedents**. Often judges and juries follow precedents when making a decision on a case before them. There are two basic categories of jurisprudence: criminal law and civil law.

Criminal Law

Criminal law governs violations of the law that are punishable as offenses against the state or government. Such offenses involve the welfare and safety of the public as a whole rather than of one individual. Criminal offenses are classified into three basic categories: misdemeanors, felonies, and treason.

Misdemeanors. A minor crime, as opposed to a felony, is called a **misdemeanor**. Such a crime is punishable by **fine** or imprisonment in a city or county jail rather than in a penitentiary. Misdemeanors vary from state to state and are often divided into subgroups or classes, such as class A, class B, or class C misdemeanors. In most states, the subgroups are divided from most serious offenses to lesser offenses. Some states have created a subcategory of misdemeanors for **infractions**, which are often called violations. Infractions are minor offenses, such as traffic tickets, which are punishable only by a fine.

Felonies. A **felony** is a major crime, such as murder, rape, or burglary, and is punishable by a more stringent sentence than that given for a misdemeanor. Federal law and most state statutes classify felonies as crimes punishable by imprisonment for more than 1 year, whereas misdemeanors are punishable by imprisonment for 1 year or less. Usually a convicted felon cannot vote, hold public office, or possess a firearm. Felonies are often divided into subgroups or degrees, such as first degree, second degree, and third degree. The first-degree offense is normally the most serious.

Treason. Treason, the most serious crime, is the offense of attempting to overthrow the government. High treason constitutes a serious threat to the stability or continuity of the government, such as an attempt to kill the president. The President of the United States has the right to declare an action against the United States to be an act of war, as opposed to an act of treason, which is considered a crime. For instance, although the terrorist attacks of September 11, 2001, were certainly a threat against the United States, they were declared acts of war.

Civil Law

Civil law is concerned with acts that are not criminal in nature, but those that involve relationships of individuals with other individuals, organizations, or government agencies. There are many types of civil law that address numerous issues. The three that most directly affect the medical profession include tort law, contract law, and administrative law.

Tort Law. Tort law provides a remedy for a person or group who has suffered harm from the wrongful acts of others. Four elements must be established in every tort action. First, the plaintiff must establish that the defendant was under a legal duty to act in a particular fashion. Second, the plaintiff must demonstrate that the defendant breached this duty by failing to conform his or her behavior accordingly. Third, the plaintiff must prove that the breach of the legal duty proximately caused some injury or damage. Fourth, the plaintiff must prove damages, the injury or loss suffered. Medical professional liability, or medical malpractice, falls into the category of tort law.

Contract Law. A contract is an agreement creating an obligation. Contract law touches our lives in many ways practically every day, but we usually do not give much thought to its influences. If a person parks a car in a parking garage for a monthly fee and signs a contract for a year, then begins parking elsewhere and refuses to pay the fee, the person may be **liable** for the fees for the duration of the entire contract. If damage occurs to the person's vehicle while it is parked in the garage, the garage may be responsible for reimbursement, if the contract does not **stipulate** otherwise. A contract does not have to be formalized in writing to be binding on the parties involved. Oral contracts are also valid in many states in most situations.

Administrative Law. Administrative law involves regulations set forth by governmental agencies. For example, the Internal Revenue Service (IRS) has thousands of regulations and codes, and the typical American does not understand all of them, which may result in errors when filing taxes. The laws that allow the IRS to collect taxes and pursue restitution are administrative laws. Other agencies that are involved with administrative law include the Social Security Administration, Immigration and Naturalization Service, and the Centers for Medicare and Medicaid Services (formerly the Health Care Financing Administration [HCFA]).

Anatomy of a Medical Professional Liability Lawsuit

A medical liability case often stems from a breach of trust or miscommunication between the physician and the patient. Even when the physician has made an error, often the level of trust between the physician and patient will determine whether a lawsuit will be pursued. First, the physician-patient relationship must be formed. Before discussing this relationship, it is important to understand what is necessary for a contract to be valid and enforceable.

There are four essential elements to a contract. First, there must be **manifestation** of **assent** or a "meeting of the minds." This element is proven by an "offer" and the "acceptance" of that offer. The parties to the contract must understand and agree on the intent of the contract. Second, the contract must involve legal subject matter. An obligation that requires an illegal action, such as a gambling contract, is not an enforceable contract. Third, both parties must have the legal capacity to enter into a contract. This means that the parties must be adults of sound mind, or an **emancipated minor**. Fourth, there must be some type of consideration. Consideration is an exchange of something of value, for example, money for the physician's time.

CRITICAL THINKING APPLICATION

Barbara works for Dr. Rebecca Patrick, who saw the patient bringing the lawsuit against the surgeon as a referral patient. Does Dr. Patrick have a contract with the patient, based on a physician-patient relationship? Why or why not?

The physician-patient relationship is generally held by courts to be a contractual relationship that is the result of three steps:
1. The physician invites an offer by establishing availability.
2. The patient accepts the invitation and makes an offer by arriving for or requesting treatment.
3. The physician accepts the offer by accepting the patient and undertaking treatment. The physician may explicitly accept the patient's offer or implicitly accept the offer by exercising their independent medical judgment on behalf of the patient.

Before accepting a patient, the physician is under no obligation, and no contract exists. However, once the physician has accepted the patient, an implied contract does exist (Figure 7-1). This implied contract assumes that the physician will treat the patient using reasonable care

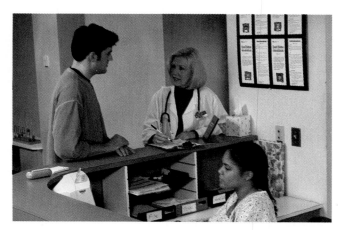

FIGURE 7-1 The physician-patient relationship is built on a strong foundation of trust, but it is also a contractual relationship.

and that the physician possesses a degree of knowledge, skill, and judgment that might be expected of any other physician in the same locality and under similar circumstances. It is extremely important that no express promise of a cure be made by anyone in the office, including the physician, because this would become a part of the contract.

The patient's responsibility in this agreement includes the liability of payment for services and a willingness to follow the advice of the physician. Most physician-patient contracts are implied contracts. Although many forms may be completed by the patient before being accepted by the physician, they do not in most cases constitute a formal contract for each specific visit to the physician.

CRITICAL THINKING APPLICATION

- If the patient does not pay for the services rendered by the physician, does this negate the physician-patient contract?
- How might Barbara, Samantha, and Lynda ensure that patients understand that they are expected to follow the advice of the physician?

After the physician-patient relationship has been established, the physician is obligated to attend the patient as long as attention is required, unless the physician or patient terminates the contract. When a physician terminates the contract, the patient must be given notice of the physician's intentions so that the patient has sufficient time to secure another physician. The physician may write a letter of withdrawal from medical care of the patient, and it should be delivered by certified mail, return receipt requested. A copy of the letter and the return receipt should be attached to the patient's chart and permanently retained.

To protect the physician against a lawsuit for abandonment, the details of the circumstances under which the physician is withdrawing from the case should be included in the patient's medical chart. The letter of withdrawal does not have to specify a reason for withdrawal unless the physician so chooses, but it should state the following:

- That professional care is being discontinued
- That the physician will provide copies of the patient's records to another physician on request
- That the patient should seek the attention of another physician as soon as possible

A patient who wishes to terminate the physician-patient relationship simply no longer seeks the physician for treatment. The patient does not have to inform the office; however, if this is done, the office manager or physician should follow up with a letter confirming notice that the patient has ended the relationship.

The Statute of Frauds

In 1677, a statute was adopted in England that was designed to reduce the occurrence of **perjured testimony** by providing that certain contracts could not be enforced if they depended on the testimony of witnesses alone and

were not evidenced in writing. The provisions of this English statute have been closely followed by statutes adopted in all 50 states in the United States.

The promise to pay the debts of another person is an example of a contract that usually must be made in writing. If a third party who is not otherwise legally responsible for a patient's medical bills agrees to pay them, the agreement cannot be enforced unless it is in writing. Or, if a physician entered into an agreement to perform a series of treatments for a given sum, and this series covered a time span of more than 1 year, the contract would have to be in writing to be enforceable.

Preliminaries of Litigation

Once a patient has decided to file a lawsuit against a physician, the first step is usually to find an attorney who will accept the case. This may be a frustration to many patients: attorneys may not wish to initiate litigation against a physician. Like physicians, an attorney does not have to accept a case he or she does not wish to pursue, and this is often because the attorney does not see enough of a financial benefit from the time it would take to work on the case. Although this sounds a bit harsh, the attorney runs a business, as does a physician, and must make good business decisions as to how his or her time is spent and invested.

CRITICAL THINKING APPLICATION

- For what reasons might a physician not wish to accept a patient?
- Must the physician treat every patient who attempts to make an appointment?
- How might Barbara tactfully explain that the physician will not accept the patient into treatment?

Lawsuits are filed in a variety of different courts, and different states have different types of courts at various levels. There are several branches of the state judiciary. At the local level, there are usually **municipal** courts. These are courts in a city or town that usually deal with ordinance violations. Municipal judges may issue search and arrest warrants. Some states also have justice of the peace courts, which have **jurisdiction** over many misdemeanors and some civil matters, as well as concurrent jurisdiction over some matters along with the municipal courts. The judges that preside over justice of the peace courts may also issue search warrants and arrest warrants. They often function as small claims courts, which the medical assistant may have contact with in cases of patients who do not pay their bills. Both municipal and justice of the peace courts are local trial courts with limited jurisdiction.

County courts are higher than municipal and justice of the peace courts. These courts handle misdemeanors and civil matters up to a certain monetary limit. District courts have unlimited jurisdiction in criminal and civil matters. They are the highest state courts, other than appellate courts. When one party of a lawsuit is dissatisfied with a lower court's decision, it has the right to

appeal to a higher court for review and possible reversal of the decision. Most states have an **appellate** court for both criminal and civil matters. The U.S. District Court handles federal matters of both a criminal and civil nature. States also have Supreme Courts that handle a limited number of appellate cases.

The U.S. Supreme Court has authority given by Article III, Section One of the Constitution, to ensure equal justice under the law (Figure 7-2). The Supreme Court interprets and guards the Constitution of the United States. There is one Chief Justice and eight Associate Justices who are appointed by the President and confirmed by the Congress. Approximately 7000 cases are on the **docket** per term, which runs from the first Monday in October to the first Monday of October in the next year.

CRITICAL THINKING APPLICATION

Samantha and Lynda are curious as to how Supreme Court decisions affect the individual physician's office. What Supreme Court decisions have affected the medical profession?

Preparing for Court

Medical professional liability suits are far from rare, and every physician faces the probability of being sued at least once during his or her career. When a suit is filed, preparation for court should start expeditiously. A medical assistant may be involved in preparing materials for court and scheduling or participating in depositions. The best advice for a medical assistant in this position is to remember to tell the truth. Attorneys will help to prepare the defense of the physician and the staff, but everyone should be truthful in the answers that are given to the court to avoid losing his or her credibility in the trial and to avoid charges of perjury (Figure 7-3).

Interrogatories

Before the trial, the physician may be requested to complete an interrogatory, which is a list of questions from each party to the other in the lawsuit. Answers to the interrogatory must be provided within a specified time, and the answers are considered to be given under oath. Only the parties named in the lawsuit may be questioned through interrogatories.

Depositions

A deposition is testimony taken from a party or witness to the litigation and is not limited to the parties named in the lawsuit. A witness who is not a party to the lawsuit may be summoned by **subpoena** for the deposition. The deposition is usually taken in an attorney's office in the presence of a court reporter and is taken under oath. The person giving the deposition is called the *deponent*. The transcribed deposition, once finished, is sent to the deponent for review, and the deponent is at liberty to request any necessary changes or corrections in the document.

CRITICAL THINKING APPLICATION

- Samantha and Lynda are anxious to hear about Barbara's experiences in testifying in court. She mentions that attorneys often advise witnesses to "answer the question, then be quiet." What might be meant by this advice?
- Discuss the phrase, "the truth, the whole truth, and nothing but the truth."

Subpoenas

A subpoena is a document issued by a court requiring a person to be in court at a specific time and place to testify as a witness in a lawsuit, either in a court proceeding or in a deposition. A *subpoena duces tecum* is a

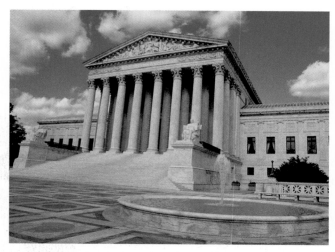

FIGURE 7-2   The U.S. Supreme Court. The Supreme Court decides cases that involve interpretation of the Constitution of the United States.

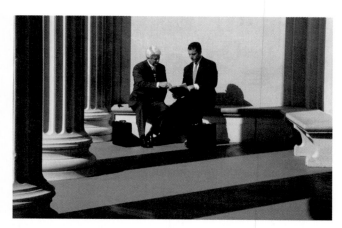

FIGURE 7-3   Preparation is of primary importance to the physician facing a medical professional liability case. A competent and experienced attorney is necessary to provide an adequate defense and present the physician's views to the court.

legally binding request to provide records or documents to appear in court and is usually issued to the person considered the custodian of the records. This may be the medical assistant or office manager. A fee may be demanded for the time spent in compiling the records and for photocopying charges, but this fee must be requested at the time the subpoena duces tecum is served, or it is considered to be waived. Physician approval must be obtained to release or copy any patient records. Original records should never be released under any circumstances.

Discovery

Discovery is the pretrial disclosure of pertinent facts or documents by one or both parties to a legal action or proceeding. Many states have extensive discovery statutes that require each side to reveal to the other the facts that they "discover" while investigating the case. Discovery is also considered the process of uncovering facts in a lawsuit before the court proceedings.

Presentation of evidence may be by **testimony**. A witness is called who has some information about an aspect of the case and is asked questions by one or both attorneys. The witness will not know about every part of the case, but something that the person knows will be **relevant** to the case.

Another type of evidence may be documentary evidence. This is any type of evidence brought before the court by document or display. It could be a patient's chart, or a letter, a lab result, or a photograph. All of these are usually entered into evidence and numbered for easy reference.

CRITICAL THINKING APPLICATION

Samantha wonders what she should do if she ever finds negative information during a medical professional malpractice case that might harm her employer's defense. What advice would you offer? Would it be considered an obligation or a choice to report the employer of wrongdoing?

Preparing Witnesses and Testifying

Attorneys will prepare witnesses who may be called to testify during the court proceedings. They will review the questions that will be asked and potential questions that the opposite side may present. The attorney will help the witness to clarify the answers that he or she gives so that they are sharp and succinct. One of the first rules that attorneys learn in law school is to never ask a question to which they do not already know the answer.

Witnesses should be certain that they know the exact location of the courthouse and to which floor and courtroom they are to report. They should always be on time for a court appearance, because the judge and jury may frown on those appearing late. That frown may also include a fine or confinement in jail for contempt of court!

When called to testify, it is critical that the witness dress conservatively and in a manner that shows respect for the court. Normal business attire should be adequate, but if there is ever any doubt, consult the attorney.

If any documents are to be referenced while testifying, the witness should review the documents before the court appearance so that the needed information will be easy to locate and discuss. The witness should speak clearly and at a volume audible to the attorneys and parties to the suit, the judge, the jury, and the court reporter. The witness should always answer each question aloud, because the court reporter must record those answers and cannot specify that the witness "nodded yes" as a response to a question.

If a question is confusing, the witness should ask the attorney to restate or repeat it. Attorneys may ask the witness to speak up, but this should not be intimidating to the witness. If the witness does not know the answer to a question or does not recall, that should be stated clearly and confidently. Above all, the parties involved are expected to tell the truth and must be seen as credible witnesses (Figure 7-4). Lying under oath constitutes perjury, which carries stiff penalties. Listening is as important as speaking, so the witness should be sure to listen to the question, and answer it, elaborating only if the attorney asks for more details.

If an attorney lodges an objection to a question, the witness should be silent until the judge rules on the objection. The objection may be sustained or overruled. Sustaining the objection means that the judge agrees with the objection and will not allow the question stated in that manner. If the judge allows the question, he or she will overrule the objection. Then the witness will be allowed to answer. The witness should never display a combative or hostile attitude and should not make sarcastic remarks while testifying in court. This is the fastest way to show

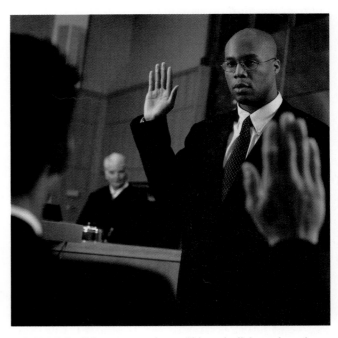

FIGURE 7-4 Witnesses must be credible and tell the truth on the stand in court to avoid charges of perjury.

disrespect for the judge, the jurors, and the court itself. No matter the circumstances, the court is no place to express discontent. The witness should be professional at all times and restrain inappropriate comments and belligerent behavior. Using "yes Sir" and "no Ma'am" is appropriate in the courtroom. Always address the judge as "your Honor."

Inside the Courtroom

It is beneficial to know the role of each person in a court of law (Figure 7-5). The person or body bringing the lawsuit to court is referred to by different terms, depending on what type of case is to be presented. In a criminal court, the government brings the case and is represented by a prosecutor. Legal documents will read, for example, "The State of Texas v. Robert Smith" in criminal cases. In this case, the fictitious Robert Smith is the defendant. In civil court, the person or group bringing the case to court is called the *plaintiff* (or *complainant* in some court systems), and the opposite party is called the *defendant* or *respondent*. A judge will preside over the case, providing instructions concerning the law to the jury, if a jury is present. If there is no jury, the judge decides the case. This is called a "bench trial." A *witness* is a person who gives testimony, knowing some pertinent information about the case (Figure 7-6). Often a court reporter takes notes of the proceedings, and a **bailiff** may be present, who assists in keeping order. All of these individuals should be treated with respect and courtesy.

Burden of Proof

In a criminal case, the burden of proof is on the prosecution, which must prove guilt beyond any **reasonable doubt**. Reasonable doubt is defined as the level of certainty a juror must have to find a defendant guilty of a crime. It is real doubt, based on reason and common

sense after careful and impartial consideration of all the evidence, or lack of evidence, in a case.

Civil cases must be proven by a **preponderance of the evidence**. This means that there must be a greater weight of evidence that points toward the defendant/respondent as being responsible for the act involved in the case.

To understand the difference between reasonable doubt and preponderance of the evidence, think of the scales of justice (Figure 7-7). For a case to be proven beyond a reasonable doubt, the scales should tip heavily toward either guilt or innocence. However, for a case to be proven by preponderance of the evidence, the scales need only tip slightly one way or the other.

To illustrate the difference in the standard of proof in criminal and civil cases, consider "The People of the State of California v. Orenthal James Simpson." In O.J. Simpson's criminal trial, although there was much circumstantial evidence, there was also enough doubt that the scales could not tip heavily toward a verdict of guilty, and Mr. Simpson was acquitted. But in the civil trial brought by family members of Nicole Brown Simpson and Ron Goldman after the criminal trial had ended, there was just enough evidence to tip the scales in favor of the families' claim that Mr. Simpson was somehow responsible for the deaths of Nicole and Ron. This is the equivalent to a preponderance of the evidence.

CRITICAL THINKING APPLICATION

The discussion of the burden of proof prompts Barbara, Samantha, and Lynda to discuss the case of O.J. Simpson. Discuss whether reasonable doubt existed in his criminal trial.

Outcome of the Case

Once both sides have presented their case to the judge or jury, usually they are given the opportunity to present a final summation of their case. After this is done, the jury retires to consider the **verdict**. This can take minutes, hours, days, or weeks. After the jury reaches a verdict, the judge may enter a judgment on that verdict or may disregard the verdict if the evidence does not support the jury's decision. The judge may also revise the verdict to comply with statutes, such as statutory limits on the amount of punitive damages. The final decision of the trial court is reflected in the judgment, signed by the judge.

Either side normally has the right to appeal the decision to a higher court. However, not all appellate courts are required to hear all cases. For instance, the U.S. Supreme Court chooses the cases that it hears each year, and it is restricted to cases that involve interpretation of the Constitution of the United States and how that interpretation affects the people it governs.

In criminal cases, when a person is found guilty of the crime with which he or she is charged, a sentencing date will be set at which the punishment will be announced. This is usually set a few weeks to a month after the verdict is announced.

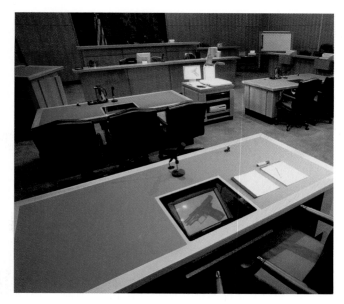
FIGURE 7-5 The inside of a typical U.S. courtroom.

HUMOR IN THE COURTROOM

Mary Louise Gilman has very possibly heard it all. As the editor of the *National Shorthand Reporter*, she collected enough courtroom bloopers to fill two books: *"Humor in the Court"* and *"More Humor in the Court."* Here are a few examples!

Q: Were you acquainted with the deceased?
A: Yes, Sir.
Q: Before or after he died?

Q: What happened then?
A: He told me, he says, "I have to kill you because you can identify me."
Q: Did he kill you?
A: No.

Q: When he went, had you gone and had she, if she wanted to and were able, for the time being excluding all the restraints on her not to go, gone also, would he have brought you, meaning you and she, with him to the station?
A: Objection. That question should be taken out and shot.

Q: And lastly, Gary, all your responses must be oral. O.K.? What school do you go to?
A: Oral.
Q: How old are you?
A: Oral.

Q: ...and what did he do then?
A: He came home, and next morning he was dead.
Q: So when he woke up the next morning he was dead?

Q: ...any suggestions as to what prevented this from being a murder trial instead of an attempted murder trial?
A: The victim lived.

Q: What is your date of birth?
A: July fifteenth.
Q: What year?
A: Every year.

Q: This myasthenia gravis–does it affect your memory at all?
A: Yes.
Q: And in what ways does it affect your memory?
A: I forget.
Q: Can you give me an example of something you've forgotten?

Q: What was the first thing your husband said to you when he woke that morning?
A: He said, "Where am I, Cathy?"
Q: And why did that upset you?
A: My name is Susan.

Q: She had three children, correct?
A: Yes.
Q: How many were boys?
A: None.
Q: Were there any girls?

Q: Doctor, before you performed the autopsy, did you check for a pulse?
A: No.
Q: Did you check for a blood pressure?
A: No.
Q: Did you check for breathing?
A: No.
Q: So, then it is possible that the patient was alive when you began the autopsy?
A: No.
Q: How can you be sure, Doctor?
A: Because his brain was sitting on my desk in a jar.
Q: But could the patient have still been alive nevertheless?
A: Yes, it is possible that he could have been alive and practicing law somewhere.

FIGURE 7-6   Humor in the courtroom. (From Gilman M, editor: *More humor in the court.* Vienna, Vir, 1985, National Shorthand Reporters Association.)

Arbitration

Arbitration is an alternative to trial that uses a third party who has been selected because of the party's familiarity with or knowledge of the law or the issues involved to hear evidence and make a decision. Arbitration is common in modern business life. It is recognized by statute in the majority of the states and is usually available to the medical profession, affording an alternative method for resolving legal disputes between physician and patient. Many physicians and attorneys see arbitration as one way to solve the crisis of litigation in this country. Court battles can take years and be extremely expensive, and much of the money will revert to the attorneys involved in the case instead of the victors of the lawsuit.

In arbitration, the patient and the physician agree to submit the dispute to an **arbitrator** in an informal hearing. The arbitrator will render a legally binding decision based on very specific rules of arbitration. Arbitration applies essentially the same rights and the same measure of damages as a court. It is fair, less expensive, faster, and more confidential than court litigation.

The staff of each medical office should know whether arbitration statutes exist in the state where the office

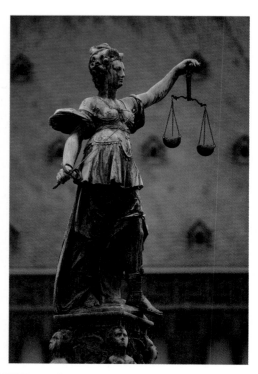

FIGURE 7-7   "Lady Justice." Justitia was the Roman goddess of justice and is the figure depicted in statues across the world, often holding both scales and a sword. Her scales imply the weighing of justice, and the blindfold represents the impartiality of justice.

conducts business. The state medical board or local medical society should be able to provide this information. An arbitration agreement is a contract and is subject to the judgment of the courts only as to the fairness of the agreement. The agreement is precisely worded by an attorney and should not be **paraphrased** when explaining it to a patient. Signing the agreement is a voluntary act by the patient, who has a grace period in which to revoke the agreement if he or she later decides against it. Likewise, a physician always has the option to decide not to care for a patient but must formally notify a patient if the decision is made to no longer render care.

If a physician elects to implement an arbitration agreement procedure with patients, every member of the physician's staff should know the details of the agreement, how and when the patient should sign up, and how to answer the patient's questions. The way that the program is presented to the patient and the willingness with which the office personnel answer the patient's questions will play a large part in whether courts will uphold the arbitration agreement as being fair and legal.

Both the patient and the physician have the opportunity to agree who will arbitrate the case, so that it does not favor one side over the other. By prior agreement, the arbitrator (or arbitrators) may be appointed by or from the American Arbitration Association, which is a neutral, private, nonprofit association dedicated to the advancement of out-of-court remedies. Its panels of arbitrators are made up of persons from business, the professions, and public interest groups.

Medical Professional Liability and Negligence

When injury results to a patient as a result of a physician's negligence, the patient may initiate a malpractice lawsuit to recover financial **damages**. However, experience has shown that the incidence of malpractice claims is directly related to the personal relationship and trust that exist between the physician and the patient. A deterioration of the physician-patient relationship is a common reason for the patient's decision to sue the physician for malpractice, even in situations where there is no real injury to the patient.

Medical professional liability, commonly called *medical malpractice*, is governed by the law of torts. The term *medical professional liability* encompasses all possible civil liability that can be incurred during the delivery of medical care. Medical professional liability is much more easily prevented than defended.

To understand medical malpractice, one must first understand the term **negligence**. Negligence, in general, implies inattention to one's duty or business, or the implication of a lack of necessary diligence or care. In medicine, negligence is defined as the performance of an act that a reasonable and **prudent** physician *would not* do or the failure to do an act that a reasonable and prudent physician *would* do. This, of course, also applies to any other healthcare professional. The standard of prudent care and conduct is not defined by law but would be left to the determination of a judge or jury, usually with the help of **expert witnesses** (Figure 7-8). Expert witnesses are members of the profession involved—in this case, medicine. To be considered an expert witness, a person usually belongs to a certifying or qualifying organization, against which the qualities of the defendant may be compared.

Professional negligence in medicine falls into one of three general classifications:

- *Malfeasance:* The performance of an act that is wholly wrongful and unlawful
- *Misfeasance:* The improper performance of a lawful act
- *Nonfeasance:* The failure to perform an act that should have been performed

A physician who performs an operation carelessly or fails to render care that should have been given may be found to have been negligent. Although a medical assistant acts as an agent of the physician in carrying out the majority of his or her duties, it is possible for the medical assistant to perform an act that can result in litigation.

For instance, if the medical assistant gives a patient the wrong medication or the wrong dosage of medication, both the physician and the medical assistant can be held liable for the error. Some states limit the scope of practice of medical assistants where medications are involved; however, if medical assistants are performing within the realm of duties for which they have received training and the physician is accepting responsibility for the actions of those in the medical office, they are usually allowed to dispense and administer medications unless prohibited by state law.

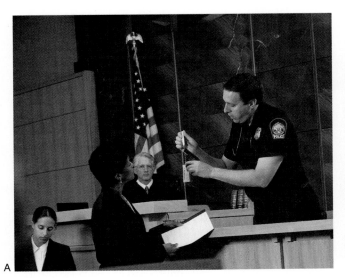

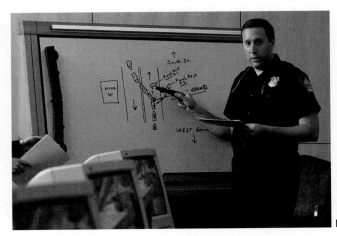

A   B

FIGURE 7-8   **A** and **B**, Expert witnesses help attorneys to prove or disprove the case in question by drawing on their experience with a given subject.

CRITICAL THINKING APPLICATION

Lynda is curious as to whether a physician is guilty of medical professional liability if he or she makes a mistake in diagnosing a patient. When might this be considered malpractice, and when might it not be considered malpractice?

What if the patient makes his or her condition worse? Is the physician then fully responsible? **Contributory negligence** exists when the patient contributes to his or her own condition and can lessen the damages that can be collected or even prevent them from being collected altogether.

The Four D's of Negligence

Negligence is not presumed—it must be proven. The Committee on Medicolegal Problems of the American Medical Association (AMA) has determined that patients must present evidence of four elements before negligence has been proven. These elements have become known as the Four *D*'s of Negligence:

1. *Duty:* Duty exists when the physician-patient relationship has been established. The patient has sought the assistance of the physician, and the physician has knowingly undertaken to provide the needed medical service.
2. *Dereliction:* Dereliction, or failure to perform a duty, is the second element required. There must be proof that the physician somehow neglected the duty to the patient.
3. *Direct cause:* There must be proof that the harm to the patient was directly caused by the physician's actions or failure to act and that the harm would not otherwise have occurred.
4. *Damages:* The patient must prove that a loss or harm has resulted from the actions of the physician.

If all four of these elements exist, then the patient may obtain a judgment against the physician in a medical professional liability case.

Types of Damages

There are several types of damages commonly seen in tort cases. They are nominal, punitive, compensatory, general, and special damages.

Nominal damages are small awards that are token compensations for the invasion of a legal right in which no actual injury was suffered. For instance, if an unauthorized medical facility employee accesses a patient's medical record and is discovered, but does not reveal any of the information in the record, the patient has not actually been harmed, but may be awarded nominal damages in a lawsuit for the invasion of the patient's privacy.

Punitive damages are designed to punish the party who committed the wrong in such a way to deter the repetition of the act, and are sometimes called exemplary damages. These damages were historically set so that the amounts would discourage intentional wrongdoings, misconduct, and outrageous behaviors. The amount of damages awarded would coincide in some percentage with the wealth of the defendant. Today there is much discussion of tort reform, which would place a cap on the amount of money that could be collected during personal injury litigation, including medical malpractice cases. Some have suggested a specific monetary figure, such as $500,000, as a limit on punitive damages, and others have suggested that plaintiffs be allowed to collect only up to three times the amount of compensatory damages.

CRITICAL THINKING APPLICATION

Samantha and Lynda disagree as to whether punitive damages should be awarded in medical professional liability cases. Samantha feels that nothing will compensate for certain losses, but Lynda feels that monetary compensation is reasonable when a loss has been suffered. Discuss both sides of the issue.

Compensatory damages are designed to compensate for any actual damages that are caused by the negligent person. They are intended to make the injured person "whole." Of course, nothing can substitute for the loss of an arm or a leg, for example, but compensatory damages help the patient or the patient's family recover from the loss.

General damages include compensation for pain and suffering, for loss of a bodily member or faculty, for disfigurement, or for other similar direct losses or injuries. The fact of the losses must be proven, but the monetary value does not.

Special damages are those injuries or losses that are not a necessary consequence of the physician's negligent act or omission. These may include the loss of earnings or costs of travel. Both the fact of these losses and the monetary value must be proven.

Standard of Care

If a physician were to be held legally responsible for every unsuccessful result occurring in the treatment of a patient, no person would undertake the responsibility of practicing medicine. The courts hold that a physician must do the following:

- Use reasonable care, attention, and diligence in the performance of professional services.
- Follow his or her best judgment in treating patients.
- Possess and exercise reasonable skill and care that are commonly possessed and exercised by other reputable physicians in the same type practice in the same or a similar locality.

Physicians who represent themselves as specialists must meet the standards of practice of their specialty. Whether or not they have met these requirements in treating a particular patient is generally a matter for the court to decide on the basis of testimony provided by an expert witness. Physicians are not required to possess extraordinary learning and skill, but they must keep abreast of medical developments and techniques, and they cannot experiment. They are also bound to advise their patients if they discover that the condition to be treated is one beyond their knowledge or technical skill.

In the worst of cases, a physician or medical facility may be faced with a wrongful death litigation. A wrongful death **allegation** is one in which the physician or medical facility is being blamed for the death of a patient as a result of error or inappropriate treatment. A wrongful death suit is usually brought by the family of the **decedent** against the physician or others involved with the patient.

A medical assistant should treat every chart touched as if it will end up in a court of law. Handwriting must be implicitly clear and legible, detailed, and leave absolutely no room for errors. Never mark out a mistake. Always draw one line through the error, then initial and date it. Nothing should be committed to memory. Remember, if it is not in the chart, it did not happen!

Consent

A physician must have consent to treat a patient, even though this consent is usually implied by virtue of the patient's appearance at the office for treatment. This **implied consent** is sufficient for common or simple procedures that are generally understood to involve little risk. A blood screen or taking vital signs are examples of procedures that usually involve implied consent. When more complex procedures are anticipated, the physician must obtain the patient's informed consent. A physician who fails to secure some formal expression of consent could be charged with the crime of **battery**.

The Health Insurance Portability and Accountability Act (HIPAA) of 1996 was designed for two major purposes. First, a standardization of electronic data exchange was sought in hopes that the efficiency of the healthcare system would be improved. Second, HIPAA was developed to protect health information and secure the contents of patient medical records. In the past, a section of the Health Insurance Claim Form (HCFA 1500) was reserved for the patient to authorize the release of medical information to the insurance company so that the claim could be evaluated and paid. Today, because of the influence of HIPAA, many medical offices are moving toward the use of a general consent form that is signed before the physician sees the patient. This form allows the physician to not only treat the patient, but also to use and submit health information to third parties for reimbursement.

Informed consent involves a deeper understanding of the patient's condition and a full explanation of the plan for treatment. Informed consent is not satisfied merely by having the patient sign a form. A discussion must occur during which the physician provides the patient or the patient's legal representative with enough information to decide whether to undergo the treatment or seek an alternative. After such discussion, the patient either consents or refuses to consent to the proposed therapy and signs a consent form. According to the AMA's standards for informed consent, the discussion should contain the following elements, at a minimum:

- The patient's diagnosis, if known
- The nature and purpose of a proposed treatment or procedure
- The risks and benefits of a proposed treatment or procedure
- Alternative treatments or procedures, regardless of the cost or the extent to which the treatment options are covered by health insurance
- The risks and benefits of the alternative treatment or procedure
- The risks and benefits of not receiving or undergoing a treatment or procedure

The discussion should be fully documented in the patient's medical record, and a copy of the signed form should be placed in the record. Treatment may not exceed the scope of the consent that the patient has given. Often the consent forms will be lengthy and mention excessive possibilities and complications. There may be language that attempts to be all-inclusive, such as "included, but not limited to" when risks are listed. It is wise to have an attorney review the forms that are used for informed consent, because those that are too broad or too specific can be detrimental to the physician in a medical professional liability case.

Patients cannot be forced to undergo any type of medical treatment or care. The ultimate decision regarding care must be left to the patient, and although medical professionals should disclose information to help the patient make a good, informed decision, the patient should never be persuaded to act in any manner or accept any treatment to which he or she does not agree. Should the patient decide not to undergo treatment that the physician feels is necessary, an informed refusal of treatment or care should be signed. This should be a statement similar to the informed consent, but will indicate that the patient has elected not to undergo treatment. Some physicians will discontinue all treatment if a patient does not participate in the care that the physician recommends. This document, once signed, should be added to the patient's medical record.

CRITICAL THINKING APPLICATION

Barbara stresses to Samantha and Lynda that there may be times in their professional career when a patient asks for their advice as to whether he or she should undergo a certain procedure or treatment. Barbara explains that patients often consider advice from the medical assistants in the office to be an extension of the physician's opinions. How might they handle such questions from patients?

Giving Consent to Medical Procedures. Mentally competent adults are certainly able to consent to medical procedures. However, if an act is unlawful, then the consent is invalid. For instance, if an abortion is performed in a state where abortion is considered illegal, then the consent to that procedure is null. Consent is also invalid if it is given by a person who is unauthorized to do so or if it is obtained by misrepresentation or fraud.

In an emergency, one may render aid or care to prevent loss of life or serious illness or injury. However, implied consent in this circumstance lasts only as long as the emergency exists, and formal consent must be obtained for further treatment as soon as the emergency has passed.

Physicians are sometimes reluctant to render aid in an emergency to someone who is not their patient for fear that they will later be charged with negligence or abandonment. In 1959, California passed the first Good Samaritan Act, which provides immunity from liability to volunteers at the scene of an accident for any civil damages as a result of rendering emergency care. Today, all 50 states have Good Samaritan statutes. As long as the emergency care is given in good faith and without gross negligence, and the healthcare worker only provides emergency care that he or she has been trained to provide, the likelihood of a successful lawsuit against that individual is very slim.

Adults who have been found by a court to be insane or incompetent usually cannot consent to medical treatment. Consent must be obtained from the guardian except in emergency situations.

Generally, when the patient is a minor, consent for surgery or treatment must be obtained from a parent, guardian, or **guardian ad litem**, except in an emergency requiring immediate treatment. If the parents are legally divorced or separated, consent should be obtained from the custodial parent, but if the child is visiting the second parent, consent may be obtained from that parent, because in this situation there is a temporary custody.

Consent is not required for minors in the following circumstances:
- When consent may be assumed, such as in a life-threatening situation
- When a certain treatment is required by law, such as a vaccination or x-ray evaluation for school entry or safety
- When a court order has been issued, as in a situation in which parents withhold consent for a necessary treatment because of religious reasons

In many states, treatment of sexually transmitted diseases, drug abuse, alcohol dependency, or pregnancy or providing birth control measures does not require parental consent.

Emancipation is defined by statute and varies from state to state. An emancipated minor is a person younger than the age of majority (usually 18 to 21 years) who meets one or more of the following conditions:
- Is married
- Is in the armed forces
- Is living separate and apart from parents or a legal guardian
- Is self-supporting

Some states include a minimum age for emancipation. Unless a statute declares otherwise, a minor who has the right to consent to treatment is entitled to the protection of his or her confidences, even from parents.

Statute of Limitations

A statute of limitations is a period of time after which a lawsuit cannot be filed. The statute of limitations varies from state to state and differs for various types of litigation. Many states have a 2-year statute of limitations for medical malpractice issues. However, in some instances, the statute of limitations may be extended because of a delay in the discovery of an injury. For example, a patient has surgery to replace a valve in the heart, and the surgery seems successful. Two years later, the patient obtains a routine echocardiogram and the physician discovers that the surgeon mistakenly replaced the aortic valve when the surgery was intended for the pulmonary valve. Although 2 years have already passed, the statute of limitations begins at the point of discovery of the injury, so the patient could now bring suit against the surgeon for the error.

Confidentiality

Confidentiality is one of the most sacred trusts that the patient places in the hands of the physician and his or her staff (Figure 7-9). Breach of patient confidentiality is grounds for immediate dismissal of a healthcare professional. The strictest care must be taken when handling patient records and discussing information about patients.

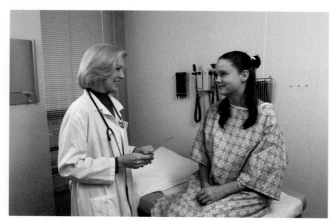

FIGURE 7-9 Patient confidentiality is the most important trust that exists between the physician and the patient.

There are many special cases in which patient confidentiality plays a vital role. A patient who is HIV positive may face discrimination if the information about his or her medical condition surfaces. Physicians who treat these patients may wish to take extra care when leaving phone messages or sending mail. Instead of leaving a message for a patient from "Dr. Watson's office," the medical assistant could say that the message is from "Terry Watson's office." This could indicate an attorney, accountant, or real estate broker. Curious co-workers or relatives may not grow as suspicious as they might if they were to encounter a message from a physician's office.

Patients who are receiving treatment for substance abuse are protected by federal statutes. Confidentiality is also of utmost importance to patients receiving treatment for mental health issues, sexually transmitted diseases, sexual **assault**, and any type of abuse.

Law and Medical Practice

Law affects the day-to-day practice of the physician. Some of the ways in which the medical assistant will encounter legal issues in the physician's offices are discussed in this section.

Legal Disclosure

The physician is charged with safeguarding patient confidences within the constraints of the law, but according to state laws, which vary somewhat throughout the nation, certain disclosures must be made. Frequently the medical assistant is involved with the responsibility for reporting these events.

Births and deaths must be reported. In some states, detailed information about stillbirths is required. Physicians must also report cases that may have been a result of violence, such as gunshot wounds, knife injuries, or poisonings. Any death from accidental, suspicious, or unexplained causes must also be reported. In some states, occupational diseases and injuries must be reported within specific time limits.

Sexually transmitted diseases are reportable in every state. All fifty states require that patients who have confirmed cases of acquired immunodeficiency syndrome (AIDS) be reported by name to the local health department. However, just over 30 states require that patients who are HIV positive be reported. Individuals are reported either by name or by unique identifiers. A continuing controversy exists as to whether the reporting prompts patients to receive care or deters patients in high-risk groups from seeking care.

Child abuse is a leading cause of death among children younger than 5 years of age, and health care professionals are required by law to report any suspected cases of child abuse. The report should be made as soon as evidence is discovered that gives the physician "cause to believe" that abuse or neglect has occurred. Even if the evidence is uncertain, the physician should report the evidence and allow the government to investigate and determine what action to take to protect the child. However, it is essential to make every attempt to ensure that the report is legitimate, because it could lead to the child's being removed from the home and placed in foster care. Cases of spousal and elder abuse are difficult, because the person being abused is often reluctant to report the situation for fear of further mistreatment. The law requires that suspected cases of abuse to children, elderly persons, or any others at risk be reported to the authorities.

Local health departments publish lists of diseases that are reportable as well as the method that should be used in reporting. Often this can be done by telephone or mail. Appropriate forms must be used for mail reporting, which are supplied by the health department or available on their websites. County and state health departments periodically issue bulletins that are sent to healthcare providers and provide information about disease outbreaks and various statistics. Local health departments should be consulted for specific procedures and reporting protocols.

Patient Self-Determination Act

The Patient Self-Determination Act of 1990 brought the term *advance directives* to the forefront of medical care. This act requires healthcare facilities to develop and maintain written procedures that ensure that all adult patients receive information about living wills, durable powers of attorney for healthcare, and advance directives. These documents place the decision-making power into the hands of the patient and the patient's family, providing them with written notification of their right to consent to or refuse medical treatment.

Patients' Bill of Rights

One of the most important contributions that President Clinton offered to America during his terms in office was his active pursuit of a Patients' Bill of Rights. Confidentiality of medical records, guaranteed access to emergency care and specialists, timely accessibility to healthcare, and an appellate process for those dissatisfied with the decisions made by healthcare providers are some of the rights that are proposed. One important aspect of this legislation deals with the rights of patients to sue their health maintenance organizations (HMOs).

Because it is a patient's right to understand his or her diagnosis, prognosis, and all aspects of care, one must take special care when dealing with a patient with whom there may be a language barrier. If the patient's ability to understand is limited, an interpreter may be needed to ensure that there is adequate communication from physician to patient.

Controlled Substances Act of 1970

On May 1, 1971, the Controlled Substances Act of 1970 became effective. In October 1973, a regulatory agency known as the Drug Enforcement Administration (DEA) became a part of the U.S. Department of Justice. The DEA works with local, state, federal, and international agencies and organizations to address and regulate the serious issues of drug use and abuse in the United States.

Before administering, prescribing, or dispensing any drugs, a physician is required to register with the regional office of the DEA. This registration is renewable every 3 years. If a physician works from more than one office, he or she must register each individual office. Regulations regarding the writing, telephoning, and refilling of prescriptions vary according to which schedule is involved.

Under the Controlled Substances Act, drugs are categorized into Schedules I, II, III, IV, and V. Drugs in Schedule I have the highest potential for abuse and addiction, and those in Schedule V have the least abuse potential.

Schedule I substances are those that have no accepted medical use in the United States. Examples include heroin and d-lysergic acid diethylamide (LSD). Only the physician who is involved in conducting research with such drugs is concerned with Schedule I substances.

Schedule II drugs have a high abuse potential, with severe risk of mental and physical dependence. They include certain narcotic, stimulant, and depressant drugs, such as opium, morphine, codeine, and methylphenidate (Ritalin). Controlled substances in Schedule II can be obtained only with a federal triplicate order form obtained from the DEA. A special inventory must be maintained on controlled substances and retained for 2 to 3 years, depending on state requirements. When a controlled substance is removed from inventory, it must be recorded. The record must show the date, the name of the drug, the dosage, and the name of the patient, physician, and employee involved. Schedule III, IV, and V substances do not require triplicate forms.

Schedule III substances have an abuse potential that is lesser than that of the first two schedules. They include compounds that contain limited quantities of certain narcotic drugs combined with nonnarcotic substances. Examples include acetaminophen (Tylenol) with codeine, hydrocodone, butalbital with aspirin and caffeine (Fiorinal), and several steroids.

Schedule IV substances have still less potential for abuse. Phenobarbital, diazepam (Valium), propoxyphene (Darvon and Darvocet), alprazolam (Xanax), chlordiazepoxide (Librium), and pentazocine lactate (Talwin) are examples.

Schedule V substances have less abuse potential than those in Schedule IV but still warrant control. They include preparations that contain moderate quantities of certain narcotics that may be found in cough medicines and antidiarrheal products.

The physician may call a prescription to the pharmacist, but the pharmacist must transcribe it in writing before filling it. With permission from the physician, the medical assistant may orally transmit a prescription for controlled substances only in Schedules III, IV, or V, and the dispensing pharmacist must put the prescription into writing before filling it. The medical assistant cannot under any circumstances orally transmit a prescription for a Schedule II drug.

Stored controlled substances must be kept in a locked cabinet or safe. Any loss of controlled drugs by theft must be reported to the regional office of the DEA at the time the theft is discovered. If a physician discovers that his or her DEA number is being used in the unauthorized prescribing of controlled substances, he or she should report the incident to the DEA, to the state regulatory agency, and to the local police authorities. This is especially important in the case of employees whose employment has been terminated and who are suspected of drug theft in the office. There have been numerous cases of retaliation by fired employees who report to the DEA exactly what they have actually taken, yet accuse the physician or other staff members of taking the controlled substances. This results in messy investigations and months of follow-up, so any suspected employee drug use or abuse should be documented and reported to the local authorities. Periodic drug testing of employees is one way to help prevent office drug abuse.

A physician who discontinues medical practice must return the registration certificate and any unused order forms and triplicate prescription pads to the nearest office of the DEA. The regional DEA office will advise the physician on the disposition of any controlled drugs still on hand.

CRITICAL THINKING APPLICATION

Barbara explains the importance of reporting any employee who is suspected of using drugs or taking drugs from the office. This may be difficult, since co-workers are often friendly and may hesitate to report such acts. Discuss ways to handle this situation.

Uniform Anatomical Gift Act

The Uniform Anatomical Gift Act was approved by the National Conference of Commissioners on Uniform State Laws in 1968. Although many states had passed laws before this time that permitted living persons to make a gift of their body or portions of it after death, the laws were so different from state to state that arrangements for a donation in one state might not be recognized in another. All states have adopted the Uniform Anatomical Gift Act or similar legislation.

Essentially, the model law for donation states the following:

- Any person of sound mind and 18 years of age or older may give all or any part of his or her body after death for research, transplantation, or placement in a tissue bank.
- A donor's valid statement of gift is paramount to the rights of others except when a state autopsy law may prevail.
- If a donor has not indicated an intent to donate during his or her lifetime, his or her survivors, in a specified order of priority, may do so.
- Physicians who accept organs or tissues, relying in good faith on the documents, are protected from lawsuits. The physician attending at the time of death, if acquainted with the donor's wishes, may dispose of the body under the Uniform Anatomical Gift Act.
- The time of death must be determined by a physician who is not involved in the transplantation, and the attending physician cannot be a member of the transplant team.
- The donor may revoke the gift, or the gift may be rejected by the proposed recipient.

The most important clause of the act permits the donation to be made by a will (without waiting for probate) or by other written or witnessed documents, such as a card designed to be carried by the person or a Uniform Donor Card (Figure 7-10). The Uniform Donor Card is considered a legal document in all 50 states. Many states now list donor preference on the driver's license as well.

The provisions of the Uniform Anatomical Gift Act are so designed that the offer is exercised only after death. Therefore donors should reveal their intentions to as many of their relatives and friends as possible and to their physician. Because the human body and its parts are not commodities in commerce, no money can be exchanged in making an anatomical donation itself. Fees are charged for performing the transplant and various procedures, but organs cannot be bought and sold. It is also important to note that family members should be prepared to receive the body of the person who has donated his or her entire body to research once the research facility has completed its study. This can often be a traumatic experience, rekindling the grief process

once again, so the procedures and final disposition of the body should be decided at the time of the donation to avoid this difficult situation.

Health Insurance Portability and Accountability Act of 1996

HIPAA was signed into law on August 21, 1996, and all healthcare providers must be in compliance by April 2003. Its history began in the Clinton healthcare reform proposals. HIPAA was designed for several purposes, with many goals in mind. Limiting administrative costs of healthcare and privacy issues, as well as prevention of fraud and abuse, are of primary importance within the HIPAA regulations.

The use of electronic transmissions would ideally lower the administrative costs of providing healthcare, but this led to problems with privacy regarding health information. Therefore the law also had to provide security and confidentiality guarantees for the individual patient. Extensive privacy rules, including the use of unique identifiers, have shaped the law.

The final regulations regarding the privacy legislation sections of HIPAA were published in December 2000, after HCFA reviewed more than 50,000 comments and concerns on this important subject. All healthcare organizations that transmit any health information electronically must comply with HIPAA, and fines as well as prison terms can be imposed on those who do not comply with the regulations.

HIPAA will have a tremendous effect on the healthcare industry. All healthcare providers, clearinghouses, and health plans that use electronic information must comply with HIPAA regulations.

Occupational Safety and Health Act and the Bloodborne Pathogens Standard

In 1970, President Nixon signed the Occupational Safety and Health Act, which created what we know today as the Occupational Safety and Health Administration (OSHA). OSHA is a division of the U.S. Department of Labor, and since its creation workplace injuries, illnesses, and fatalities have been significantly reduced. OSHA's mission is to ensure workplace safety and a healthy environment within the workplace.

Although OSHA is commonly thought of as the regulatory agency that requires steel-toed boots and hard hats, the medical industry moved into the OSHA spotlight in the late 1980s, when the threat of HIV infection extended to healthcare workers. Hepatitis and other pathogens were already of concern to healthcare workers, but when HIV, the virus that causes AIDS, was identified, action was needed to better protect the individuals who cared for patients with these infectious diseases. OSHA's Final Ruling on Bloodborne Pathogens became fully effective in July 1992, and since that time, various additions have been made to update the regulations in light of new information learned about bloodborne pathogens.

The law requires medical facilities to comply with the Bloodborne Pathogens standard and to be able to prove

FIGURE 7-10 Organ donation card.

that compliance to OSHA inspectors if necessary. The actual standard can be found in the 29 **Code of Federal Regulations (CFR)** 1910.1030. The following information details the legal requirements of the OSHA Standard as it pertains to the physician's office.

General Duty Clause. No law can cover every single situation that may arise in the course of daily living. Because of this, OSHA's general duty clause is a catch-all regulation that fits almost any situation not specified in any other section of the law. The general duty clause simply states that a workplace must be free of any hazard that might cause serious harm or death. For example, one breach of the general duty clause is the "failure of a facility to provide reasonable security procedures at a retail store." Although not a specific breach of any regulation, this fits nicely into the general duty clause.

OSHA Regulations as Performance-Based Standards. OSHA regulations are considered performance-based standards. This means that adequate compliance depends largely on what happens in the facility. For instance, the same regulations may not apply to two offices located right next to each other. Would it be possible that a family practitioner could be fined for not having sharps containers, and then the same OSHA inspector goes next door to a surgeon's office and does not fine the surgeon for not having sharps containers? It is possible if the surgeon does not perform any invasive, surgical, or any other procedures in the office that involve blood!

This is one reason that employees must be trained in their individual facilities. Even if training was done 1 month before a job change, the employee must be trained again in the new facility. Offices and procedures are different from place to place, and the employee must have adequate training to function successfully in the medical office.

OSHA inspectors can recommend fines when a facility is found to be out of compliance with an OSHA standard. One of the most common infractions is that the facility has an Exposure Control Plan in the facility but is not using it or following the procedures and policies set forth within it. This could lead to an inspector's declaring the facility to be *willfully negligent.* Willful negligence exists when "an employer representative was aware of the requirements of the [OSHA] Act, or the existence of an applicable standard or regulation, and was also aware that the condition or practice was in violation of those requirements, and did not abate the hazard." Fines for noncompliance can quadruple for willful negligence.

COMMON OSHA VIOLATIONS

- No eyewash facilities available
- No labeling or improper labeling of hazardous chemicals
- No MSDS for each hazardous chemical
- Storage of contaminated laboratory coats with clean ones
- Not communicating hazards to employees
- No documentation of initial employee training
- No documentation of annual employee training
- No annual hazard assessment performed
- Having an Exposure Control Plan but not following it
- No proof of destruction of hazardous waste
- No Emergency Action Plan in the facility
- No Written Exposure Control Plan
- OSHA Form 300A not posted during required period
- No records of hepatitis B vaccinations or declination forms

Exposure Control Plan. The Exposure Control Plan can be a part of the regular safety plan written for the medical facility or may be a stand-alone document, but it must cover all of the elements required by OSHA. This plan must be in writing and be reviewed annually, and there must be written documentation that the plan was reviewed and updated or revised, if needed. A hard copy must be provided to employees on their request within 15 working days, and the plan must be available at all times in the workplace.

The plan must delineate the tasks that employees perform where there is risk of blood exposure. It must also classify jobs within the facility according to the likelihood of exposures. For instance, some job duties would always expose the employee to blood or **other potentially infectious materials (OPIM)**, often on a daily basis. Some duties would only occasionally expose the employee, and other duties would never expose the employee to blood or OPIM. Employees must be told which category they are a part of, and what duties they will perform that could lead to exposures.

The Exposure Control Plan must contain a Waste Management section that details how waste is removed from the facility and destroyed. Most medical offices contract with companies that specialize in removing and destroying medical waste. The office must keep the receipts given by the company that prove that the waste was taken away from the facility and then incinerated or otherwise destroyed.

The plan must also contain a section on Hazardous Materials Communication, which explains what substances in the facility are hazardous and how to handle a spill or exposure to those products. Only the manufacturer of a chemical can determine whether it is hazardous, and Material Safety Data Sheets (MSDS) must be kept on almost all chemicals and reagents in the facility. Recent rulings have exempted some chemicals, but without the MSDS information, a medical assistant could not determine what type of health, reactivity, flammability, or other risks the chemical could have.

If the facility has equipment for x-ray studies, a Radiation Safety Plan must also be written and followed. All facilities should have an Emergency Action Plan in place, which provides procedures in case of tornadoes, fires, floods, or any other type of emergency that might occur in the office. This plan should contain floor plans of the facility, diagrams depicting the most efficient exits from the building, and the chain of command in an emergency. Diagrams with exit routes should be posted in every room of the medical office. At least annually, a hazard assessment must be performed on the entire facility. The hazard assessment is an inspection for problem areas in which the facility might be out of compliance. The facility must have documentation that the hazard assessment was done.

OSHA Recordkeeping Regulations. An injury or illness is considered to be work related when an event or exposure in the work environment contributed or caused the condition or significantly aggravated a preexisting condition. OSHA made several changes in the regulations concerning work-related injury recordkeeping to simplify forms, protect employee privacy, encourage employee involvement, and enable computer usage for meeting OSHA requirements. The revised rules took effect on January 1, 2002. Three basic forms are now used to keep records regarding injuries, accidents, and illnesses related to the workplace. The forms are as follows:

* *OSHA Form 300—Log of Work-Related Injuries and Illnesses* (Figure 7-11): Information is posted on form 300 regarding work-related deaths and every work-related injury or illness that involves loss of consciousness, restricted work activity or job transfer, days away from work, or medical treatment beyond first aid. An OSHA Form 301 (Injury and Illness Incident Report) should be completed for each entry on the log.
* *OSHA Form 300A—Summary of Work-Related Injuries and Illnesses* (Figure 7-12): Form 300A must be completed even if no injuries or illnesses occurred during the year that were work related. It must be posted in a common area for viewing by all employees, and provides the total number of accidents, illnesses, and injuries in the facility for the previous year. The length of time that this information must be posted has increased from 1 month to 3 months, specifically from February 1 to April 30 each year. An additional change is the certification of the form. A company executive must examine the document and certify that it is accurate.
* *OSHA Form 301—Injury and Illness Incident Report* (Figure 7-13): Form 301 is used to report what actually happened when an employee suffers a work-related injury or illness. This form, or an acceptable substitute, such as a state worker's compensation form, must be completed within 7 calendar days after notification of the illness or injury. The form should be completed as quickly as possible so that an exact recollection of events can be documented. Now that the new recordkeeping regulations have become effective, employees are guaranteed access to their OSHA 301 forms for the first time.

The log and summary forms must be kept on file for a minimum of 5 years. Only the Summary should be posted during the specified time period from February 1 to April 30 each year, reflecting information from the previous calendar year. The forms are not sent to OSHA unless specifically requested.

CRITICAL THINKING APPLICATION

Barbara quickly realizes that the office is using older versions of OSHA Forms 300 and 301. Where might she look or go to find updated information and copies of forms?

It is wise to keep a communication log of calls to OSHA in which questions were asked or information verified. Note the day and time called, the first and last name of the person spoken to, the person's title, and the question asked and response given. Take detailed notes while discussing the issue on the phone. This log could be invaluable if a question ever arises about a subject discussed with a local OSHA official. It may make the difference when an OSHA inspector suggests a hefty fine. If the medical facility can show documentation that a certain procedure was discussed with an OSHA official and decisions were made based on that discussion, the facility may have sufficient evidence that the law was considered and the facility did its best to comply.

Needlestick Safety and Prevention Act. An estimated 600,000 to 800,000 injuries occur annually among healthcare workers. One third of these injuries happen during the disposal process. In an effort to reduce these injuries that can lead to exposure to HIV, hepatitis B virus (HBV), or other bloodborne pathogens, OSHA revised its Bloodborne Pathogens standard to comply with the Needlestick Safety and Prevention Act, which became law on November 6, 2000. The new regulations became effective on April 18, 2001.

Employers are now required to involve employees in the selection of needle safety devices. The facility must be able to prove that consideration was given to various types of devices that promote needle safety, what led to the decision to choose the device currently in use, and which employees were involved in these decisions. A list should be kept of which employees contributed to the selection decisions. Minutes from meetings, copies of employee response forms, and the forms used to solicit input are good methods of proving that employees were involved in the selection process.

CRITICAL THINKING APPLICATION

Barbara needs input about the needle safety devices being used in the facility. Should she call a meeting of the entire office, or are there specific employees that should be present? If so, discuss who should have input in these decisions.

A needlestick and sharps injury log must also be kept in the medical facility. At a minimum, the log must include the following information:

OSHA's Form 300

Log of Work-Related Injuries and Illnesses

Attention: This form contains information relating to employee health and must be used in a manner that protects the confidentiality of employees to the extent possible while the information is being used for occupational safety and health purposes.

U.S. Department of Labor
Occupational Safety and Health Administration

Form approved OMB no. 1218-0176

Year 20____

You must record information about every work-related death and about every work-related injury or illness that involves loss of consciousness, restricted work activity or job transfer, days away from work, or medical treatment beyond first aid. You must also record significant work-related injuries and illnesses that are diagnosed by a physician or licensed health care professional. You must also record work-related injuries and illnesses that meet any of the specific recording criteria listed in 29 CFR Part 1904.8 through 1904.12. Feel free to use two lines for a single case if you need to. You must complete an Injury and Illness Incident Report (OSHA Form 301) or equivalent form for each injury or illness recorded on this form. If you're not sure whether a case is recordable, call your local OSHA office for help.

Establishment name _____
City _____ State _____

Identify the person

(A) Case no.
(B) Employee's name
(C) Job title (e.g., Welder)

Describe the case

(D) Date of injury or onset of illness
(E) Where the event occurred (e.g., Loading dock north end)
(F) Describe injury or illness, parts of body affected, and object/substance that directly injured or made person ill (e.g., Second degree burns on right forearm from acetylene torch)

Classify the case

Using these four categories, check ONLY the most serious result for each case:

| Death (G) | Days away from work (H) | Remained at work Job transfer or restriction (I) | Remained at work Other recordable cases (J) |

Enter the number of days the injured or ill worker was:

| On job transfer or restriction (K) | Away from work (L) |
| days | days |

Check the "Injury" column or choose one type of illness:

| (M) Injury (1) | Skin disorder (2) | Respiratory condition (3) | Poisoning (4) | All other illnesses (5) |

Page totals ▶

Be sure to transfer these totals to the Summary page (Form 300A) before you post it.

Page ____ of ____

Public reporting burden for this collection of information is estimated to average 14 minutes per response, including time to review the instructions, search and gather the data needed, and complete and review the collection of information. Persons are not required to respond to the collection of information unless it displays a currently valid OMB control number. If you have any comments about these estimates or any other aspects of this data collection, contact: US Department of Labor, OSHA Office of Statistics, Room N-3644, 200 Constitution Avenue, NW, Washington, DC 20210. Do not send the completed forms to this office.

FIGURE 7-11   OSHA Form 300—Log of Work-Related Injuries and Illnesses. (Source: US Department of Labor, Occupational Safety and Health Administration.)

OSHA's Form 300A

Summary of Work-Related Injuries and Illnesses

Year 20____

U.S. Department of Labor
Occupational Safety and Health Administration

Form approved OMB no. 1218-0176

All establishments covered by Part 1904 must complete this Summary page, even if no work-related injuries or illnesses occurred during the year. Remember to review the Log to verify that the entries are complete and accurate before completing this summary.

Using the Log, count the individual entries you made for each category. Then write the totals below, making sure you've added the entries from every page of the Log. If you had no cases, write "0."

Employees, former employees, and their representatives have the right to review the OSHA Form 300 in its entirety. They also have limited access to the OSHA Form 301 or its equivalent. See 29 CFR Part 1904.35, in OSHA's recordkeeping rule, for further details on the access provisions for these forms.

Number of Cases

Total number of deaths	Total number of cases with days away from work	Total number of cases with job transfer or restriction	Total number of other recordable cases
___(G)	___(H)	___(I)	___(J)

Number of Days

Total number of days of job transfer or restriction	Total number of days away from work
___(K)	___(L)

Injury and Illness Types

Total number of . . .
(M)
(1) Injuries ___
(2) Skin disorders ___
(3) Respiratory conditions ___
(4) Poisonings ___
(5) All other illnesses ___

Establishment information

Your establishment name _____

Street _____
City _____ State ____ ZIP ____

Industry description (e.g., Manufacture of motor truck trailers) _____

Standard Industrial Classification (SIC), if known (e.g., SIC 3715) __ __ __ __

Employment information (If you don't have these figures, see the Worksheet on the back of this page to estimate.)

Annual average number of employees _____

Total hours worked by all employees last year _____

Sign here

Knowingly falsifying this document may result in a fine.

I certify that I have examined this document and that to the best of my knowledge the entries are true, accurate, and complete.

_____   _____
Company executive   Title

(___) _____   ___/___/___
Phone   Date

Post this Summary page from February 1 to April 30 of the year following the year covered by the form.

Public reporting burden for this collection of information is estimated to average 50 minutes per response, including time to review the instructions, search and gather the data needed, and complete and review the collection of information. Persons are not required to respond to the collection of information unless it displays a currently valid OMB control number. If you have any comments about these estimates or any other aspects of this data collection, contact: US Department of Labor, OSHA Office of Statistics, Room N-3644, 200 Constitution Avenue, NW, Washington, DC 20210. Do not send the completed forms to this office.

FIGURE 7-12   OSHA Form 300A—Summary of Work-Related Injuries and Illnesses. (Source: US Department of Labor, Occupational Safety and Health Administration.)

OSHA's Form 301
Injury and Illness Incident Report

U.S. Department of Labor
Occupational Safety and Health Administration

Form approved OMB no. 1218-0176

Attention: This form contains information relating to employee health and must be used in a manner that protects the confidentiality of employees to the extent possible while the information is being used for occupational safety and health purposes.

This *Injury and Illness Incident Report* is one of the first forms you must fill out when a recordable work-related injury or illness has occurred. Together with the *Log of Work-Related Injuries and Illnesses* and the accompanying *Summary*, these forms help the employer and OSHA develop a picture of the extent and severity of work-related incidents.

Within 7 calendar days after you receive information that a recordable work-related injury or illness has occurred, you must fill out this form or an equivalent form. Some state workers' compensation, insurance, or other reports may be acceptable substitutes. To be considered an equivalent form, any substitute must contain all the information asked for on this form.

According to Public Law 91-596 and 29 CFR 1904, OSHA's recordkeeping rule, you must keep this form on file for 5 years following the year to which it pertains.

If you need additional copies of this form, you may photocopy and use as many as you need.

Completed by _____

Title _____

Phone (____) ____ - ____   Date ___/___/___

Information about the employee

1) Full name _____

2) Street _____
   City _____ State _____ ZIP _____

3) Date of birth ___/___/___

4) Date hired ___/___/___

5) ☐ Male
   ☐ Female

Information about the physician or other health care professional

6) Name of physician or other health care professional _____

7) If treatment was given away from the worksite, where was it given?
   Facility _____
   Street _____
   City _____ State _____ ZIP _____

8) Was employee treated in an emergency room?
   ☐ Yes
   ☐ No

9) Was employee hospitalized overnight as an in-patient?
   ☐ Yes
   ☐ No

Information about the case

10) Case number from the Log _____ (Transfer the case number from the Log after you record the case.)

11) Date of injury or illness ___/___/___

12) Time employee began work ____ AM / PM

13) Time of event ____ AM / PM   ☐ Check if time cannot be determined

14) **What was the employee doing just before the incident occurred?** Describe the activity, as well as the tools, equipment, or material the employee was using. Be specific. *Examples:* "climbing a ladder while carrying roofing materials"; "spraying chlorine from hand sprayer"; "daily computer key-entry."

15) **What happened?** Tell us how the injury occurred. *Examples:* "When ladder slipped on wet floor, worker fell 20 feet"; "Worker was sprayed with chlorine when gasket broke during replacement"; "Worker developed soreness in wrist over time."

16) **What was the injury or illness?** Tell us the part of the body that was affected and how it was affected; be more specific than "hurt," "pain," or sore." *Examples:* "strained back"; "chemical burn, hand"; "carpal tunnel syndrome."

17) **What object or substance directly harmed the employee?** *Examples:* "concrete floor"; "chlorine"; "radial arm saw." *If this question does not apply to the incident, leave it blank.*

18) **If the employee died, when did death occur?** Date of death ___/___/___

Public reporting burden for this collection of information is estimated to average 22 minutes per response, including time for reviewing instructions, searching existing data sources, gathering and maintaining the data needed, and completing and reviewing the collection of information. Persons are not required to respond to the collection of information unless it displays a current valid OMB control number. If you have any comments about this estimate or any other aspects of this data collection, including suggestions for reducing this burden, contact: US Department of Labor, OSHA Office of Statistics, Room N-3644, 200 Constitution Avenue, NW, Washington, DC 20210. Do not send the completed forms to this office.

FIGURE 7-13   OSHA Form 301—Injury and Illness Incident Report. (Source: US Department of Labor, Occupational Safety and Health Administration.)

- Description of the incident
- The type and brand of device used when the incident took place
- Location of the incident

The regulations that took effect in 2001 require all needlestick and sharps injuries to be reported and documented, not just the ones that result in injury or illness.

OSHA Training Requirements. All employees, including full-time, part-time, and temporary employees with a risk of occupational exposure, must receive training within the facility in which they are employed at two very specific times. Initial training must be conducted before commencement of any work-related duties by a new employee. In addition, training must be conducted on an annual basis to update and inform employees on new regulations and procedures related to OSHA compliance. The initial training requirement is one of the most frequently breached regulations, yet is critical for the safety of the employee.

Training must include the following:

- Making accessible a copy of the regulatory text of the standard and explanation of its contents
- General discussion on bloodborne diseases and their transmission
- Universal precautions and body substance isolation
- The Exposure Control plan
- Engineering and work practice controls, including handling of needles and sharps
- Personal protective equipment
- Hepatitis B vaccine
- Response to emergencies involving blood
- Potential sources of infection and tasks that might preempt exposure
- Written schedules for cleaning
- Handling contaminated laundry
- How to handle exposure incidents and spills
- The postexposure evaluation and follow-up program
- Reading Materials Safety Data Sheets (MSDS), signs, labels, and color-coding (Figure 7-14), and locations of these items

There must be an opportunity for questions and answers, and the trainer must be knowledgeable in the subject matter. Documentation of the training sessions should be kept in each employee's personnel file or a special file for OSHA-related information.

CRITICAL THINKING APPLICATION

Barbara reviews the employee files and finds that neither Samantha nor Lynda received OSHA training when they were initially hired. How might Barbara rectify this and what documentation would be helpful?

Hepatitis B Vaccination. The hepatitis B vaccination series must be offered to employees at risk of occupational exposures at no cost to the employee. The employee cannot be asked to pay in advance for the vaccination and be reimbursed, nor can the employee be asked to put the vaccination series on his or her personal health insurance policy. It must be made available to the employee within 10 working days of initial hire or assignment. The vaccination series can be declined by the employee, who must sign a declination form. If at any time the employee decides to receive the vaccination series, this must still be offered at no cost. The employee does not have to offer a reason for the declination. Prescreening or postvaccination serological tests cannot be required.

The vaccination series is completed within a 6-month period. The second vaccination is given 1 month after the first, and the third 5 months after the second. Documentation should be provided to the employee for each vaccination received. Currently a booster dose of the hepatitis B vaccination is not required. However, if a routine booster is recommended by the U.S. Public Health Service in the future, it must be made available at no cost to employees.

CRITICAL THINKING APPLICATION

Lynda has not disclosed to anyone at the facility that she has had a case of hepatitis. Should she discuss this matter with Barbara? Is Lynda required to discuss this matter with Barbara? Is Lynda placing her patients at risk? If Lynda declines the hepatitis vaccination, must she explain why on the declination form?

Clinical Laboratory Improvement Act. The Clinical Laboratory Improvement Act (CLIA) was a result of the Congressional investigation of **physician office laboratories (POLs)** and the deficiencies in the quality of the services and results provided by these laboratories. A set of minimum standards for laboratories was established, which involved quality improvement in test procedures. Quality control and assurance, as well as personnel and proficiency testing, are of utmost importance to the facility complying with CLIA.

CLIA regulations set the minimum standard for laboratory practice and quality. Remember that CLIA is not a governmental agency, but a law. CLIA is enforced by the Department of Health and Human Services (DHHS). OSHA is a law (Occupational Safety and Health Act), but also an agency (Occupational Safety and Health Administration). This is an important difference between the two.

Some tests conducted in the laboratory are exempt from CLIA standards. These tests include the following:

- Nonautomated dipstick or tablet urinalysis
- Fecal occult blood
- Ovulation using visual color comparison
- Urine pregnancy using visual color comparison
- Erythrocyte sedimentation rate
- Hemoglobin by copper sulfate method
- Spun microhematocrit
- Blood glucose using certain devices cleared by the FDA for home use
- Specialized self-contained hemoglobin tests

Material Safety Data Sheets communicate hazards to employees about the products and chemicals used in the medical office. They also inform the employee as to what to do in case of an exposure. OSHA requires that MSDS sheets are kept on all hazardous chemicals, unless exempted. Only the manufacturer can determine if a product is hazardous. MSDS sheets can be obtained from either the manufacturer or the medical supply company from which the product was ordered. They must be provided after requested from the manufacturer within 30 days. Keep copies of requests to prove that an attempt has been made to obtain the MSDS information.

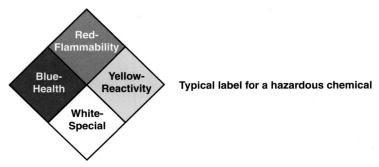

Typical label for a hazardous chemical

The appropriate number should be placed inside each box that applies in the figure above. Most offices use the National Fire Protection Association Rating System. Many MSDS sheets provide the labeling information on the sheet. Others must be read thoroughly to determine how the labels should be completed. If the MSDS says that a chemical has a "moderate to high" hazard, label it high. If it says "low to moderate," label it moderate. Never guess at the numbers used for the label—always consult the MSDS. If individual containers are labeled, the facility is said to always be out of compliance, because it is easy to miss a container that may have just arrived in a shipment. Many medical facilities place labels on a permanent fixture next to where the product is stored, but it must be permanently stored in that area.

Simple Rating Guide
0—no hazard
1—slight hazard
2—moderate hazard
3—high hazard
4—extreme hazard

NFPA Rating Summary

Health (Blue)			Reactivity (Yellow)		
4	Danger	May be fatal on short exposure. Specialized protective equipment required.	4	Danger	Explosive material at room temperature.
3	Warning	Corrosive or toxic. Avoid skin contact or inhalation.	3	Danger	May be explosive if shocked, heated under confinement, or mixed with water.
2	Warning	May be harmful if inhaled or absorbed.	2	Warning	Unstable or may react violently if mixed with water.
1	Caution	May be irritating.	1	Caution	May react if heated or mixed with water but not violently.
0		No unusual hazard.	0	Stable	Not reactive when mixed with water.
Flammability (Red)			**Special Notice Key (White)**		
4	Danger	Flammable gas or extremely flammable liquid.	W		Water reactive.
3	Warning	Flammable liquid flash point below 100° F.	Oxy		Oxidizing agent.
2	Caution	Combustible liquid flash point of 100° to 200° F.			
1		Combustible if heated.			
0		Not combustible.			

FIGURE 7-14   Labeling and the National Fire Protection Association (NFPA) Rating System. (Courtesy the National Fire Protection Association.)

Offices that only perform these tests may obtain a certificate of waiver and will not be routinely inspected for CLIA compliance. Tests of moderate or high complexity must be performed by trained personnel with education and experience in the test areas in which they are working. A list of the moderate- and high-complexity procedures can be found in the July 26, 1993, issue of the Federal Register, and updates are periodically published that detail any changes in the list or regulations regarding testing procedures. Laboratories apply for a CLIA certificate through their local health departments and will be periodically inspected for compliance.

Physician Licensure and Registration

A graduate of a medical school must be licensed before beginning the practice of medicine. Licensure is regulated by state statutes through the Medical Practice Acts. It is important for a medical assistant to understand licensing and other laws and regulations that are intended to protect patients, physicians, medical assistants, and other healthcare workers.

Medical Practice Acts

Medical practice acts existed as early as colonial days. However, these acts were later repealed, and in the mid-nineteenth century practically none of the states had laws governing the practice of medicine. As one might expect, a rapid decline in professional standards followed. The general welfare of the people was endangered by medical **quackery** and inadequate care. By the beginning of the twentieth century, medical practice acts were established by statute and were again in effect in every state. The purpose of the medical practice acts is as follows:

- To define what is included in the practice of medicine within that state
- To govern the methods and requirements of licensure
- To establish the grounds for suspension or revocation of license

Licensure

A doctor of medicine (MD), doctor of osteopathy (DO), or doctor of chiropractic (DC) degree is conferred on graduation from medical or chiropractic school. The license to practice medicine or chiropractic is granted by a state board, frequently known as the State Board of Medical Examiners or Board of Registration. Licensure may be accomplished by examination, reciprocity, or endorsement.

Examination. Every state requires medical doctors to pass a written examination. The Federation of State Medical Boards and the National Board of Medical Examiners agreed in 1990 to establish a single licensing examination—the Federation Licensing Examination (FLEX)—for graduates of accredited medical schools. Medical graduates in the United States must pass either the FLEX examination, the U.S. Medical Licensing Examination (USMLE), or the National Board of Medical Examiners' Examination (NBME). Osteopathic physicians pass the National Board of Osteopathic Medical Examiners' Comprehensive Osteopathic Medical Licensing Examination (COMLEX).

Reciprocity. Some states grant the license to practice medicine by reciprocity; that is, they automatically recognize that the requirements of the state in which the license was granted meet the standards required by the second state.

Endorsement. Most graduates of medical schools in the United States have been licensed by endorsement of the National Board certificate. To explain in simpler terms, a state will offer a license to a physician based on the examinations taken to grant the license, not by virtue of the license granted from another state. Licensure by endorsement is granted on a case-by-case basis. Graduates who have not been licensed by endorsement are required to pass a state board examination.

In all states graduates of foreign medical schools who are seeking licensure by endorsement must meet the same requirements as graduates of medical schools in the United States, in addition to various other qualifying factors.

Exemptions. Some graduates may not wish to engage in the practice of medicine; their interests may lie in research or administration, or even in the practice of law with a special interest in medical liability. In such instances licensure is not required. Licensed physicians in the Armed Forces, Public Health Service, or Veterans Administration facilities need not be licensed in the state in which they are employed. However, the Department of Defense is encouraging states to require full licensure of military personnel.

Registration and Reregistration

After a license is granted, periodic reregistration is necessary annually or biennially. A physician can be **concurrently** registered in more than one state. The issuing body notifies the physician when reregistration is due. A medical assistant can aid the physician by being aware of when the registration fees are due, thus preventing a possible lapsing of the registration.

Many states require proof of continuing education besides payment of a registration fee. Continuing education units (CEUs) are granted to physicians for attending approved seminars, lectures, scientific meetings, and formal courses in accredited colleges and universities. A total of 50 hours per year is the average requirement for a license renewal. A medical assistant may be expected to help the physician arrange for completing the required units for license renewal.

Revocation or Suspension

Under certain conditions, the license to practice medicine may be revoked or suspended. Grounds for revocation or suspension of the license to practice medicine fall within one of three categories:

1. *Conviction of a crime:* This may include felonies such as murder, rape, larceny, and narcotic violations.
2. *Unprofessional conduct:* Failure to uphold the ethical standards of the medical profession may be indicated by betrayal of patient confidence, giving or receiving rebates, and excessive use of narcotics or alcohol.
3. *Personal or professional incapacity:* Such incapacity is difficult to label or prove. For example, advanced age or an injury may reduce the apparent capacity of some physicians. Certain illnesses can affect the memory or judgment necessary to practice medicine.

A physician studies many years to learn the profession before becoming licensed by the state to practice medicine. A medical assistant is not licensed to practice medicine and must never prescribe or attempt to diagnose a patient's ailment. This is the illegal practice of medicine. For this reason, a medical assistant must use great care in discussing the patient's complaints and treatment with them because patients identify the medical assistant's remarks as being the opinion of the physician.

Closing Comments

The majority of patients never entertain the thought of taking legal action against their physicians, and a medical assistant should not develop an attitude of skepticism. However, a medical assistant can play an important role in preventing medical claims.

Give scrupulous attention to the needs of each patient and avoid leaving them alone for long periods. This especially applies to young children and elderly patients. Always avoid criticism of other physicians or healthcare facilities. Never give out any information about the patient without written consent and verify the identity of anyone asking for information about a patient.

Use discretion in phone and office conversations. One never knows who is standing just around the corner. Be aware of tone of voice and attitude during spoken conversations. Communicate office policies and procedures to patients clearly in advance of treatment whenever possible.

Keep accurate records that show exactly what was done to the patient and when it was done. Make no promises as to the outcome of treatment. Record cancelled and no-show appointments and record the facts if a patient discontinues treatment.

Check office equipment often to ensure that it is working properly. Keep drug samples and prescription pads out of sight. Never diagnose, prescribe, or offer a prognosis. Perform only the tasks for which you are trained and keep abreast of new findings and procedures in healthcare. Correctly follow all federal and state regulations.

Play a positive part in the prevention of medical liability claims. Take care of the patient in a compassionate and competent way, and malpractice will not be a frequent issue in the medical facility.

Patient Education

Perhaps the most important detail to remember with regard to patient education and law is patience. Many medical forms are complicated, and regulations change often. Patients are not usually as well educated as the medical assistant on matters concerning legal policies and procedures. Often patients become frustrated with the number of changes that they are expected to contend with, and they may unintentionally project this frustration onto the medical assistant. Remain calm and answer questions, offering as much assistance to the patient as possible.

Legal and Ethical Issues

Generally, the law holds that every person is liable for the consequences of his or her own negligence when another person is injured as a result. In some situations this liability also extends to the employer. Physicians may be held responsible for the mistakes of those who work in their healthcare facility, and sometimes they must pay damages for the negligent acts of their employees.

Under the doctrine of respondent superior, physicians are legally responsible for the acts of their employees when the employees are acting within the scope of their duties or employment. Physicians are also responsible for the acts of assistants who are not their own employees if they commit acts of negligence in the presence of the physician while under the physician's immediate supervision. *Respondeat superior* is a Latin term meaning "let the master answer." When physicians practice as partners, they are liable not only for their own acts and those of their partners, but also for the negligent acts of any agent or employee of the partnership. A medical assistant, while acting within the scope of the employment contract, is considered an agent of the employer.

Medical assistants who are guilty of negligence are liable for their own actions, but the injured party generally sues the physician, because there is a better chance of collecting damages. However, even an assistant who has no money can still be liable for any negligent action. This fact illustrates the continuing importance of exercising extreme care in performing all duties in the professional office.

SUMMARY OF SCENARIO

Barbara is enthusiastic about her new job and duties. She is confident about appearing in court to represent Dr. Patrick and discuss the contents of the medical record of the patient suing his surgeon. Dr. Patrick is not a party to the lawsuit but has a physician-patient relationship with the patient just the same. An offer existed, as well as the acceptance of that offer. The relationship was based on legal subject matter, and the physician and the patient had the legal capacity to enter into a contract. Consideration existed as well, because the patient paid for services and the physician treated the patient. Both received something of value. Samantha and Lynda would like to accompany Barbara to the court proceedings to watch and learn.

Even if a patient does not pay for treatment, a contract still exists. The physician may elect to terminate the physician-patient relationship if the patient does not pay, but the trust that the patient places in the physician can be considered a thing of value. Patients should understand their role in their treatment, and their responsibilities to the physician. Often this information is communicated in the patient policy brochure or may be verbally discussed with the patient. Physicians are not required to accept all patients; for instance, not all physicians deliver babies. Some physicians do not treat patients with worker's compensation claims. The physician does have the right to see the types of patients he or she wishes and is competent to treat but should never discriminate on the basis of race, sex, or any other protected status. A physician may not always be correct in his or her diagnoses, but this does not mean that the physician has committed malpractice. However, if expert witnesses feel that the physician should have made a different diagnosis based on the case, then the physician might be held liable for negligence. If an employee has information about a case that is damaging to the physician, he or she is ethically obligated to report the information, but rarely legally liable to speak up unless a law has been broken.

Samantha and Lynda have learned many new concepts about law from Barbara and are anxious to watch the court proceedings. They will learn more by seeing the actual process of law at work. Barbara looks forward to sharing more knowledge with the employees as they continue to work together.

SUMMARY OF LEARNING OBJECTIVES

- Different types of laws and regulations affect us, depending on the origination of the law. Acts are introduced at the federal level and must be passed by Congress. State legislative bodies develop statutes, and local governments create ordinances.

- Criminal law governs violations that are punishable as offenses against the state or government. Civil law is concerned with acts that are not criminal in nature, but those that involve individual relationships and relationships between others, groups, or government agencies.

- Misdemeanors are minor crimes, punishable by a fine or imprisonment in a city or county jail. Felonies are major crimes, such as rape, murder, or burglary. Most felonies carry punishment of imprisonment for at least one year, and they are divided into subgroups, usually first-, second-, and third-degree felonies. Treason is an attempt to overthrow the government. High treason constitutes a serious threat to the stability of the government, for example, an attempt on the life of the President.

- Tort law is the division of civil law that deals with medical professional liability. Tort law provides relief for those who have suffered harm from the actions of others. The plaintiff must establish duty, breach of duty, damages as a result of the breach of duty, and the extent of the damages suffered.

- Four elements are essential to a valid, legal contract: (1) there must be a "meeting of the minds" or manifestation of assent; (2) the contract must involve legal subject matter; (3) the parties to the contract must have the legal capacity to enter into a contract; and (4) some type of consideration must be offered.

- Interrogatories are lists of questions directed from each party of a lawsuit to the other. Interrogatories are answered under oath and only directed to the parties actually named in the lawsuit. Depositions, however, can be taken from any witness or party to the lawsuit. They are also taken under oath, and often witnesses are subpoenaed to offer a deposition.

- Testifying in court can sometimes be an intimidating experience, but good preparation beforehand will alleviate many anxieties. Discussing potential questions with the attorney will help prepare the witness for giving testimony. Always tell the truth to avoid charges of perjury. Speak clearly and distinctly and do not hesitate to ask the attorney to repeat a question. There is no harm in a brief pause to think about an answer. Dress conservatively, know the location and room of the court in advance, and always arrive on time. Credibility is critical in a medical professional liability trial.

- Arbitration is a popular alternative to court trials. It involves the use of a third party familiar with law or the issues at hand. It is recognized by statute in most states and provides a faster, confidential, fair, and less expensive resolution to a dispute.

- Malfeasance, misfeasance, and nonfeasance are types of negligence often involved in medical professional liability cases. Malfeasance is performing an act that is completely wrong or unlawful. Misfeasance, comparable to a mistake, is the improper performance of a lawful act. Nonfeasance is the failure to perform some act that should have been performed.

- Informed consent gives the patient a full understanding of the condition that has been diagnosed, including what could happen if the patient undergoes treatment, refuses treatment, or delays treatment. It provides the patient with information on the advantages and risks of a medical procedure and alternative treatments that the patient may wish to consider. Informed consent places the control in the hands of the patient, who is given the opportunity to make the decisions about his or her healthcare. Patients can never be forced to undergo any type of procedure or treatment.

- Several disclosures must be made by the physician with regard to a patient's health that do not require patient consent. Information about births and deaths, injuries or illnesses as a result of violence, accidental or suspicious deaths, sexually transmitted diseases, and any type of abuse are examples of legal disclosures that must be made by healthcare professionals.

- Passage of the Health Insurance Portability and Accountability Act of 1996 offered the healthcare profession extensive privacy rules and regulations concerning the electronic transfer of information. The Act also limited administrative costs by supporting the use of electronic transfer of information, and presented fraud and abuse prevention guidelines. The privacy issues that surround HIPAA, however, have been the most discussed and debated topics related to this law.

- The Occupational Safety and Health Administration is an agency and a division of the U.S. Department of Labor. More than 2300 employees work for OSHA, and the agency runs on an annual budget of approximately $443 million as of 2002. Twenty-six states have their own OSHA programs, which adds an additional 3100 employees. The Occupational Safety and Health Act of 1970 created this agency to ensure safety in the workplace. The Clinical Laboratory Improvement Act is a law that regulates the quality of services provided by laboratories. CLIA is enforced by the Department of Health and Human Services.

■ Physicians may receive a license to practice medicine through examination, reciprocity, or endorsement. FLEX, USMLE, and NBME are all designed for graduates of accredited medical schools. Some states recognize the requirements of another state in which a license was granted, and through reciprocity will give a physician a license to practice medicine. Endorsement is the method of obtaining a license by recognition of the passed examinations, instead of by virtue of the license obtained in another state. Most physicians in the United States are licensed by endorsement, because they take the examination after graduating from medical school

and this prompts the receipt of the license, after proper application and providing all required documentation. Practicing medicine without a license is illegal.

■ A physician may lose his or her license to practice medicine if convicted of a crime, found guilty of unprofessional conduct, or as a result of personal or professional incapacity. An arrest will not cause the physician to lose the license, since this is an allegation not yet proven in court. Unprofessional conduct is usually determined by local medical societies or other organizations, such as a hospital, with which the physician is affiliated.

INTERNET CONNECTIONS

- American Medical Association
  www.ama-assn.org
- Department of Health and Human Services
  www.os.dhhs.gov
- Occupational Health and Safety Administration
  www.osha.gov
- United States Supreme Court
  www.supremecourtus.gov

UNIT two

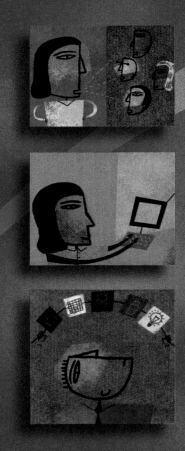

Administrative Medical Assisting

CHAPTER 8

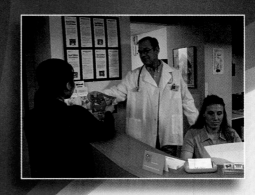

Scenario

Dr. Michael Bouchard is aware of the advantages of networking his office computers and having Internet access to meet the needs of his facility. Every day he sends and receives many important email messages to and from patients and colleagues. His staff members use the computer for communications and to access sources of online information. Patient tracking, accounting functions, and health information retrieval are immensely faster on a computer than with the use of a paper-based system. One other distinct advantage to Dr. Bouchard is the scheduling features of his software. Because the schedule is shared, everyone in the office knows the doctor's schedule and avoids double-booking and miscommunications. Dr. Bouchard sends his staff members for regular computer training so that all of them can use the computers in the best and most efficient ways possible.

Computers in the Medical Office

Learning Objectives

- Define and spell the terms listed in the vocabulary.
- List several ways that the computer can be effective in a medical office.
- Explain the basic functions that a computer performs.
- Explain the basic parts of a computer.
- List the three elements that differentiate microprocessors.
- Discuss the differences among various types of printers.
- Explain the importance of a motherboard.
- Explain and give examples of peripheral devices.
- List and discuss several types of file formats.
- Explain the concept of computer networking.
- Define the function of browsers.
- Discuss the importance of computer security.

National Curriculum Competencies

TRANSDISCIPLINARY COMPETENCIES

4c. Utilize computer software to maintain systems
Computer terminology and overview of
computer concepts
Knowledge of basic computer commands and
functions

Vocabulary

applications software Software programs designed to perform specific tasks.

artificial intelligence The aspect of computer science that deals with computers taking on the attributes of humans. One such example is expert systems, which are capable of making decisions, such as software that is designed to help a physician diagnose a patient, given a set of symptoms. Game-playing programs and programs that are designed to recognize human speech are other examples.

ASCII codes Acronym for American Standard Code for Information Interchange; a code representing English characters as numbers where each is given a number from 0 to 127.

backup Any type of storage of files to prevent their loss in the event of hard disk failure.

banners Advertisements often found on a web page that can be animated to attract the user's attention in hopes that he or she will click on the ad, be redirected to the advertiser's home page, and purchase from the site or gain information from the site.

bit The smallest unit of information inside the computer, represented by either the digit "0" or "1"; eight bits equal one byte.

byte A unit of data that contains eight binary digits, or bits.

cache A special high-speed storage that can either be a part of the computer's main memory or can be a separate storage device. One function of a cache is to store websites visited in the computer memory for faster recall the next time the website is requested.

CD burner A device that is capable of "writing" data onto a blank compact disk (CD) or copying data from one CD to a blank CD.

computer A machine that is designed to accept, store, process, and give out information.

cookies Messages sent to a web browser from a web server that identify users and can prepare custom web pages for them, possibly displaying their name on return to the site.

cursor A symbol appearing on the monitor that shows where the next character to be typed will appear.

cyberspace Describes the nonphysical space of the online world of computer networks in which communication takes place.

database A collection of related files that serves as a foundation for retrieving information.

device driver The program or commands given to a device connected to a computer that enable the device to function. For instance, a printer may come equipped with a software program that must be loaded onto the computer first, so that the printer will work.

digital subscriber line (DSL) High-speed, sophisticated modulation scheme that operates over existing copper telephone wiring systems; often referred to as "last-mile technologies," because DSL is used for connections from a telephone switching station to a home or office, and not from between switching stations.

digital versatile disk or digital video disk (DVD) An optical disk that holds approximately 28 times more information than a CD; a DVD is most commonly used to hold full-length movies. Compared with a CD, which holds approximately 600 megabytes, a DVD has the capacity to hold approximately 4.7 gigabytes.

disk A removable device with a magnetic surface that is capable of storing computer programs, stored in a hard plastic square; also called diskettes, and early versions were called "floppy disks."

disk drives Devices that load a program or data stored on a disk into the computer.

ecommerce An abbreviation for *electronic commerce*; used to describe the sale and purchase of goods and services over the Internet; doing business over the Internet.

email Communications transmitted via computer using a modem.

environment The state of a computer, usually determined by the programs that are running as well as hardware and software characteristics.

fax Abbreviation for *facsimile*; also, a document sent using a facsimile (fax) machine.

flash Animation technology often used on the opening page of a website to draw attention, excite, and impress the user.

font A design for a set of type characters; a combination of typeface, spacing, pitch, and other qualities. Fonts are named; examples include Times Roman, Arial, and Garamond.

format To magnetically create tracks on a disk where information will be stored, usually done by the manufacturer of the disk.

gigabyte Approximately 1 billion bytes; abbreviated GB.

hard copy The readable paper copy or printout of information.

HTML Acronym for HyperText Markup Language, which is the language used to create documents for use on the Internet.

HTTP Acronym for HyperText Transfer Protocol, which defines how messages are formatted and transmitted over the Internet. When a URL is entered into the computer, an HTTP command tells the web server to retrieve the requested web page.

hub A common connection point for devices in a network containing multiple ports, often used to connect segments of a LAN.

icon A picture, often on the desktop of a computer, that represents a program or an object. By clicking on the icon, the user is directed to the program.

input Information entered into and used by the computer.

Java A commonly used object-oriented high-level programming language that is well suited for the Internet.

megabyte Approximately 1 million bytes; abbreviated MB.

megahertz The measuring device for microprocessors, abbreviated MHz. A megahertz is 1 million cycles of electromagnetic currency alternation per second and is used as a unit of measure for the clock speed of computer microprocessors. The hertz is a unit of measure named after Heinrich Hertz, a German physicist.

MIDI Acronym for Musical Instrument Digital Interface; a MIDI interface allows computers to record and manipulate sound.

modem A device that allows information to be transmitted over telephone lines, at speeds measured in bits per second (bps); short for modulator-demodulator.

monochromatic Having or consisting of one color or hue.

multimedia The presentation of graphics, animation, video, sound, and text on a computer in an integrated way, or all at once. CD-ROMs are the most effective multimedia devices.

output Information that is processed by the computer and transmitted to a monitor, printer, or other device.

queries Requests for information from a database.

router A device used to connect any number of LANs, which communicate with other routers and determine the best route between any two hosts.

scanner Device that reads text or illustrations on a printed page and can translate the information on that page into a form that the computer can understand.

search engines Programs that search documents for keywords and return a list of documents containing those words.

server A computer or device on a network that manages shared network resources.

sound card Device that allows a computer to output sound through speakers that are connected to the main circuitry board, or motherboard.

switch In networks, a device that filters information between LAN segments and decreases overall network traffic and increases speed and bandwidth usage efficiency.

systems software The operating system and all utility programs that allow the computer to function and perform operations.

TCP/IP Acronym for Transmission Control Protocol/Internet Protocol; a suite of communications protocols used to connect users or hosts to the Internet.

telecommunication The science and technology of communication by transmission of information from one location to another via telephone, television, telegraph, or satellite.

URL Acronym for Uniform Resource Locator; specifies the global address of documents or information on the Internet. The URL provides the IP address and the domain name for the web page, such as *microsoft.com*.

virtual reality An artificial environment presented to a computer user that feels as if it were a real environment, often using special gloves, earphones, and goggles to enhance the experience.

Zip drive A small, portable disk drive that is primarily used for backing up information and archiving computer files. A 100-megabyte Zip disk will hold the equivalent of about 70 floppy disks.

Computers in the New Millennium

Nearly 60 years ago, in 1946, the first electronic computer (ENIAC) was completed after $2\frac{1}{2}$ years in the making. It weighed 30 tons, required a space of 15,000 square feet, and cost more than $1 million. Since that time, a computer explosion has taken place, and today our lives are affected by computers on a daily basis. Personal computers, laptop or notebook computers, and even cell phones that send and receive **email** are commonplace. Our world is now one of enhanced **telecommunications**, where faster processing of information is both needed and expected. Most people venture into **cyberspace** on a daily basis, where a world of information is waiting with the simple click of a mouse!

For many years computers have been used in medical facilities, including physicians' offices. The development of software, the decrease in the cost of computer hardware, and the time savings that the computer brings to the office make it well worth the investment. Computers are now standard equipment in healthcare facilities (Figure 8-1). A medical assistant must have more than computer literacy—a good understanding of the way computers work and their capabilities is essential in a medical office.

Computers in the Medical Office

Getting Started

Even with some basic knowledge of computer components and of what computers can do, without hands-on knowledge, the beginner may have some initial fear of the unknown. However, the computer is only a machine that takes its direction from the person operating it. It will perform the tasks that it is told to do. A computer cannot really think or make decisions (yet); it will wait for commands that will prompt it to act. Computers assist workers in medical offices in some of the following ways:

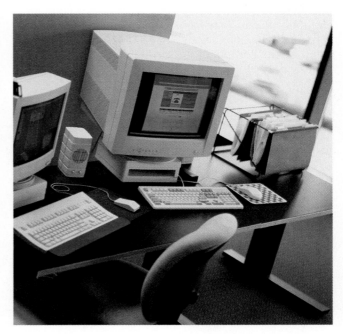

FIGURE 8-1 Computers are an invaluable tool for today's medical office.

- Performing repetitive tasks
- Reducing errors
- Speeding up production
- Recalling information on command
- Saving time
- Reducing paperwork and storage space
- Allowing for more creative and productive use of workers' time

The more familiar a medical assistant becomes with the computer, the better skilled he or she will become in its use. Occasionally errors will be made, and the computer may respond with an error message. However, the monitor screen normally indicates what to do next. The computer will usually allow the operator the opportunity to figure out the correct information and input that information into the computer. A help menu can always be accessed, or the instruction manual can be consulted; help lines and technical support are available as well when problems occur. The problem may be with the software, or with the computer itself. Usually it is fairly easy to determine which is causing the problem.

Rarely will the computer "break," although this is a common fear among new users. It is unlikely that records will be destroyed by accident; usually very specific commands are needed to delete stored information. However, a medical assistant must take care not to shut off the computer without saving the information that has been entered. By using a computer in the classroom and practicing at home or at a library, if possible, the medical assistant will gain familiarity with computer operation and confidence that it can be mastered. Mastery is accomplished only through practice.

With a knowledge of computer terms, the ability to follow step-by-step instructions, and reasonable expertise with a keyboard, a medical assistant can rapidly learn and use almost any computer system. Although the computers and the software may vary from facility to facility, basic computer operation is similar, and if the instructions given by the computer are carried out, the user should be successful in the tasks attempted.

Computer Basics

A **computer** is a machine that is designed to accept, store, process, and provide information (Figure 8-2). Computers serve the following basic functions:

- *Input:* **Input** includes any information that enters the computer. It can take a variety of forms, from commands that are entered from the keyboard to data from another computer or device, such as a scanner. The device that feeds data into a computer is called an *input device*, such as a mouse, scanner, or keyboard.
- *Processing:* Processing is the act of manipulating the data that are currently inside the computer to carry out a certain task.
- *Output:* **Output** is anything that exits the computer. Output can appear in many forms, such as binary numbers, characters, pictures, printed pages, or a simple image on the monitor. Output devices include monitors, speakers, and printers.
- *Storage:* The act of retaining data or applications is called storage. Data can be stored on disks, on CDs, or on separate drives, such as a **Zip drive**.

CRITICAL THINKING APPLICATION

Dr. Bouchard plans to send two of his employees to a training class on using a new software program designed to perform all computer functions needed for his practice. Although he can only send two employees, how can the others learn the system?

Would it be beneficial or detrimental to close the office for a day to educate the other employees about the system? What should the physician consider before losing a day of patient visits?

Parts of the Computer

A medical assistant must understand the function of the different parts of a computer. The physical pieces that can be touched and seen are called hardware. Computers

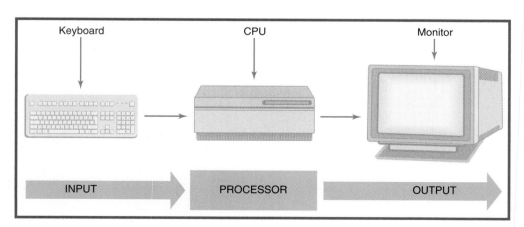

FIGURE 8-2   Input devices allow data to be entered into the computer, where they are processed; output is available in several different forms.

using Windows software have an option in the control panel for adding hardware. This shortcut makes adding new equipment easy and provides instruction all along the way. Hardware provides the medium on which software can be used. Most personal computers (PCs) have a microprocessor, monitor, keyboard, mouse, and printer.

Microprocessor

Inside the casing of the main computer hardware, the microprocessor is housed. The microprocessor is the central unit of the computer that contains the logic circuitry, which carries out the instructions of a computer's programs. It is considered the most important piece of hardware in a computer system. Microprocessors act as the brain of the computer and interpret instructions from a program. Microprocessors, sometimes called *central processing units*, are differentiated by three basic elements:

- *Bandwidth:* Bandwidth describes how much information can be sent over a connection at one time, or how many bits can be processed in one single instruction. **Bits,** short for binary digits, are the smallest pieces of information on the computer. Eight bits make up one **byte**.
- *Clock speed:* Clock speed determines how many instructions per second that the processor can handle. Clock speed is measured in **megahertz** (MHz). One megahertz equals 1 million cycles per second, so a processor that operates at 300 MHz executes 300 million cycles per second.
- *Instruction set:* The instruction set is the set of instructions that the microprocessor can execute.

The higher the bandwidth and clock speed, the faster and more powerful the microprocessor. For instance, a 32-bit microprocessor that runs at 50 MHz is more powerful than a 16-bit microprocessor that runs at 25 MHz.

A microprocessor contains memory consisting of electronic and magnetic cells, each of which contains information. There are two kinds of memory: read-only memory (ROM) and random access memory (RAM). ROM is internal memory that contains a portion of the operating system and computer language. This is sometimes known as *main memory*. Data that have been "burned" onto a ROM chip cannot be removed and can only be read, similar to a CD-ROM, unless the CD is a "rewriteable" type. With this permanent memory, much less information has to be transferred from a disk to start the computing process. ROM cannot be overwritten and is not erased when the power is shut off. RAM can be thought of as an internal scratch pad for the computer. It contains the program instructions and the data that are currently processing. RAM is normally erased when the power is shut off.

CRITICAL THINKING APPLICATION

A colleague of Dr. Bouchard's has mentioned that he knows about a website that has several software programs online that can be downloaded free of charge. Dr. Bouchard investigates the site and realizes the software has been pirated. What concerns could this cause if he uses the software in his office? What would happen if any of this software malfunctioned?

Monitor

A monitor, which looks very much like a television screen, is a device used to display computer-generated information. A few are **monochromatic,** but most monitors today are color, capable of being adjusted for brightness, sharpness, and other settings of the user's choice. Color monitors allow for a high quality display, and the more advanced models have resolutions capable of reproducing quality pictures good enough for viewing a **digital video disk** (DVD). By viewing the monitor, the user receives instant feedback on entries into the computer. Monitors are sometimes referred to as *displays* and are considered output devices.

Keyboard

For most computers, the keyboard is the primary text input device. Keyboards contain special function keys, such as the escape key, tab key, cursor movement keys, numeric keys, shift keys, and control keys. Additional function keys, numbered *F1* to *F12,* are used to perform specific word processing or other computer-related operations. Used alone, a function key may create bold print, underline, indent, or call up a help screen. Used in conjunction with the *Ctrl, Alt, or Shift* keys, the function keys can produce other desired results, such as activating the printer, inserting the current date into a document, retrieving a file, or moving a designated block of text.

Mouse

The mouse first became a widely used computer tool when Apple Computers made it a standard part of the Apple Macintosh computer. It resembles a mouse because of its shape and the cord, which attaches it to the microprocessor. The mouse is a pointing device with a ball on the bottom that is moved by rolling it on a flat table top or mouse pad. Some computers, especially laptops, have a built-in device called a *trackball* that is moved with the finger or thumb and serves the same function as a mouse. Other computers have a touchpad or a track-point that is manipulated to control the cursor. The **cursor** is a pointer or flat bar appearing on the monitor that shows where the next character will appear, which is the insertion point. The mouse allows the user to navigate around the screen quickly and click on links to access websites.

Printer

Printers are output devices. Documents appearing on the monitor may be directed to a printer to produce a printout or **hard copy** of a document. Many printers are bidirectional, which means they print both from left to right and from right to left. The type of printer used should depend on the job being performed.

Dot matrix printers are inexpensive and produce a moderate-quality hard copy. They form letters or shapes that they are directed to print by arranging patterns of dots on the paper. They operate faster than letter-quality machines, but the print lacks the clarity generally desired for a professional look.

Ink jet printers use an ink cartridge that feeds an array of nearly microscopic tubes, each of which has a heating element that is energized during the printing process. The ink cartridge may be black-and-white or color. Ink jet printers cost less than laser printers, but the ink cartridges they use are fairly expensive and increase the operating cost.

Laser printers use xerographic technology similar to that in photocopiers, so the laser printer is able to produce an almost limitless variety of forms and sizes as well as complex graphics. One disadvantage of ink jet and laser printers is that they are incapable of producing multiple copies with carbon sets or multicopy forms, which are often used by insurance companies for their filing forms.

Some printers today are multifunctional, serving as a printer, **fax, scanner,** and copier. Although these are excellent for home offices, they may not be the best investment for offices that will use these machines often during the day.

> ### CRITICAL THINKING APPLICATION
>
> Dr. Bouchard has asked his office manager to perform a cost comparison on a printer for three of the office computers. He prefers that they have scanning and fax capability. What are some of the features that the office manager will be interested in knowing about these machines?

Inside the Computer

Basic knowledge of the parts of a computer and their function will help a medical assistant to deal with minor technical issues and give him or her the ability to speak with technical support personnel with more ease.

Motherboard

A motherboard is the main circuit board for the computer, to which other devices can be attached. Usually it contains the processor, the memory, and other controllers and devices that allow the system to operate and function.

Disk Drives

Today's computers have various **disk drives** on which information can be stored or accessed. The hard disk or hard drive is a magnetic disk inside the computer that holds from approximately 10 **megabytes** to several hundred **gigabytes** of information (Figure 8-3). Application

software is normally saved to the hard disk and stored there on the computer for use when needed. This is commonly called the C drive.

Floppy disks or diskettes are normally used in the computer's A drive, although the drives can have different names or labels, depending on the brand of computer. Floppy disks were so named because the original $5^{1}/_{4}$-inch variety was housed in a soft plastic cover that would "flop" if waved up and down. The $3^{1}/_{2}$-inch diskettes are less frequently used now, because CDs have a higher capacity for holding information. However, diskettes are still in use and are easily portable.

> ### CRITICAL THINKING APPLICATION
>
> Dr. Bouchard mentions that he noticed CD-R disks on sale over the weekend. The price that he saw was $30 for 100 CD-Rs. One of the medical assistants noticed a 30-pack of CD-Rs for $9.99. Which is the better buy?

CD-ROM

Most of today's personal computers are equipped with CD-ROM drives, which allow the storage of data on a compact disc. CDs hold much more information than floppy disks. A single CD can store as much information as approximately 700 floppy disks, which is the equivalent of about 300,000 text pages (Figure 8-4). A CD-RW is one on which data can be written, erased, and rewritten. Computers that have a **CD burner,** or CD-R drive, can take information from one CD or another source and write it to another CD. The computer must also have software that enables the burner to work. Software that is installed on a computer to allow a hardware device to function is called a **device driver**.

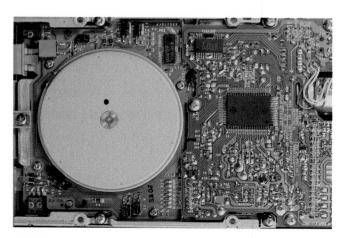

FIGURE 8-3 Hard drives store data and applications for fast and effective access and retrieval. Although a program installed on a hard drive can be removed, most programs are placed there for permanent use, such as Microsoft Office or Peachtree Accounting.

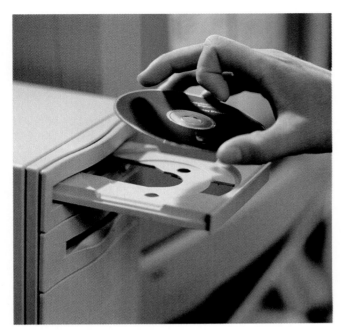

FIGURE 8-4 CD-ROMs allow the user to store and retrieve large amounts of information. Many computers are now equipped with CD-ROM burners, which allow copying of information from one CD to another, or from Internet files to CD-ROMs.

Expansion Boards

Expansion boards are devices that are inserted into a computer that give the computer added capabilities. For example, a **sound card** may be installed so that music or **MIDI** files can be heard from the unit. Other expansion boards are video adapters, internal modems, and graphics accelerators.

Software

Software encompasses the programs and utilities that are loaded onto or inside the computer and used to carry out the work performed by the machine. There are two types of software: systems software and applications software. **Systems software** serves as the operating system of the computer and allows it to run and carry out the functions that the computer performs. For instance, Windows XP, Linux, and the now somewhat antiquated DOS are all types of operating systems software. **Applications software** refers to the programs loaded onto the computer that carry out the work for the actual users of the computer. Examples of applications software are Microsoft Office, MediSoft, and Medical Manager. Applications programs are designed to perform specific tasks, such as word processing, billing, accounting, appointment setting, insurance form preparation, payroll, and **database** management. Many software applications are available for complete medical practice management.

Modems

A **modem,** short for modulator-demodulator, is a device over which data can be transmitted via telephone lines and other media, such as a coaxial cable. Modems can be internal or external. An internal modem is built or added to the inside of the computer casing. A cable modem operates over cable TV lines, and uses the coaxial cable to provide faster Internet access. **Digital subscriber line** (DSL) modems operate over phone lines like normal modems, but they use a different frequency; thus the telephone can be used while the computer is accessing the Internet. Often a filter is attached to the phone that removes other frequencies wherein the DSL is working, avoiding interference with the telephone line operation.

Speakers and Microphones

Some computers have external speakers to provide a higher quality sound from the computer. Many computers also have built-in speakers that provide a fair quality of sound. Microphones can be built-in or attached, so that the user can speak directly into the computer, even to someone on the other side of the world!

Peripheral Devices

Peripheral devices are those that are not essential to the operation of the computer. For instance, the computer will operate without a modem, although a modem is necessary to access the Internet. A mouse is even considered a peripheral device, because everything that the mouse can access can also be reached by certain buttons on the keyboard, although often multiple keys have to be pressed at once. This section discusses some of the peripheral devices in use today.

Scanner

Scanners read text, illustrations, or photos printed on paper and put them into a **format** that the computer can understand. Photographs can be placed into the scanner, saved on the computer, and then used in a document.

Digital Cameras

Digital cameras use a charge-coupled device (CCD) to convert light into electrical charges. Digital cameras do not use film. Light strikes the surface of a photosite inside the camera, and then filters add color and create the digital image. Many digital cameras can be attached directly to a computer and photos can be downloaded from the camera to the computer. Other cameras use a disk to put the pictures into the computer.

CRITICAL THINKING APPLICATION

How might a digital camera be of use to a physician in his or her medical practice? What care should be taken when using the camera with a patient?

Zip Drives

A Zip drive is a disk drive that has a very high storage capacity and is attached externally to a computer. It is usually used as a **backup** device for important data that should not be lost. Zip drives can hold between 100 and 250 megabytes of data and can even be stored somewhere other than the facility so that they are safe in case of fire or other destructive event.

Adding a Program to a Computer

Adding or loading a program onto a computer is relatively easy. Most programs today come in the form of a CD-ROM. The program will contain instructions as to how it should be loaded onto the computer. Watch the monitor for steps to complete and information concerning the user's preferences, then follow all of the directions given.

In a Windows **environment,** the control panel provides an option called *add/remove programs*. Once clicked, this will allow the program in the CD disk drive to be loaded onto the computer. At several points the computer may ask the user questions about his or her preferences for the program. Often the computer may need to be restarted after installation.

When removing a program from the computer, the "add/remove programs" **icon** should be accessed and directions followed for removal of the program. This may be the only way to completely remove the program from the computer system.

File Formats

A file is a collection of data. There are many types of files that are related to computers. A text file, for example, contains some type of text, which is the main body of printed words or written matter on a page. Often an extension exists at the end of the file name that designates what type of file the document is. A file named manual.com might indicate that the file is some type of command file. A few of the common file extensions include the following:

- *JPEG:* JPEG stands for Joint Photographic Experts Group and is a format often used for photographs.
- *GIF:* GIF stands for Graphics Interchange Format, which supports color and is often used for scanned images and illustrations rather than photographs.
- *DOC:* A file that includes the extension *.doc* is usually a file created by a word processor or word processing software, and stands for *document*.
- *TXT:* A text file usually has the extension .txt after its name. Characters in a text file are represented by their **ASCII codes**.
- *RTF:* RTF stands for Rich Text Format. This type of file combines ASCII codes with special commands that distinguish variations, such as a certain **font**.
- *BMP:* Bit-mapped graphics are indicated by the extension *.bmp*. These are compiled by a graphics image that is set in rows or columns of dots.

A medical assistant who is familiar with these types of files will be able to save and open them correctly and use the computer to the fullest advantage in the medical office.

Computer Networking

A network is a group of two or more computer systems that are linked together. There are several types of networks:

- *LAN:* A LAN is a Local-Area Network, or a computer network spanning a relatively small area. Most LANs are contained in a single building or group of buildings and are connected by a **router**, but LANs can be connected to other LANs even at a distance. A **hub** is a device that connects several computers or networks together, and a **switch** is designed to help the LAN run more efficiently by controlling local network traffic.
- *MAN:* MAN stands for Metropolitan-Area Network. A MAN spans an area that does not exceed a metropolitan area or city and connects several LANs together.
- *WAN:* A WAN is a Wide-Area Network, which spans a relatively large geographic area. Typically, a WAN consists of two or more LANs or MANs. These networks can be connected through public networks, such as a telephone system, or through leased lines or satellites. The largest WAN that exists is the Internet.
- *HAN:* A HAN is a Home-Area Network, which connects computers inside a user's home.
- *CAN:* A CAN is a Campus-Area Network, often used on college campuses and sometimes on military bases.

Servers

A **server** is important to the network, because it is the computer that manages the shared network resources. There are several types of servers. When many computers are connected to one printer, often a print server manages these printers. File servers are used for file storage, and database servers are used to process database **queries.** Some servers are considered to be dedicated servers, meaning they only perform tasks as a server, although a server may also operate as a normal computer.

Clients

A client is a computer that is configured to request access to resources from a server. Server applications, like access to the Internet, network printing, or email access, can run on a server and are accessed by the clients so that they can accomplish these tasks.

The Internet

The Internet is a global network that connects millions of computers together. This fascinating structure has made the world a smaller place (Figure 8-5). Through chat programs, one can talk with individuals literally on the other side of the world and be introduced to cultures that 20 years ago would never have been understood. Through web pages we can visit different parts of the world and learn and see many things that previously were impossible for the average person to experience. **Ecommerce** allows us to shop on the net, from the most exclusives shops in Beverly Hills to the corner grocery store. The Internet has changed the way we learn, do business, communicate, and entertain ourselves.

Each computer connected to the Internet is called a *host* and is independent of all the others. The users of each computer determine which services to make available to other users on the Internet. Often a company or organization also has an Intranet, which is a local network that uses Internet technology within a company or single location but does not have access to the Internet directly.

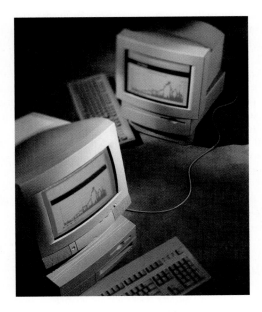

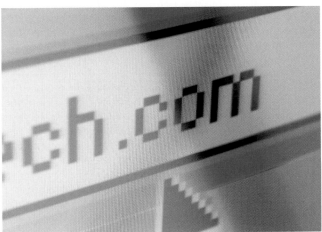

FIGURE 8-5 Computers in today's businesses can speak to each other from across the room or across the world.

Internet service providers (ISPs) are companies that provide access to the Internet. Examples include America Online, Mindspring, Verizon, Earthlink, and Yahoo. ISPs issue each user an IP (Internet Protocol) address, which is a unique identifier for that user's particular computer on a **TCP/IP** network. An IP address is a 32-bit number written as four numbers separated by a period. Each number can be zero to 255, so a valid IP address could be 10.145.32.254. Messages are defined and transmitted over the Internet when a **URL** is entered into the browser and an **HTTP** command tells the web server to retrieve the requested web page.

Domain names identify one or more IP addresses, such as *microsoft.com* or *ama-assn.org*. There are a limited number of top-level domains to which a domain name can be attached. Some of these top-level domains include .com (familiarly called *dot-com*) for commercial businesses; .org for organizations, usually nonprofit; .edu for educational institutions; .gov for government agencies; and .net for network organizations. Most Internet sites use a language called **HTML,** which was one of the first and is still one of the most popular languages used to create web pages. **Java** is another popular language used in website creation.

Many physicians and health organizations offer a website with information about their services. In today's data-driven society, this is an excellent way to educate the public about the services the organization offers and to provide all types of information to the audience that the organization wishes to reach. To obtain a domain name, one must pay a small fee to have the name registered and added to a central database, if the desired name is available. Companies such as *register.com* or *verisign.com* offer domain name registration services.

Websites often contain **banners,** which attract the eye of the user and tempt a click of the mouse, taking the user to a new website. They are similar to internet commercials. These sites usually contain advertisements or surveys and can track the number of times a user views the site. These views are called "hits." Banners and website home pages sometimes use **flash,** which is designed to grab the interest of the user with multimedia and encourage further exploration of a website.

Browsers

Web browsers are software applications that allow the user to locate and display web pages. The most commonly used browsers are Netscape Navigator and Microsoft Internet Explorer. These browsers are able to display graphics as well as text and can also present **multimedia** information, the quality of which is dependent on the computer system in use and the Internet connection speed. Browsers also have a bookmark capability that allows the user to mark a certain web page and then easily return to it by clicking on its link in a drop-down box in the browser's menu. The **cache** allows quick retrieval of previously viewed sites because the computer remembers and saves the information on the hard drive. **Cookies** store information about individual users, like screen names and passwords.

Browsers and other websites also contain **search engines.** These are programs in which a topic, word, or group of words can be entered, and the engine will search the Internet for matches. A listing of those matches will appear, and the user can click on each match to reference information and complete research. Information on just about any subject can be found through using search engines.

POPULAR SEARCH ENGINES

www.alltheweb.com	www.netscape.com
www.altavista.com	www.search.aol.com
www.excite.com	www.search.msn.com
www.google.com	www.webcrawler.com
www.hotbot.com	www.yahoo.com
www.lycos.com	

CRITICAL THINKING APPLICATION

Dr. Bouchard likes that all employees have Internet access at his office, but is still concerned that there will be occasional misuse of the computer. He does not want the staff to use the computer for personal business, but does not mind if they check their personal email on a break or at lunch. What are some reasonable policies for office Internet usage?

The Computer as a Co-Worker

The computer is a valuable tool in the medical office. It can assist in filing insurance claims by sending information from the computer in the office to the computers at the insurance company using a modem. Electronic processing of insurance claims not only saves time but also provides immediate information as to whether a claim will be accepted. Errors in coding or procedure are immediately evident, and many rejections can be avoided even before the claim is transmitted. Many insurance companies give preferential treatment to providers who file claims electronically.

The demographics about a patient will appear on computerized patient ledgers, listing name, address, telephone number, and insurance information. As services are rendered, charges are entered into the computer and payments will be displayed as well. This helps the medical facility to maintain an accurate balance of all patient accounts.

At the appropriate time each month, the computer can print a patient's billing statement, which shows detail of charges, payments, adjustments, and the current balance. Additionally, the computer can be programmed to age the accounts according to any criteria selected and to include this information on the billing statement. A series of collection letters can be developed and personalized for individual patients as they are needed.

Database software makes it possible to organize a large volume of information that can be used in a number of ways. One of the most practical uses is the organization of identifying information on each patient. The computer can also store clinical information about patients using much less space and with greater security than papers in a patient's chart. Access to records can be limited with passwords.

The computer has virtually replaced the appointment book in many medical offices today. Software for appointment-setting ranges from relatively simple programs to very sophisticated systems. An advantage to computer scheduling is that more than one person can access the system at one time, and the same information is available to all users.

Computers are even being used as marketing tools and virtual secretaries in some modern medical offices (Figures 8-6 and 8-7). Computers can be programmed to call all patients with appointments for the next day to remind them to visit the doctor, or perhaps call all patients due for a 6-month eye or dental examination. As a marketing tool, computers can be programmed to call all phone numbers in a certain area code with a prerecorded message about a new procedure available at the office or a new physician in the area. Although many individuals are annoyed at the telemarketing concept and being called by a computer, the success rate is good. Computers can call thousands upon thousands of phone numbers, relay a message, and track replies within a matter of hours. This could never be accomplished in the same time period by humans. These methods of using the computer open all kinds of doors for the medical practice of the future.

The medical office should routinely perform a file backup to be sure that valuable data can be retrieved in the event of a system failure. Many medical office software programs have an automatic backup function, but some must be done manually. It is wise to keep backup copies of the database and other critical documents off the premises in case of fire or other tragedy.

Computer Security

Patients are entitled to the utmost confidentiality with respect to their medical records and the release of any information of a personal nature. Computer technology allows the accumulation and storage of a vast amount of data that may be accessible to a variety of individuals, making it imperative that guidelines be set up for the protection of that data.

Encryption is the translation of data into a code that is not readily understood by most users. It is one effective way to achieve data security. To access or read an encrypted file, the user must have a password that enables the code to be decrypted. Once the code is decrypted, it is then useable by the application. Encrypted data are called *cipher text.*

Some individuals attempt to access information in a computer without the owner's consent. These people may intend to use the information just for fun or may have a malicious intent, such as to steal or corrupt the data. Although these people are commonly called *hackers,* computer enthusiasts insist that the correct term for

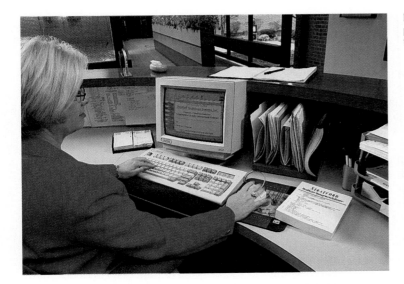

FIGURE 8-6   Computers assist the staff members and physicians of the medical office in numerous ways, making the office run in a more efficient manner.

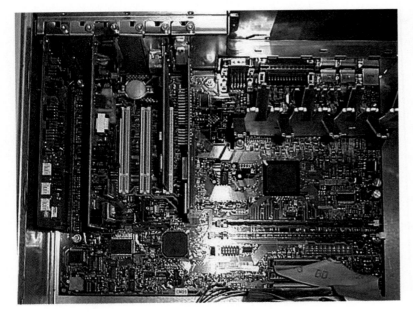

FIGURE 8-7   Inside a computer. Today's microprocessors are designed so that memory, additional drives, and other hardware can be easily added to the system.

individuals who break into computers with dishonorable intent is *crackers*. The term hacker originally simply described a person who enjoyed learning about using computers and becoming proficient in that use.

There are various ways to protect computers and data from unauthorized access. Firewalls are systems designed for just such a purpose and can be implemented into both the hardware and the software of the computer. Firewalls are often used to prevent individuals from accessing private networks. Each message sent and received is examined and the firewall blocks those that do not meet specific security criteria.

Viruses are programs or pieces of code that are loaded onto a computer, usually without the owner's knowledge, that can act like a physical virus in that they can make the computer "sick." Viruses can replicate themselves, copying themselves over and over again, and then be passed to other computers through emails, usually without the sender's knowing that a virus was passed along. Even

simple viruses can quickly use all available memory and bring the system to a standstill; some can completely corrupt the computer's hard drive. More dangerous types of viruses can transmit over networks, bypassing security systems and destroying valuable data. This is why antivirus software is an important part of any computer system.

Electronic Signatures

A recently introduced convenience option is the electronic signature. Electronic signature programs are offered both as stand-alone products and as part of computerized medical record systems. After dictated reports are transcribed, a physician can use a password and personal identification number (PIN) to electronically "sign" the document by clicking on an icon after it has been reviewed for accuracy. Once the document has been signed, it cannot be altered—only addenda are allowed.

Computers and Ergonomics

The increased use of computers in the workplace has underscored the need to choose comfortable, safe furniture and equipment. Repetitive strain injury (RSI) accounts for the majority of work-related injury claims. This includes a number of conditions that are caused by repeatedly straining certain nerves, muscles, or tendons. Carpal tunnel syndrome is one example of RSI.

To avoid such injuries, office staff should use posture chairs that support the lumbar section of the back, with a correct angle of the knee and the feet resting on the floor. Of the many designs for keyboards available, one should be chosen that allows the correct angle at the elbow and the wrist to be held in a neutral position.

Eyestrain is another danger arising from continuous use of a computer. The monitor should be just below eye level and at an arm's length away. At least once each hour, the user should take a break from looking at the monitor.

Closing Comments

Computers should be thought of as additional workers in the office. A medical assistant who learns how best to use the computer and discovers as many of its capabilities as possible will be a valuable employee.

Read the manuals that accompany equipment and programs and try new applications for old procedures. Computers are designed to save time, so look for ways to make the day's workload lighter by taking full advantage of the computer.

The future promises more rapid technological advances, since computer equipment can become archaic in as short a time as 6 months after purchase. **Artificial intelligence,** voice recognition, **virtual reality,** and retinal scanning, seen mostly in the movies, will become commonplace in our homes and businesses. These tools will make the work environment even faster and more efficient, as the world becomes a smaller place.

Patient Education

The evolution of computers will continue to bring about changes in medical facilities of the future. Medical staffs will find themselves educating their patients about computer use, because there are numerous programs in development that will allow patients to "check in" once they arrive at the office and verify their identity. A medical assistant will need patience to instruct these procedures and assure the patients that these new methods will increase their security as well as the protection of their medical records.

With the growing number of medical databases online, physicians can now use information on the Internet to help educate their patients about the illnesses that they are facing. While consulting with the patient, with a few clicks of the mouse, the physician can print out excellent information, often that will assist the patient with referrals to help agencies and suggestions for better healthcare.

Legal and Ethical Issues

Concerns about confidentiality continue to be a top priority among patients, and some feel that computers are not as secure as paper-based record-keeping. However, computers can promote a higher degree of accuracy. Some physicians even use computers inside the treatment room to immediately record findings and diagnoses. Care must be taken to ensure that only authorized personnel can access computer-based patient information at all times.

SUMMARY OF SCENARIO

Dr. Bouchard is a progressive physician who believes that the use of technology will assist him in the care of his patients. He understands the need to train his staff and keep them up to date on the latest versions of their computer software. His willingness to close his office for staff-wide training demonstrates his commitment. He is cost conscious and looks for the best available equipment for the investment he is willing to make.

Dr. Bouchard often uses digital camera equipment to take "before" and "after" pictures of his patients, but only with their special written consent. He also uses the computer to send his patients a monthly email newsletter with health information and special news about the practice.

He monitors his staff's Internet usage but is reasonable about allowing them a small degree of personal access on breaks and at lunch.

He is very interested in new developments for healthcare facilities, such as those that will allow his patients to check in themselves and gain access to limited information about their own medical record. He has a vision that one day his patients will be able to download their statement or perhaps their child's immunization records from their home computers, reducing the staff's workload and providing instant access to some information for his patients. Insightful physicians like Dr. Bouchard will see the computer as a co-worker in the medical facility.

SUMMARY OF LEARNING OBJECTIVES

■ The computer can be an effective tool in the medical office. It performs repetitive tasks, reduces errors, speeds up production, recalls information on command, saves time, reduces paperwork, and allows for more creative and productive use of workers' time.

■ The computer performs four basic functions, which are input, processing, output, and storage. Input includes information that is put into the computer, and output is information that comes out of the computer. Processing is in-between, and is the actual manipulation of data. Storage is the retention of data inside the computer or on storage medium.

- There are several basic parts that make up a computer system. The microprocessor is the brains of the system that interprets the instructions given to it by an application program. The monitor allows the user to see immediate output on a screen, and printers allow the output to be printed to a hard copy. The keyboard and mouse serve as input devices.

- Three elements differentiate microprocessors. The bandwidth describes the amount of information that can be sent over a connection at one time, while the clock speed determines the number of instructions per second that the processor can handle. The instruction set is the instructions that the microprocessor can execute.

- There are three main types of printers in use in today's medical offices. Dot matrix printers produce output of moderate quality but are inexpensive. Ink jet printers use a cartridge and a heating element to produce an image on a page. A laser printer uses technology similar to a photocopier.

- The motherboard is the main connection board to which all other devices are connected inside the computer. It contains all of the essential wiring and expansion devices needed to operate the computer, as well as the battery that keeps the clock and calendar running when the computer is turned off.

- Peripheral devices, such as scanners, Zip drives, and other devices, are not necessary to the function of the computer but perform special functions.

- File format refers to the extension just after the file name, which describes the method used to save the file. This also helps to identify the type of file on the computer. For example, a JPEG file is often used for photographs, a GIF file is used for scanned illustrations or images, and a TXT file is usually specifically for text for a printed page.

- Computer networks are groups of two or more computers linked together. These networks can be local or cover a city or wide geographic area. Some are limited to a few buildings. Networks often share resources, such as printers.

- Browsers are software applications that allow a user to find information on the Internet. They are able to show graphics, and often multimedia, such as videos. The most commonly used browsers are Internet Explorer and Netscape Navigator.

- Computer security is critical, especially because confidential patient information is stored on computers in medical facilities. There are several ways to enhance computer security, such as the use of firewalls and antivirus programs. Restrictions as to who may log in and the use of passwords also will assist the facility to ensure that only authorized individuals have access to confidential information.

INTERNET CONNECTIONS

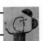

- Webopedia—an Online Computer Dictionary
  www.webopedia.com

CHAPTER 9

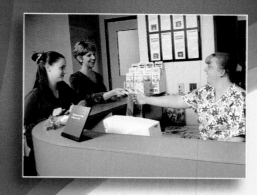

Scenario

Ashlynn McDowell is a recent graduate of a medical assisting program and has begun her first position as a receptionist in an obstetrician's office. It has been Ashlynn's lifelong goal to work with pregnant women, and she is determined to perform to the best of her abilities. However, Ashlynn has never held a job in a professional office. She knows that she will need to practice all of the skills she learned in school with regard to being an effective receptionist.

The physician Ashlynn works for, Dr. Stella Frank, is customer service oriented and wants her patients to feel special and well cared for. She insists that they be treated as important and that their concerns be taken seriously. Ashlynn is anxious to build trust with the patients and offer help to them with the problems they encounter. She knows that she will be required to speak clearly and distinctly and be adept at follow-up skills. She plans to dress professionally each day, so that she projects the right image to the patients with whom she comes in contact. Ashlynn will strive to be the type of employee who presents a willingness to learn, an ability to adapt, and a heart with compassion for the patient. She is a team player who sincerely wishes to cooperate with other staff members that might need her help.

Dr. Frank is pleased that she has found such an eager person to add to her staff and will provide assistance and guidance to her as she learns how to make her patients feel a part of her clinic family. Ashlynn's self-esteem has increased because she feels she is making a great contribution to healthcare.

Telephone Techniques

National Curriculum Competencies

TRANSDISCIPLINARY COMPETENCIES

1b. Recognize and respond to verbal communication
1d. Demonstrate telephone techniques

2a. Identify and respond to issues of confidentiality
3a. Explain general office policies
3e. Identify community resources

Vocabulary

clarity The quality or state of being clear.

competent Having adequate abilities or qualities; having the capacity to function or perform in a certain way.

cultivate To foster the growth of; to improve by labor, care, or study.

diction The choice of words especially with regard to clearness, correctness, or effectiveness.

enunciation Utterance of articulate, clear sounds.

inflection A change in pitch or loudness of the voice.

invariably Consistent; not changing or capable of change.

jargon The technical terminology or characteristic idiom of a particular group or special activity.

monotone A succession of syllables, words, or sentences in one unvaried key or pitch.

multitasking Performing multiple tasks at the same time.

pitch The property of a sound, especially a musical tone, that is determined by the frequency of the waves producing it; the highness or lowness of sound.

provider Individual or company that provides medical care and services to a patient or the public.

salutation An expression of greeting, goodwill, or courtesy by words or gestures.

screen Something that shields, protects, or hides; to select or eliminate through a screening process.

stat Medical abbreviation for immediately; at this moment.

tactful Having a keen sense of what to do or say to maintain good relations with others or to avoid offense.

tedious Tiresome because of length or dullness.

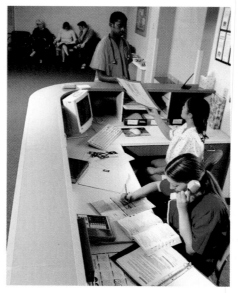

FIGURE 9-1 The telephone plays a vital role in the success of a medical practice.

Effective Use of the Telephone

Active Listening

Although great emphasis is placed on rules for speaking, the importance of active listening is often overlooked. The same attention should be given a telephone conversation that would be given a face-to-face conversation. Concentration is not always easy for a medical assistant who is juggling several duties at once in the medical office, so he or she must practice focusing on the call at hand. Effective active listening also provides vital information about the nature of the call—whether the caller is distressed and agitated or has a concern that needs to be addressed immediately.

Developing a Pleasing Telephone Voice

Individuals who call a physician's office should hear a pleasant, friendly voice when they are greeted. It is a common sales technique to be sure that the caller "hears a smile." Customer service is critical in today's medical offices, and this technique is quite useful for medical assistants, who are likely to be the caller's first point of contact with the practice. Be sure to enunciate words clearly, pronouncing them separately and distinctly. **Diction, pitch,** and **clarity** are important as well. Avoid speaking in a **monotone;** instead, use **inflection,** or a change in the pitch and loudness of the voice when speaking. This helps the speaker to emphasize certain points during the conversation.

When a telephone call is received from a stranger, one usually tries to visualize that person's appearance and perhaps will form an opinion of his or her personality. The caller may sound mature, somewhat worried, well educated, or frantic. As discussed in Chapter 5, communication is a two-way street, so the caller will be forming an impression of the person answering the phone at the

The telephone is the lifeline of a medical practice as well as a powerful public relations tool. The majority of patients who are seen in a medical facility make their initial appointments by telephone. When used appropriately, the telephone can help build a medical practice from its beginning and throughout its life (Figure 9-1). If used inappropriately, it can destroy even a flourishing practice. Medical assistants must remember that the voice on the other end of the line is that of the patient, and telephone calls can never be considered an interruption of the work day.

Most incoming calls are from these sources:
- Established patients calling for appointments or to ask questions
- Individuals reporting emergencies
- Other physicians who are making referrals
- Laboratories reporting vital information regarding a patient
- New patients making a first contact with the physician's office

same time. Sometimes these impressions are incorrect, but much can be assumed by what is heard on the telephone.

Always use a friendly and warm tone of voice and project confidence when speaking with patients. Be courteous and **tactful** and choose words carefully. Every caller should be made to feel that the medical assistant has time to attend to his or her wishes. A small mirror, placed near the telephone, will serve as a reminder to smile. If the medical assistant is rushed to pick up the telephone, he or she should wait a few seconds until able to answer graciously without seeming breathless or impatient.

Be alert and interested in the person who is calling. Always give full attention to the caller and do not allow distractions from the conversation. Build a pleasant, friendly image for the office. Talk naturally and avoid repetition of mechanical words or phrases, such as "uh huh" and "you know." Avoid the use of professional **jargon,** such as referring to *otalgia* when the patient is reporting an *earache.* Using correct grammar adds to the caller's favorable impression. Speak distinctly; clear pronunciation and **enunciation** are vital. Move the lips, tongue, and jaw freely. Talk directly into the mouthpiece. Never answer the telephone when eating, drinking, or chewing gum. A well-modulated voice carries best. Use a normal tone of voice, neither too loud nor too soft. Talk at a moderate rate, neither too quickly nor too slowly. Be expressive and vary the tone of voice. This will bring out the meaning of sentences and add color and vitality to what is said.

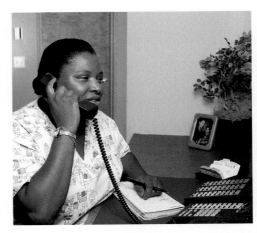

FIGURE 9-2   The handset should be held in the center, with the mouthpiece about 1 inch in front of the lips.

Speak directly into the telephone immediately after removing it from its cradle. When turning to face another part of the room, make sure the handset moves, too; otherwise, the voice will be lost. A medical assistant who speaks too fast, enunciates poorly, or fails to speak directly into the transmitter may not be easily understood by the person on the other end of the receiver.

Maintaining Confidentiality

Keep in mind that all communications in a healthcare facility are confidential. If others are nearby, use discretion when mentioning the name of the caller. Be careful about being overheard when repeating any symptoms or other information received by telephone. Never use a speaker phone to listen to voice mail or hold a phone conversation within the hearing range of others.

CRITICAL THINKING APPLICATION

Ashlynn has a tendency to speak a little fast in her normal conversations. How will she need to adjust as she is answering phones in the medical office? She is also a friendly person and enjoys talking on the phone. What precautions should she take so that this does not become an issue on the job?

CRITICAL THINKING APPLICATION

Ashlynn hears two employees speaking on the intercom in a derogatory manner about a patient who just left the office. How should she handle this situation? Who should Ashlynn report this activity to, if anyone, and why? What problems could be caused when staff members are overheard talking in this manner?

Holding the Telephone Handset Correctly

A medical assistant must develop professional telephone habits in the medical office and correct the more casual habits that are used at home. Consider how the handset is held. It should be placed so that the medical assistant's voice is relayed distinctly and accurately. Practice holding the handset around the middle, with the mouthpiece about 1 inch from the lips and directly in front of the teeth (Figure 9-2). Never hold it under the chin. Check the proper distance by taking the first two fingers and passing them through sideways in the space between the lips and the mouthpiece. If the fingers just squeeze through, then the lips are the correct distance from the telephone and the voice will go over the line as close to its natural tone as possible. When using a headset, speak directly into its mouthpiece, positioning it the same distance from the mouth as a regular telephone.

Thinking Ahead

It is always helpful to think ahead when there is an important call to make. Have the patient's chart or the bill in question at hand before dialing the phone. Write down a list of questions to ask or goals for the conversation. Keep the call short and simple, then free the line for other calls.

Most offices keep a list of frequently called phone numbers to offer patients for referrals. A list of local pharmacies and hospitals and their departments is also very helpful. All of these are time-savers that will help the medical assistant to better serve patients.

PROCEDURE **9-1**

Answering the Telephone

GOAL: To answer the telephone in a physician's office in a professional manner and respond to a request for action.

EQUIPMENT AND SUPPLIES

- Telephone
- Message pad
- Pen or pencil
- Appointment book
- Notepad

PROCEDURAL STEPS

1 Answer the telephone by the third ring, speaking directly into the mouthpiece, which should be positioned one inch from the mouth.

Purpose: Answering promptly conveys interest in the caller. Proper positioning of the handset allows for audible tone and carries the voice well.

2 Speak distinctly with a pleasant tone and expression, at a moderate rate, and with sufficient volume for the calling party to understand every word.

3 Identify the office and/or physician and yourself.

Purpose: The caller will know that the correct number has been reached and the identity of the staff member.

4 Verify the identity of the caller.

Purpose: To confirm the origin of the call.

5 Triage the call, if necessary.

Purpose: To determine if the caller has an emergency and needs immediate attention, or a referral to the emergency department of a hospital.

6 Determine the needs of the caller, and provide the requested information or service, if possible. Provide the caller with excellent customer service. Be as helpful as possible.

Purpose: The medical assistant can handle many calls and conserve the time and energy of the physician or other staff members.

7 If unable to assist the caller, transfer the call to the appropriate person. Before transferring the call, provide the person to whom the call is being transferred with as much information as possible about the caller and his or her needs.

Purpose: To provide good customer service and be as helpful to the caller as possible.

8 Take a proper message for further action, if required.

Purpose: Not all calls can be responded to immediately.

9 Terminate the call in a pleasant manner and replace the receiver gently. Always allow the caller to hang up first.

Purpose: To promote good public relations, provide excellent customer service, and ensure that the caller has no further questions.

Techniques for Incoming Telephone Calls

Many incoming calls will be received in the medical office during the course of a single day. Each one deserves the medical assistant's complete and **competent** attention (Procedure 9-1).

Answering Promptly

Whenever possible, answer the telephone on the first ring, and always by the third ring. If the facility has several incoming lines or more than one telephone, it will sometimes be necessary to interrupt a conversation to answer another call. It is considered courteous to say, "Pardon me just a moment; the other line is ringing." Answer the second call and determine who is calling. If it is not an emergency, ask that person to hold while the first

call is completed. Do not make the mistake of continuing with the second call while the first caller waits. Return to the first call as soon as possible and apologize briefly for the interruption.

Think of what would happen during a face-to-face conversation. A second person who approaches people involved in a conversation would not expect to interrupt and be heard at length. However, if the second call is an emergency, take a moment to return to the first line and alert the caller that he or she will have to be kept waiting or be called back.

Never answer a call by saying, "Please hold" without first finding out who is calling. It could be an emergency, and it is extremely discourteous. It takes only a moment to be polite, and this practice could save a life.

Keep the focus on the call. Attempting **multitasking** while answering the telephone will take attention away from the patient. Treat the phone call just as if the patient were standing in the office face-to-face.

Identifying the Facility

The response to an incoming call should be to first identify the facility and then the person answering the phone. Numerous telephone greetings can be used. Discuss which are best with the physician or office manager. Examples of telephone greetings include the following:

- "This is Dr. Frank's office, Miss McDowell speaking. How may I help you?"
- "Frank Maternal Health Clinic, this is Miss McDowell. How may I help you?"
- "Stella Frank's office, this is Miss McDowell. How may I help you?"

Some physicians avoid using the title "Doctor" so that they may protect their patient's confidentiality. For instance, if a physician needs to call and leave a message for a patient, that patient's curious co-workers might attempt to investigate what type of physician is being seen. Dropping the "Doctor" when leaving messages and when answering the telephone can be an effective means of protecting the patient's privacy.

Merely saying "Hello" is unsatisfactory. The caller will **invariably** ask if he or she has reached the physician's office, so time is wasted, and the opportunity to create a favorable impression of your facility has been lost.

The use of a **salutation** in telephone identification is optional. Sometimes the addition of "Good morning" or "Good afternoon" to the identification is awkward. A rising inflection or a questioning tone in your voice indicates interest and a willingness to assist and eliminates the need for an additional greeting.

When you have decided on the greeting to be used, practice it until you can say it easily and smoothly without having to think about what you are saying. It is critical that the greeting not be rushed so that all callers can easily understand exactly what is being communicated.

CRITICAL THINKING APPLICATION

Most offices dictate how the phone is to be answered. What should Ashlynn do if she is very uncomfortable with the way she is being asked to answer the phone? Who should ultimately make the decision as to how the phone is answered?

Identifying the Caller

If the caller does not identify himself or herself, ask who is calling. Repeat the caller's name by using it in the conversation as soon as possible. Name repetition assures the patient that he or she has been correctly identified and is pleasing to the patient. Try to use the person's name at least three times during the call, and remember other courteous expressions, such as "thank you," "please," and "you're welcome" as often as possible. However, if other patients are within the range of your voice, remember that the caller's privacy should be respected.

Occasionally a caller will refuse to identify himself or herself to the medical assistant and may be quite insistent on speaking with the physician. The individual could be a patient, and the medical assistant should make every attempt to identify the patient and assist his or her needs. Such callers may also be salespersons who are fully aware that if their identity is revealed, they will never get the opportunity to speak to the physician. These people may be firmly told, "Dr. Frank is busy with a patient and has asked that we take messages for her. If you will not leave a message, you may wish to write a letter to her and mark it 'personal.'"

Screening Incoming Calls

Most physicians expect the medical assistant to **screen** all telephone calls. The physician and office manager will provide guidance as to the type of calls that should be routed to the physician and those that he or she will want to return at a later time. The medical assistant should become familiar with their preferences and also use good judgment, much of which comes with experience, in deciding whether to put a call through to the physician (Figure 9-3).

If it is the policy of the office, put calls from other physicians through at once. If the physician is busy and cannot possibly come to the telephone, explain this briefly and politely and then say that the physician will return the call as soon as possible.

Many callers will ask, "Is the doctor in?" or "May I speak to the doctor?" Avoid answering this question with a simple "Yes" or "No" or by responding with the question, "Who is calling, please?" If the physician is not in, say so *before* asking the identity of the caller. Otherwise, the impression may be created that the physician is just not willing to talk with this person.

STAYING IN CONTROL OF CALLS

The Dartnell Corporation publishes a newsletter entitled "Effective Telephone Techniques" that is an excellent tool for building good customer relations while using the phone. One issue suggests ways to control calls and keep them from becoming too lengthy. Try the tips below to keep callers on track and make all phone time productive.

- Ask the caller, "How may I help you today?"
- If the caller becomes sidetracked, say "You were describing the pain in your side?"
- When making a call, get right to the purpose of it after the initial greeting by saying "I was calling you about..."
- Keep explanations short and direct.
- Type information directly into the database, if used, while speaking on the phone.
- Keep personal and friendly comments to a minimum, or only one per call.
- Once the business is concluded, say "If there are no other questions..." and bring the conversation to a close.

FIGURE 9-3 Several tips to stay in control of the telephone calls in the medical office.

If the physician is away from the office, the rule of offering assistance still holds. The medical assistant may say, "No, I am sorry, Dr. Frank is not in. May I take a message?" or "No, I am sorry, but Dr. Frank will be at the hospital most of the morning. May I ask her to return your call after 1 o'clock?"

If the physician is in and is available for telephone calls, a typical response would be, "Yes, Dr. Frank is in; may I say who is calling, please?"

When physicians prefer to keep telephone calls to a minimum, say, "Yes, Dr. Frank is here, but she is not free to come to the phone. May I take a message, please?" By responding in this way, the physician is not committed to taking the call.

During the time that a physician is examining a patient, he or she will not wish to be interrupted with a routine call. In such cases you might say, "Yes, Dr. Frank is in but is with a patient right now. May I help you?" or "Yes, Dr. Frank is in but is with a patient right now. Is there anything you would like me to ask her?"

Try to guard against being overprotective. A patient should be able to talk with the physician when necessary; but unless it is an emergency, the patient is probably willing to do so at the convenience of the physician. The medical assistant who answers the telephone acts as a screen, not a roadblock.

CRITICAL THINKING APPLICATION

Ashlynn answers the phone and a male pharmaceutical representative who has been visiting the clinic for several months is on the phone. She cheerfully greets him and asks if he is calling to make an appointment. He states that he wants to make an appointment with Ashlynn—for a date. How should she handle this call? What problems could arise if this were a patient and Ashlynn accepted the date?

Find out exactly how calls are to be handled when the physician is out of the office and under what circumstances he or she can be interrupted when the physician is on the premises. **Cultivate** a reputation for being helpful and reliable. Medical assistants will save the physician many interruptions if patients develop confidence in their ability to help them and have faith in their promises to take their messages and deliver them properly.

Minimizing Wait Time

When a call cannot be put through immediately, ask, "Would you prefer to wait, or shall I call you back when Dr. Frank is free?"

If the caller elects to wait, remember that waiting with a silent telephone can be irritating and **tedious**. The waiting time always seems long, no matter how brief it really is. Many of today's phones are equipped with timers that tell the caller exactly how long they have been waiting on hold. The longer they wait, the more irritated they may become. Let no more than 1 minute pass without breaking in with some reassuring comment. For instance: "I'm sorry, Dr. Frank is still busy."

If the wait is longer than expected, the caller may wish to reconsider and call back at another time or have the call returned. By going back on the line at frequent intervals, the caller has an opportunity to express such concerns. Ask the caller if he or she wishes to continue waiting. The medical assistant could say, "I'm sorry to keep you waiting so long, Ms. Hughes. Would you prefer to have me return your call when Dr. Frank is free?"

Try to give the caller some estimate of when he or she may expect the return call. In any event, be considerate and remember that irritation can be lessened each time the medical assistant returns to the call by saying, "Thank you for waiting, Ms. Hughes."

When it is necessary to leave the telephone and obtain information, ask the caller, "Will you please wait while I get the information?" Listen for a reply. If it will take longer than a few seconds to get the information, give some estimate of the time required and offer to call back. When returning to the telephone, always thank the caller for waiting. Requests that might require pulling the patient's chart from the files are best handled with a call back to the patient.

Remember that leaving a person on hold ties up one of the physician's telephone lines, and an emergency call could be coming through, or new patients might be attempting to call. The majority of phone calls that come in to a physician's office during the day are important, so the lines should be kept clear as much as possible.

Transferring a Call

Always identify the person who is calling when a call is transferred to the physician or another person in the facility. Always ask the patient's permission to place him or her on hold and to transfer the call. It is considered poor customer service to simply transfer the call to a co-worker's voice mail without warning the caller that the person is not available. Any person who refuses to give a name should not be put through unless the medical assistant has been specifically instructed to do so. If the person is not immediately available, ask the caller whether he or she would prefer to be put through to voice mail. Some callers simply believe their call will receive more attention if a human takes the message. If the caller insists, take a written message and deliver it to the proper person as soon as possible.

One very important skill that all medical assistants should learn is "who does what" in the medical facility. Knowing about the functions of the office and which person is responsible for which areas will make a significant difference in the customer service provided to the patient. To illustrate: suppose that the medical office employs one insurance receptionist, named Sarah, and three insurance billers. Opel handles names that begin with A through G, David handles names that begin with H through P, and Andrea handles names that begin with Q through Z. If a call comes to the office and the patient has an insurance question, the medical assistant could put the call through to Sarah. However, better customer service dictates that the medical assistant ask the name of the patient and put the call through to the person who handles that patient's particular claims. If the patient's name is Rebecca Whitehead, the medical assistant should call Andrea and ask if she may transfer Ms. Whitehead's call to her. The fewer times the caller is transferred, the happier the caller.

When the caller is a patient, the physician will probably need the patient's chart at hand during the conversation. If there is no concern about others hearing the conversation, the medical assistant can announce the caller's name on the intercom and tell the physician that the chart is on its way back to his or her office. Remember that it is vital to protect the patient's right to privacy. If there are others within hearing range, take the chart to the physician and say, "Dr. Frank, this patient is waiting on the telephone to speak with you."

Ending a Call

When a caller's requests have been satisfied, do not encourage inappropriate chatting or permit the call to monopolize your time unnecessarily. The telephone lines should be cleared for other calls. Allow the person who placed the call to hang up first, and be sure to thank him or her for calling. Close the conversation with some form of "good-bye" and replace the telephone on its cradle gently.

Taking a Telephone Message

Always have a pen or pencil in hand and a message pad nearby when answering the telephone. Several calls may be answered before there is an opportunity to relay a message or carry out a promise of action. The *written message* is vital (Procedure 9-2).

There are numerous types of message pads available today (Figure 9-4). An ordinary spiral-bound stenographer's notebook is inexpensive, sturdy, and well proportioned; lies flat on a desk; and can be filed for future reference if desired. Never use small scraps of paper for messages; they are too easily lost. Bear in mind that the message book should be kept indefinitely in the medical office, because it could be used as evidence in a court of law. Messages should also be added to the patient's chart once acted on, or at a minimum, noted in the chart.

Date the bottom of the first blank page in the notebook at the beginning of each day. This creates a permanent record that can be referred to later if the need arises. Check off each message in the log as it is delivered or taken care of. This creates a good reminder system.

A minimum of seven items are needed to take a telephone message correctly:
1. The name of the person to whom the call is directed
2. The name of the person calling
3. The caller's daytime and/or evening telephone number
4. The reason for the call
5. The action to be taken
6. The date and time of the call
7. The initials of the person taking the call

Messages that are to be transmitted to another person may be rewritten on individual message slips and delivered or posted on a message board later. Impression-sensitive message pads that provide a copy of each page ensure that no message will be forgotten and are the best way to keep track of messages. The nature of the message will determine whether it should be reported immediately. The person who completes the call must sign and date it. If the call is from a patient and relates in any way to the medical history, or if any instructions were given or queries answered, this information should be placed in the patient's chart. Message forms are available that have a self-adhesive backing and can be placed permanently in the patient's case history.

Taking Action on Telephone Messages

The message procedure is not complete until the necessary action has been taken. Notations on the memo pad should be carried over to the following day if they have not been completed, but this should be a rare occurrence. Do not trust to memory messages that were not attended to from previous days; always carry them forward in writing.

Make brief notations of patients' reactions while talking to them on the telephone. The physician does not require a character study, but it is helpful to know when a patient appears fearful, apprehensive, or nervous. If a patient shows such symptoms, it may be wise to consult with or transfer the call to the physician.

When the employer is talking to another physician about a referral, the medical assistant may be requested to take down a brief outline of the patient's case history while listening on the extension telephone. This information can be typewritten and incorporated with the patient's chart and handed to the physician before the patient is seen.

Retaining Telephone Records

Each office must develop a policy regarding retention of telephone message records. Many offices elect to keep message pads for the same period that the statute of limitations exists for medical professional liability cases. Remember, phone records would include telephone bills, especially those that detail long-distance charges. Keeping these records can be of assistance in proving any number of claims, including the number of times that patients called the office and the fact that calls to the patient were returned. Be sure that accurate telephone records are kept to ensure good patient care and customer service

Typical Incoming Calls

One reason for having a medical assistant answer incoming calls is to spare the physician unnecessary interruptions during visits with patients. Many calls relate to the administrative aspects of the office and can actually be better handled by the medical assistant. The policy regarding how calls are to be handled should be clearly set forth in the office procedures manual.

Some of the kinds of calls that can be handled by the medical assistant in most offices will be discussed next.

PROCEDURE **9-2**

Taking a Telephone Message

GOAL: To take an accurate telephone message and follow up on the requests made by the caller.

EQUIPMENT AND SUPPLIES

- Telephone
- Message pad
- Pen or pencil
- Notepad

PROCEDURAL STEPS

1 Answer the telephone using the guidelines in Procedure 9-1.
Purpose: Answering promptly and courteously conveys interest in the caller and promotes good customer service.

2 Using a message pad or notepad, take the phone message, obtaining the following information:
- The name of the person to whom the call is directed
- The name of the person calling
- The caller's daytime and/or telephone number
- The reason for the call
- The action to be taken
- The date and time of the call
- The initials of the person taking the call
Purpose: Accurate information allows the staff member to address the caller's issues quickly and efficiently.

3 Repeat the information back to the caller after the message is recorded on the message pad.

Purpose: To verify that all information taken has been recorded accurately.

4 Provide the caller with an approximation of the time and date that he or she will be called back, if possible.
Purpose: To be considerate of the patient's time, and keep him or her from sitting next to the phone awaiting a call.

5 End the call and wait for the caller to hang up first.

6 Deliver the phone message to the appropriate person. Separate trays or slots for each staff member are helpful.

7 Follow up on important messages.
Purpose: To make certain that important issues are addressed in a timely manner.

8 Keep old message books for future reference. Carbonless copies will allow the facility to keep a permanent record of phone messages.
Purpose: To have a permanent source of messages in case a number is needed after the paper message has been discarded.

9 File pertinent phone messages in the patient's chart.
Purpose: To keep a permanent record of important information in the patient's chart.

New Patients and Return Appointments

Procedures for handling appointments for new patients and scheduling return appointments are discussed in the chapter on appointment scheduling. In general, provide excellent customer service to the caller. Remember that the routine questions that may be asked should be answered in a polite and cheerful manner. Follow the designated office procedure as to what information should be gathered and recorded when appointments are made.

Directions

Each office should have a clear set of directions written out that can be read to the caller when there is a request for directions. Prepare directions from various points in the area; for instance, one set would guide a patient who is coming from the north, and another set will be for a patient coming from the south. Place these directions close to the telephone so that all employees can access them easily. Not all employees live close to the clinic or are familiar with all areas, so the written set of directions

will be helpful to all staff members and those who call the facility.

Inquiries About Bills

A patient may ask to speak with the physician about a recent bill. Ask the caller to hold for a moment while the ledger is pulled. If nothing irregular is found on the ledger, return to the telephone and say, "I have your account in front of me now. Perhaps I can answer your question." Most likely, the caller will have some simple inquiry, such as whether the insurance has paid, or may wish to delay making a payment until the next month. Not all patients realize that the medical assistant usually makes such decisions and is the best person with whom to discuss these matters.

A patient may have a question about a statement that was received in the mail. If billing matters are handled by another employee, tell the patient that you will transfer his or her call to the billing office. If you are responsible for billing, politely ask the patient to hold the line while you pull the patient ledger. When you return to the line, thank the patient for waiting and explain the charges carefully. If

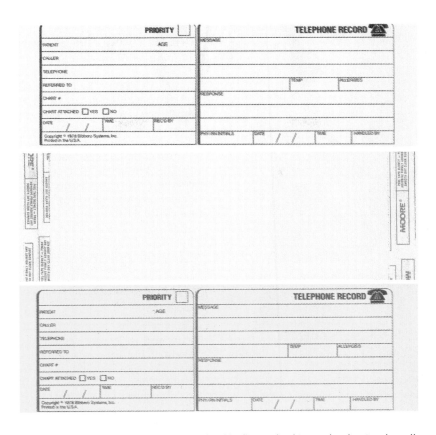

FIGURE 9-4   Phone message forms with self-adhesive backing make charting the call easier and more time efficient. (Courtesy Bibbero Systems, Inc., Petaluma, CA 94654.)

there is an error, apologize and say a corrected statement will be sent out at once. Always remember to thank the patient for calling. If patients are properly advised about charges at the time that services are rendered, the number of these calls will be considerably reduced.

Inquiries About Fees

Fees vary widely in each medical office, and it is very difficult to quote an exact fee before the patient is seen by the physician. However, a good range should be given to the patient as to what they should expect to pay, especially on the first visit. Asking a patient to just appear at the office without having any idea of the cost is unreasonable. Discuss with the physician or office manager what range should be quoted to the patient and then follow your quotes with the statement that the fees will vary, depending on the patient's condition and tests that the physician orders. If fees are regularly discussed on the telephone, write a suggested script in the policy manual. Do not be evasive. Have a schedule of fees available.

Participating Provider

Patients may call the office to inquire as to whether the physician is a participating **provider** with their particular insurance plan or managed care organization. The physician should keep a carefully updated list of which plans are valid. This is important, because insurance benefits vary for participating and nonparticipating providers.

Requests for Assistance With Insurance

In today's environment of managed care, copays, Medicaid, and Medicare, insurance claims will more than likely be completed and filed by the healthcare facility. Nevertheless, patients may call to inquire about their coverage or ask whether there has been any response to the filing of the claims. A medical assistant or member of the staff whose responsibility is the filing of insurance claims will have the knowledge to answer these inquiries (Figure 9-5). Be patient with these inquiries, because insurance is a difficult subject to understand, even for those who are trained and familiar with the various forms and procedures to use. Some patients, especially elderly ones, are quite confused when dealing with these insurance companies. Help them as much as possible so that they can collect the benefits to which they are entitled.

Radiology and Laboratory Reports

Laboratory and radiological findings may be telephoned to the physician's office on the day the procedures are performed, when their results are urgently needed. The medical assistant can take these reports and relay them to the physician. More often, the report is faxed to the physician if it is a **stat** report. Original reports will be delivered by mail for the permanent record. Some facilities are equipped to receive laboratory results directly from the laboratory by computer.

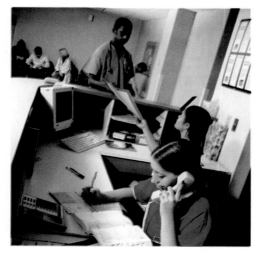

FIGURE 9-5 Many of the calls that come into the medical office are insurance questions, with which the medical assistant will assist the caller.

Satisfactory Progress Reports From Patients

Physicians sometimes ask patients to phone the office to report on their conditions a few days after their office visit. The medical assistant can take such calls and relay the information to the physician if the report is satisfactory. Assure the patient that you will inform the physician about the call.

Routine Reports From Hospitals and Other Sources

There may be routine calls from a hospital and other sources reporting a patient's progress. If it is only a normal reporting procedure, take the message carefully, make sure that the physician sees it and then place the message in the patient's medical record.

Office Administration Matters

Not all calls concern patients. There may be calls from the accountant or auditor or calls regarding banking procedures, office supplies, or office maintenance, most of which the medical assistant can handle or refer to the appropriate person. For some of these calls the medical assistant may need to gather additional information and return the call.

Requests for Referrals

Physicians who are liked and respected by their patients frequently will be called for referrals to other specialists. If the physician has furnished the medical assistant with a list of practitioners for this purpose, these inquiries can usually be handled without consulting the physician. However, the physician should always be informed of such requests.

Some managed care organizations require a physician referral before a patient may see a specialist. This referral should come from the physician, unless he or she has authorized automatic referrals. Handle these calls as quickly as possible so that the patient may make an appointment to see the referral physician.

Prescription Refills

Pharmacies will periodically call the physician's office to obtain approval for a patient to refill a prescription. Most prescriptions have a specific notation as to the number of times the prescription can be refilled. However, the physician may have noted in the chart that a certain medication is to be taken for 6 months, but the prescription was only written for 1 to 2 months. Any prescription refills should be authorized only with the physician's approval. Tell the pharmacist that you will have to check with the physician and call back. Be sure that state regulations and procedures are followed any time the medical assistant deals with prescription refills or calls (Procedure 9-3).

Special Incoming Calls

Patients Refusing to Discuss Symptoms

Occasionally patients will call and wish to talk with the physician about symptoms that they are reluctant to discuss with a medical assistant. Patients do have a right to privacy, but the physician cannot be expected to take numerous calls from patients who do not wish to speak to the medical assistant. If the patient refuses to discuss any symptoms, suggest that he or she make an appointment with the physician to discuss the problem in person.

Unsatisfactory Progress Reports

If a patient under treatment reports that he or she is still not feeling well or that the prescription the doctor provided is not helping, do not try to practice medicine by giving the patient medical advice. Make detailed notes about the patient's comments, then present them to the physician. He or she will make the decision as to whether the patient should return to the office or may make a medication change. Follow up with the patient and convey the physician's instructions.

Requests for Test Results

When the physician orders special tests for the patient, the patient may be told to call the office in a couple of days for the results. Never assume that the patient will call for results. It is ultimately the responsibility of the physician to notify the patient of test results. Be certain that the physician has seen the results and has given permission before sharing the results with the patient. Patients do not always understand that the medical assistant does not have the privilege of giving out information without the permission of the physician. If the result is unfavorable, the physician should be the one to inform the patient and give further instructions. This call must be handled tactfully; otherwise, the patient may feel as if the staff is concealing information.

Most physicians prefer that medical assistants only provide normal test results to the patients. However, the medical assistant may provide abnormal test results to the patient if authorized by the physician. For example, when a patient has a questionable Pap smear, the medical

PROCEDURE 9-3

Calling the Pharmacy With New or Refill Prescriptions

GOAL: To call in an accurate prescription to the pharmacy for a patient in the most efficient manner.

EQUIPMENT AND SUPPLIES

- Prescription
- Notepad
- Patient chart
- Telephone

PROCEDURAL STEPS

1 Receive the call from the patient requesting a prescription, using appropriate telephone technique.
Purpose: To provide consistently good customer service when speaking with callers.

2 Obtain the following information from the patient:
  - Patient's name
  - Telephone number where he or she can be reached
  - Patient's symptoms and current condition
  - History of this condition
  - Treatments the patient has tried
  - Pharmacy name and telephone number
Purpose: To have the information the physician will need to make a determination as to whether a prescription will be called in for the patient, or whether he or she needs to come to the office to be seen by the doctor.

3 Write in the patient's chart the prescription that the physician wishes the patient to have. Be very careful to transcribe the information correctly. Read it back to the physician.
Purpose: To have a permanent record of the prescription in the chart, and make certain that the prescription is exactly what the physician wants the patient to take, eliminating errors in medication name and dosage.

4 If the prescription is a refill, give the physician the patient's chart with the message requesting a refill attached, along with the information in procedure step two as listed above.
Purpose: To have the patient's chart as reference and provide the physician with the information needed to determine if the medication requested should be refilled.

5 Note the comments that the physician writes in the chart. If the prescription is written or a refill is approved, call the patient's pharmacy and ask to speak to a member of the pharmacy staff.

6 Ask the pharmacy staff member to repeat the prescription back to you.
Purpose: To verify that the pharmacy staff member took the prescription down accurately.

7 Note the date and time that the prescription was called to the pharmacy in the chart.
Purpose: To provide a permanent record of the medication being called to the pharmacy, along with the correct dosage amounts and frequency of doses.

8 Call the patient to notify him or her that the prescription has been called in. Provide any information regarding the prescription doses, frequency, etc. that is requested by the physician. Tell the patient when to return to the office, if necessary. Ask the patient to write this information down.
Purpose: To inform the patient as to the dosage and frequency, so that if an error is made by the pharmacy, the patient will notice a discrepancy and the error can be corrected prior to taking any dosages of the medication.

---

assistant is usually the person who calls the patient with the results and further instructions from the physician. If the patient then has any questions about the test results, he or she must then be referred to the physician. The medical assistant will need good communication skills to relay information such as this without crossing the lines of practicing medicine without a license. HIV test results should never be given on the telephone, and the physician should always inform the patient when a HIV test returns as being positive.

Patients who call the office for results of tests must be appropriately identified before the results are given. Some offices use a special code that is written in the chart, and knowledge of this code or password gives the person access to the information. Make sure the right individual is on the line before offering test results. Especially be careful in situations in which the family includes a "Senior" and "Junior." If the medical assistant calls and asks for Robert Smith, the elder Mr. Smith may answer, whereas the younger Mr. Smith is the one who came to the office for tests. Awkward situations can be created when the office staff do not accurately identify the patient.

Requests for Information From Third Parties

The patient must give written permission before any member of the physician's staff can give information to third-party callers. This includes insurance companies, attorneys, relatives, neighbors, employers, and any other third party.

Complaints About Care or Fees

A medical assistant may be able to offer a satisfactory explanation to a patient who complains about the care he or she received or the fee charged. If a patient seems angry, offer to pull the chart, research the problem, and if needed, discuss it with the physician. Four magic words often calm the angry patient: "Let me help you." This reassures the patient that someone is willing to talk about the problem. However, if you are unable to appease the patient easily, the physician or office manager may prefer to talk directly to the patient.

Calls From the Physician's Family and Friends

Personal calls to the physician from family members or friends are handled in accordance with instructions from the physician. If the physician does not wish to take the calls, the medical assistant must tactfully tell the caller that the physician cannot be disturbed at that time.

Calls From Staff Members' Family and Friends

The telephone lines should never be burdened with an excess of personal calls to the staff. A call is necessary in emergencies, but staff members should never monopolize the telephone for personal business and conversations. Emergency calls could be coming through, and the lines must be clear. Keep these calls to an absolute minimum.

Handling Difficult Calls

Angry Callers

No matter how efficient you are on the telephone or how well liked your employer may be, sooner or later there will be an angry caller on the line. There may be a legitimate reason for the anger, or the caller's irritation may have resulted from a misunderstanding. It is a real challenge to handle such calls. First, take the required action—even if it is to say that the matter will be discussed with the physician as soon as possible and the patient will be called back later. If answers are not readily available, a friendly assurance that the situation is important and that every attempt will be made to find the answer quickly will usually calm the angry feelings.

The medical assistant may find that lowering the tone of voice and volume of speech may force the angry caller to do the same in order to hear. This method does not always work, but it is usually true that when dealing with an angry person, calm promotes calm. There are always those who will misread this method and become even angrier, thinking that their complaint is not being taken seriously. Human relations are so critical when dealing with other individuals, because the more skilled the medical assistant becomes, the better able he or she is to deal with multiple types of personalities.

Always avoid getting angry in response, and try to get to the root of the real problem. Express interest and understanding, take careful notes, and follow through with the problem to the most appropriate resolution. Never

"pass the buck" by saying, "That isn't my job," or "I am not the person who filed that insurance claim." No matter whose fault the problem is, it is best to deal with it and find a solution instead of placing blame.

CRITICAL THINKING APPLICATION

An angry caller raises his voice at Ashlynn over an issue that happened before she began to work at the facility. She suggests that he speak with the office manager, but he refuses and continues to berate Ashlynn. What choices does she have in this situation and should she simply hang up on the patient?

Aggressive Callers

Aggressive callers insist that they receive whatever action *they* feel is necessary, and they usually insist on action immediately. Treat these callers with a calm, poised attitude, but do not allow the caller's aggression to initiate inappropriate action. Reassure the caller that the concern being shared is valid and will receive the full attention of the right person. Explain when they can expect a response from the office, and be sure to follow up that the appropriate action was taken on the call.

Unauthorized Inquiry Calls

Some individuals call the physician's office requesting information to which they are not entitled. These callers must be told politely but firmly that such information cannot be provided to them because of privacy laws. Insistent callers should be referred to the office manager or physician.

Sales Calls

Sales calls are often thought of as an interruption to the physician's busy day, but some salespersons may have important information on products, equipment, or services that the office uses regularly. Do not completely disregard salespersons, but do not allow them to monopolize time or telephone lines, either. Keep these calls quick and to the point. Most professional salespersons realize that the physician's and the staff's time is extremely valuable and will respect this. Developing a good rapport with representatives ("reps") from the companies whose products are frequently used in the practice may result in discounted prices and first news of sales and promotions. In turn, these people rarely waste the time of office personnel.

Physician Shopping

Some calls will be from prospective patients seeking information about the office and the types of illnesses or conditions that the physician treats. Consider these callers to be future patients, or as those who may refer patients to the office. Always be polite and answer questions respectfully. Remember, even if the caller does not become a patient, he or she may share his or her impressions of the practice with another prospective patient.

Complaints

For callers with a complaint, use an approach similar to the one used with angry callers. Do not make an attempt to blame, and never argue with the patient. Find the source of the problem and then present the options to the caller as to how the situation can be resolved. It is very important to remember to treat callers in the same manner that one would wish to be treated. A complaint may seem small and insignificant to the office staff, but to the patient, it could be paramount. Provide good customer service to patients, and complaints will be few and far between.

Emergency Calls

Many emergency calls require judgment on the part of the person answering the phone in the medical practice. Good judgment comes from experience and proper training by the physician in what constitutes a real emergency in each type of practice and how such calls should be handled. If the physician is not immediately available, what should the staff do? The person answering the telephone should first determine whether the call is truly urgent.

If the physician is in, the call should probably be transferred immediately. All offices should have a written plan of action for the times that the physician is not physically present in the office to handle the call. The physician and medical assistant may also jointly develop typical questions to ask the caller to determine the validity and disposition of an emergency. Some examples of questions to ask would include the following:

- At what telephone number can you be reached?
- What are the chief symptoms?
- When did they start?
- Has this happened before?
- Are you alone?
- Do you have transportation?

If the call is such that an ambulance is dispatched, the policy in most offices is to stay on the line until the paramedics or police arrive on the scene.

Triage Guidelines

In the facility with multiple employees, the physician may designate one individual as the triage nurse or assistant. Within the environment of managed care, every physician would be wise to have a written telephone protocol for handling urgent situations and emergencies. The protocol should state that the employees are bound by the written guidelines and that any giving of advice by unauthorized personnel may be grounds for dismissal.

A special sheet of instructions listing specific medical emergencies such as chest pain, heavy bleeding, fainting, seizure, and poisoning should be posted by each telephone. The phone numbers for the nearest poison control center, hospital, and ambulance should be listed. Such calls should be routed to a physician immediately. Additional instructions should include what action to take if no physician is available (e.g., sending the patient to an emergency department or calling an ambulance or 911). Most offices have some means of constant contact with the physician, whether by pager, cell phone, or another method.

Getting the Information the Physician Needs

As the medical assistant gains experience and knows the physician better, he or she will begin to have a sense of the questions that the physician will have for patients that call the facility. For instance, the physician will be interested in how long the patient has had symptoms, what makes the symptoms better or worsens them, what remedies have been tried, what has worked and not worked, and other specifics about the condition the patient is experiencing. If the patient complains of painful urination, the medical assistant will learn to ask about pain in the back, blood in the urine and/or stool, and cramping. One way to learn about questions to ask is to listen to the physician carefully as he or she questions patients about their symptoms. This will help the medical assistant to learn more about signs and symptoms, and will enable him or her to be a better assistant to the physician.

Remember to always be "patient with your patients." Those who call the medical office for help are almost never at their best. When feeling ill, people are often short-tempered and even display poor manners. Some can be verbally abusive. Care for patients as if they were family members, and they will feel care and compassion in the medical facility.

Telephones in the Millennium

Voice Mail

Voice mail is widely used in today's business offices, because it affords an around-the-clock method for receiving patient messages. Yet it can prove frustrating to many who find themselves speaking to an electronic device more often than talking with a human being. Voice mail allows the caller to hear a recorded message that may also provide information about what to do in case of an emergency. Voice mail is similar to an answering machine and will record a caller's message that can later be retrieved. Often voice mail allows special temporary greetings when the user is away from the office. Keep patients happy by answering voice mail messages promptly.

Answering Machines

Answering machines do the same job as voice mail, but a machine is attached to the telephone rather than being an integral part of the office phone system. With the inexpensive cost of voice mail, most businesses have retired their answering machines and have chosen more modern methods of message-taking.

Answering Services

Because a physician's telephone is an all-important tool of the practice, there must be someone to answer it at all times—day and night, weekends and holidays. This presents no problem during weekdays, but nights and weekends require special attention. Most physicians subscribe to telephone answering services that provide round-the-clock coverage. Answering services normally provide an operator (rather than a recording device) to answer the phones, and this is often preferred over standard voice mail. There are two types of operator-answered services. With the first type, physician-subscribers leave messages with, or obtain patients' messages from, a service whose number appears in the local telephone directory after the physician's number, with a notation to call the second number after hours. This form of service is somewhat inconvenient for the patient but is far better than no coverage at all. In the second type, the answering service has a direct connection with the office telephone. When the telephone rings in the physician's office or at home, it also signals on the switchboard of the answering service. As long as the telephone is ringing, it will continue to signal at the answering service. If no one answers within a certain agreed-on number of rings, the answering service operator takes the call. This method provides continuous live telephone coverage.

Even during the day, such an answering service can function effectively. There may be times when the staff are assisting the physician and not available to answer the telephone. Not answering the telephone is extremely poor policy, so if the office has an agreement with the answering service, its operators will accept calls in such situations. With this direct-wire answering method, the operator answers the telephone in the same manner as the regular staff.

The answering service will greatly appreciate receiving a call every day from a member of the physician's staff before leaving the office with information as to where the physician will be during the evening or other special messages. The next morning, a staff member should call the service and ask for any messages they may have taken. Usually there will be messages from patients who called after office hours but whose calls were not urgent enough to merit an emergency call to the physician. An answering service can act as a buffer for the physician and help eliminate too frequent, unnecessary calls during the late evening or night hours.

Automatic Call Routing

In automatic call routing, a call is answered by an automated operator's message that presents a list of options, such as "If you are calling about your account, press 1; to make an appointment, press 2;" and so forth. The impersonal nature of automation does not lend itself well to answering the telephone in a private physician's office, but the medical assistant will encounter it frequently when placing outgoing calls.

Call Forwarding

Call forwarding allows the user to forward calls to another designated number, such as a cellular phone. Usually a code is entered, then the phone number to which the calls should be forwarded. This keeps the user from missing important calls when away from the main telephone.

Caller ID

Caller ID allows the user to see who is calling before picking up the handset to answer the phone. The caller's phone number and name appear on a screen, and the user can decide whether to take the call. If the user subscribes to call-waiting services, another benefit called *call-waiting caller ID* is often available. Call-waiting caller ID allows the user to see who is calling even when the user is already on the phone.

Cellular Phones

Considered a luxury item only 10 years ago, cellular (or cell) phones have become commonplace in today's world (Figure 9-6). Many people no longer have a home phone because of the expense of having two phones, and the cell phone is usually the better buy for the money. Several of the more popular cell phone companies offer free long-distance calls in the United States and may provide users free night and weekend minutes as a bonus. Some of today's advanced cell phones will even allow the user to access the Internet through the telephone, and the user can check email.

Pagers

The popularity of pagers has dwindled somewhat with the growth of cell phones. However, pagers are quite useful in reaching individuals to notify them that they are needed quickly. Physicians often carry pagers with them at all times.

Fax Machines

A fax machine can be a great time and labor saver in conveying patient information from physician to physician or from physician to hospital. It allows its user to send and receive copies of printed documents over telephone lines to other facilities that have fax machines (Figure 9-7). Most offices find this machine indispensable.

CELL PHONE RULES OF ETIQUETTE

1. *Hang Up and Drive:* Take care when using the phone and driving. It is best to pull over and talk on the phone instead of trying to manipulate the car and carry on a conversation.
2. *Turn Off the Phone at the Right Time:* Never leave the phone on during meetings or at public events like movies and formal dinners.
3. *Respect Personal Space:* Most people do not want to hear personal or business conversations while they are in line for a movie or eating dinner. Step away when speaking on the cell phone in public.
4. *The Phone Is Not a Human:* Nothing is more rude than having dinner with a friend and taking a casual call on the cell phone. Pay attention to the human and turn the phone off until later.
5. *Keep it Charged:* It is very frustrating to speak to someone on a cell phone who can not hear. Keeping the phone charged will cause less periods of static and more clarity when in use.

FIGURE 9-6   Etiquette rules for cellular phones.

Unless precautions are taken to ensure security of information arriving by fax, there is the danger of loss of confidentiality. When sending sensitive material, it is wise to telephone ahead to alert the receiver that this information will be arriving so that the appropriate person will be on hand to receive it.

Headsets

In today's world of multitasking, the headset helps a medical assistant to keep hands free while speaking on the phone. A popular headset is a very lightweight plastic earphone and microphone combination that allows the wearer to move about the room and to have the hands free (Figure 9-8). One brand name is StarSet. Originally designed for astronauts, it weighs less than 1 ounce and is worn behind the ear or clipped to the wearer's glasses. The headset can be equipped with a cord up to 10 feet long for easy mobility. It also has an optional quick-disconnect feature that allows the user to separate the headset even during a call without breaking the connection.

Using Long Distance and Special Services

Long-distance calls are simple to place, usually inexpensive, and efficient. When information is needed in a hurry, it is much more expedient to telephone rather than wait for an exchange of letters. Before placing a long-distance call, have the correct number ready. This number

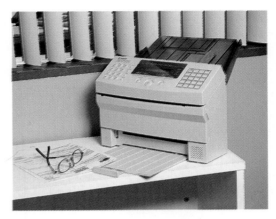

FIGURE 9-7   Fax machines allow the transfer of written data from one place to another with the simple dial of a telephone number.

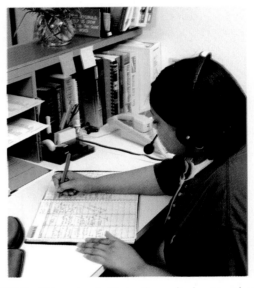

FIGURE 9-8   Using a headset helps the medical assistant keep hands free while using the telephone and is better ergonomically.

often may be obtained from a letterhead or from other records. If you do not have the number, you may obtain directory assistance by dialing the area code of the party you are calling, followed by 555-1212. In some areas you must dial 1 before the area code. Directory assistance is now an automated service in many regions, and you will be asked for the name of the city and the person you are calling. There is often a charge for using directory assistance.

One alternative to directory assistance is using the Internet to find phone numbers. A search for the business or physician the medical assistant is looking for may yield the information needed. There are also Internet services that allow the user to call long distance, and sometimes even internationally, through the computer with absolutely no long-distance charges.

Time Zones

The continental United States is divided into four standard time zones: Pacific, Mountain, Central, and Eastern

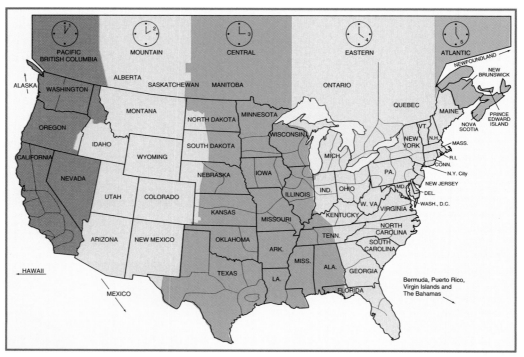

FIGURE 9-9 Time zones across the United States.

(Figure 9-9). When it is noon Pacific time, it is 3 PM Eastern time. When calling from San Francisco to New York, plan to make the call no later than 2 PM if the call is to a business or professional office. When it is 2 PM on the West Coast, it is 5 PM on the East Coast. Only Arizona, Hawaii, and a part of Indiana do not observe Daylight Saving Time.

International Service

International Direct Distance Dialing (IDDD) is available in many areas. International dialing codes are the same for all companies offering IDDD. Depending on your long-distance company, additional numbers or codes may preface the international access, country, and city codes. IDDD is still not available in all areas. If it is available, you may place international station-to-station calls by dialing in sequence:

1. International code 011
2. Country code
3. City code
4. Local telephone number
5. The pound sign (#) button if your telephone is Touch-Tone

After dialing any international code, allow at least 45 seconds for the ringing to start.

Wrong Numbers

One slip in direct distance dialing can mean a call to Los Angeles or New York instead of Dallas. If you reach a wrong long-distance number, be sure to obtain the name of the city and state that was called. Report this information promptly to the local operator, so the facility will not be charged for the call. If you are cut off before terminating a call, report this as well. The operator will either reconnect the call or make an adjustment of the charge.

Conference Calls

Conference telephone service is of great value to the medical profession in notifying and explaining to a family how a patient is progressing. It has exceptional value in family conferences, at which a quick decision by the entire family regarding a patient's condition is required.

This service can connect from 3 to 14 points for a two-way conference in which each person can hear or talk to all others participating. Conference calls may be local or long distance. Charges are added for the number of places connected, the mileage, and the length of the conversation.

Conference calls can be set up by a normal long-distance operator or through conference call services. To schedule a call, contact either an operator or the calling service and relay the pertinent information about time, date, and the individuals who are to be included in the call. Many businesses have conference call capabilities on their phone or computer systems. Notify everyone participating in the call of the time, date, number to call, and subjects to discuss. If prior arrangements are made with all parties, there is a better chance of reaching everyone and having a successful conference.

Operator-Assisted Calls and Services

Operator-assisted calls include calls such as:

- Person-to-person
- Billing to a third party
- Collect calls

- Requests for time and charges
- Certain calls placed from hotels
- Credit for wrong numbers
- Conference calls
- Some international calls

There is an initial charge and a service charge for operator-assisted calls provided through most phone service providers.

Office Telephone Equipment Needs

Number and Placement of Telephones

Familiarity with a multiple-line telephone system is a must for medical assistants. Few healthcare facilities can get along with just one telephone line. Two incoming lines along with a private outgoing line with a separate number for the physician's exclusive use is the minimum recommended.

One medical assistant can handle no more than two incoming lines, so the addition of more lines may also involve additional staffing (Figure 9-10). If there is a staff member assigned solely to dealing with insurance and billing, a separate line and listing in the telephone directory for this service may considerably lessen the load on the main incoming lines.

Telephones should be placed where they are accessible but private. Rather than placing telephones in the examining rooms, many practices have a wall telephone placed near a stand-up desktop outside the examining room.

Some facilities also place a telephone in the reception room for the convenience of patients and to prevent their asking to use the facility's phones. However, recent trends suggest that a separate telephone line with a limited calling area for the convenience of patients who need to call out may be preferable. This telephone should not be in the reception room but in an area available to patients on request. It should be placed low enough for use by patients in wheelchairs. Wherever possible, other telephones should be placed on the wall to conserve desk space.

Equipment Selection

Selection of telephone equipment and services offers many options. The *six-button key set*, with several incoming lines, an intercom line, and a hold button, has been the standard business phone for decades. It is still being used in many offices. Lights within the buttons flash slowly for incoming calls and blink rapidly to remind of calls being held; a steady light indicates that the line is in use.

A popular modern system is the two-line speaker phone that has distinctive ringing and flashing indicators that reveal which line is receiving a call. It also has other features:

- Last number redial
- Volume control on the receiver, ringer, and speaker
- Memory for frequently dialed numbers
- Intercom paging

Another available feature, *ring back on hold*, allows the caller who dials a busy number to place it on hold. When the called line is free, the connection is completed and the caller is reminded.

Larger facilities tend to select small switchboard-type equipment. One system can start with as few as 2 lines and 6 extensions and expand to a maximum of 8 outside lines and 24 extensions.

Using a Telephone Directory

The primary purpose of the telephone directory, of course, is to provide lists of those who have telephones, their telephone numbers, and, in most cases, their addresses. Additionally, the directory is an aid in checking the spelling of names and in locating certain types of businesses through the yellow pages. Some directories are color coded, with residence listings on white pages, business numbers on pink pages, and business by categories and advertisements on yellow pages. Often, federal, state, county, and city government listings are included as blue pages. Directories are usually organized into three sections:

- Introductory pages
- Alphabetical pages (white pages)
- Yellow pages

The introductory pages are sometimes entirely overlooked by subscribers. This section precedes the white alphabetical pages and provides basic information concerning the telephone services in the area, including the following:

- Emergency services (fire, police, ambulance, and highway patrol)
- Service calls
- Dialing instructions for local and long-distance calls
- Area codes for some cities

The introductory pages may also include the following:

- A survival guide
- Community service numbers
- Prefix locations
- Rates
- International calling information
- Time zones

Government Listings

Some directories include ZIP code maps for the local area. Take a few moments to become familiar with the local directory; then use it frequently for getting information fast.

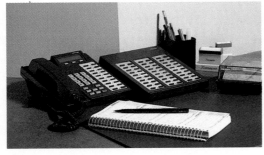

FIGURE 9-10 Multiline telephones allow numerous calls to come into the office at once. Each call deserves the same kind of attention and care from the medical assistant.

The white pages are an alphabetical listing of telephone subscribers with their telephone numbers and, in most cases, their addresses.

The yellow pages directory, sometimes published separately, contains listings for businesses arranged by the product or services they sell. Physicians are listed alphabetically, usually under the heading *Physicians and Surgeons*, and have the option of another listing by type of practice.

In some metropolitan areas, a street address telephone directory is published that is arranged by street address, followed by the name and telephone number of the person or business at that address.

Organizing a Personal Phone Directory

Organize telephone numbers in a tabbed 3- × 5-inch desktop file or a rotary file. Binders with clear sheet protectors also work well as personal phone directories. Emergency numbers might be typed on a colored card or flagged with a color tab. A personal directory of telephone numbers should include all the numbers that are frequently called.

Closing Comments

A telephone can be a tool to build a physician's practice, or one to break it apart. Medical assistants must become proficient in good telephone technique and must ensure that the caller hears compassion and patience in the voice of the medical assistant, even over the phone. A medical assistant must convey a genuine sense of caring for the patients that call the facility, just as if they were standing in the office face-to-face. By keeping this in mind, the medical assistant will play a major role in patient satisfaction, and the patients will find their medical care a pleasant process.

Patient Education

Today's telephone systems allow physicians to educate patients while they are on hold; recordings may be played that offer health information on subjects from *A* to *Z*. These messages can be professionally recorded or custom designed by the physician and staff. Special events may be announced, with the option to press a certain number for more information about the event.

Some phone directories offer listings of health information in the introductory pages. A patient may call a main number and then press a second number to reach the subject of his or her choice. Such features help to address the needs of today's more information-oriented consumers of health care, who have an interest in healthy lifestyles and in gaining useful information immediately.

Legal and Ethical Issues

The guidelines for medical confidentiality apply equally to telephone conversations, and care must be taken to ensure that no one overhears sensitive information. Use discretion when mentioning the name of a caller or a patient.

Placing and receiving personal phone calls should be avoided during work hours. This is a facet of professional behavior for the medical assistant and will probably be addressed in the office's employee procedures manual. The telephone is a business line and should be reserved for calls from patients or others conducting business with the office. The medical assistant should encourage friends and family to call him or her at home, so that all patient calls may get through to the office.

Telephone and message records may be brought into court as evidence, so be sure that all messages are complete and legible. Most offices should keep these records for at least the same amount of time as the statute of limitations in their state.

SUMMARY OF SCENARIO

Ashlynn is quickly becoming a part of the team at Dr. Frank's office and developing into a well-liked asset to the staff. She has learned to slow down when speaking on the phone and to adjust her volume and pitch, depending on the patient with whom she is speaking. Although she tends to be quite talkative, she is balancing just the right amount of friendly chat with the business at hand. Dr. Frank is very pleased with her performance.

Ashlynn takes care when she speaks to patients and others on the phone so that she does not breach confidentiality in any way. She has become comfortable with the way she is to answer the telephone. The pace of her speech and the wording are now a habit. Ashlynn is determined to maintain a professional relationship with all of the people related to her work environment. She is adept now at handling calls from angry patients and can maintain control with even the most aggressive callers. She shows much promise for a long and rewarding career in the medical field and is satisfied with the track her career is on at the present time. As she continues to settle into her position, she looks forward to learning more about efficiency and time management. Her good attitude and desire to learn will only enhance her performance at work and make her an employee worth promoting and of great value in the facility.

SUMMARY OF LEARNING OBJECTIVES

■ Incoming calls to a physician's office come from a wide variety of sources. Established or new patients may be calling to set appointments. Insurance companies may be seeking information about a claim. Hospitals, nursing facilities, or other healthcare units may need to report the progress of a patient. Laboratory results may be coming in for a patient who is very ill. Routine sales calls and telemarketing calls also come to the office, in addition to personal calls to the physician and staff members.

■ A pleasing telephone voice is one that is friendly and conveys a favorable impression of the physician's practice. Enunciate words and pronounce them clearly and distinctly. Vary the pitch of your voice, avoiding a monotonous or droning manner. Always be courteous and use tact.

■ The telephone handset should be held around the middle of the shaft, with the mouthpiece situated approximately 1 inch from the lips, in front of the teeth. Talk directly into the handset so the caller can clearly hear what is being said. Do not hold the mouthpiece beneath the chin, because the voice may not be heard clearly. Do not lean the head downward to hold the phone between the ear and the shoulder to avoid sore muscles and neck problems.

■ It is vital to be courteous to patients and other callers. First impressions are important, and a medical assistant's phone manner sets the tone for the caller's perception of the physician's practice. Customer service is important to today's physician, because many patients have choices among their healthcare providers as to which physician provides their care, and the attitude of staff members may play a large part in such a decision. Good customer care to patients means that they will not only continue to see the provider, but they will also refer other patients to the physician. This is one of the best ways to help a practice grow.

■ The physician's time is valuable but is also centered around his or her patients. It would be physically impossible for the physician to take all of the calls from those who wished to talk each day. Therefore the medical assistant must screen the physician's calls and make decisions about which ones should be put through to the physician. The medical assistant should offer to take a message and attempt to find out exactly what the caller's needs are and how they can be resolved. The patient should not feel that the physician is totally inaccessible, but must also understand that the patient in the office must have his or her full attention.

■ Seven distinct items are needed when taking a phone message, including the name of the person to whom the call should be directed and the name of the person calling. The caller's telephone number must be noted as well as the reason for the call. The

medical assistant should describe the action to be taken. The date and time of the call should always be noted, as well as the initials of the person taking the call, so that if there is any question, that person can be identified and asked.

■ Never return anger when a caller is angry. Remain calm and speak in tones that are perhaps slightly quieter than those of the caller. This often prompts the caller to lower his or her tone of voice. Offer to help the angry person, and ask questions to gain control of the conversation, moving it toward solution. Do not argue with angry callers.

■ Callers who have a complaint should be handled in a similar way as angry callers. Remain calm and offer to help. Take a serious interest in what the caller has to say. Let the caller know that his or her concerns are important to the staff and the physician. Find the source of the problem and determine exactly what the caller wants or expects toward its resolution. Always follow up with complaints and be sure that they were resolved as much to the caller's satisfaction as possible.

■ Several questions should be asked when an emergency call comes to the medical office. First, obtain a phone number at which the caller can be reached in case there is a sudden disconnection. Ask about the chief symptoms and when they started. Find out if the patient has had similar symptoms in the past and what happened in that situation. Determine whether the patient is alone, has transportation, or needs an ambulance dispatched to the location. In cases of severe emergencies, do not hang up the phone until the ambulance or police arrive.

■ The introductory pages of the telephone book contain several sections of useful information, such as area codes, emergency service information, long-distance calling information, time zones, government listings, and community service numbers. It may be helpful to tear these pages out and place them in clear sheet protectors, then add them to a binder for easy reference.

INTERNET CONNECTIONS

- The Dartnell Corporation
www.dartnellcorp.com

CHAPTER 10

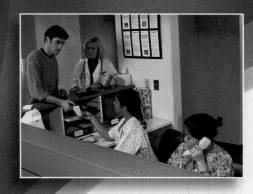

Scenario

Ramona West is the medical assistant in charge of scheduling appointments for Dr. Charlotte Brown. Ramona is an extremely organized person who thinks quickly and creatively. One of her professional goals is to ensure that the office stays on schedule throughout each day and that patient wait time is kept to an absolute minimum. She is fortunate that Dr. Brown is cooperative and time oriented, so they work well together to reach this common goal.

Ramona usually arrives at work at least 15 minutes early to begin her preparations for the day. She pulls patient charts each evening for the next day, so that they are easily accessible each morning. Throughout the course of her duties, she pays particular attention to the patients that arrive in the office. Ramona greets each patient by name. She often makes a short note in the patient chart about what events are happening in the life of each patient. With a quick glance, she remembers that a certain patient has a new granddaughter, or another patient just returned from a weeklong Caribbean cruise. Ramona uses this information to carry on a brief but cordial conversation with the patient. Patients appreciate that she goes the extra mile to remember something about them, and this promotes excellent patient relations.

Ramona leaves a little time in the morning and afternoon for emergency appointments. She calls to confirm patient appointments in advance or emails them, and this increases her show rate. Her friendly and caring attitude make her a favorite among the patients, and Dr. Brown is pleased with the relationship-building skills that Ramona has developed.

Scheduling Appointments

National Curriculum Competencies

ADMINISTRATIVE COMPETENCIES

1a. Schedule and manage appointments
1b. Schedule inpatient and outpatient admissions and procedures

TRANSDISCIPLINARY COMPETENCIES

1b. Recognize and respond to verbal communication
1d. Demonstrate telephone techniques
2d. Document appropriately
3a. Explain general office policies
3b. Instruct individuals according to their needs
4a. Utilize computer software to maintain office systems

Vocabulary

disruption An unexpected event that throws a plan into disorder; an interruption that prevents a system or process from continuing as usual or as expected.

established patients Patients who are returning to the office who have previously been seen by the physician.

expediency A means of achieving a particular end, as in a situation requiring haste or caution.

integral Essential; being an indispensable part of a whole.

interaction A two-way communication; mutual or reciprocal action or influence.

intermittent Coming and going at intervals; not continuous.

interval Space of time between events.

matrix Something in which a thing originates, develops, takes shape, or is contained; a base on which to build.

no-show A person who fails to keep an appointment without giving advance notice.

prerequisite Something that is necessary to an end or to carry out a function.

proficiency Competency as a result of training or practice.

socioeconomic Relating to a combination of social and economic factors.

triage Process of evaluating the urgency of medical need and prioritizing treatment.

The most valuable asset within a medical practice is the physician's time. The person responsible for scheduling this time must understand the practice, be familiar with the working habits of the physicians, and have clear guidelines for time management within the practice.

Appointment scheduling is the process that determines which patients will be seen by the physician, the dates and times of appointments, and how much time will be allotted to each patient based on his or her complaint, as well as the physician's availability. Time management involves the realization that there will always be unforeseen interruptions and delays. Most providers of medical care find that efficient scheduling of appointments is one of the most important factors in the success of the practice. There are many approaches to scheduling, and each facility must find what suits it best.

Guidelines for Appointment Scheduling

One of the most common complaints that patients have is the amount of money they pay for such short visits with the physician. A patient may say, "I only saw the doctor for 5 minutes and could not even remember all the questions I wanted to ask!" The patient must feel confi-dent that the physician took enough time to understand his or her concerns. Well-planned scheduling and adherence to that schedule will allow the physician to do more than run in and out of examination rooms, leaving little time for the patient to talk with the physician.

Some medical offices stick to a strict schedule, with little room for maneuvering, whereas many are more flexible in scheduling to meet the needs of the patients and the providers. The key to good scheduling is organization and teamwork in the office. Without these, even the best-planned schedule will not succeed.

The person who is scheduling appointments must learn the physician's habits and desires. If the physician suggests scheduling patients every 15 minutes but always spends 20 to 25 minutes with a patient, the schedule must be adjusted. Talk with the physician and/or office manager and compromise so that the schedule is a workable one. Some physicians need prompting to end the patient visit and move to the next patient. The medical assistant who is assisting in the examination room can help the physician remain on schedule.

Guides for Scheduling

The scheduling system must be individualized to each specific practice. The following guidelines are general and can be applied to any practice, whether paper-based or computer-based. Three items must be considered when scheduling—patient need, physician preference and habits, and available facilities.

Patient Need

A major consideration in determining office hours and appointment times is the **socioeconomic** status of the area being served. The office staff should answer the following questions:

- Is the office located in a busy metropolitan area or a rural agricultural community?
- Are the patients young, middle-aged, or retirement age?
- Is the area more industrial or residential?
- What type of patients are seen?
- Are evening and weekend appointments essential for most of the patients served?

After these items are considered, the scheduler must allot time based on the patient needs for each individual office visit. These needs can be assessed by determining:

- What is the purpose of this visit?
- What is the age of the patient?
- Will the patient require the physician's time for the entire visit, or will another staff member perform all or part of the service?
- Is the patient a young mother who prefers to schedule her appointments while her children are at school?
- Does the patient object to traveling after dark?
- Is the patient a day worker who cannot take time off?
- Is the patient a child whose parents are both working during the day?

The office should make every attempt to meet the patient's needs, while balancing the physician's preferences and available facilities.

Physician Preferences and Habits

The preferences and habits of the physicians in the practice must be considered before a scheduling plan can be established and followed. Consider the following:

* Does the physician become restless if the reception room is not packed with waiting patients?
* Does the physician worry if even one patient is kept waiting?
* Is the physician methodical and careful about being in the facility when patient appointments are scheduled to begin?
* Is the physician habitually late?
* Does the physician move easily from one patient to another?
* Does the physician require a "break time" between a few patients?
* Would the physician rather see fewer patients and spend more time with each one, or schedule more patients each day?

All of these preferences and habits become an **integral** part of the scheduling process (Figure 10-1). Keep in mind that the physician cannot spend every moment of the day with patients. There are telephone calls to make and receive, reports to examine and dictate, meetings to attend, mail to answer, and many other business items that require the physician's attention. An experienced staff can handle many—but not all—of these tasks.

CRITICAL THINKING APPLICATION

Ramona has noticed that Dr. Brown is taking a little longer with patients than normal and that she is running consistently behind schedule by about 5 to 15 minutes. How can she help to rectify this situation?

Discuss ways of approaching the physician when he or she is the cause of the delays in the schedule. What opening remarks can the medical assistant use to start the discussion in a positive way?

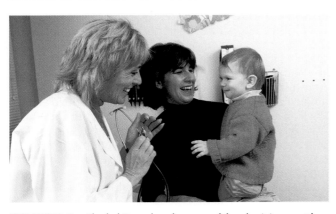

FIGURE 10-1   The habits and preferences of the physician must be considered when scheduling appointments for patients.

Available Facilities

There is no point in getting a patient into the office at a time when no facilities are available for the services needed. For example, suppose that in a two-physician office there is only one room that can be used for minor surgery. You would not schedule two patients requiring minor surgery for the same time block even though both doctors could be available. If there is only one electrocardiograph, you would not book two electrocardiograms at the same time. As the medical assistant gains **proficiency** in scheduling, patient needs will be paired with the available facilities, according to the physician's preference.

Selecting the Method of Appointment Scheduling

The two most common methods of appointment scheduling are using an appointment book and computer-based scheduling. There are advantages and disadvantages with each, and the physician's office should weigh the benefits and choose the method that best suits the physician and the staff.

Appointment Books

Office suppliers carry a variety of appointment book styles. There are certain basic features to consider when choosing an appointment book:

* The size should conform to the desk space available.
* It should be large enough to accommodate the practice.
* It should open flat for easy writing and reference.
* It should allow space for writing when, who, and why.

Some appointment books show an entire week at a glance, and many are color coded, with a special color for each day of the week (Figure 10-2). This is very helpful when the physician asks the patient to return, for instance, in 2 weeks. If Wednesdays are colored yellow, the medical assistant can flip quickly to the correct day and schedule the appointment. Multiple columns may be available to correspond with the number of doctors in a group practice, and the time can be divided according to their preferences.

Computer Scheduling

The computer has replaced the appointment book in many practices. Software for appointment scheduling ranges from relatively simple programs that merely display available and scheduled times to more sophisticated systems. Many programs can display such information as the length and type of appointment required and day or time preferences. The computer can then select the best appointment time based on the information entered into the computer.

The computer can also be used to keep track of future appointments. For example, when a patient calls and inquires about an appointment, the system can search

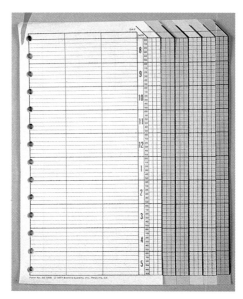

FIGURE 10-2   Color-coded appointment book pages help a medical assistant to flip to the right day of the right week quickly. Appointments for multiple physicians can be color-coded in the book.

by his or her name to find the time and date. Printouts can also run to show the physician's daily schedule, including the patients' names and telephone numbers and the reason for the visit. Multiple copies of these schedules can be made, according to the needs of the practice.

One advantage of computer scheduling is that more than one person can access the system at one time, and the information is available to all operators. The medical assistant can generate a hard copy of the next day's appointments before leaving each evening. In some facilities, employees still maintain an appointment book as a backup to computer scheduling.

Self-Scheduling

The future of appointment scheduling includes *self-scheduling*, which is a method by which a patient can log on to the Internet and view a facility's schedule, then schedule his or her own appointment (Figure 10-3). Software is available that will allow the patient to self-schedule through secure links to the physician's appointment book. The software or internet site for the physician's office should give the patient guidelines as to the amount of time needed for certain appointments, or should only allow a certain length of time to be self-scheduled, such as 15 minutes. These systems will reduce calls to the office and are available to the patient 24 hours a day. Some of these systems will also send an automatic email reminder to the patient the day before the appointment, requesting a reply to confirm. These systems are less frustrating to patients, who do not have to wait on hold to speak to the person who does scheduling for the office. Appointments that are more lengthy or complicated should be scheduled through the office staff.

Advance Preparation

Having chosen an appropriate method of appointment setting, some advance preparation should be done. This is sometimes called *establishing the* **matrix** (Procedure 10-1). Block off time slots when the physician is routinely not available to see patients, such as days off, holidays, time for hospital rounds, and meetings. In the space in which a patient's name would normally be placed, note the reason the time is blocked off. Always try to account for every time period in each day. The medical assistant should also make a note of social or family engagements to help the physician remember these obligations. Because time is a valuable commodity for the physician and the office staff, the schedule is the tool that assists in making certain that the day runs smoothly.

Types of Appointment Scheduling

Different types of appointment scheduling are used to meet the various needs of the medical facility, the providers, and the patients served. Several methods are discussed next. Some offices use a combination of methods to create the right mix of activity during the day.

Open Office Hours

Few healthcare facilities in metropolitan areas have open office hours with no scheduled appointments, but this system is still found in some rural areas, where the way of life is governed not so much by the clock as by the needs of the people in the area. Many freestanding emergency clinics also offer open office hours. With open office hours, the facility is open at given hours of the day or evening, and the patients are "scheduled" by the physician by mentioning to the patient that he or she should return "in a couple of weeks" for follow-up. At **intermittent** times the patients come in, knowing in advance they will be seen in the order of their arrival. Physicians who use this method say that it eliminates the annoyance of broken appointments and of the office running behind schedule. The open office hours method has also been referred to as *tidal wave scheduling.*

There can be many disadvantages to open office hours. The office may already be crowded when the physician arrives, resulting in an extremely long wait for some patients. Patients may arrive in waves throughout the day,

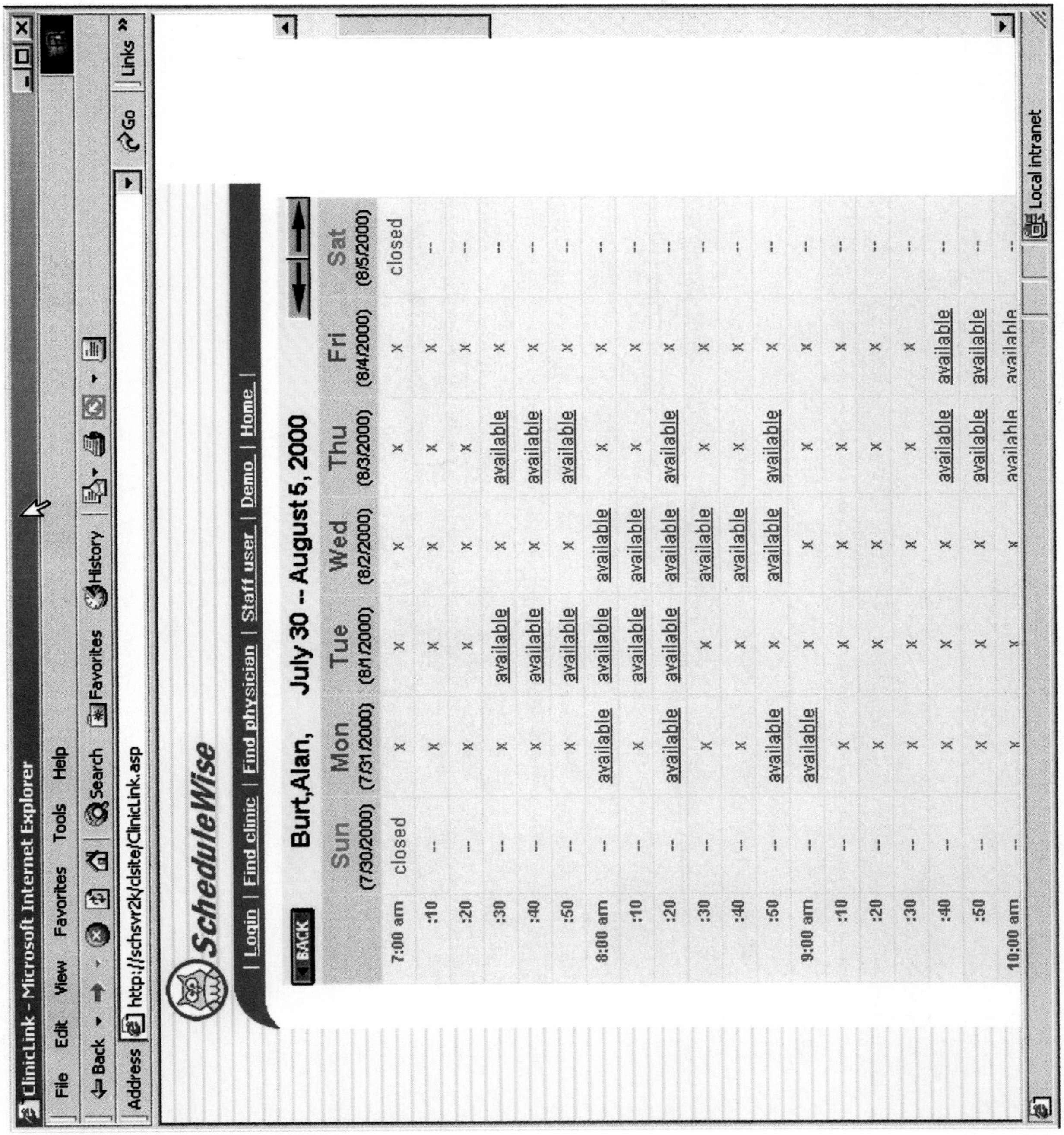

FIGURE 10-3   New computer scheduling programs allow patients to access the physician's schedule over the Internet and schedule their own appointments.   *continued*

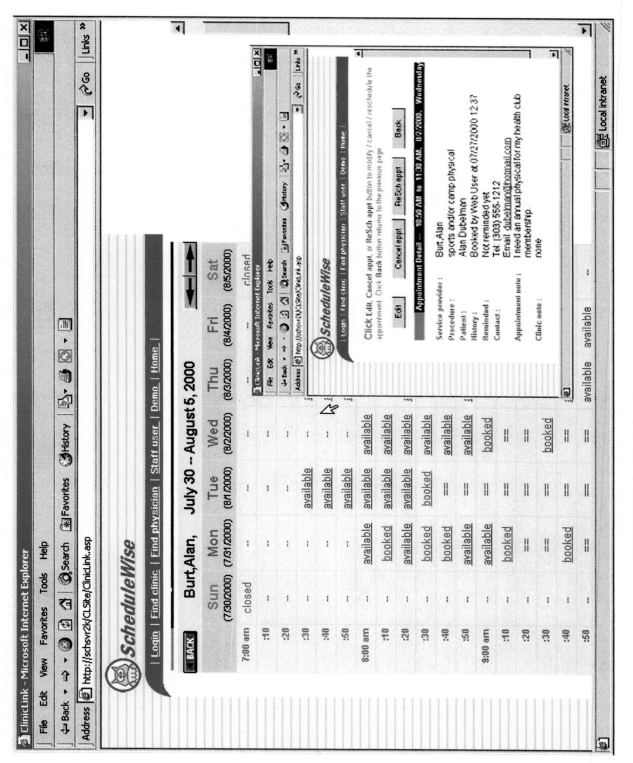

FIGURE 10-3—Cont'd For legend see previous page.

PROCEDURE **10-1**

Preparing and Maintaining the Appointment Book

GOAL: To establish the matrix of the appointment page, arrange appointments for 1 day, and enter information according to office policy.

EQUIPMENT AND SUPPLIES

- Page from appointment book
- Office policy for office hours and doctors' availability
- Clerical supplies
- Calendar
- Description of patients to be scheduled

PROCEDURAL STEPS

1 Determine the hours that a physician will not be available.
   Purpose: To block out those hours on the appointment page for the day.

2 Establish the matrix of the appointment page for the day.
   Purpose: To leave available only those time slots that can be used for patient appointments.

3 Identify each patient's complaint.
   Purpose: This information is necessary in allotting time and space for the appointment.

4 Consult guidelines to determine the length of time necessary for each patient.

5 Allot appointment time according to the complaint and facilities available.

6 Enter information in the appointment book.
   Note: A telephone number must follow the patient's name. If the patient is new, add the letters *NP* (new patient) after his or her name.

7 Allow buffer time in the morning and afternoon.
   Purpose: To allow the physician and staff a short rest period and catch-up time.

---

which causes parts of the day to be very busy and parts to be slow. This makes it difficult to get other office duties accomplished. Without planning, the facilities and staff can be overburdened.

Other types of practices that have open office hours include emergency centers, many of which are open 24 hours a day. Although called emergency centers, most of these facilities deal with general practice cases.

Scheduled Appointments

Studies have shown that practitioners are able to see more patients with less pressure when their appointments are scheduled. Unfortunately, the skill required for scheduling appointments is often not fully appreciated by the practitioner or office manager, resulting in the responsibility being delegated to the least qualified medical assistant. Although the skill and attitude of the assistant who manages the appointment schedule is very important, the ultimate success of the system lies in the cooperation of the physicians.

Flexible Office Hours

Most scheduling practices are carryovers from the days when expectant mothers of families with young children relied on one wage earner. Today families commonly have two working parents. As a result, many healthcare providers are turning to extended-day and flexible office hours. Staff hours are affected by these schedules, but this flexibility works to the advantage of the employee and the employer. For instance, if a medical assistant has decided to continue his or her education, morning class hours become available if he or she agrees to work evening hours. Scheduling evening and weekend hours may increase the size of the practice because of the convenience offered to patients.

CRITICAL THINKING APPLICATION

Dr. Brown would like to implement evening appointments one night each week and open the office every other Saturday morning. She feels this will better serve her patients with children who have difficulty making daytime appointments. If this is her primary goal, should other types of patients be seen during these time slots? Why or why not?

Wave Scheduling

Many office schedules lack flexibility, and wave scheduling is an attempt to create short-term flexibility within each hour. Wave scheduling assumes that the actual time needed for all of the patients seen will average out over the course of the day. Instead of scheduling patients at each 20-minute interval, wave scheduling places three patients in the office at the same time, and they are seen in the order of their arrival. Thus, one person's late arrival will not disrupt the entire schedule.

Modified Wave Scheduling

There are several ways to modify the wave schedule. One method is to have two patients scheduled to come in at, for example, 10:00 AM, and a third at 10:30 AM. This hourly cycle is repeated throughout the day. Another application would have patients scheduled to arrive at given intervals during the first half of the hour, and none scheduled to arrive during the second half of the hour. Physicians can modify wave scheduling to best suit the clinic's needs.

Double Booking

Booking two patients to come in at the same time, both of whom are to be seen by the physician, is poor practice. Of course, if each appointment is expected to only take 5 minutes, there is no harm in telling both to come at the same time and reserving a 15-minute period for the two. This is simply one method of wave scheduling. However, if each patient requires 15 minutes, two will require 30 minutes. This must be reflected in the scheduling. It is not considered double booking if a patient comes to the office to receive a treatment by someone other than the physician, such as a patient receiving a physical therapy modality or an allergy injection.

Grouping Procedures

Another method of scheduling that appeals to many practitioners is the grouping or categorizing of procedures. For instance, an internist might reserve all morning appointments for complete physical examinations or well-baby visits. A surgeon might devote one day each week to seeing only referral patients. Obstetricians often schedule pregnant patients on different days than gynecology patients. The physician and staff can experiment with different groupings until the plan that works best for the practice eventually becomes evident. In applying a grouping system of appointments, the medical assistant may find it helpful to color-code the sections of the appointment book being reserved for designated procedures.

Advance Booking

Often appointments are made months in advance. When any appointment is made, an appointment card should be completed and given to the patient. All appointment cards should mention that patients must give 24 hours' notice if they are unable to keep the time reserved for them. Most offices have some type of confirmation procedures by which patients are called the day before to verify that they will keep the appointment.

Time Patterns

When booking appointments, a medical assistant should make it a policy to leave some open time during each day's schedule, so that if a patient calls with a special problem that is not an immediate emergency, there will be some time available to book the patient for at least a brief visit. It is also wise to keep one time slot available in the morning and afternoon specifically for emergencies. A busy physician will always be able to fill these open slots of time, and having them in the schedule will cause the least amount of **disruption** during the day. If possible, time should be set aside in the morning and afternoon for a break. Even 15 minutes will give the physician time to return calls from patients, verify prescription calls, or answer questions.

Studies have shown that in the average medical practice, Mondays and Fridays are the most hectic days of the week. Patients may have been waiting the whole weekend to call for an appointment and expect to be seen immediately on Monday. Similarly, toward the end of the week, small problems that could magnify if left unattended over the weekend may prompt the patient to be anxious to see the physician on Friday. Incorporating more buffer time on these 2 days may be worthwhile.

Patient Wait Time

Be conscious about the amount of time that the patient sits in the reception area. Ideally, the patient's name will be called to go to the examination room precisely at the scheduled appointment time (Figure 10-4). However, the scheduling has failed if the patient then waits in the back office for 30 minutes to see the physician. Make it clear to the patient whether he or she is free to leave the office when the physician has finished the examination. Some patients mistakenly wait in the room until told they are free to leave, when they could have left several minutes sooner.

If a patient has waited more than 15 minutes in the reception area, the medical assistant should briefly explain the delay and offer to reschedule the appointment. The longer patients sit and wait, the more anxious and frustrated they become. Remember, some patients are there to see the physician for test results or may be expecting a negative diagnosis. Do not make their visit more stressful by forcing them to wait for a long time.

Of course, some delays are unavoidable. The physician may be delayed as a result of unforeseen circumstances, or there could be a patient with an emergency. Occasion-

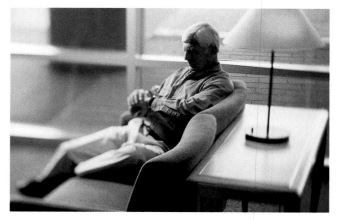

FIGURE 10-4 One of the most common patient complaints is the time spent in the reception area.

ally a physician becomes ill or must be unexpectedly absent from the office. Briefly explain the situation to the patient and allow him or her to decide whether to wait or reschedule. If a delay is forthcoming, attempt to call patients who may be en route to the office and inform them that there will be a delay. Again, offer to reschedule, or allow the patient to come in and wait to see the physician. Always ask for the patient's cell phone number for just such events.

CRITICAL THINKING APPLICATION

Ramona offers to reschedule patient appointments if the schedule ever falls more than 15 minutes behind. If a patient becomes belligerent about the delays, how can Ramona handle the situation in a professional manner?

Telephone Scheduling

It is just as important for a medical assistant to be pleasant and express a desire to be helpful on the telephone as it is when meeting face-to-face. This is especially true when making appointments, because the telephone contact may be the patient's first impression of the facility. Often the manner in which the booking is made makes more of an impact than the convenience of the appointment time.

Be especially considerate if the time requested for an appointment must be refused. Briefly explain why the time is not available and offer a substitute date and time. Comply with the patient's desires as much as possible and do not show any annoyance if the patient does not understand the scheduling process. Most people, however, understand the need for a well-managed office and are willing to cooperate.

Many offices offer the patient a choice when scheduling the appointment, and let the patient decide which option is best for him or her. For example, the following dialog might take place during the scheduling call:

- "Mrs. Thomas, Dr. Stern is available to see you in the office next Tuesday or Wednesday, January 6 or 7. Which day is better for you?"
  "I will be working on Wednesday, so I would like to come on Tuesday."
- "Do you prefer a morning or afternoon appointment?"
  "The afternoon is best for me."
- "Great. Would 1:30 or 3:30 be a better time?"
  "I can be there at 1:30."
- "Then Dr. Stern will see you at 1:30 next Tuesday, January 6. Thank you for calling, Mrs. Thomas. We'll see you then!"

These small courtesies will give patients the feeling that they are in control of their time. Always repeat the time to reinforce the appointment, and do not hesitate to ask the patient if he or she has a pen with which to jot down the time and date. While repeating the information to the patient, check the appointment book or computer screen to ensure that it was posted correctly.

Write legibly when using an appointment book. These records could be called to court, and the medical assistant must be able to read his or her own writing if asked to testify. Form the habit of entering the patient's daytime telephone number after every entry. It may become necessary to cancel or rearrange the schedule in a hurry, and many precious minutes can be saved if the telephone number is handy. Cell phone numbers are also quite useful when tracking down a patient quickly.

Scheduling Appointments for New Patients

Arranging the first appointment for a new patient requires time and attention to detail (Procedure 10-2). This first encounter provides the first impression of the office and may set the tone for all subsequent visits. Tact, courtesy, and professionalism are extremely important. During the conversation with the new patient, request preliminary information to assist in deciding how much time to allot for the visit on the appointment schedule. The physician may also expect the medical assistant to give general instructions to patients seeking care for specific complaints. For example, the patient may be required to bring a urine specimen or to make certain that laboratory tests are completed before the appointment. Some offices obtain enough information to build a patient chart before the office visit; others wait until the patient actually arrives to construct the chart.

After the necessary information has been recorded, offer the first available appointment to the patient. Whenever possible, offer the patient choices between two dates and times. Ask the patient if he or she knows the directions to the office, or offer the physical address for those who wish to obtain exact directions from one of the many Internet sites, such as Mapquest. Tell the patient whether there are any special parking conveniences and whether the office will provide a token or parking validation. The options that the patient will have for the first payment should also be discussed. If payment is expected immediately, inform the patient. The office staff should expect patient concerns about the amount of the first bill and address this issue in advance of the appointment so that there are no surprises or misunderstandings. Before ending the conversation, repeat the appointment date and time, then thank the patient for calling.

Some medical offices mail an information packet about their facility to new patients, especially if the appointment is several days away. With today's technology and the patient's email address, such information can also be sent via the Internet. This information should tell the patient about the nature of the practice, introduce the medical staff, and explain appointment policies and financial arrangements.

If another physician has referred the patient, the medical assistant may need to call the referring physician's office to obtain additional information before the patient's appointment. This information should be printed out and given to the attending physician in advance of the patient's arrival.

PROCEDURE **10-2**

Scheduling a New Patient

GOAL: To schedule a new patient for a first office visit.

EQUIPMENT AND SUPPLIES

- Appointment book
- Scheduling guidelines
- Appointment card
- Telephone

PROCEDURAL STEPS

1 Obtain the patient's full name, birth date, address, and telephone number.
Note: Verify the spelling of the name.

2 Determine whether the patient was referred by another physician.
Purpose: You may need to request additional information from the referring physician, and your physician will want to send a consultation report.

3 Determine the patient's chief complaint and when the first symptoms occurred.
Purpose: To assist in determining the length of time needed for the appointment and the degree of urgency.

4 Search the appointment book for the first suitable appointment time and an alternate time.

5 Offer the patient a choice of these dates and times.
Purpose: Patients are better satisfied if they are given a choice.

6 Enter the mutually agreeable time in the appointment book followed by the patient's telephone number.
Note: Indicate that the patient is new by adding the letters *NP*.

7 If new patients are expected to pay at the time of the visit, explain this financial arrangement when the appointment is made.
Purpose: The patient will be aware of the payment policy and can come prepared to pay at the time of the visit.

8 Offer travel directions for reaching the office as well as parking instructions.
Purpose: To relieve any anxiety about being able to find the medical facility.

9 Repeat the day, date, and time of the appointment before saying good-bye to the patient.
Purpose: To verify the patient understands the date and time of the appointment.

Many offices call each patient the day before the appointment as a reminder and a courtesy. This can be a time-consuming procedure, but most patients appreciate this service, and it may open appointments for others if the original patient cannot keep the scheduled time slot. Email can also be programmed to send reminders to patients of their appointments the day before if the email address is obtained. This procedure can run automatically, taking no time away from the medical assistant's other duties.

Scheduling Appointments for Established Patients

In Person

Most return appointments for **established patients** are arranged when the patient is leaving the office. It is a good policy for all patients to stop by the front desk before leaving, in case there is any information needed from the patient or any outside scheduling to do. The patient's chart can be reviewed to see whether the physician ordered any laboratory tests or procedures, and these

can be scheduled and discussed with the patient. When making a return appointment, follow the same procedures as scheduling any appointment by phone, offering the patient choices in the day and time slots. If a certain time is not available that the patient specifically requests, offer two alternatives. Always give the patient an appointment card and any necessary instructions at this time, along with a bright smile. Never forget to provide excellent customer service to the patient.

By Telephone

Usually it is only necessary to determine when the patient is required to return and then to find a suitable time on the schedule. Established patients do not usually need directions and parking information, unless the office has recently moved. If there has been a lengthy **interval** since the patient's last visit, the medical assistant should recheck certain information and enter any changes on the patient's chart. Be sure to ask whether insurance companies or benefits have changed, and it is always a good idea to verify the address and phone numbers of the patient. If an email address is not on file, obtain one for quick and easy notification of appointments and other events.

Scheduling Other Types of Appointments

There are other appointments that a medical assistant will make and that will appear on the appointment schedule, such as surgeries the physician will be performing at a hospital or other facility, hospital rounds and consultations, appointments and meetings, and even house calls if the physician performs them. The physician must also have time to get from one location to another, so driving time must be considered when arranging all appointments.

Surgeries

When scheduling a surgery, call the facility where the procedure will be performed as soon as the operation is planned. Most surgical departments and centers have a surgical secretary that makes these arrangements. Provide all necessary information as well as any special requests that the physician may have, such as the amount of blood to have available for the patient. The secretary may want all of the patient's insurance information and will certainly want a phone number so that the patient could be contacted before the surgery if necessary. Be sure that all of this information is handy before placing the call.

Some hospitals request that the patient complete a preadmittance form so that all records can be processed before the patient is admitted. In such cases it may be the medical assistant's responsibility to see that this is done. These are general guidelines only, because procedures will vary in different areas and hospitals.

Outside Visits

If the physician regularly makes house calls or visits patients in skilled nursing facilities, a special block of time will need to be reserved in the appointment schedule. The physician will need demographic information, such as addresses, room numbers, and the best route to each home or facility. Remember to allow for travel time. Although most physicians never make house calls because of the ease of seeing patients in the office, they may be necessary in certain situations. The physician's medical bag should always be prepared and well-stocked before he or she has to make any outside visits.

Outside Appointments

A medical assistant is often requested to arrange laboratory or radiography appointments for patients. Before calling the facility to schedule the appointment, be sure all necessary information is handy. When the patient is informed of the time and place for the appointment, relay any special instructions that may be necessary. Then, note these arrangements in the patient's chart. Some offices will make a reminder call to the patient, or a reminder email message can be sent.

Outpatient testing is common, because most physicians do not have extensive x-ray or laboratory equipment in their offices. MRIs, CT scans, numerous x-ray evaluations, ultrasonography, and simple blood tests all may need to be scheduled (Procedure 10-3). Provide the patient with the name, address, and phone number of the facility where the tests will be performed.

Some patients may require a series of appointments, such as at weekly intervals. Try to set up these appointments on the same day of each week at the same time of day. This considerably reduces the risk that the patient will forget an appointment.

In some cases, the medical assistant may be responsible for scheduling inpatient admissions or inpatient surgical procedures (Procedures 10-4 and 10-5). This is similar to scheduling outpatient testing, but the medical assistant must coordinate with the hospital instead of with an outside facility.

Special Circumstances

Late Patients

Probably every medical practice has a few patients who are habitually late for appointments. This seems to be a problem for which no cure has been found. Emergencies and small delays can happen to anyone, but a patient who constantly arrives late can place a strain on the practice. Such patients can be booked as the last appointment of the day. Then, if closing time arrives before the patient does, there is no obligation to wait. Some medical assistants tell the patient to come in 30 minutes before the appointment time that is actually scheduled. Make an attempt to work with patients who have occasional difficulties arriving on time, but do not allow the schedule to be constantly disrupted by late patients.

CRITICAL THINKING APPLICATION

Seth Jones is always late for his appointments. How might Ramona approach him about this? What can Ramona do to assist Mr. Jones in arriving for appointments on time?

Rescheduling Canceled Appointments

Changes sometimes must be made in the appointment schedule. Unexpected conflicts might arise that force a patient to change the appointment time. When rescheduling an appointment, be sure that the first appointment day and time is removed from the appointment book or database, and then set the new appointment. Otherwise, the patient will be expected in the office on 2 days, and time will be wasted with calls and follow-up, only to find out that the appointment was rescheduled.

Emergency Calls

Periodically, emergency or urgent calls will come to the office and an appointment will need to be scheduled. To some extent, all calls that come to the office go through a **triage** process, and emergencies are prioritized to evaluate

PROCEDURE 10-3

Scheduling Outpatient Admissions and Procedures

GOAL: To schedule a patient for outpatient admission or procedure within the time frame needed by the physician, confirm with the patient, and issue all required instructions.

EQUIPMENT AND SUPPLIES

- Diagnostic test order from physician
- Name, address, and telephone number of diagnostic facility
- Patient demographic information
- Patient chart
- Test preparation instructions
- Telephone
- Consent form

PROCEDURAL STEPS

1 Obtain an oral or written order from the physician for the exact procedure to be performed.
Purpose: To have a documented order for the procedure to be performed.

2 Precertify the procedure with the patient's insurance company, if necessary.
Purpose: To make certain that expected insurance benefits are valid and the procedure will be covered by the patient's insurance policy.

3 Determine the physician and patient availability.
Purpose: To be certain that the patient will be able to comply with the arrangements for the test and that the physician is available, if he or she must be present for the procedure. The urgency of the needed test results affects the time and date of the appointment needed.

4 Telephone the diagnostic facility and schedule the procedure or test.
- Order the specific test needed.
- Provide the patient's diagnosis.
- Establish the date and time.
- Give the name, age, address, and telephone number of the patient.
- Provide the demographic information for the patient, including insurance policy numbers and addresses for filing claims.

- Determine any special instructions for the patient or special anesthesia requirements.
- Notify the facility of any urgency for test results.
Purpose: To schedule the procedure or admission and provide needed information.

5 Notify the patient of the arrangements, including:
- Name, address, and telephone number of the diagnostic facility.
- Date and time to report for the test.
- Instructions concerning preparation for the test (e.g., eating restrictions, fluids, medications, enemas).
- Tell what preadmission testing will be necessary, if any.
- Ask the patient to repeat the instructions.
Purpose: To be certain that the patient understands the preparation necessary and the importance of keeping the appointment. If time permits, issue written instructions to the patient.

6 Have the physician review the consent form with the patient. The patient should sign the consent form and a copy should be placed in the chart. Note arrangements on the patient's chart.
Purpose: To make certain that the patient understands the risks, benefits, and alternatives to the procedure. To ensure follow-up on diagnosis and/or treatment.

7 Place reminder on the physician's tickler or desk calendar, if needed. Be sure the information is listed on the office schedule. Check the postsurgical status of the patient. Follow up if results are not received in a timely manner.
Purpose: To check whether the appointment was kept and a report was received from the testing facility.

---

the urgency of the need to see the physician. Triage is an extremely important function that requires experience and knowledge of signs and symptoms, as well as tact.

Emergencies may include emotional crises as well as the more obvious physical problems. Patients with emergencies should be seen the same day. The urgency of the call can be initially determined by having a list of questions prepared for reference with the help of the physician. The physician should determine what is con-

sidered urgent. The patient may need to be referred directly to the emergency department of a hospital, or the physician may want to see the patient that day in the office. In many cases, the caller will consider the situation more urgent than his or her responses to the medical questions may indicate. Skillful handling of these situations requires considerable tact. Maintaining a caring and reassuring response will frequently alleviate the fear evidenced by the caller.

Scheduling Inpatient Admissions

GOAL: To schedule a patient for inpatient admission within the time frame needed by the physician, confirm with the patient, and issue all required instructions.

EQUIPMENT AND SUPPLIES

- Admission orders from physician
- Name, address, and telephone number of inpatient facility
- Patient demographic information
- Patient chart
- Any preparation instructions for the patient
- Telephone
- Admission packet for the patient

PROCEDURAL STEPS

1 Obtain an oral or written order from the physician for the admission.
   Purpose: To have a documented order for the admission.

2 Precertify the admission with the patient's insurance company, if necessary.
   Purpose: To make certain that expected insurance benefits are valid and the admission will be covered by the patient's insurance policy.

3 Determine the physician and patient availability if the admission is not an emergency.
   Purpose: To be certain that the patient will be able to comply with the arrangements for the admission and that the physician is available to care for the patient during the admission. The urgency of the admission affects the time and date of the appointment needed.

4 Telephone the diagnostic facility and schedule the admission.
   - Order any specific tests needed.
   - Provide the patient's admitting diagnosis.
   - Establish the date and time.
   - Convey the patient's room preferences.
   - Give the name, age, address, and telephone number of the patient.

   - Provide the demographic information for the patient, including insurance policy numbers and addresses for filing claims.
   - Determine any special instructions for the patient.
   - Notify the facility of any urgency for test results.
   Purpose: To schedule the admission and provide needed information.

5 Notify the patient of the arrangements, including:
   - Name, address, and telephone number of the facility.
   - Date and time to report for admission.
   - Instructions concerning preparation for any procedures, if necessary (e.g., eating restrictions, fluids, medications, enemas).
   - Tell what preadmission testing will be necessary, if any.
   - Ask the patient to repeat the instructions.
   Purpose: To be certain that the patient understands the preparation necessary and the importance of admittance. If it is your office policy to do so, give an admission packet to the patient that contains the orders and basic instructions for the admission.

6 Note arrangements and the admission on the patient's chart.
   Purpose: To ensure follow-up on diagnosis and/or treatment.

7 Place reminder on the physician's tickler or desk calendar, if needed. Be sure the information is listed on the office schedule. If the physician keeps a list of all inpatients, add the patient's name to that list.
   Purpose: To keep a record of the number of days the patient was seen in the hospital by the physician during rounds for insurance billing purposes.

Acutely Ill Patients

There is sometimes a fine line between an emergency patient and an acutely ill patient, but the latter should be seen as soon as possible. At the very least, let the physician decide whether an appointment should be made for another day. For example, a patient may report having had flu symptoms for several days and now has an elevated temperature. The physician will probably want more information before deciding whether the patient should be seen immediately or whether some other course of action is appropriate. The 15- to 20-minute breather time saved in the middle of the morning may rescue the schedule and provide the needed time for the patient. Escort these patients to the exam room upon their arrival if possible. Patients with symptoms of infection should be placed so as to prevent cross-contamination.

Physician Referrals

If another physician telephones and requests that a patient be seen today, most offices will honor that request if at all possible. It is important to keep a schedule that will not be intolerant of this type of request.

PROCEDURE **10-5**

Scheduling Inpatient Surgical Procedures

GOAL: To schedule a patient for inpatient surgery within the time frame needed by the physician, confirm with the patient, and issue all required instructions.

EQUIPMENT AND SUPPLIES

- Orders from physician
- Name, address, and telephone number of inpatient facility
- Patient demographic information
- Patient chart
- Any preparation instructions for the patient
- Telephone
- Consent form

PROCEDURAL STEPS

1 Obtain an oral or written order from the physician for the admission.
Purpose: To have a documented order for the admission.

2 Precertify the admission with the patient's insurance company, if necessary.
Purpose: To make certain that expected insurance benefits are valid and the admission will be covered by the patient's insurance policy.

3 Determine the physician availability if the surgery is not an emergency. Another physician may be the surgeon. If this is the case, the surgery will need to be coordinated with his or her office as well.
Purpose: To be certain that the physician is available to care for the patient during the admission and the surgery. The urgency of the surgery affects the time and date of the appointment needed.

4 Telephone the hospital surgical department and schedule the procedure.
- Order any specific tests needed.
- Provide the patient's admitting diagnosis.
- Establish the date and time.
- Give the name, age, address, and telephone number of the patient.
- Provide the demographic information for the patient, including insurance policy numbers and addresses for filing claims.
- Determine any special instructions for the patient.
- Notify the facility of any urgency for the surgery.

Purpose: To schedule the surgery and provide needed information to the facility.

5 Notify the patient of the arrangements, if the patient is not already admitted to the hospital. Include:
- Name, address, and telephone number of the facility.
- Date and time to report for admission.
- Instructions concerning preparation for any procedures, if necessary (e.g., eating restrictions, fluids, medications, enemas).
- Tell what preadmission testing will be necessary, if any.
- Ask the patient to repeat the instructions.

Purpose: To be certain that the patient understands the preparation necessary and the importance of surgery. If it is your office policy to do so, give an admission packet to the patient that contains the orders and basic instructions for the surgery.

6 The physician should review the consent form with the patient. Have the patient sign a consent for the surgical procedure. Keep the original consent in the patient's chart and give a copy to the patient.
Purpose: To ensure that the patient understands the risks, benefits, and alternatives to the surgical procedure.

7 Note arrangements on the patient's chart.
Purpose: To ensure follow-up on diagnosis and/or treatment.

8 Place reminder on the physician's tickler or desk calendar, if needed. Be sure the information is listed on the office schedule. If the physician keeps a list of all inpatients, add the patient's name to that list. Follow up with the hospital after the procedure regarding the patient's condition as required by the physician.
Purpose: To check on the patient's status and keep a record of the number of days the patient was seen in the hospital by the physician during rounds for insurance billing purposes.

Patients Without Appointments

There must be a policy agreed on by the physician and then carried out by medical assistants for patients without appointments. A patient who requires immediate attention will most likely be accommodated into the schedule somehow. If the patient does not need immediate care, a brief visit with the physician and a scheduled appointment at a later time may be the answer. The medical assistant may simply have to turn down the request. Follow established office policy.

The medical assistant should always make it clear, even when accommodating patients without appointments, that the office runs on an appointment basis. Try to convey the message that appointments save not only the physician's time but also the patient's time. Emphasize that the physician is able to give the patient full attention and more time if an advance appointment is made.

Failed Appointments

Why do patients fail to keep appointments? Some are simply forgetful. Once this tendency is detected in a patient, form the habit of telephoning or emailing a reminder the day before the appointment, or send a postcard timed to arrive 1 or 2 days in advance.

A patient who has been pressed for a payment may stay away because of his or her inability to pay for medical services. Do not make the mistake of classifying all such patients as "deadbeats." Many have every desire to pay, but they cannot afford to and feel embarrassed about their situation, so they avoid their appointments.

If the office consistently runs behind schedule, some patients may not be willing to waste any time waiting to see the physician. Time is a valuable commodity for patients as well, and every effort must be made to get patients in at their appointment time and out quickly.

One other reason for failed appointments that is often overlooked is a patient's state of denial regarding his or her condition. For instance, if a patient has been recently diagnosed as HIV positive, he or she may avoid doctor appointments, because going to see the physician forces the patient to face the reality of the disease. Take special care with such patients, and if denial is suspected, discuss this with the physician, who may wish to refer the patient for counseling.

It is important to determine the reason for failed appointments and do whatever is possible to remedy the situation. Telephone the patient to be sure there is no misunderstanding. If the patient's health is such that medical care must continue, write a letter and explain this to the patient. Send the letter by certified mail, with return receipt requested. Keep the letter in the patient's chart for legal protection.

No-Show Policy

Some patients may not realize the importance of keeping their appointments. The patient who does not arrive for a scheduled appointment or reschedule it is called a **no-**show. A busy practice must have a very specific policy on appointment no-shows and enforce it effectively. The first time a patient fails to show, note the fact on the medical chart and/or ledger card. The second time, warn the patient, and if a third no-show occurs, consider dropping the patient by using the customary methods that provide legal protection for the physician.

The physician may wish to charge patients for not showing up or rescheduling the appointment. Be understanding whenever possible, but do not let a patient take advantage of the physician's time. The office policy manual must state that patients may be charged for missed appointments, especially if the time slot could not be filled with another patient. Many physicians do not press this issue, but it is an available tool if needed.

Recording the Failed Appointment

When a patient fails to keep an appointment, a notation should be made in the patient's chart as well as in the appointment book or database. If the patient is seriously ill, the physician should also be told about the failure to show. In some cases, it may be necessary to call or write the patient to remind that a missed appointment may have serious effects on the patient's health.

Increasing Appointment Show Rates

Everyone benefits from a full schedule of appointments that are kept. There are several ways to increase appointment show rates.

Appointment Cards

Most healthcare facilities use appointment cards to remind patients of scheduled appointments, as well as to eliminate misunderstandings about dates and times (Figure 10-5). Make a habit of reaching for an appointment card while writing an entry in the appointment book. After the date and time have been written on the card, double-check with the book to see that the entries agree.

Confirmation Calls

Patients who have made appointments in advance may appreciate a confirmation call to remind them that they have a time set aside to see the physician. Always note the phone number that the patient prefers the office use for such calls. Many individuals now have a home phone, cell phone, and work number; however, they may wish calls from the physician to go only to their home phone. The preferred phone number can be highlighted in the chart or on the computer. The office must use caution in making calls to patients because of the significance of privacy guidelines and standards. Some offices may wish to prepare a release form in which the patient grants the office staff permission to contact the patient. Many physicians insist that messages left on voice mail not mention the term "doctor" for confidentiality reasons. The medical assistant might say:

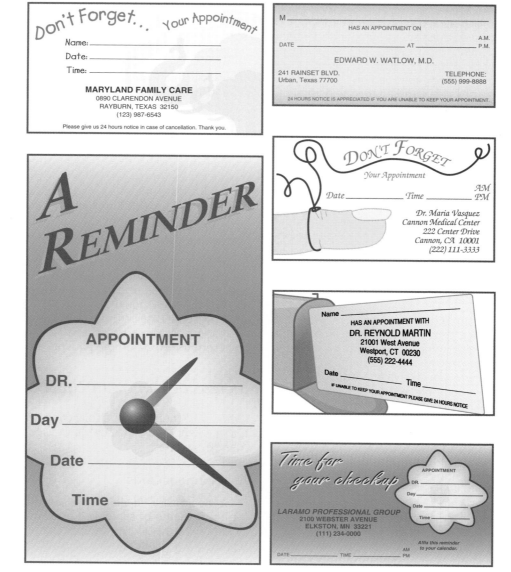

FIGURE 10-5   Examples of appointment cards.

"This is Pam at Robert Welch's office confirming your appointment tomorrow at 2:00 pm. Please call us if you cannot make the appointment. Our number is 555-212-0909. Thank you!"

Email Reminders

Many computer scheduling programs have the capacity to send an email to patients to remind them of appointments the day before. This is a great time-saver for the office staff, because no time is taken to perform this duty, other than the original scheduling of the appointment.

Mailed Reminders

Mailed reminder cards may be sent to patients by the office staff. This method is a bit time consuming, but worth the effort if the patients show for their appointments.

A patient who is due for an appointment but has not yet arranged a date and time may be sent a reminder. A simple way of handling this is to have a supply of postcards on hand, and while patients are still in the office, have them write their name and address on the postcard. Then place the card in a file box under the date it is to be mailed.

Innovative Ideas

Knowing that time is valuable to patients as well as the physician, many of today's offices try to make the time spent at the office as productive as possible for the patient. Some reception areas are equipped with computers, televisions, and even video games and movies for children. Often a small desk with a phone will allow the patient to do a limited amount of work, if needed, while waiting to see the physician. Keeping the patient's needs in mind makes the patient less likely to break an appointment.

Handling Cancellations and Delays

When the Patient Cancels

Inevitably, some cancellations will occur. If a list is kept of patients with advance appointments who would like to come in sooner, the medical assistant can begin calling to try to get one of them in to fill the available opening. By placing a colored dot beside their names in the appointment book where the first appointment was made, the medical assistant can readily identify which patients to call to fill the vacancy.

When the Physician Is Delayed

There will be days when the physician is delayed in reaching the office. If there is advance notice of the delay, start calling patients with early appointments and suggest that they come later. If some patients have already arrived before the office learns of the delay, explain that an emergency has detained the physician.

Show concern for the patient but avoid being overly apologetic, which might imply some degree of guilt. Most patients realize that a physician has certain priorities. The patient who is in the office may be inconvenienced, but it is not a life-or-death matter. If this kind of situation occurs frequently, however, consider devising a different scheduling system.

When the Physician Is Called for Emergencies

Physicians are conscious of their responsibilities for responding to medical emergencies, and most patients will be sympathetic to such occurrences if the medical assistant takes the time to explain what has happened. The medical assistant may say:

"Dr. Wright has been called away to answer an emergency. She asked me to tell you she is very sorry to keep you waiting. There will be at least a 1-hour delay."

Ask the patient:

"Do you wish to wait? If it is inconvenient, I'll be glad to give you the first available appointment on another day. Or perhaps you'd like to have some coffee or do some shopping and return in an hour."

As quickly as possible, call the patients who are scheduled for a later hour. In many offices, especially those of obstetricians, surgeons, and general practitioners, it sometimes is necessary to cancel a whole day's appointments. For this reason, it is particularly important to have the daytime telephone number of each patient available so that the appointment can be rescheduled. If it is at all possible, cancel appointments *before* the patient arrives in the office to find that the physician is not available. The **expediency** of the office staff in contacting the patients who will be affected by an emergency will be most appreciated.

When the Physician is Ill or Out of Town

Physicians get ill, too, and the patients who are scheduled to be seen during the course of the physician's expected recovery period must be informed of this. They need not be told the nature of the illness. When the physician is called out of town for personal or professional reasons, the appointments will have to be canceled or rescheduled. It is customary to give the patient the name of another physician, or possibly a choice of several, who will be providing care during such absences. For security reasons, it is best to merely state that the doctor is unavailable. Stating over the telephone that the physician is out of town could lead to attempted burglary or other unauthorized intrusion of the premises.

Other Types of Appointments

There will be a wide range of other unscheduled callers with whom the physician will need to meet. Handle all of these individuals with care and courtesy.

Physicians

Another physician dropping in to the facility should be ushered in to see the physician as soon as possible, regardless of the appointment schedule. If the physician is seeing a patient, explain the situation and, if possible, take the visiting physician into a private room to wait. Then notify your employer as soon as possible. Visits from other physicians are usually brief and do not appreciably affect your schedule.

Pharmaceutical Representatives

Also known as *detail persons* or *reps*, representatives from pharmaceutical houses are frequent visitors to physicians' offices and are generally welcomed when the schedule permits. They are well trained and bring valuable information on new drugs to the physician. The medical assistant is often expected to screen such visitors and turn away those whose products would not be used in that practice. If the representative or the pharmaceutical company is unknown to the office, ask for a business card, then check with the physician, who will decide whether to see the caller.

Specialists usually limit their conferences with pharmaceutical representatives to their line of practice. The medical assistant, together with the physician, can prepare a list of the representatives with whom the physician is willing to spend time, and then let the list be the determining factor in future conferences. The medical assistant can say whether the physician will be available that day and give an estimate of the waiting time or suggest a later time at which to return. The caller can then make a decision regarding whether to wait or return later. The pharmaceutical representative is usually quite understanding and cooperative and is willing to wait patiently a long while for just a brief visit with the physician. The medical assistant should in turn treat the representative with courtesy, showing as much cooperation as possible.

In some cases, the representative will just leave literature or materials for the physician with the medical assistant. The detail person who is not on the calling list for a particular physician will also appreciate the saving in time by knowing this in advance. Most representatives say they would rather be told outright if the physician does not wish to see them than to be given some evasive reply.

Salespersons

Salespersons from medical, surgical, and office supply houses call regularly at physicians' offices. Sometimes they will want to see the physician, but the office manager or the medical assistant who is in charge of ordering supplies usually is able to handle these calls.

Unsolicited salespersons can sometimes present a problem in the professional office. If the physician does not wish to see such callers, the medical assistant must firmly but tactfully send them away. Suggest that they leave their literature and cards for the physician to study and say that the physician will contact them if further information is desired.

Miscellaneous Callers

From time to time, other callers appear in the medical office. Some are civic leaders seeking the physician's aid in community projects. Others may be church leaders, insurance representatives, solicitors for fund drives, and so forth. A general policy regarding seeing such callers should be established so that each incident does not require a separate discussion and decision.

Civic leaders should be treated with courtesy and consideration when they telephone or come into the office. Most physicians feel a responsibility to take an active part in community affairs, but no one can participate in all activities. The responsibility for accepting or refusing such community appointments is sometimes delegated to the office manager or medical assistant. In this event, one should use discretion and exercise great tact and courtesy. Turning away community leaders with a blunt refusal does not create good medical public relations.

When it is necessary to refuse requests for community projects, the medical assistant can explain that the physician is already participating in such community projects as, for example, the Boy Scouts, Girl Scouts, Kiwanis, and the Health Council and cannot accept additional responsibilities at this time. The practice of tact, courtesy, and consideration applies to every caller in the healthcare facility.

Planning for the Next Day

Before leaving at the end of the day, look over the appointments scheduled for the next day. Review the charts for scheduled patients. If laboratory tests or other procedures were scheduled on the patient's last visit, determine that the reports are available in the chart. If the patient is scheduled for specific procedures on this visit, make certain that everything that will be needed for the procedure is on hand and available. Planning can save many precious moments at the time of the patient visit.

Closing Comments

The person charged with the responsibility for scheduling appointments will have a huge impact on the efficiency of the medical office. A friendly and helpful attitude is a prerequisite for cordial interaction with patients and the ability to make compromises that will benefit both the physician and the patient. The office that runs smoothly and stays on schedule is an indication of professionalism and competence and will be greatly appreciated by all who come into contact with the medical office.

Patient Education

Providing patients with an information booklet about the office will help to acclimate them to the policies and procedures of the office. Many physicians compile an extensive booklet that even provides tips as to when the physician should be called immediately, listing symptoms and signs of emergencies.

Educating the patient regarding office policies will help the facility to run smoothly from day to day. All patients should be familiar with the policies about appointments. This leads to fewer misunderstandings and conflicts over bills that might include a charge for a missed appointment.

If the facility offers web-based appointment scheduling, patients will have to be taught how to use the system. A printed pamphlet or information sheet will be helpful in providing instruction to the patient. It would be wise to have a special phone number that patients could call who have problems with the scheduling system. Choose a program that is simple to use and easy to understand for best results.

Legal and Ethical Issues

The appointment schedule may be used as a legal record and could be brought by subpoena into a court of law. Be sure that all handwriting in the book is completely legible and that information is routinely collected in a consistent manner for each entry. Do not fail to note a no-show in the patient's chart as well as the appointment schedule. This is often helpful when a physician must prove that the patient did not follow medical advice or that the patient contributed to his or her poor condition by missing appointments. Old appointment schedules should be kept for a time equal to the statute of limitations in the state in which the practice exists.

SUMMARY OF SCENARIO

Ramona is an asset to the medical office, because her dedication and customer service skills help her to interact with patients in a positive way. She genuinely cares about the patients and makes every effort to meet their needs while following the preferences of her physician. She has found that her bright smile is a valuable tool to use when patients have been waiting and are growing restless.

Ramona cooperates with other staff members to get the patients seen as quickly as possible and minimize wait time. She is flexible and can change the order of the patients seen, if needed, to maximize the use of time and facilities in the office. Because she is so cheerful and friendly, patients do not seem to mind when she asks for their cooperation. She keeps current phone numbers and cell phone information so that she can notify a patient quickly if Dr. Brown is running behind schedule. Ramona's proficiency on the computer also is an asset, and she makes frequent use of email to take care of patient problems or rescheduling desires.

Because of the cooperation she receives from staff and patients alike, Ramona successfully runs an efficient office.

SUMMARY OF LEARNING OBJECTIVES

- When scheduling appointments, a medical assistant must consider the patients' needs, the physician's preferences, and the available facilities. Make every attempt to schedule a patient at his or her most convenient time. This will help to avoid no-shows. The physician will outline preferences, which should be of high priority to the medical assistant. However, most physicians are flexible and will make adjustments according to the needs of the office. The availability of facilities within the office are perhaps the most inflexible. If a certain room or piece of equipment is being used for one patient, it usually cannot be used for another.

- When choosing an appointment book, all of the needs of the office should be considered. If there are multiple physicians, the book should be arranged so that each physician is readily identified. Books that open flat on the surface of the desk are much easier to handle, but if there is not enough space to open the book entirely, another style might be better. The book should also provide enough space to write all of the patient information needed in the various time slots, such as the name, phone number, and reason for the visit.

- Computerized scheduling programs are in demand today because they are easy to operate, simplifying scheduling appointments and making changes to the schedule. The computer can find the first available time much more quickly than scanning through an appointment book. Most programs can prepare reports and even notify patients automatically by email of the impending appointment. Web-based self-scheduling programs are becoming popular: these allow a patient to see the physician's available appointments and book his or her own date and time.

- Self-scheduling would vastly reduce calls to the office, because a high number of everyday calls are requests to schedule appointments. Patients could make an appointment at midnight, if they desired.

- Open office hours allow patients to come to the physician's office when it is convenient and wait in turn to see the physician. Scheduling specific appointments is the most popular method of seeing patients. Flexible office hours allow patients to see the physician during the evening and often on weekends. Many of today's medical offices have some flexible scheduling, because most families now consist of two working parents. Wave scheduling brings two or three patients to the office at the same time, and they are seen in the order of their arrival. This type of scheduling can be modified in many ways to suit the needs of the facility. Other scheduling methods include double booking and grouping of like procedures.

- When the office is running 15 minutes behind schedule, the medical assistant should briefly explain the delay to the waiting patients and then offer to reschedule their appointments. Keep the patients informed of wait times until the schedule resumes.

- Giving a patient a choice in appointment times to better meet his or her needs is a part of good customer service. Offering the patient a choice of 2 days, morning or afternoon, and two times helps to ensure that the patient will keep the appointment.

- Because the appointment schedule might be called into a court of law, it is vital that the handwriting in the book be completely legible. Even if the book is 5 years old, the person charged with testifying in court should be able to clearly read all entries. Scribbled, messy handwriting implies incompetence and reflects on the practice.

- Patients who are habitually late for appointments might be told to arrive 15 minutes before the time written in the book. Some offices book these patients as the last appointment of the day, so that if they do not arrive promptly, they do not see the physician. Usually talking with the patient and gaining an understanding of why the patient arrives late will improve the situation. The office can work with the patient to choose the best times that will result in a show appointment.

- Some patients accidentally forget the appointment with the physician, and some are habitually careless about remembering their scheduled time. Small emergencies often come up, and in today's busy business world, some patients just cannot get away from their own offices or other obligations to visit the physician. In some cases patients do not keep appointments because they do not want to deal with a health issue confronting them.

INTERNET CONNECTIONS

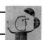

- Schedule Wise
  http://www.schedulewise.com

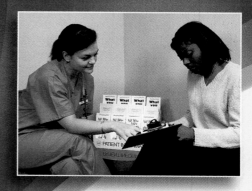

CHAPTER 11

Scenario

Most people enter the healthcare field for very specific reasons. One medical assistant, Georgina Robertson, recalls being in a serious car accident when she was about 6 years old, and as a result her vision was temporarily impaired. She remembers seeing a woman in a white uniform who offered words of comfort. She seemed to have a haze around her, which when combined with the lights, made her look as if she had wings. This vision of an "angel" never left her thoughts and led her into the medical field.

Today Georgina works for Dr. Stuart Wade, a cardiologist in a metropolitan city near Detroit. Georgina is a seasoned medical assistant, and she enjoys getting to know her patients. She makes notes on the chart that remind her of special events in the lives of the patients that visit Dr. Wade's office. The patients feel that she truly cares about them, aside from her duties at the clinic. Although she is efficient and time conscious, she always has a moment to share a warm smile or hear about a new grandchild. Georgina is a valued member of the medical team in her office. She is currently attending a state college in the evening hours, gaining credits toward her bachelor's degree. She plans to continue her education and perhaps apply to medical school one day.

Patient Reception and Processing

Learning Objectives

- Define and spell the terms listed in the vocabulary.
- Explain the purpose of the office mission statement.
- List several patient amenities and why these are important additions to the medical office.
- Describe how to prepare for patient arrivals.
- Explain why it is important to use the patient's name as often as possible.
- Discuss how the medical assistant may help the patient prepare for an examination.
- List and explain two methods of chart placement.
- Discuss how the medical assistant might deal with talkative patients.
- Explain how the medical assistant can recall closing duties.
- Discuss ways to make the patient feel at ease and comfortable in the medical office.
- Correctly prepare charts for registered patients who are scheduled.
- Demonstrate the correct way to register a new patient.

National Curriculum Competencies

TRANSDISCIPLINARY COMPETENCIES

2c. Establish and maintain the medical record
3b. Patient instruction

Vocabulary

amenity Something conducive to comfort, convenience, or enjoyment.

demographic The statistical characteristics of human populations (as in age or income) used especially to identify markets.

depleted To lessen markedly in quantity, content, power, or value.

fervent Exhibiting or marked by great intensity of feeling.

flagged Marked in some way as to remind or remember that specific action needs to be taken.

harmonious Marked by accord in sentiment or action; having the parts agreeably related.

immigrant A person who comes to a country to take up permanent residence.

intercom A two-way communication system with a microphone and loudspeaker at each station for localized use.

mnemonic A device, such as a sentence or rhyme, used as a memory aid (e.g., Roy G. Biv for remembering the colors of the spectrum: red-orange-yellow-green-blue-indigo-violet).

perception A quick, acute, and intuitive cognition; a capacity for comprehension.

phonetic Constituting an alteration of ordinary spelling that better represents the spoken language, that employs only characters of the regular alphabet, and that is used in a context of conventional spelling.

progress notes Notes used in the patient chart to track the progress and condition of the patient.

sequentially Of, relating to, or arranged in a sequence.

The patient reception area should be an inviting place in which patients feel comfortable. Visits to the physician can be times of great stress, so the office staff must do everything possible to make the experience pleasant for patients. A patient usually has a choice of healthcare providers and should be treated with excellent customer service. Good patient relations will result in referrals to the physician, and this helps the practice grow. When patients have a good experience with a physician, they are likely to tell others. When the office staff are committed to making the patient feel welcome and the focus is on care of the patient, the success of the practice is inevitable.

The Office Mission Statement

Healthcare providers often have a **fervent** reason for entering the medical field. One physician remembers the heritage his **immigrant** grandfather left in his heart. The physician has fond memories of his grandfather's pride and thankfulness for the opportunities he found in America, after coming to the United States with nothing but the clothes on his back. The grandfather's dream was to see his grandson become a physician, and that is exactly what he did. Even on the most trying days, he could step into his office and see the picture of his grandfather and find the strength and determination to care for his patients.

The office mission statement reflects this deep-seated desire by expressing the reasons for the existence of the practice (Figure 11-1). The physician may develop the mission statement alone or may consult the office staff for input. Many offices display the mission statement prominently in the reception area and on printed material, such as patient information booklets. Whatever the contents, each employee of the facility should be familiar with the statement and have a personal commitment to promoting the mission statement ideas in everyday practice.

The Reception Area

A first impression is lasting. Nowhere is this more important than in the healthcare facility, where the environment must appear orderly and faultlessly clean. The facility may be a physician's office, a hospital, a health maintenance organization, an insurance company, or one of the many other healthcare sources. No matter what facility is involved, the appearance of the reception room and the front desk, and a cordial greeting by the receptionist, influence a patient's **perception** of the entire facility and the care that he or she will receive.

The reception area is just that—a place to receive patients. The area should be planned for the patients' comfort, made as attractive and cheerful as possible, and kept clean and uncluttered (Figure 11-2). Often a medical assistant has the opportunity to assist in the design and decoration of this very important area.

WADE CARDIAC CLINIC MISSION STATEMENT

The mission of the Wade Cardiac Clinic is fourfold:
- The staff of the clinic promotes the highest standards of ethical medical practice.
- The physician and staff members commit to serving their patients with respect and courtesy.
- All staff members shall promote a healthy lifestyle and preventative measures for the patients that present to the clinic.
- The clinic will support medical patient education, scientific research and development, community service, and community health promotion.

It is our desire to give the best customer service to our patients and care for them as if they were members of our own families.

FIGURE 11-1 The mission statement should be presented to all employees early in their tenure, and the staff should strive to meet the mission every day.

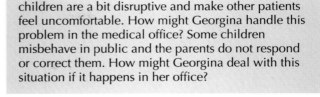
Fresh, **harmonious** colors and cleanliness are the basis of an attractive room (Figure 11-3). Add comfortable furniture that is adequate to accommodate the peak load of patients seen each day and arrange it in conversational groups. Individual chairs are best (Figure 11-4); people sometimes prefer to stand rather than sit next to a stranger on a sofa. Provide good lighting, ventilation, and a regulated temperature for additional comfort, and the essentials are in place for an attractive reception area. A place to hang coats, rainwear, and umbrellas helps reduce reception room clutter. Professional designers can be consulted regarding reception room décor and improvements or when there is a problem area that inhibits office traffic.

Most physicians' offices are well supplied with recent magazines and pictorial travel books. Publications with short items of popular interest are favorites. Some offices have a book share program, where patients bring paperback books to the office and can trade them for another. The next time the office is visited, the paperback is returned and another can be taken. The reception room, incidentally, is not the place for the physician's professional journals.

A writing desk with writing paper in the reception area for the convenience of patients is a nice touch, as is restful music from a concealed speaker. A lighted aquarium or an educational display of some sort will enhance the attractiveness and individuality of the reception area of the professional practice. Patients are often interested in health-related brochures. The physician may also have a videotape or healthcare book library, which allows patients to check out items of interest to them.

Additions such as a television and VCR or DVD player will help the time pass much faster, especially in pediatric offices. Children enjoy Disney movies and cartoon programs, and these hold their interest until it is time to see the physician. A children's corner equipped with small-scale furniture and some playthings works well (Figure 11-5). Youngsters who might otherwise get into mischief are kept pleasantly occupied. Toys should be easily cleanable; plastic washable items are especially good. Take extra care to ensure that no toy has sharp corners that could injure a child and that there are no small parts that could be swallowed. In selecting toys, make certain that they will not stimulate the child toward noisy activity. And no rubber balls, unless there is time to chase them around the room!

Many of today's modern offices offer a computer for patient use while waiting to see the physician. This is a wonderful **amenity**, because the patient can make good use of his or her time while in the reception area. An amazing amount of work can be done just by checking office email, so providing Internet access to patients is also helpful. A telephone in the reception area is an asset and can be programmed by the phone company not to allow long-distance calls.

Periodically, take an objective look around the reception room. Could it use a little brightening or freshening up? Try to look at it as if you were seeing it for the first time. The receptionist is partly responsible for the appearance of the area by making certain that the room remains neat and orderly throughout the day. Check the temperature and lighting for comfort. Scan the room at various intervals during the day to ensure that the room is in order.

If the medical assistant's desk is in the reception area or in open view of the patients, it should be free of clutter. In particular, patients' charts and financial records should not be in sight. Computer monitors should not be in view of patients, to protect the confidentiality of records. Personal articles, coffee cups, and so forth should not be on the receptionist's desk.

Preparing for Patient Arrival

Advance preparation helps to make the day go smoothly and contributes toward a more relaxed atmosphere for all concerned. Some offices prepare for the next day on the evening before, whereas others prepare each morning. The office should be consistent and always perform the same routine.

Readying the Patient Charts

Pull the charts for the day (or the next day if this is done in the evenings), and check off the patient's name on a copy of the appointment schedule to be sure that all charts have been located and are ready (Figure 11-6). Occasionally

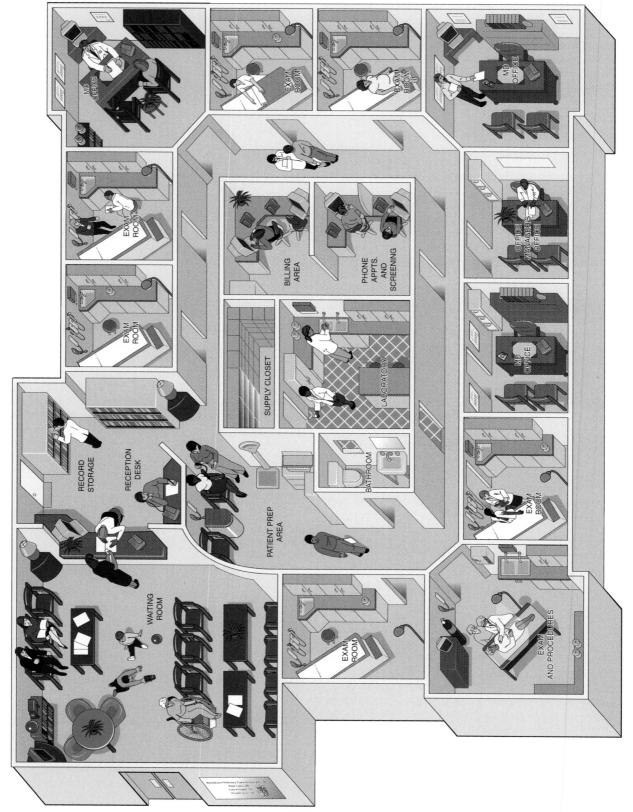

FIGURE 11-2 The medical office should be arranged so that the flow of traffic is conducive to the movement of patients throughout the office.

more than one patient may have the same or a similar name. Review each chart to verify that any recently received information, such as laboratory reports and radiograph readings, has been correctly entered, permanently attached to the chart, and that each chart is current (Procedure 11-1). Arrange the charts **sequentially** in the order the patients are scheduled to be seen. The medical assistant may be expected to place the charts of all the patients to be seen that day on the physician's desk, but it is more likely that the physician will prefer to receive a patient's chart just before seeing him or her. Be sure that there is enough space on the **progress notes** for the physician to write in the chart. A new sheet may need to be added.

Replenishing Supplies

Supplies at the reception desk need to be replenished regularly. Stationery, appointment cards, charge slips,

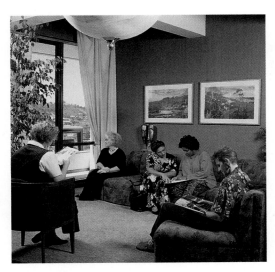

FIGURE 11-3 Patients appreciate cleanliness, restful colors, good ventilation, and light to read by when waiting in the reception area.

sharpened pencils, and any items likely to be needed during the day should be on hand when the day begins. Discovering that supplies are **depleted** during a busy day can seriously interrupt the flow of patient care. One person should be in charge of checking the inventory of supplies on a regular basis and ordering as necessary.

In a multiple-employee practice, a clinical assistant usually has the responsibility of checking clinical supplies and preparing the patient rooms. However, in a small practice there may be only one assistant in charge. Before patients start arriving, everything should be ready for the day so that the physician and medical assistant can give undivided attention to the patients' needs.

Greeting the Patient

Every patient has the right to expect courteous treatment in a physician's office. No matter what the patient's economic or social status may be, each individual who enters the reception room should receive a cordial, friendly greeting (Figure 11-7). Using a personal touch in receiving patients is important.

Patient Check-in

The reception desk is usually placed for a clear view of all visitors who come into the office. If there is only one medical assistant, it is sometimes impossible for each new caller to be welcomed personally. In this situation, some announcement system must be worked out. The patient who enters an empty reception room does not know whether to sit down, knock on the glass partition, or try to announce his or her presence in some way. A bell at the desk or window that the patient can ring is one solution. Sometimes a sign is placed in the reception room that reads, "Please sit comfortably. The receptionist will be with you shortly."

The receptionist should check the reception area each time he or she has been away from the desk to see if additional patients have arrived. These patients should

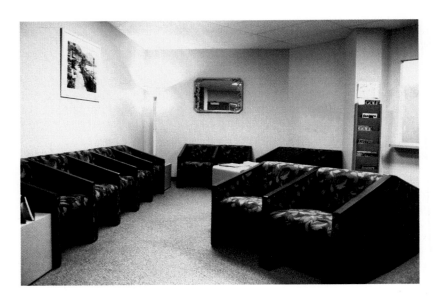

FIGURE 11-4 Patients tend to prefer individual seating. Comfortable seating helps patients relax and be at ease while waiting to see the physician. (Courtesy August Incorporated, Centerville, Ohio.)

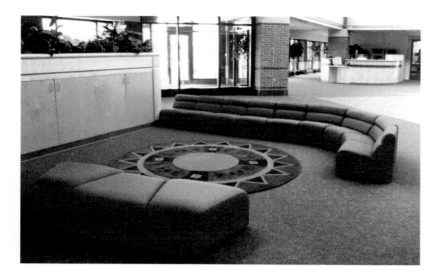

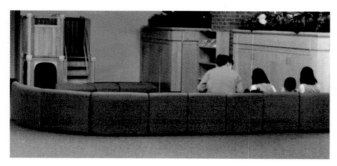

FIGURE 11-5 Furniture in a pediatrician's office should be durable and fun, child sized, and able to withstand the most active children. (Courtesy August Incorporated, Centerville, Ohio.)

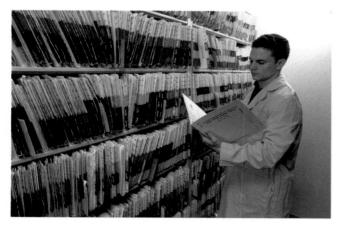

FIGURE 11-6 Charts should be pulled in advance for the patients arriving for appointments. Each chart should be checked to see whether it has adequate forms and is in good order for the physician's use.

CRITICAL THINKING APPLICATION

Everyone forgets someone's name on occasion. How might Georgina and her staff members remember names? What special tips or techniques assist in remembering names? Eventually a patient will come to the clinic whose name just cannot be recalled. How can the staff determine who the patient is without offending him or her?

Knowing the Patients

Cultivate the habit of greeting each patient immediately in a friendly, self-assured manner. Establish eye contact and smile while introducing yourself to the patient. For example, "Good morning, I'm Elizabeth Parr, Dr. Wade's medical assistant."

Patients like to be acknowledged when they arrive. All staff members should review the day's schedule in the morning to be prepared to greet patients by name and to know whether the patient is new or established (Figure 11-8). Learn how to pronounce each patient's name correctly, because incorrect pronunciations may offend and irritate some people. If the name is unusual, write the **phonetic** spelling on the record for reference. Using the patient's name often also ensures that the correct patient is being treated.

also be greeted by name. The office staff should avoid having a sign-in register that stays at the patient reception window, because patient confidentiality is violated when others can read the register. It is preferable to hand the register to the patient if a sign-in sheet is used. Patients should not be expected to provide details of the reason for their visit in a public area. Remember to ask about the patient before asking about insurance.

PROCEDURE 11-1

Preparing Charts for Scheduled Patients

GOAL: To prepare patient charts for the daily appointment schedule and have them ready for the physician before the patients' arrival.

EQUIPMENT AND SUPPLIES

- Appointment schedule for current date
- Patient files
- Clerical supplies (e.g., pen, tape, stapler)

PROCEDURAL STEPS

1 Review the appointment schedule.

2 Identify full name of each scheduled patient.

3 Pull patients' charts for files, checking each patient's name on your list as each is pulled.
Purpose: To determine that the correct charts have been pulled and that no charts have been omitted.

4 Review each chart.
Purpose: To reaffirm that:
- The correct patient chart has been pulled

- Any previously ordered tests have been performed
- The results of the tests have been mounted or entered in the chart
- Forms have been replenished inside the chart, such as progress notes, and so forth

5 Annotate the appointment list with any special concerns.
Purpose: To alert the physician regarding matters that should be checked or discussed with the patient.

6 Arrange the charts sequentially according to each patient's appointment.

7 Place the charts in the appropriate examination room or other specified location.

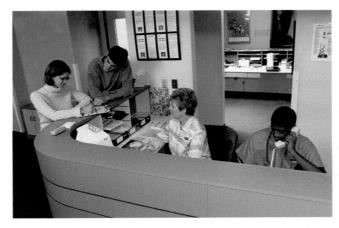

FIGURE 11-7 Greet all patients with a warm smile and assist them with forms they need to complete for the chart.

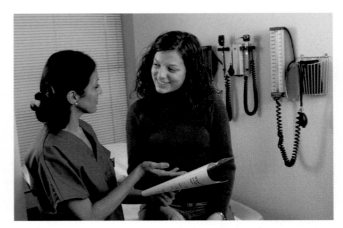

FIGURE 11-8 The medical assistant should develop a good relationship with the patient and be a caring advocate.

It is helpful to make brief notes in the chart about the current events in the patient's life. With this information, the medical assistant and the physician can read those notes before entering the examination room, and share a short dialog with patients at the beginning of their visits. An example follows:

Georgina: Hello, Mrs. Williams, how are you today?
Mrs. Williams: I am doing very well, Georgina, how are you?
Georgina: I'm fine. How was the cruise you took with your husband last month?

Mrs. Williams: It was wonderful! The water was the bluest I have seen!
Georgina: You went to Grand Cayman and Cozumel, didn't you?
Mrs. Williams: Yes, we did! I'm surprised you remember as many patients as you see each day!

This brief chat will confirm that the staff cares about the individual patients because they take an interest in their personal lives (Figure 11-9). Because the medical assistant or physician looked at the notes before entering the patient room, the patient assumes that the informa-

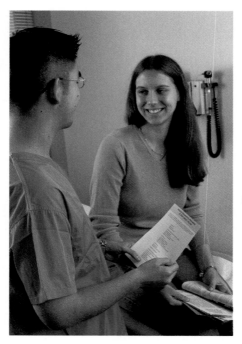

FIGURE 11-9 Patients appreciate being called by name and remembered from visit to visit.

tion is being recalled from memory, and that is an impressive customer service technique. Most patients appreciate the interest of the physician and the staff in their families, hobbies, and work.

Registration Procedures

Certain registration procedures are required on a patient's first visit to the facility (Procedure 11-2). Most physicians use a patient information form to gather **demographic** information about the patient. The form may be attached to a clipboard and handed to the patient with instructions to complete all parts of the form, with assurance that the assistant is ready and willing to answer any questions (Figure 11-10). The patient's name should appear prominently at the top of the form, followed by other pertinent facts in logical order. Most information sheets contain the following information:
- Patient's name and date of birth
- Responsible person's name
- Relationship to patient
- Address and telephone number
- Name, address, and telephone number of spouse
- Occupation

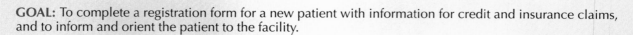

PROCEDURE 11-2

Registering a New Patient

GOAL: To complete a registration form for a new patient with information for credit and insurance claims, and to inform and orient the patient to the facility.

EQUIPMENT AND SUPPLIES
- Registration form
- Clerical supplies (pen, clipboard)
- Private conference area

PROCEDURAL STEPS

1 Determine whether the patient is new.

2 Obtain and record the necessary information:
- Full name, birth date, name of spouse (if married)
- Home address, telephone number (include ZIP and area codes)
- Occupation, name of employer, business address, telephone number
- Social Security number and driver's license number, if any
- Name of referring physician, if any
- Name and address of person responsible for payment
- Method of payment
- Health insurance information (photocopy both sides of insurance ID card)
- Name of primary carrier

- Type of coverage
- Group policy number
- Subscriber number
- Assignment of benefits, if required
Purpose: This information is necessary for credit and insurance claims.

3 Review the enter form and confirm patient eligibility for insurance coverage.
Purpose: To verify that the given information is complete and legible.

4 Determine that required referrals have been received, if applicable.
Purpose: Insurance coverage may not be valid without referral.

5 Explain medical and financial procedures to patients.
Purpose: The patient develops a comfort level and knows what to expect.

6 Collect co-payments or balance payment charges.
Purpose: Keeps accounts current and prevents the necessity of mailing statements.

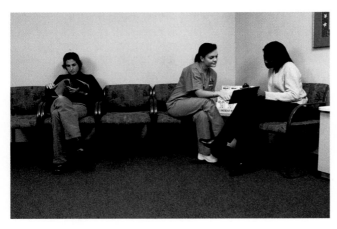

FIGURE 11-10   The medical assistant should take the time to explain forms that the patient does not understand and always be willing to answer questions.

- Place of employment
- Social Security number
- Driver's license number
- Nearest relative not living with patient, and his or her relationship
- Source of referral, if any

When the completed form is returned to the medical assistant, it must be checked carefully to verify that all the necessary information has been included.

CRITICAL THINKING APPLICATION

Often some time is needed to complete patient forms when a new patient arrives in the office. How might Georgina keep the office on schedule when new patients arrive, necessitating chart construction and form completion? What are some ways to trim time from these activities?

Obtaining a Patient History

The personal and medical history, and the patient's family history, may be obtained by asking the patient to complete a questionnaire; the physician can augment this information during the patient interview. The experienced medical assistant may be expected to conduct the interview for the patient's personal and medical history, family history, and chief complaint. This is a very specialized procedure, and the interviewer must be specifically trained for the individual practice.

Consideration for Patients' Time

Once the preliminaries have been completed, the patient will expect to see the physician or practitioner at the appointed time. The medical assistant should get the patient in for treatment or consultation as near the appointment time as possible or explain any potential delay to

the patient. All patients want to be kept informed about how long to expect to wait. Almost all patients will respond positively when the physician or the assistant comes to the reception area to apologize for any delay. Consideration for the patient's time is essential.

Most experts will agree that in a solo or small practice, there should seldom be more than three to five patients in the reception room. Wait time is one of the most frequently heard criticisms of the medical profession. The patient who complains about medical fees or the care received may actually be complaining about the long wait or discourteous service. Most patients are fearful and tense, but the medical assistant can often put them in a better frame of mind with just a friendly smile and a show of concern.

A crowded reception room is not always an indication of a physician's popularity. It may simply mean that the physician or the assistant is inefficient in scheduling patients. Business people, for example, who are in the habit of making the most of their time, are particularly displeased at what may appear to them to be inefficient scheduling of appointments. Any delay of longer than 10 to 15 minutes should be explained to the person waiting. Some personal attention, such as offering a drink of water, a cup of coffee, or a new magazine, may help to calm a patient who appears irritated with the delay. However, be sure that the patient is allowed caffeine before offering coffee. Be careful that the refreshment offered does not go against the physician's orders or would interfere with scheduled blood testing or other procedures.

Patients With Special Needs

Some patients will be physically challenged, some very ill, and some severely uncomfortable. There may be language or cultural barriers. Observe the patient's appearance and behavior. Is the patient pale or drawn looking? Do the eyes or voice reflect pain or discomfort? Find out how the patient is feeling before you suggest that he or she be seated to wait for the physician. The patient may need to lie down in a cool room or perhaps should be seen as an emergency.

The patient who is in a wheelchair or using a walker or crutches may need personal attention. Some patients may need help in disrobing even when a disability is not obvious. Ask if the patient needs assistance. The medical assistant must use good judgment in helping disabled patients, perhaps even bypassing some of the usual routines.

Escorting and Instructing the Patient

Sometimes we become so accustomed to our own surroundings that we forget that a stranger to the practice's environment may be confused or disoriented by all the hallways, doors, and rooms. Uncertainty creates anxiety. Take the time to personally escort the patient to the appropriate examination or treatment room (Figure 11-11). This is usually the responsibility of a clinical medical assistant. If a urine specimen is to be obtained, direct the patient to the rest room.

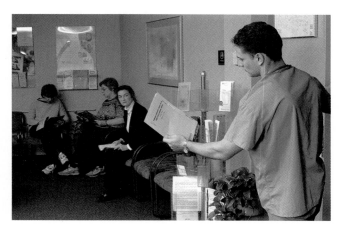

FIGURE 11-11   Pronounce the patient's name correctly and use it often. This promotes good customer service and pleases the patient.

If the patient is to disrobe, explain what garments, if any, can be left on, whether shoes are to be removed, that he or she must remove jewelry if an x-ray film is to be taken, and so forth. If a gown is to be worn, specify whether the opening should be in the front or back and tell the patient where he or she can hang up clothes if this is not obvious. An examination table should never be placed in such a position that the patient is exposed to passersby in the hallway if the door is opened. Imagine a patient ready for a Pap smear, facing the door as the physician enters! Allow patients a sense of modesty at all times and make all instructions crystal clear. Do not assume that patients will know what is expected of them. Be equally clear when the examination has been completed. Tell the patient whether he or she should go to the physician's office for consultation, or return to the reception area to wait, or whether he or she is free to check out with the front office and leave.

The medical assistant can help keep the schedule operating smoothly by immediately tidying each examination room and moving the next patient in so that the physician need have no idle moments waiting for a patient to be prepared. Try not to place a patient in an examination room just to clear out the reception area. It is especially inconsiderate to keep the patient waiting after being gowned, draped, and positioned on the examining table. A magazine rack on the wall of the treatment room is a welcome addition in some practices.

Chart Placement

Patient charts should never be left in the examination room to be picked up and read by a patient. This can cause misunderstandings because patients often do not know medical terms and abbreviations. Physicians have different methods of being signaled that a patient is ready to be seen. Often there are chart holders on the doors of the examination rooms, where the chart can be placed horizontally when the patient is ready to be seen. Then the physician can signal the medical assistant that he or she is finished examining the patient by placing the chart in an upright position on leaving the examination room.

Some offices have call systems, by which a physician can press a button to call the medical assistant for help with the examination. Today's physicians often prefer a second person in the room during examinations to avoid claims of sexual assault or harassment.

Other offices place patients in exam rooms in a certain order, and the physician knows, for instance, that when he or she has finished with the patient in room 1, the next patient will be waiting in room 2. The office should develop a method that allows the most efficient use of time while providing quality care to the patients.

Problem Situations

Talkative Patients

There can be certain problem patients in any professional office. Talkative patients, for example, take up far more of the physician's time than is justified. An alert medical assistant can usually spot this tendency during the initial interview. The patient's history can be **flagged** with a symbol to alert the physician. A prearranged agreement to contact the physician on the **intercom** at the end of the allotted time with the message that the next patient is waiting gives the physician an opportunity to conclude the interview. Once you have learned which patients take extra time, you can book them for the end of the day or simply allow more time for them.

CRITICAL THINKING APPLICATION

Georgina has one patient who insists on sitting close by her desk and attempting to chat the entire time she is waiting to see the physician. What is worse, she comes to her appointments at least an hour early. How might Georgina subtly deal with this patient?

Children

Children frequently present special management problems. It is sometimes advisable to escort younger patients into the treatment room without the parent. Of course, this should be at the discretion of the physician and must be with the permission of the parent. The physician cannot force the parent to leave the examination room by any means. Although this practice of separating children from their parents to treat their needs is not always feasible, it sometimes can be applied with great success. In some offices a token of the physician's friendship, such as a trinket or toy, is given to the child at the completion of the visit.

Angry Patients in the Reception Area

Every medical assistant at some time will be confronted by an angry patient. The anger may simply be a reflection of the patient's pain or fear of what the physician may discover on the examination. If possible, invite the patient into another room out of the reception area. Usually it is best to let the patient talk out his or her anger. A calm attitude on the part of the medical assistant, with a few remarks interjected in a low voice, will often pacify the patient. Under no circumstances should the assistant return the anger or become argumentative.

Patient Relatives

A patient will sometimes be accompanied by a relative or well-meaning friend who may become restless while waiting for the patient and attempt to discuss the patient's illness. The medical assistant should sidestep any discussion of a patient's medical care, except by direction of the physician. Also avoid a too casual attitude, such as "I'm sure there's nothing to worry about." A show of moderate concern and offering reassurance that "the patient is in good hands" usually takes care of the situation.

Patient Check-out

When the patient has been referred back to the front office for check-out, he or she should be greeted with a friendly smile and called by name. It is wise to form the habit of asking the patients if they have any questions once again. Then the chart must be checked to see when the physician wishes the patient to come back to the office. Most physicians will note this information on the encounter form. Make the return appointment, remembering the technique of giving the patient choices as to which day they wish to come, morning or afternoon, and specific time. Then ask the patient for their payment, using phrasing such as, "Your co-pay today is $15, Mrs. Williams. Will you be writing a check or would you like to charge this visit to your Visa?"

Be sure to thank the patient for coming, and wish him or her well as they leave the office (Figure 11-12).

The Friendly Farewell

As soon as the visit with the physician has been completed the medical assistant should be ready to take charge by assisting the patient in dressing, if necessary, and

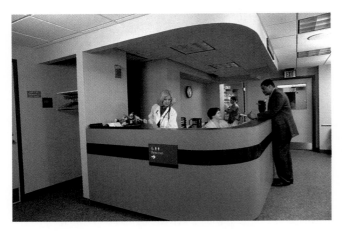

FIGURE 11-12   Always thank the patient for coming and wish him or her well.

by making sure that any questions that the patient may have are answered. In a small practice, this may be the responsibility of the administrative medical assistant.

If the patient has questions that the assistant can capably and ethically answer, the assistant should answer them clearly and note this on the patient's chart. Some questions can be answered only by the physician; in such cases the assistant can offer to get answers for the patient. Remember, patients view the medical assistant as an extension of the physician and the medical assistant must be very careful to avoid accusations of practicing medicine without a license.

The assistant can help convey a sense of caring by terminating the patient's visit cordially. If the patient is returning for another visit, the assistant can say something like "We'll see you next week." If it is the patient's last visit, a pleasant "I certainly hope you'll be feeling fine from now on" is appropriate. The assistant may wish to tell a patient on a last visit that he or she has been a fine patient and that it has been a pleasure to make his or her acquaintance. Whatever words of good-bye are chosen, all patients should leave the facility with the feeling that they have received top-quality care and were treated with friendliness, respect, and courtesy.

Leaving the Office for the Day

Each office should have a specific routine when it is time to leave the office for the day. Patient file cabinets must be locked and secure to help prevent breaches in patient confidentiality. Lab specimens may need to be placed in a lockbox outside the office for pickup. General housekeeping duties are often performed at the end of the day and certain reports may need to be generated for accounting purposes daily, weekly, or monthly. These are usually done at the close of the business day. The phones will usually need to be turned over to the answering service or voicemail.

Those responsible for closing the office should have a method in place for remembering each closing duty. For instance, if the medical assistant knows that five specific things must be done before leaving the office, it may help to devise a **mnemonic** device to jog the memory and ensure that each task is completed. For instance:

Leave lab specimens outside
Close patient file cabinets
Lock safe
Lock file room door
Turn off lights
Set alarm

The mnemonic that the staff member remembers could be "*Loose cats leave lots to steal.*" The more nonsensical, the easier to remember. This trick can help the medical assistant recall every closing duty every day.

Closing Comments

A personal touch is vital to projecting a sense of care to the patients seen in the physician's office. Many medical offices are not concerned enough about the customer service aspect of the business. Patients talk about their experiences with their friends and relatives and may be an excellent source of referrals if they are treated with dignity and courtesy. If they have had a good experience, they will tell several people. If they have a poor experience, they tend to tell everyone they know! Be sure to have a part in each patient feeling a sense of satisfaction as they leave the office. All patients should feel that their time and money were well spent.

Patient Education

Offering a patient education center in the reception area is an effective way to provide up-to-date information about healthcare issues to patients. Brochures and information sheets can be displayed, and if the office is equipped with a VCR in the reception area, videotapes that deal with health topics can be available for viewing while the patient is waiting to see the physician.

Both the physician and the medical assistants caring for patients should ask if the patient has any questions during his or her visit to the office. Patients often complain that they did not have a chance to speak to the physician long enough to have their questions answered sufficiently. Be sure that this is not the case, and prompt the patient to ask about anything he or she is unclear on while the physician is still in the examination room.

Legal and Ethical Issues

A medical assistant must take care not to offer medical advice to a patient unless specifically instructed to do so by the physician. The patient sees the medical assistant as an extension of the physician and tends to weigh advice and comments by the medical assistant with the same validity as if they came from the physician. Provide only information that the physician has approved or is included in the office policy and procedure manuals.

When a patient complains, listen carefully and attempt to resolve the problem or assure the patient that the issue will be discussed with the appropriate staff member to find a solution. If someone other than the patient asks for information about the patient, refrain from discussion unless the patient or physician has authorized the release of information.

SUMMARY OF SCENARIO

Georgina is a person who truly makes a difference in the healthcare profession. She takes her role seriously as a patient advocate and strives to make her patients feel comfortable in her physician's office. She keeps the mission statement posted close to her desk and rereads it often to keep her focus clear. She shares the vision with the other staff members, who are supportive and in agreement with the purpose for which the office exists.

Dr. Wade promotes continuing medical education and encourages his staff members to participate in courses and seminars that will assist them in being more effective

patient advocates. The office sends birthday and Christmas cards to the patients in their database, and at their annual Christmas Party, the staff hand-signs each Christmas card. Georgina sends a monthly newsletter to the patients, some by mail and some by email, to keep the patients up to date on office policies and interesting health information. All of these activities indicate a strong caring attitude toward the patients. Georgina considers each one a customer of the clinic, and she is determined that they receive excellent customer service.

Wait times are at a minimum in Dr. Wade's office. Cell phone numbers and email addresses are gathered at registration and updated frequently so that the staff can quickly contact patients. Georgina offers new patients a form for evaluation of the office, so that they can provide input about the experience they had as a new patient. All of these efforts promote a trusting, caring relationship among physician, staff, and patients.

SUMMARY OF LEARNING OBJECTIVES

■ The office mission statement is the philosophy of why the office exists. Often physicians develop the mission statement themselves, which outlines their vision and reasons for entering medical practice. Some physicians allow the office staff to assist in its development. All employees should become familiar with the mission statement and promote its ideas to all patients and visitors.

■ Patient amenities include such things as a VCR, television, computer, telephone, and a desk where patients can sit and balance a checkbook or review work while away from the office. These features turn the time spent in the physician's office into productive minutes instead of wasteful ones.

■ Some offices prepare for patient arrivals the evening before, and some in the morning. Patient charts must be pulled and should be reviewed, checking for completed laboratory tests, posting of results, and to ensure that there are ample progress notes for this visit. Rooms should be checked and inventoried to make certain there are enough supplies on hand and that they present a clean, neat appearance.

■ People like hearing their own names; a better relationship is built between the staff and patients when the names are used often. Patients feel that the office staff care enough about them to acknowledge them, and this custom adds a personal touch.

■ The medical assistant should escort the patient to the examination rooms and other areas of the office. Always tell the patient when to disrobe and exactly what should be removed. Offer to assist with disrobing if the patient needs extra help. Take care that the patient's purse or wallet is in a secure place. Be sure that doors do not open and expose the disrobed patient. Instruct the patient as to whether he or she may leave or should wait after seeing the physician. Ask whether the patient has any questions.

■ Some medical offices place patient charts in a door file, which alerts the physician that the patient is ready to be seen. The chart may be placed horizontally or vertically, one placement meaning that the patient is ready for the physician, and the other meaning that the doctor is finished with the patient. Other offices place the charts in door files in a certain order. For example, if examination rooms 1, 2, and 3 are available, patients are seen in that order by the physician.

■ Patients who are talkative may be lonely and enjoy the social interaction of their visits to the physician's office. Be as courteous as possible with talkative patients, expressing to them when necessary that another patient is waiting or the physician needs assistance. When said with a smile, most patients understand.

■ Closing duties can be easily remembered by creating a mnemonic device, associating each duty with the first letter of each task, then making a nonsense sentence to prompt recollection of those duties. Lists posted close to the door will help, or developing a checklist of closing duties will help the medical assistant recall what to do before leaving for the day.

■ The personal touch will help the patient to feel at home and comfortable in the office. An attractive reception area with various patient amenities will provide a warm atmosphere. Using the patient's name often and a gentle touch will impart a sense of caring as well.

INTERNET CONNECTIONS

- August Incorporated
  www.augustinc.com

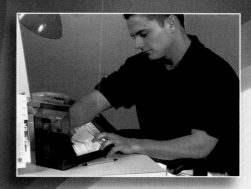

CHAPTER 12

Scenario

Brandon Tipps is a medical assistant working with his father, Dr. Rick Tipps. Brandon has considered continuing his education to become a doctor, but he is not sure whether he would like to be a medical doctor, an osteopathic physician, or a chiropractor. He decided to spend his summer off from college working in his father's family practice so that he could get a close look at the inner workings of a physician's office.

Brandon assisted with every procedure in the clinic, including the administrative skills required in the front office. The staff has been overwhelmed with Brandon's ability to do any task, no matter how small, as if it was the most important task of the office. He continuously moves from employee to employee to ask what he can do to help. When the administrative medical assistant working in the front office, Darla Grover, was injured in a car accident and had to be off work for a while, Brandon stepped right in to her job and learned her duties quickly. His help meant that the office continued to run smoothly even with one employee absent for several weeks.

Brandon has an excellent command of the English language and types at speeds of about 60 wpm. He is organized and efficient, so he is able to handle the enormous amount of incoming and outgoing mail with very little assistance from the office manager. He is also able to answer phones and schedule appointments. He speaks clearly and is an expert at customer service. Many of Dr. Tipps' patients have come to know him during his time in the office. The patients and staff alike will certainly miss him once he returns to college.

Written Communications and Mail Processing

National Curriculum Competencies

COMMUNICATION COMPETENCIES

1a. Respond to and initiate written communication

OPERATIONAL COMPETENCIES

4a. Perform an inventory of supplies and equipment
4b. Utilize computer software to maintain office systems

Vocabulary

academic degree A title conferred by a college, university, or professional school on completion of a program of study.

annotating To furnish with notes, which are usually critical or explanatory.

archaic Of, relating to, or characteristic of an earlier or more primitive time.

archived To have filed or collected records or documents.

bond A durable, formal paper used for documents.

categorically Placed in a specific division of a system of classification.

clauses A group of words containing a subject and predicate and functioning as a member of a complex or compound sentence.

collect on delivery (COD) Method of payment used when an article or item is delivered and payment is expected before it is released.

concise Expressing much in brief form.

continuation pages The second and following pages of a letter.

curt Marked by rude or peremptory shortness.

disseminate To disperse throughout.

domestic mail Mail that is sent within the boundaries of the United States and its territories.

flush Directly abutting or immediately adjacent, as set even with an edge of a type page or column; having no indention.

girth A measure around a body or item.

grammar The study of the classes of words, their inflections, and their functions and relations in the sentence; a study of what is to be preferred and what avoided in inflection and syntax.

international mail Mail that is sent outside the boundaries of the United States and its territories.

intrinsic Belonging to the essential nature or constitution of a thing; indwelling, inward.

portfolio A set of pictures, drawings, documents, or photographs either bound in book form or loose in a folder.

ream A quantity of paper being 20 pounds or, variously, 480, 500, or 516 sheets.

recipient The receiver of some thing or item.

stationers Sellers of stationery.

substance number A number based on the weight of a ream of paper containing 500 sheets.

superfluous Exceeding what is sufficient or necessary.

watermark A marking in paper resulting from differences in thickness usually produced by the pressure of a projecting design in the mold or on a processing roll and visible when the paper is held up to the light.

Entrepreneur and co-founder of the Amway Corporation, Rich de Vos, believed in a simple principle regarding the many business papers that crossed his desk on a daily basis. He believed that each paper should be handled only once. Whatever the news, information, or action required, the paper should be dealt with immediately, and this resulted in the most efficient use of his time. This is an excellent concept that is beneficial in any business, including the medical office.

Correspondence and mail processing can consume a large part of the administrative medical assistant's day. Many physicians, when queried about the skills they most desire in an administrative assistant, have said that a person who can spell accurately and write a good letter is a valuable addition to the medical office. When a physician delegates the responsibility of composing letters or reports that have the potential to reflect positively or negatively on the practice, he or she is expressing confidence in the medical assistant.

Importance of Written Communications

Written communications offer the perfect opportunity for making a good impression on others, but they do not just happen. They require thought, preparation, skill, and a positive attitude. Written communications take many forms in the medical office. The medical assistant should be skilled in creating various forms of communication.

Written communications include original letters, memorandums, replies to inquiries, responses to requests for information, telephone messages, email, transcriptions, orders for supplies, instructions for patients, and a variety of other forms. These communications should be courteous to the reader, correct in content, and concise without being curt. Communication is truly an art as well as a skill. The ability to communicate effectively is extremely important to the administrative medical assistant who wishes to succeed and advance in his or her career.

CRITICAL THINKING APPLICATION

Brandon has just found a small backlog of correspondence that accumulated during the first 3 days that Darla was out of the office. A large amount of mail comes to the office each day. How can Brandon manage the daily mail and clear the pile of communications that accumulated over those 3 days?

Written Communication as a Public Relations Tool

Public relations involves "telling the organization's story." The public relations department or director of any organization exists to present a business in the best possible light and to communicate to the public and other interested parties all of the positive aspects of a business. With this understanding, it is easy to see why written communications are so important. These documents can present a professional image or a very poor image to the receiver. Although individual medical offices rarely employ public relations professionals, each member of the staff must be conscientious about the documents and materials that are present within and that leave the office. An envelope addressed carelessly or a patient information sheet that has been photocopied over and over insinuates that the office personnel are not concerned about the appearance of documents that leave the office. If the staff is careless in this respect, many patients will assume that the staff is careless with everything, including patient care!

Reflection on the Physician

Everything that happens in the medical office is a reflection on the physician or physicians who practice there. Letters with misspelled words or errors will give the reader a negative impression of the physician and the practice itself. Great care must be taken to ensure that each document in the office and sent from the office is well written and grammatically correct. Table 12-1 lists proofreader's marks, while Tables 12-2 and 12-3 list frequently misspelled and misused words.

Equipment and Supplies

To create a favorable impression with letters, the medical assistant must use good equipment and quality supplies. Whatever kind of equipment is available, it is the medical assistant's responsibility to know how to use it to the best advantage and to keep it in good working condition. If the equipment manual is available, study it and keep it handy for reference when problems occur. Know how to maintain equipment so that the effort made in composing the correspondence results in a quality appearance.

Equipment

Computers. Computers have made composing correspondence simple. Various letters and documents may be saved and reused time after time by changing the name and basic information contained within the text. Computers can add graphics to text, compute figures, and use multimedia in communications—all of which enhance the appearance and effectiveness of the document.

Word Processors. Word Processors are used mainly for letter writing and simple documents. The word processor has taken a backseat to today's desktop and notebook computers.

Typewriters. Most typewriters use correctable film ribbons that pass through the spool only one time. However, if the typewriter uses a cotton or silk ribbon that becomes lighter with use, be sure to change the ribbon before the resulting type impression becomes too light. The typewriter keys need to be cleaned frequently in typewriters that use a cotton ribbon. Typewriters, too, are all but **archaic** compared with the versatility of the computer.

Copiers. When a typewriter is used to compose a document, a copier may be used for making any necessary copies of the original. Here, too, maintain the copier so that copies are crisp and clear. The toner must be changed when needed and can be expensive. Multiple copies of documents are usually made on a copier rather than printed from the computer.

Scanners. Occasionally, documents are scanned and sent by email. Scanners provide high resolution and can produce images of written text and photos. Scanners are often used to create images so that older documents can be stored, much like the microfiche systems of the past.

Supplies

Stationery. The quality of paper unquestionably affects the reader's total impression of the communication. **Stationers** or printing companies are qualified to advise on the selection of paper, which can range from all-sulfite (a wood pulp) to all-cotton fiber (sometimes called *rag*). Letterhead paper is usually on **bond** with a 25% or higher cotton fiber content.

The weight of paper is described by a **substance number**. This number is based on the weight of a **ream** consisting of 500 sheets of 17×22-inch paper. The larger the substance number, the heavier the paper. If the ream weighs 24 pounds, the paper is referred to as *Sub 24* or *24-pound weight*. Letterhead stationery and matching envelopes are usually 16-, 20-, or 24-pound weight. This is often abbreviated as *16#, 20#,* or *24#.*

Sizes and Types of Letterhead Paper. Letterhead paper is available in four basic sizes:

Standard or letter	$8^{1}/_{2} \times 11$ inches
Monarch or executive	$8^{1}/_{4} \times 10^{1}/_{2}$ inches
Baronial	$5^{1}/_{2} \times 8^{1}/_{2}$ inches
Legal	$8^{1}/_{2} \times 14$ inches

Standard letterhead is used for general business and professional correspondence. Monarch is often used by professional people for informal business and social correspondence. Baronial, which is a half-sheet of standard, is used for very short letters or memoranda. Legal, as its name indicates, is used for the lengthy documents presented in court or of a legal nature. Each size of letterhead should have its matching envelope.

Letterhead should be well designed and of a high-quality paper. The letter represents the sender, and the letterhead paper should be carefully chosen to promote the image that the sender wishes to convey. The paper itself makes a strong statement about the business or person it represents and can help the receiver form an impression of the professionalism of the business.

Bond paper has a felt side and a wire side. When a sheet of letterhead is picked up and held to the light, a design or letters can be read from the printed side. This design is called a **watermark** and is an indication of quality. The side from which the watermark can be read is the felt side of the paper and is the side on which printing or typing should be done. The watermark should always read across the page in the same direction as the typing.

Paper with a linen finish is so named because it is similar to fine cloth, with finely spaced lines crossing each other at right angles. Wove is a smooth paper that is normally inexpensive. Antique finish has a semismooth texture, and laid has a finish similar to that of corduroy. All of these paper finishes can make a very professional, impressive letterhead.

TABLE 12-1	Proofreader's Marks		

Proofreader's Mark		Draft Copy	Finished Copy
ss [	Single space	ss [Read a good book / every day	Read a good book / every day
ds [	Double space	ds [Where will you go / on your vacation?	Where will you go / on your vacation?
2	Indent two spaces	His address is / 2 450 Newport Avenue	His address is / 450 Newport Avenue
⊙	Insert period	Mr⊙ Herbert Hoover	Mr. Herbert Hoover
⋀	Insert comma	Marysville⋀Indiana	Marysville, Indiana
⊙	Insert colon	Dear Mr. Adams⋀	Dear Mr. Adams:
;/	Insert semicolon	letter of March 6⋀your question	letter of March 6; your question
?/	Insert question mark	Will he come⋀	Will he come?
˅/	Insert apostrophe	the captains ship	the captain's ship
˅˅	Insert quotation marks	his remark,⋀don't be late⋀	his remark, "don't be late"
=/	Insert hyphen	a one⋀time thing	a one-time thing
#	Insert space	townhouse⋀	town house
⋀	Caret—to mark exact position of error	Insert caret to⋀show error #	Insert caret to show error
℘	Delete	℘ It may ~~not~~ be yours	It may be yours
◠	Close up	Cl◠ose	Close
℘	Delete and close up	Me◠erry Christmas	Merry Christmas
¶	Begin new paragraph	¶ At the time	At the time
no ¶	No paragraph	no ¶ This is correct	This is correct
//	Align vertically	// Ellen Peters / Alice Brown	Ellen Peters / Alice Brown
=	Align horizontally	Dear Doctor ⌐Roberts	Dear Doctor Roberts
⌐	Move right	$10,000 ═══	$10,000
⌐	Move left	⌐ Read a book	Read a book
⊓	Move up	Mo⊔ve	Move
⊔	Move down	Mo⊓ve	Move
⌐⌐	Center	⌐$10,000⌐	$10,000
∼	Transpose	resile(i)nt	resilient
(sp)	Spell out	③ years ago	three years ago
stet	Let it stand	They were ~~very~~ sad	They were very sad
lc	Lower case	It is a B̸ig house	It is a big house
≡	Upper case	Robert birch	Robert Birch
sc	Set in small capitals	Regional	REGIONAL
ital	Set in italic	special	*special*
bf	Set in bold	federal government	**federal government**
wf	Wrong font	invest**m**ent⋀	investment
˅	Superscript	reference number ˅3	reference number[3]
⋀	Subscript	reference number ⋀7	reference number[7]
⌢	Ligature Æ	ae̼sop	æsop

TABLE 12-2	150 Frequently Misspelled or Misused English Words			
absence	corroborate	inimitable	persistent	ridiculous
accede	definitely	inoculate	personal	sacrilegious
accessible	description	insistent	personnel	seize
accommodate	desirable	irrelevant	possession	separate
achieve	despair	irresistible	precede	siege
affect	development	irritable	precedent	similar
agglutinate	dilemma	judgment	predictable	sizable
all right	disappear	labeled	predominant	stationary
altogether	disappoint	led	predominate	stationery
analyses (pl.)	disastrous	leisure	prerogative	subpoena
analysis (s.)	discreet	license	prevalent	succeed
analyze	discrete	liquefy	principal	suddenness
anoint	discriminate	maintenance	principle	superintendent
argument	dissatisfaction	maneuver	privilege	supersede
assistant	dissipate	miscellaneous	procedure	surprise
auxiliary	drunkenness	mischievous	proceed	tariff
balloon	ecstasy	misspell	professor	technique
believe	effect	necessary	pronunciation	thorough
benefited	eligible	newsstand	psychiatry	tranquility
brochure	embarrass	noticeable	psychology	transferred
bulletin	exceed	occasion	pursue	truly
category	exhilaration	occurrence	questionnaire	tyrannize
changeable	existence	oscillate	rearrange	unnecessary
clientele	February	paid	recede	until
committee	forty	pamphlet	receive	vacillate
comparative	grammar	panicky	recommend	vacuum
concede	grievous	parallel	referring	vicious
conscientious	height	paralyze	repetition	warrant
conscious	incidentally	pastime	rheumatism	Wednesday
coolly	indispensable	perseverance	rhythmical	weird

TABLE 12-3	Frequently Misspelled Medical Words			
abscess	defibrillator	intussusception	parietal	pruritus
additive	desiccate	ischemia	paroxysmal	psoriasis
aerosol	ecchymosis	ischium	pemphigus	pyrexia
agglutination	effusion	larynx	percussion	respiratory
albumin	epididymis	leukemia	perforation	rheumatic
anastomosis	epistaxis	malaise	pericardium	roentgenology
aneurysm	eustachian	malleus	perineum	sagittal
anteflexion	fissure	melena	peristalsis	sciatic
arrhythmia	flexure	mellitus	peritoneum	scirrhous
bilirubin	glaucoma	menstruation	petit mal	serous
bronchial	gonorrhea	metastasis	pharynx	sessile
cachexia	graafian	neurilemma	pituitary	sphincter
calcaneus	hemorrhage	neuron	plantar	sphygmomanometer
capillary	hemorrhoids	occlusion	pleura	squamous
cervical	homeostasis	optic chiasm	pleurisy	staphylococcus
chromosome	humerus	oscilloscope	pneumonia	suppuration
cirrhosis	idiosyncracy	osseous	polyp	trochanter
clavicle	ileum	palliative	prophylaxis	venous
curettage	ilium	parasite	prostate	wheal
cyanosis	infarction	parenteral	prosthesis	xiphoid

CRITICAL THINKING APPLICATION

Brandon realizes that his father's office does not have a method of inventory and supply ordering in place. The employees simply order more when they see that a certain supply is getting low, but there is no formal system. This often causes them to run out of certain supplies, especially stationery and envelopes. How might this issue be resolved?

Continuation Pages. The second and continuing pages of a letter are placed on plain bond that matches the letterhead in weight and fiber content. The stationery used for continuation pages should be an exact match to the letterhead, only without the letterhead printing. It is considered unprofessional to use different paper for the continuation pages.

Envelopes. Envelopes are usually made of the same paper as the letterhead stationery. Just as the continuation pages should be the same type of paper as the letterhead, so should the envelopes.

Envelopes also come in the following basic sizes:

* No. 10
* No. 6³/₄
* Window

No. 10 envelopes are the general business size used for letter and legal stationery. No. 6³/₄ envelopes and window envelopes are often used for statements.

Letter Styles

A business letter is usually arranged in one of three styles: block, modified block or standard, or modified block indented. A fourth style, called *simplified*, is occasionally used. The block and modified block styles are most commonly used in the physician's office.

Block Letter Style

When block letter style is used, all lines start **flush** with the left margin (Figure 12-1). This style is considered the most efficient but is less attractive on the page.

Modified Block Letter Style

The dateline, the complimentary closing, and the type-written signature all begin at the center when typing in modified block letter style. All other lines begin at the left margin (Figure 12-2).

Modified Block Letter Style With Indented Paragraphs

The modified block letter style with indented paragraphs is identical to the block style except that the first line of each paragraph is indented five spaces (Figure 12-3).

Simplified Letter Style

With the simplified letter style, all lines begin flush with the left margin (Figure 12-4). The salutation is

---

Elizabeth Blackwell, M.D.
223 Orange Avenue, N.W.
Cottonwood, UT 84121

January 26, 20—

Mr. Richard Fluege
3678 North Willow Avenue
Palm Beach, FL 33480

Dear Mr. Fluege:

Please send me full particulars on the professional suites you expect to offer for sale or rent in the Medical Arts Professional Annex.

In about six months, I will be ready to open my practice, and I am interested in locating in Florida. My preference is a street-level suite of approximately 2,000 square feet.

After I have had an opportunity to study the information you send me, I will write or telephone you if I have further questions.

Very truly yours,

Elizabeth Blackwell, M.D.

EB:mek

FIGURE 12-1 Block letter style.

MEDICAL ARTS PROFESSIONAL ANNEX
3678 North Willow Avenue
Palm Beach FL 33480

January 29, 20—

Elizabeth Blackwell, M.D.
223 Orange Avenue, N.W.
Cottonwood, UT 84121

Dear Doctor Blackwell:

We have two remaining street-level suites available for occupancy about July 1. These are marked on pages 3 and 4 of the enclosed descriptive brochure. If one of these suites appeals to you, we will be pleased to customize it for your practice.

Please feel free to call me collect at the number on the brochure for further discussion of your needs.

Sincerely yours,

Richard Fluege
Business Manager

RF:ab
Enclosure

FIGURE 12-2   Modified block letter style.

WILLIAM OSLER, M.D.
1000 South West Street
Park Ridge, NJ 07656

January 26, 20—

Robert Koch, M.D.
398 Main Street
Park Ridge, NJ 07656

Dear Doctor Koch:

Mrs. Elaine Norris

Thank you for referring your patient, Mrs. Elaine Norris, for consultation and care. She was examined in my office today.

FINDINGS: The patient complained of pain in the left lower quadrant and some abdominal tenderness. She had a temperature of 100.2 degrees.

RECOMMENDATIONS: The patient was placed on a soft, low-residue, bland diet, antibiotics, and bed rest for a few days. Upper and lower gastrointestinal x-rays will be performed next week.

TENTATIVE DIAGNOSIS: Diverticulitis of large bowel.

Mrs. Norris has been asked to return here for reevaluation in about ten days.

Sincerely yours,

William Osler, M.D.

WO:gm

FIGURE 12-3   Modified block letter style with indented paragraphs.

ROBERT KOCH, M.D.
398 Main Street
Park Ridge, NJ 07656

January 30, 20—

William Osler, M.D.
1000 South West Street
Park Ridge, NJ 07656

ANNABELLE ANDERSON

You will be pleased to know, Bill, that Mrs. Anderson is progressing nicely. Her wound is healing. Her temperature has returned to normal, and she is beginning to resume her usual activities.

Mrs. Anderson has an appointment to return here for one more visit next week. At that time, I will ask her to return to you for any further care.

ROBERT KOCH, M.D.

RK:hb

FIGURE 12-4 Simplified letter style.

replaced with an all-capital subject line on the third line below the inside address. The body of the letter begins on the third line below the subject line. The complimentary closing is omitted. An all-capital typewritten signature is entered on the fifth line below the body of the letter.

Types of Punctuation

Traditionally, the punctuation pattern is selected on the basis of letter style. Normal punctuation is always used within the body of a business letter. The other parts use either standard or open punctuation.

When standard punctuation is used, a colon is placed after the salutation, and a comma is placed after the complimentary closing. This is the punctuation pattern most commonly used. It is appropriate with the block or modified block letter styles.

When open punctuation is used, no punctuation is used at the end of any line outside the body of the letter unless that line ends with an abbreviation. This pattern is always used with the simplified letter style.

Spacing and Margins

Generally, a letter centered on a page is the most attractive. Accomplishing this is easy with today's computer programs, such as Microsoft Word or WordPerfect. Business letters are almost always single spaced. If a letter consists of only a few lines, double-space both the inside address and the message and indent the first line of each paragraph five spaces.

The first typed entry, which is the date, is usually placed on the third line below the letterhead or on line 13 if there is no letterhead. Continuation pages begin 1 inch from the top.

On standard letterhead, the side margins are usually $1^1/2$ to 1 inches on each side. The appearance of a very short letter is improved by increasing the width of all margins.

A 1-inch bottom margin is the minimum. This can be increased if the letter is to be carried over to a second page. Never use a second page to type only the complimentary closing and signature. Carry over a minimum of two lines of the body of the letter.

Parts of Letters

The structure of a letter and its placement on a page have been fairly well standardized into the following main parts:
- Heading
- Opening
- Body
- Closing

Heading

The heading includes the letterhead and the dateline. The printed letterhead is usually centered at the top of the page and includes the name of the physician or group and the address. It may include the telephone number and the medical specialty or specialties. In a group or corporate practice, the names of the physicians may also be listed. Occasionally, the heading also includes the name of an office manager.

The dateline consists of the name of the month written in full, followed by the day and year. The date should not be abbreviated, nor should ordinal numbers (e.g., 1st, 2nd, and 3rd) be used after the name of the month.

Opening

The opening consists of the inside address, the salutation, and the attention line, if there is one. The inside address has two or more lines, starts flush with the left margin, and contains at least the name of the individual or firm to whom the letter is addressed and the mailing address. When the letter is addressed to an individual, the name is preceded by a courtesy title, such as *Dr.*, *Mr.*, *Mrs.*, *Miss*, or *Ms.* When addressing a letter to a physician, omit the courtesy title and type the physician's name followed by his or her **academic degree**, such as *Rick P. Tipps, MD.* Do not use both a courtesy title and a degree that mean the same thing, as in *Dr. Rick P. Tipps, MD.*

CRITICAL THINKING APPLICATION

Brandon has noticed that some of the correspondence leaving the office is signed incorrectly, with "Dr. Rick P. Tipps, MD" in the typed signature line. This is an uncomfortable situation because Brandon realizes that the person who is typing the signature this way is the office manager.

- How might he approach her so that the mistake can be corrected?
- Is it wise to approach the office manager, or should Brandon go to his father? Why or why not?

The salutation is the letter writer's introductory greeting to the person being addressed. It is typed flush with the left margin on the second line below the last line of the address and is followed by a colon unless open punctuation is used. The words in the salutation vary depending on the degree of formality of the letter.

The attention line, if used, is placed on the second line below the inside address. If the name of the person for whom the letter is intended is known, that person's name is used in the inside address and he or she is addressed personally. If the letter is being addressed to a company or organization and directed to a division or department within the company, the division or department name is placed on the attention line.

Body

The body of a letter includes the subject line, if one is used, and the message. In medical office correspondence, the subject of a letter is frequently a patient. The patient's name is used as the subject line. Because the subject line is considered to be a part of the body of the letter, it is placed on the second line below the salutation. It may start flush with the left margin or at the point of indentation of indented paragraphs, or it may be centered. The word *subject*, followed by a colon, may be used or omitted entirely.

Begin typing the message on the second line below the subject line or on the second line below the salutation if there is no subject line. The first line of each paragraph may be indented five spaces or may start flush with the left margin, depending on the chosen letter style.

Closing

The closing includes the complimentary closing, the typed signature, the reference initials, and any special notations.

The complimentary closing is the writer's way of saying good-bye. It is placed on the second line below the last line of the body of the letter and is followed by a comma unless open punctuation is used. Only the first word is capitalized. The words used are determined by the degree of formality in the salutation. For example, if the salutation is *Dear Herb*, the closing might be *Cordially*, *Very truly yours*, or *Sincerely yours* with consistent punctuation. If the letter is addressed to a business, the complimentary closing most used is *Sincerely*.

A typewritten signature is a courtesy to the reader, especially if the name does not appear on the printed letterhead or if the personal signature is difficult or impossible to decipher. The typewritten signature is placed on the fourth line directly below the complimentary closing.

Reference initials that identify the typist are placed flush with the left margin on the second line below the typewritten signature. If the writer's name is included on the signature line, the writer's initials need not be included in the reference block unless desired. The writer's initials, if used, should precede the typist's initials and are separated by a colon or diagonal line. Examples include *mek*, *GB:mek*, or *GB/mek*.

Special notations are sometimes needed to indicate that enclosures are included with the letter or that copies of the letter are being distributed to others. If the letter indicates an enclosure, type the word *Enclosure* or *Enc.* on the first line below the reference initials. If there is more than one enclosure, specify the number (e.g., *Enclosures 3*). If copies are to be sent to others, type this notation in the same manner as the enclosure notation or after it if both notations are needed. The copy notation is usually written as *c:* or *copy to:* followed by the name or names of those to whom a copy will be sent. If the person to whom the letter is addressed is not to know that copies are being distributed to others, use the notation *bc:* for "blind copy" on all copies *except* the original. Place this notation either in the upper left of the letter at the margin or below the last notation at the lower left margin.

Postscripts

Although a postscript may sometimes be used to express an afterthought, it is often used to place emphasis on an idea or statement. Begin the postscript on the second line below the last special notation. Follow the style of the letter, indenting the first line if paragraphs were indented in the body of the letter or starting at the margin if indentation was not used in the letter.

Continuation Pages

If the letter requires one or more **continuation pages**, the heading of the second and subsequent pages must contain the following three items of information:

- The name of the addressee
- The page number
- The date

The heading should begin on the seventh line from the top of the page. Continuation of the body of the letter begins on the tenth line or the third line below the heading. There are three accepted forms for the continuation page heading, as shown below:

Rick P. Tipps, M.D.
Page 2
July 5, 2003

Rick P. Tipps, M.D.
Page 2
July 5, 2003
Subject: Susan Clemmons

Rick P. Tipps, M.D.   -2-   July 5, 2003

Signing the Letter

Some physicians prefer to compose and sign all letters that leave their offices. The majority are more than pleased to delegate to a competent assistant the responsibility of composing and signing letters of a business nature. Although not all authorities agree on the form to be followed, most recommend that a woman's typewritten signature includes a courtesy title (Miss, Mrs., or Ms.) and that the title not be enclosed in parentheses. It is not necessary to include the courtesy title in the handwritten signature.

In general, the physician signs all of the following:

- Letters that deal with medical advice to patients
- Letters to officers or committees of the medical society
- Referral and consultation reports to colleagues
- Medical reports to insurance companies
- Personal letters

The medical assistant usually composes and signs letters dealing with the following matters:

- Routine matters such as arranging or rescheduling appointments
- Orders for office supplies
- Notification to patients about surgery or hospital arrangements
- Collection of delinquent accounts
- Letters of solicitation

CRITICAL THINKING APPLICATION

One of the employees has brought an urgent letter to Brandon that his father neglected to sign before leaving the office for the day. The letter is to another physician reporting his findings on a referred patient. The employee asks Brandon to sign the letter. What should he do? What are some ways to resolve this situation, if the letter must leave in the mail today?

Writing Skills and Composing Tips

Business letters are much different than the social letters that the medical assistant may have written. Social letters tend to be long and chatty and do not necessarily follow any organized plan. Most business letters should be less than one page in length and carefully organized (Procedure 12-1). This takes practice and preparation.

The medical assistant should carefully read the letter to be answered. Make note of or underline any questions asked or materials requested. Then decide on the answers to the questions and verify the information. This is called **annotating**. Draft a reply, and then rewrite for clarity (Procedure 12-2). Keep most of the sentences short. Put only one idea in each sentence, and eliminate **superfluous** words. Be careful about using medical terms in correspondence with patients. Instead, use language that the reader will easily understand. Every person who writes letters develops his or her own personal style.

Most physicians conform to a highly professional and formal style in their dictation. The medical assistant who is given the responsibility of composing correspondence for the medical office should strive for the same degree of formality used by the physician. It would be inappropriate for the assistant to write in a breezy, informal style when acting as the representative of an employer who is more formal in his or her approach. The principal point to remember is that every letter produced in your office should project the image of the physician regardless of who composes or signs the letter.

Grammar Review

Good **grammar** is essential to writing effective, professional business letters. The medical assistant should have an understanding of the elements of acceptable grammar and writing skills.

Parts of Speech

Nouns. A noun is a person, place, or thing. Nouns can also be a thought, an idea, or a concept, as in *freedom* or *courage*. Common nouns name general persons, places, or things, such as *teacher* and *city*. Proper nouns are specific, such as *Mrs. Roberts* and *New York City*.

PROCEDURE 12-1

Composing Business Correspondence

GOAL: To compose a letter that will convey information in an accurate and concise manner, and that is easy to comprehend by the reader.

EQUIPMENT AND SUPPLIES

- Computer or word processor
- Word processing software
- Draft paper
- Letterhead
- Printer
- Pen or pencil
- Highlighter
- Envelope
- Correspondence to be answered
- Other pertinent information needed to compose a letter
- Electronic or hard cover dictionary and thesaurus
- Writer's handbook
- Portfolio

PROCEDURAL STEPS

1 Read through any correspondence to be answered and highlight the specific questions that should be addressed.

Purpose: To make certain that all of the issues raised in the correspondence are answered.

2 Make any necessary notes on the letter or a copy of the letter. A scrap sheet of paper may be used.

3 Prepare a draft of the letter using good grammatical skills and save it in the computer or word processor.

Purpose: To put the thoughts on paper for later revision and make the letter easy to understand for the reader.

4 Proofread a printed copy of the letter, using proofreader's marks to make corrections.

Purpose: To see the document as it will look once printed, and speed the process of writing by using proofreader's marks.

5 Make any necessary corrections.

6 Allow the physician or other interested parties to proofread the letter, if the medical assistant is not the person whose signature will appear at the bottom.

Purpose: To give the physician an opportunity to correct the letter and add additional thoughts, if desired.

7 Make any final changes, then print the letter on stationery. Allow the person whose name appears at the bottom to sign the letter.

8 Address the envelope using OCR guidelines and place the letter and any supporting documents inside. See Procedure 12-5 for using USPO OCR guidelines.

9 Mail the letter using correct postage.

Purpose: Using incorrect postage or guessing can delay the arrival time of the document.

Pronouns. Pronouns replace nouns and provide the writer with shortcuts so that proper nouns do not have to be constantly repeated. Pronouns include words such as *it, you, he, she, her, his, them, mine, you, yours, its, ours,* and *theirs.*

Verbs. Verbs are action words that express movement, such as *runs, drove,* or *type.* Linking verbs express a condition or state of being and include *am, are, was, be,* and *been.* Linking verbs also express the senses, as in *smell, hear, taste, touch, feel,* and *look.*

Adjectives. Adjectives are words that describe nouns and pronouns or may show which one, how many, and what kind of. *A, an,* and *the* are special types of adjectives called *articles.* Examples of adjectives include a *golden* sunset, a *mangy* dog, and a *crooked* nose.

Adverbs. Just as adjectives describe nouns, adverbs describe verbs, adjectives, or other adverbs. Adverbs specify when, where, to what extent, or how. Examples include *unusually* warm, *never* won, and *quite* cold.

Prepositions. Connecting words that show a relationship between nouns, pronouns, or other words in a sentence are called *prepositions.* Examples of prepositions include *by, from, of, to, in, at, with, into,* and *on.*

Conjunctions. Conjunctions join words or phrases. These helpful words include *and, or, nor,* and *but.*

Interjections. Interjections show strong feeling. They are often followed by an exclamation point and sometimes by a comma. *"Ouch! That really hurt!"* is a sentence that uses an interjection.

Making Sense of Sentences

Sentence structure is important when writing a professional letter or document. The medical assistant should know the basics of good sentence structure so that written documents will make sense and represent the medical facility and staff in a positive way.

PROCEDURE **12-2**

Proofreading Written Correspondence

GOAL: To compose a clearly written, grammatically correct business letter that is easily understood by the reader, and to eliminate spelling errors.

EQUIPMENT AND SUPPLIES

- Stationery
- Computer or typewriter
- Correspondence to be answered or notes

PROCEDURAL STEPS

1 Place the stationery into the printer or typewriter.

2 Scan through the letter to be answered or the notes about the correspondence to be written and highlight any questions that should be answered or points to be made.
Purpose: To ensure that the goals of the correspondence are fulfilled and no important points are omitted.

3 Write the letter using grammatical guidelines.

4 Print a draft copy of the letter. Read it carefully and highlight changes to be made or note any additions to be made. Use proofreader's marks.

Purpose: Seeing a hard copy of a letter is more conducive to finding errors and grammatical mistakes.

5 Revise the letter using the notes.

6 Read the letter once again on the screen. Complete spell and grammar checks if those tools are available on the computer.
Purpose: To locate any missed errors or misspelled words.

7 Print a final draft. Read the letter word for word and check once again for errors.

8 Have another person proofread especially important correspondence.
Purpose: Often another person can locate missed errors quickly.

9 Complete the final preparations for mailing the letter. Address the letter using guidelines for OCR and fast processing at the post office.

Types of Sentences. There are four basic sentence types, as follows: declarative, interrogative, imperative, and exclamatory. Declarative sentences make a statement, whereas interrogative sentences ask a question. Imperative sentences state a command or request. Exclamatory sentences express strong feeling. An example of each type is listed below.

Declarative	*She was the last person here.*
Interrogative	*Are we going to the fair today?*
Imperative	*Clean your room before dinner.*
Exclamatory	*I am so excited for you!*

Sentence Structure. Sentences, when written correctly, follow certain patterns. There are three very basic patterns that are used in constructing sentences. These patterns are:

- Subject-predicate
- Subject-object
- Subject-complement

The subject of a sentence is usually a noun and is the word or group of words in a sentence that acts, is acted on, or is described by the verb. The predicate is the part of the sentence that contains the verb and tells what the subject is doing or experiencing or what is being done to the subject. The object is a noun, pronoun, or group of words functioning as a noun or pronoun that receives the action of the verb. The complement is a word or group of words in the predicate of a sentence that renames or describes a subject or object in that sentence.

Sentence Errors. Three main sentence errors plague most writers. These include the sentence fragment, the run-on sentence, and the comma splice.

A sentence fragment is an incomplete thought or a portion of a sentence that is punctuated as though it were a complete sentence. An example follows:

Although the doctor had seen the patient.

A run-on sentence contains independent **clauses** without a semicolon, comma, or conjunction between them. These sentences are also called *run-together* or *fused sentences*. An example follows:

The office was clean when the staff left on Friday the doors were locked.

A comma splice is a sentence in which a comma alone joins independent clauses. An example follows:

The storm grew worse, it began to snow.

More Types of Written Communications

There are many types of written communications other than a business letter. One of the most common types of written communication in the medical office is the telephone message. Seven items must be recorded when taking a phone message, including the following:

- The name of the person to whom the call is directed
- The name of the person calling
- The caller's daytime and/or cell phone number
- The reason for the call
- The action to be taken
- The date and time of the call
- The initials of the person taking the call

Email is a very popular way to send written communications in today's computer-literate society. Email messages can be saved, printed for the patient's chart, and **archived** for storage.

Faxes are another form of written communication. All faxes should have a cover sheet that states that the information contained within it is of a confidential nature and is intended only for the person to whom the fax was sent (Procedure 12-3).

Most offices **disseminate** various memorandums throughout the business week (Figure 12-5). These written documents must also be clear, concise, and grammatically correct.

CRITICAL THINKING APPLICATION

- Email is used more and more often to communicate with employees. Brandon has noticed that there are very few printed memos that circulate throughout the office. What are the advantages and disadvantages of communicating through email with employees?
- The office manager has given Brandon information to disseminate to all of the employees of the clinic. She did not specify whether to give out the memo by hand or by email but did state that the information was very important. Which would be the best method?

Personal Tools

Competent handling of written communications requires a basic knowledge of composition. A personal reference library that includes an up-to-date standard dictionary, a medical dictionary, a composition handbook, an English-language reference manual, and a thesaurus will be a tremendous help.

For those who have difficulty with spelling, keep a small loose-leaf indexed notebook or card index of words that are troublesome. When it is necessary to look up a word in the dictionary for spelling, record it in the notebook or card index for quick reference. The physician or a medical assistant who is familiar with the practice might compile a basic list of frequently used medical terms and abbreviations as a reference for the trainee.

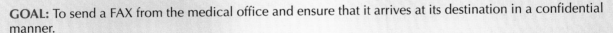

PROCEDURE 12-3

Preparing a FAX for Transmission

GOAL: To send a FAX from the medical office and ensure that it arrives at its destination in a confidential manner.

EQUIPMENT AND SUPPLIES

- FAX machine
- FAX cover sheet
- Correspondence to be sent

PROCEDURAL STEPS

1 Fill out a FAX cover sheet. Include the name of the person sending the FAX and that person's phone number. List the name of the person to receive the FAX and the FAX number where the document is being sent. Use cover sheets that contain a confidentiality statement.
Purpose: To identify a FAX that has been misdirected and to ensure that it goes to the right person when it arrives.

2 Note the number of pages that are being sent, including the cover page.
Purpose: To ensure that all pages are received.

3 Turn the last page upside down and write the fax number on the top of the document. Many machines require the documents to be in place prior to starting the fax. This allows the user to see the number without having to memorize it and make an error.
Purpose: To see the FAX number clearly once the pages have been placed in the FAX machine.

4 Follow the instructions for individual FAX machines.

5 Be sure the machine is set to provide a verification that the fax went through. Print the verification and attach it to the fax. Verify the arrival of critical FAX documents on the phone.
Purpose: To document that the fax arrived at its destination.

6 File the fax and verification sheet in the appropriate location.
Purpose: To maintain a record of information sent via FAX.

INTEROFFICE MEMORANDUM

TO   All Staff

FROM   Office Manager

DATE   December 1

SUBJECT   Holiday Schedule

Our entire facility will be closed on December 24, December 25, December 31, and January 1. The office will be on reduced staff during the days of December 26, 27, 28, 29, and 30. Assignments will be based on seniority of staff members. Please submit your preferences as soon as possible.

A

FIGURE 12-5 **A** and **B**, Examples of memoranda. Memos are intended to be short, specific, and to the point.

MEMO TO: George Walker

FROM: Stanley Barr

DATE: February 8

SUBJECT: Office rental

We are experiencing unexpectedly rapid growth in our business office and will soon need additional space for our increased number of employees. Do you have a larger facility available in this building? If so, I would like to hear from you regarding the location, square footage, and anticipated rental costs.

B

Developing a Portfolio

Letter composition can be sped up by developing a **portfolio** of sample letters to suit the various situations that frequently arise. As the physician approves letters, add them to the office portfolio. Suppose, for instance, a letter is needed for a patient who wishes to change an appointment. Compose a letter that is clear, concise, and courteous—and make an extra copy to place in the portfolio of letters. Alternatively, if using a computer, store the letter on a disk or on the computer's hard drive. If letters and other documents are stored on the hard drive, be sure to back the files up on disk or a zip drive. Do this each time a new kind of letter is written. Soon, the medical assistant will be able to select a letter from the portfolio and change it slightly to suit the current situation. This will make letter writing in the medical office quick and easy.

Mail Processing

Incoming Mail

Each day, a great variety of mail comes into the professional office and must be processed. Common items in the daily mail include the following:
- General correspondence
- Payments for services
- Bills for office purchases
- Insurance claim forms to be completed
- Laboratory reports
- Hospital reports

- Medical society mailings
- Professional journals
- Promotional literature and samples from pharmaceutical houses
- Advertisements

In large clinics and medical centers, the mail is opened by specially designated people in a central department to speed up this daily task. In the average medical office, however, a medical assistant opens the mail using the ordinary letter-opener method.

Opening the Mail

Before opening any mail, the medical assistant should have an agreement with the physician as to what procedure to follow regarding incoming mail—in other words, what letters should be opened and what pieces, if any, the physician prefers to open personally. For example, the physician may prefer to open any communications from an attorney or accountant, even when they are not marked *personal*. If there is any doubt in regard to opening an envelope, do not open the item and forward it to the person to whom it is addressed. Even a simple procedure such as opening the daily mail can be done with more efficiency if a good system is followed (Procedure 12-4).

Annotating

Annotating the mail is an additional service the medical assistant can perform. By reading each letter through, underlining the significant words and phrases, and noting

PROCEDURE 12-4

Opening the Daily Mail

GOAL: To sort through the mail that arrives in the medical office on a daily basis in an efficient way.

EQUIPMENT AND SUPPLIES
- Computer or word processor
- Draft paper
- Letterhead stationery
- Pen or pencil
- Highlighter
- Staple remover
- Paper clips
- Letter opener
- Stapler
- Transparent tape
- Date stamp

PROCEDURAL STEPS

1 Have a clear working space on the desk or countertop.

2 Sort the mail according to importance and urgency:

- Physician's personal mail
- Ordinary first-class mail
- Checks from insurance companies and patients
- Periodicals and newspapers
- All other pieces, including drug samples

3 Open the mail neatly and in an organized manner.

4 Stack the envelopes so that they are all facing in the same direction.

5 Pick up the top one and tap the envelope so that when you open it you will not cut the contents.

6 Open all envelopes along the top edge for easiest removal of contents.

7 Remove the contents of each envelope and hold the envelope to the light to see that nothing remains inside.

8 Make a note of the postmark when this is important.

9 Discard the envelope after you have checked to see that there is a return address on the message contained inside. Some offices make it a policy to attach the envelope to each piece of correspondence until it has received attention.

10 Date-stamp the letter and attach any enclosures.

11 If there is an enclosure notation at the bottom of the letter, ensure that the enclosure was included. If it is missing, indicate this on the notation by writing the word *no* and circling it. This may be as far as your employer will want you to proceed with handling the correspondence.

---

in the margin any action required, taking action on the mail is much easier. If the letter needs no reply, code it for filing at this time. A highlighter that does not photocopy may be used for annotating. When mail refers to previous correspondence, obtain this from the file and attach it or a copy. If the patient's chart is needed when replying to an inquiry, pull the chart and place it with the letter.

There should be a specific place for placing the opened and annotated mail in the medical office. This will probably be some area on the physician's or office manager's desk. After sorting, opening, and annotating the mail, place those items that the physician will wish to see in the established place, with the most important mail on top. Personal mail, of course, is to remain unopened. If a piece of personal mail addressed to the employer is opened in error, fold and replace it inside the envelope, and write across the outside *opened in error*, followed by the initials of the person who opened the mail. Use the same procedure with a piece of mail addressed to another office that may have been opened in error. In such cases, reseal the envelope with transparent tape and hand it to the mail carrier.

Responding to the Mail

In some offices, the physician and the medical assistant go over the mail together. Once the medical assistant gains confidence, he or she will find it easy to draft a reply to most inquiries. Usually, the physician is very pleased to delegate this responsibility, especially on matters that do not relate to patient care.

Letters of referral from other physicians should be carefully noted so that an answer may be sent after the patient has been seen and the physician can give a report. If considerable time may pass before such information can be sent, it is a courteous gesture to write a letter to the referring physician advising that a detailed report will follow. Some physicians send printed cards expressing thanks for referrals; others prefer to write thank-you letters to professional colleagues.

Mail Requiring Special Handling

Payment Receipts. Payments from patients and insurance companies will come to the office on a daily basis. All payments should be separated and recorded immediately in the day's receipts. If the patient requests a receipt, it should be mailed. Otherwise, the receipt may be placed in the patient's chart for delivery on a future office visit.

CRITICAL THINKING APPLICATION

Brandon notices that Mrs. Attaway, a widow and long-time patient of his father's, sent in a check for $125 for a bill. However, her insurance company had already paid $112 toward the bill. Brandon knows that Mrs. Attaway must be very careful with her money and has always paid her bills quickly. The policy of the office is to route the overpayment through the system, but refund checks are cut only once per month. What should Brandon do in this situation?

Insurance Information. Insurance information should be put in a predetermined place for handling by the billers. Documents relating to insurance should be passed to the appropriate person immediately to avoid delays and time limitations that might cause the claim to go unpaid.

Drug Samples. Sample drugs and related literature are usually delivered by pharmaceutical representatives, and may occasionally arrive in the mail. Determine from the physician what types of literature and samples should be saved. Most physicians keep pertinent new samples in a sample storage area, along with the accompanying literature for immediate reference. Other drug samples are **categorically** stored. Drugs should never be tossed into the trash.

Vacation Mail. When the physician is away from the office, it is generally the responsibility of a medical assistant to handle all mail. In this event, all pieces should be examined carefully. The medical assistant can then decide how to handle each piece based on the following questions:

- Is this important enough that I should phone or fax the physician?
- Shall I forward this for immediate attention?
- Shall I answer this myself or send a brief note to the correspondent, explaining that there will be a slight delay because the physician is out of the office?
- Can this wait for attention until the physician returns without appearing negligent?

If the medical assistant is unable to contact the physician or to forward important mail, he or she should always answer the sender immediately, explaining the delay and requesting cooperation. Instead of forwarding an original piece of mail and risking possible loss, make a copy for forwarding. Then, if the physician wishes the letter answered, notations can be made on the copy and returned without defacing the original letter.

When the physician is traveling from place to place, the envelope on each communication should be numbered consecutively. Doing this enables the physician to easily determine whether any mail has been lost or delayed. By keeping a record of each piece of mail sent out, with its corresponding number, anything that might be lost can be identified and remailed if necessary.

Correspondence not requiring immediate action that the medical assistant is unable to answer until the physician returns should be placed in a special folder marked *Requires Attention* and placed on top of other accumulated mail. Mail that the medical assistant can compose but that requires the physician's approval before mailing should be put into another special folder marked *For Approval*. When the physician returns, these letters can be rapidly checked and signed.

Any letters marked *Personal* may be acknowledged to the return address on the envelope. The brief acknowledgment should state that the physician is out of town for a certain length of time and will attend to the letter immediately on returning. This acknowledgment should also offer help in any way possible in the meantime.

Discard any mail that would ordinarily not be brought to the physician's attention. Some promotional literature falls into this category. Make certain that mailings from professional organizations are saved.

There may be rare periods when the entire facility is closed. In such cases, the post office can be contacted to hold mail until the facility reopens. The postal carrier cannot accept an oral request, so a formal request must be made. Never leave mail unattended to gather outside a mailbox or clutter up a doorway in a hall. Even mail slots may become filled or magazines may become stuck in them, causing important mail to pile up outside the slot. Far too much money and mail of a confidential nature are sent to physicians' offices to take chances on mail theft or destruction.

Outgoing Mail

Folding and Inserting Letters. Standard ways of folding and inserting letters are used so that the letter fits properly into the envelope and so that it can be easily removed without damage (Figure 12-6).

No. 10 Envelope. Bring the bottom third of the standard-sized letter up and make a crease. Fold the top of the letter down to within about $3/8$ inch of the creased edge and make a second crease. The second crease goes into the envelope first.

No. $6^3/4$ Envelope. For a standard-sized letter, bring the bottom edge up to within about $3/8$ inch of the top edge and make a crease. Then, folding from the right edge, make a fold a little less than one third of the width of the sheet and crease it. Folding from the left edge, bring the edge to within about $3/8$ inch of the previous crease. Insert the left creased edge into the envelope first.

Window Envelope. To fold a letter for insertion into a window envelope, bring the bottom third of the letter up and make a crease, then fold the top of the letter back to the crease you made before. The inside address should now be facing forward. This method is often followed for mailing statements.

Addressing the Envelope

Mailing Addresses. The U.S. Postal Service attempts to have all mail in standard-sized envelopes read, coded,

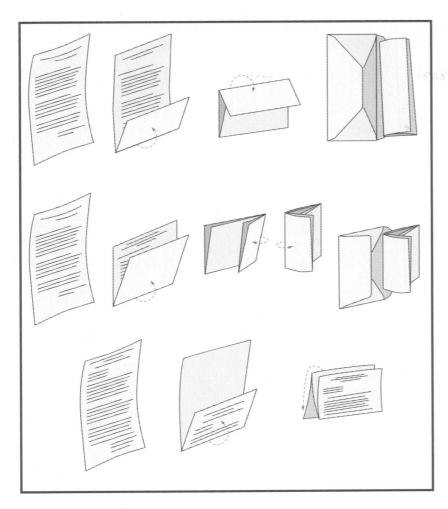

FIGURE 12-6   Correct methods of folding letters.

sorted, and canceled automatically at regional sorting stations where mail can be processed at a rate of 30,000 letters per hour. The success of automatic sorting depends on the cooperation of mailers in preparing envelopes in a format that can be read by automatic equipment (Procedure 12-5).

KEY POINTS FOR ADDRESSING ENVELOPES

- Use dark type on a light background; black on white is best.
- Do not use script or italic type; an electronic scanner cannot read these.
- Type all addresses in block format and in the area on the envelope that the scanner is programmed to read.
- Capitalize everything in the address.
- Eliminate all punctuation in the address.
- Use the standard two-letter state code instead of the spelled out name of the state.

- The last line of the address must contain the city, state code, and ZIP code, and it must not exceed 27 characters in length.
- The characters should be distributed so that they will not exceed the following limits:

Allowance for city name	13
Space between city name and state code	1
Allowance for state code	2
Space between state code and ZIP code	1
Space for basic ZIP code	5
Space for hyphen and four additional characters	5

If a city name contains more than 13 characters, you must use the approved code for that city as shown in the Abbreviations Section of the National Zip Code Directory.

MEDICAL ASSOCIATES INCORPORATED
4444 AVENIDA WILSHIRE
SAN CLEMENTE CA 92672-1500

HENRY B TURNER MD
PO BOX 845
JACKSONVILLE FL 32232-9950

PROCEDURE 12-5

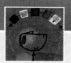

Addressing Outgoing Mail Using U.S. Post Office OCR Guidelines

GOAL: To correctly address business correspondence so that the mail arrives and is processed by the U.S. Post Office as efficiently as possible.

EQUIPMENT AND SUPPLIES

- Envelopes
- Computer or typewriter
- Correspondence

PROCEDURAL STEPS

1 Place the envelope into the printer or typewriter.

2 Enter the word processing program, such as Microsoft Word, and check the "Tools" section for envelopes. If this is not available in the word processing program, or a typewriter is being used, judge the area on the envelope that can be read by the optical character reader (OCR). The address block should start no higher than 2¾ inches from the bottom. Leave a bottom margin of at least ⅝ inch and left and right margins of at least 1 inch. Nothing should be written or printed below the address block or to the right of it.

Purpose: To ensure the correct placement of the address for accurate reading by the OCR.

3 Use dark type on a light background, no script or italics, and capitalize everything in the address.

Purpose: To ensure that the OCR can read the address.

4 Type the address in block format, using only approved abbreviations and eliminating all punctuation.

5 Type the city, state, and zip code on the last line of the address.

6 No line should have more than 27 total characters, including spaces.

7 Leave a ⅝-inch by 4¾-inch space blank in the bottom right corner of the envelope.

Purpose: To allow for bar code scanning (BCS).

8 Mail addressed to other countries includes the city and postal code on the third line, and the name of the country on a fourth line.

The Postal Service provides three special sets of abbreviations: (1) state names; (2) long names of cities, towns, and places; and (3) names of streets and roads and general terms, such as University or Institute. The information can be obtained from the Postal Service, or a program can be purchased for the computer. When these abbreviations are used, it is possible to limit the last line of any domestic address to 27 strokes. The next-to-last line in the address block should contain a street address or post office box number.

The address block should start no higher than 2³/₄ inches from the bottom. Leave a bottom margin of at least ⁵/₈ inch and left and right margins of at least 1 inch. Nothing should be written or printed below the address block or to the right of it.

The regulations for addressing envelopes were developed mainly for volume mailers with computerized mailing lists (Figure 12-7). Some exceptions are acceptable to the Postal Service and its scanning equipment. For example, the traditional style of typing an address in lower case with initial capital letters is readable by the optical scanners. Also, if the ZIP code cannot fit on the line with the city and state, it can be placed on the line immediately below.

Return Addresses. Always place a complete return address on the envelope. The U.S. Postal Service will not deliver mail without postage. If there is no stamp on the

envelope or if the stamp falls off and there is no return address, it will go to the dead letter office. There, the postal employees will open the mail in an attempt to identify the sender, but huge time delays may make the mail useless on delivery. If an address is found for the sender, the mail will be returned in an official envelope with a notice of postage due. If an address is not found for the sender, the mail is destroyed.

Notations. Any notations on the envelope directed toward the addressee, such as *Personal* or *Confidential*, should be typed and underlined on line 9 or on the third line below the return address, whichever is lower. Align it with the return address on the left edge of the envelope.

Any notations directed toward the postal service, such as *special delivery* or *certified mail*, should be typed in all capital letters on the upper right side of the envelope immediately below the stamp area. If an address contains an attention line, it should be typed above the organization line or on the line immediately above the street address or post office box number.

Sealing and Stamping Hints. Here's a suggestion for speeding up the sealing of a number of envelopes; at statement time, for example, many envelopes go into the mail at one time:

- Fan out unsealed envelopes, address side down, in groups of six to ten.

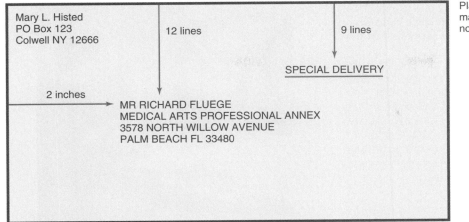

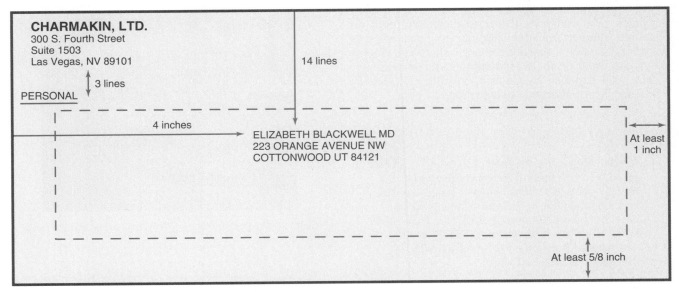

FIGURE 12-7   Addressing envelopes.

• Draw a damp sponge over the flaps, and starting with the lower piece, turn down the flaps and seal each one.

Do not use too much moisture because this may cause the glue to spread and several envelopes to stick together. A similar process simplifies stamping several letters at one time if not using a postage meter. If possible, purchase stamps by the roll. Tear off about ten stamps from the roll. Fanfold the stamps on the perforations so that they separate easily. Fan the envelopes address side up. Wet a strip of stamps with the sponge and, starting at one end of the fanned envelopes, attach the stamp at the end of the strip, tear it off, and proceed to the next envelope. Automated sealers and stampers are also available to make this procedure easier and more efficient.

Cost-Saving Mailing Procedures

Using ZIP Codes. The ZIP code is a very important part of an address, just as the area code is a very important part of a telephone number. ZIP codes start with the number 0 on the East Coast and gradually increase to number 9 on the West Coast and Hawaii.

The five-digit ZIP code was introduced in 1961. The first three digits identify a major city or distribution point, and all five digits identify an individual post office, zone of a city, or other delivery unit. The Postal Service later developed the nine-digit ZIP code, consisting of the original five digits followed by a hyphen and four additional digits that further identify the addressee's street location. The ZIP code is electronically transformed into a bar code. The office computer may have this capability. The Postal Code claims that the ZIP-plus-4, when used with the automated letter-sorting machinery, can eliminate 20 mail-handling steps and result in considerable savings. This saving is passed on to bulk mailers on mailings of 250 or more pieces that have typewritten addresses in machine-readable format along with the nine-digit ZIP code.

Presorting. Bulk mailers can get a discount on postage for presorting their mail. A discounted presort rate is charged on each piece that is part of a group of 10 or more pieces sorted to the same five-digit code or a group of 50 or more pieces sorted to the same first three-digit ZIP code.

Using Correct Postage. Although mailing fees are still one of our better bargains, the mailing costs for even a small office are a sizable item in the annual budget, and carelessness can cause them to soar. If the facility does not have a postage meter that dispenses postage exactly, then be sure that you are not putting too many stamps on your outgoing mail. Use an accurate postage scale and remember that only the first ounce requires the base rate; additional ounces are at a lower rate.

Getting Faster Mail Service

Postage Meters. The postage meter is the most efficient way of stamping the mail in a large business office (Figure 12-8). It can print postage onto adhesive strips that are then placed onto the envelopes or packages, or it can print the postage directly onto an envelope. Metered mail does not have to be canceled or postmarked when it reaches the post office. This means that it can move on to its destination faster. Meters vary in size and capabilities. Consult an office equipment dealer for information on postage meters.

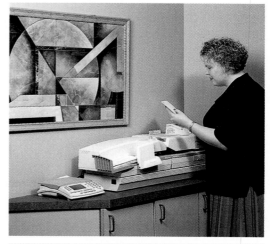
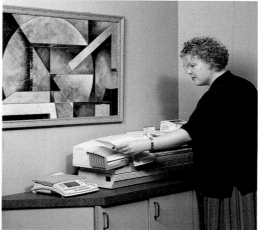

FIGURE 12-8 Postage meters help the mail processing run more efficiently.

> ## CRITICAL THINKING APPLICATION
>
> - Brandon knows that the mail processing would go much faster if the office invested in a postage meter. The office manager states that she has mentioned this to Brandon's father several times, but he did not purchase a meter. How might Brandon approach his father about this issue?
> - What should Brandon do before discussing the postage meter with his father?

Mailing Practices. For large mailings, local letters should be separated from out-of-town letters. Letters or packages that need to be rushed should be taken directly to the post office for mailing. Others can be placed in street boxes or the building's mail chute for pickup. Packages should always be taken to a post office and weighed for proper postage. Place a letter tray on the desk or some other convenient place so that all outgoing mail is kept together until it is ready to leave the office.

Classifications of Mail

Mail is classified according to *type*, *weight*, and *destination*. The ounce and pound are the units of measurement. **Domestic mail** is that which is sent within the United States and its territories, and **International mail** is that which is sent outside the United States. Letters to distant points of the globe are in almost all cases sent by air and can be expected to reach their destination within a few days. The rates for international mail are based on increments of $1/2$ ounce. A table of rates can be obtained from the post office.

Express Mail. Express Mail is available 7 days per week, 365 days per year for items weighing up to 70 pounds and measuring 108 inches in combined length and **girth**. Service features include the following:

- Noon delivery between major business markets
- Merchandise and document reconstruction insurance
- Express mail shipping containers
- Shipment receipt
- Optional return receipt service
- Optional **collect-on-delivery (COD)** service
- Waiver of signature option
- Collection boxes
- Optional pickup service

First-Class Mail. First-class mail includes sealed or unsealed handwritten or typed material, such as letters, postal cards, postcards, and business reply mail. Postage for letters weighing 11 ounces or less is based on weight, in 1-ounce increments. Envelopes larger than the standard No. 10 business envelope should have the green diamond border to expedite first-class delivery.

Priority Mail. First-class mail weighing over 11 ounces is classified as Priority Mail, and the postage is calculated on the basis of weight and destination, with the maximum weight being 70 pounds.

Second-Class Mail. Regular and preferred second-class rates are available only to newspapers and periodicals that have been authorized to receive second-class mail privileges. Copies mailed by the public are charged at the applicable Express Mail, Priority Mail, or single-piece first-, third-, or fourth-class rate.

Third-Class Mail. Third-class mail includes such items as catalogs, circulars, books, photographs, and other printed matter. Pieces should be sealed or secured so that they can be handled by machine but must be clearly marked as third class.

Fourth-Class Mail. Fourth-class mail consists of merchandise, books, and printed matter that are not included in first or second class and that weigh 16 ounces or more but do not exceed 70 pounds. There are size limitations on fourth-class mail; check with the post office regarding regulations on very large parcels.

Special Services

Insured Mail. Insurance for coverage against loss or damage is available for Priority Mail, first-class mail, or parcel post.

Registered Mail. Mail of all classes, particularly that of unusually high value, can be additionally protected by registering it. The sender may request evidence of its delivery. Registering a piece of mail also helps to trace delivery, if necessary.

When sending a registered letter, it is necessary to go to the post office and fill in the required forms. All articles to be registered must be thoroughly sealed with U.S. Postal Service tape. Cellophane tape is not permitted. On receipt of the item, the **recipient** is required to sign a form that acknowledges delivery. A registered letter may be released to the person to whom it is addressed or to his or her agent. For an additional fee, a personal receipt may be requested (Figure 12-9). This ensures that the letter will be released only to the individual to whom it is addressed. Such pieces bear the label *To Addressee Only*.

Registered mail is accounted for by number from the time of mailing until the time of delivery and is transported separately from other mail under a special lock. In case of loss or damage, the customer may be reimbursed up to certain limits, provided that the value of the registered article has been declared at the time of mailing and that the appropriate fee has been paid.

Postal Money Orders. Postal money orders are a convenient way of mailing money, especially for the individual who does not have a personal checking account. They may be purchased in amounts as high as $700.

Special Delivery. Mail of any class that has been marked *special delivery* is charged at the special-delivery rate. Such pieces may be regular first- or second-class, registered, insured, or COD pieces. The special-delivery designation generally does not speed up the normal travel time between two cities but does ensure immediate delivery of the item when it arrives at the designated post office.

Special Handling. Third- and fourth-class mail sent by special handling receives the fastest service and ground transportation practicable—about the same as that for first-class mail. The special-handling fee is in addition to required postage and is determined according to weight. This fee does not include insurance or special delivery at the destination, but special delivery, if desired, is available at an added cost. If a parcel is sent by Priority Mail, special handling is of no additional advantage because it is already traveling at the greatest possible speed.

Certified Mail. Any piece of mail without **intrinsic** value and on which postage is paid at the first-class rate will be accepted as certified mail. Such items as contracts, deeds, mortgages, bank books, checks, passports, insurance policies, money orders, and birth certificates that are not themselves valuable but that would be difficult to duplicate if lost should be certified. Certified mail is also often used as an aid in debt collection.

Regular postage in addition to a certified mail fee must be affixed. For an additional fee, a receipt verifying delivery can be requested (Figure 12-10). Certified mail can be sent special delivery if the prescribed fees are paid. A record of delivery of certified mail is kept for 2 years at the post office of delivery; however, no record is kept at the post office of origin. Furthermore, this type of mail does not provide insurance coverage.

The medical assistant should keep a supply of certified mail forms and return receipts on hand. These may be obtained at any post office. Full instructions are included on the forms. Fees and postage may be paid using ordinary postage stamps, meter stamps, or permit imprints. Certified mail can be mailed at any post office, station, or branch or can be deposited in mail drops or in street letter boxes if specific instructions are followed.

Certificate of Mailing. If a sender needs proof of mailing but is not especially concerned with proof of receipt of an item, the most economic method is to obtain a certificate of mailing. Obtain this form at the post office and fill in the required information. Attach a stamp for the current fee and hand the form to the postal clerk along with the piece of mail. The clerk will postmark the receipt, initial it, and hand it back as acknowledgment of having received the piece of mail at the post office. This is sometimes used when mailing tax reports or other items that must be postmarked by a certain date.

Private Delivery Services

Not all mail is delivered by the U.S. Postal Service. Many private services pick up and deliver mail overnight. Among these are Federal Express, United Parcel Service, Emery, Airborne Express, and DHL. These services are highly advertised and competitive. All large cities and many smaller communities have centralized points where packages can be dropped off for the service of the sender's choice. Pickup service is also available in many communities.

CRITICAL THINKING APPLICATION

- The office has always used FedEx for sending packages. However, Brandon is curious as to whether FedEx offers the best rates. How might he gather this information?
- What should be considered when choosing a private delivery service?

Handling Special Situations

Forwarding and Obtaining a Changed Address. By marking a piece of mail with the notation *Forwarding Service Requested*, the U.S. Post Office will forward mail to the new address if it is sent within 12 months of the change or if the receiver has left a forwarding order with the post office. At that time the forwarding order is expired unless the receiver requests that it be continued. Between 12 and 18 months, the piece will be returned to the sender with the new address noted. After 18 months, mail is usually returned with the reason for nondelivery noted. There is no charge for forwarding when priority or first-class mail is used.

If the mailer wants to know an addressee's new address, this service can be obtained from the post office by placing the words *Address Correction Requested* beneath the return address on the envelope. This can be hand-written, stamped, typewritten, or printed. The new address will be noted on a sticker and returned to the sender, and there is no charge for this if the item is sent priority or first-class mail. The post office charges a weighted fee for this service for standard mail and packages. If the envelope is marked *Change Service Requested*, the post office will dispose of the piece of mail and return a card to the sender showing the forwarding address of the addressee. If the piece was sent priority or first class, there

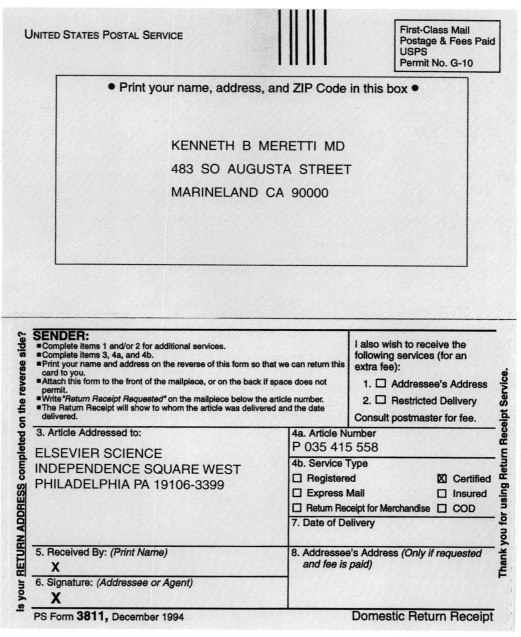

FIGURE 12-9   Delivery receipts for certified, registered, and insured mail. Attach to the back of the article, and endorse the front with the phrase *return receipt requested* adjacent to the article number.

FIGURE 12-9, Cont'd   For legend see opposite page.

is no charge for the service unless the notification is sent electronically, and then there is a small charge.

Recalling Mail. If a letter has been dropped in the mailbox by mistake, do not ask the mail collector to give it to you; he or she is not permitted to do so. However, mail can be recalled by making written application at the post office, together with an envelope addressed identically to the one being recalled. If the letter has already left the local post office, the postmaster, at the sender's expense, can notify the postmaster at the destination post office to return the letter. However, there is no guarantee that the letter will be retrieved.

Returned Mail. If a letter is returned to the sender after an attempt has been made to deliver it, it cannot be mailed again without new postage. It is best simply to prepare a new envelope with the correct address, affix the proper postage, and place in the mail.

When mail is returned to the medical office, be sure to correct the database, indicating that mail has been returned on a certain patient, so that postage is not wasted sending mail to that address again.

Tracing Lost Mail. Receipts issued by the post office, whether for money orders, registered mail, certified mail, or insured mail, should be retained until receipt of the item has been acknowledged. If, after an adequate time elapses, no acknowledgment of receipt

for such mailing arrives, notify the post office to trace the letter or package. Regular first-class mail is not easily traced, but the post office will make every attempt to find it for you. In tracing a lost letter or package, the post office requires that a special form be filled out; data from any original receipt should be written along with any other identifying information on this form.

Closing Comments

Remember that every letter sent from the medical office should project a professional image. Use neat handwriting when correspondence is not typed or generated on a computer. All of the office staff must be able to read items written years ago. It is worth the time and effort to brush up on English skills so that writing documents becomes as comfortable as setting an appointment or assisting in a procedure.

Patient Education

Medical offices often use brochures and printed material for the education of their patients. It is critical that these

```
        P 268 875 363

US Postal Service
Receipt for Certified Mail
No Insurance Coverage Provided.
Do not use for International Mail (See reverse)
```

Sent to ELSEVIER SCIENCE	
Street & Number INDEPENDENCE SQUARE WEST	
Post Office, State, & ZIP Code PHILADELPHIA PA 19106-3399	
Postage	$
Certified Fee	
Special Delivery Fee	
Restricted Delivery Fee	
Return Receipt Showing to Whom & Date Delivered	
Return Receipt Showing to Whom, Date, & Addressee's Address	
TOTAL Postage & Fees	$
Postmark or Date	

PS Form **3800**, April 1995

```
Fold at line over top of envelope to
the right of the return address

        CERTIFIED

       P 268 875 363

            MAIL
```

FIGURE 12-10 Receipt for certified mail. Attach the bottom portion of the receipt to the top of the envelope, just to the right of the return address.

materials look professional and reflect a positive image for the physician and the facility. Be sure that copied material is clean without streaks and that it looks attractive to the eye. If the information is written by an office staff member, make certain that correct grammar is used and that several office members proofread the work for errors and proper use of the English language. It is wonderful to make a good first impression, but every impression in the medical office is an important one.

Legal and Ethical Issues

A copy should be kept of all communications leaving the office that relate to patient care. If any information is handwritten, it must be completely legible to the patient. Certainly, everyone should be able to read his or her own handwriting, even years later.

Since the appointment book is also considered a communications tool, the information entered by hand in the book must also be clear and easy to read. Take enough time to write legibly so that there is no confusion when the document is referred to at a later date. In legal battles, all written documentation must be concise and must not promote questions about the content.

SUMMARY OF SCENARIO

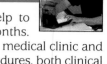

Brandon has been a tremendous help to the office staff over the summer months. He has learned about every area of the medical clinic and has mastered several of the office procedures, both clinical and administrative. He has a greater understanding now of the business aspect of the medical office.

His duties as a temporary administrative medical assistant have opened his eyes to the value and importance of the administrative personnel. He can easily see that from the receptionist to the scheduler to the insurance billers—all play a vital role in the smooth operation of the facility.

Toward the end of the summer, the office staff honored Brandon with a going-away party. He announced with a smile that he had decided, based on his experience in his father's family practice, that he wished to become a pediatrician. He expressed to the staff that he planned to hire them all away from his father! Then on a serious note, he thanked all the employees for their patience and for their willing spirit to let him learn from them. Everyone expects Brandon to be a complete success.

SUMMARY OF LEARNING OBJECTIVES

■ The medical assistant is responsible for making certain that equipment is in good working order. Warranties should always be mailed when new equipment is purchased, and the correct maintenance procedures should be followed to keep machines working at an optimal level. Supplies should be ordered before they run out, and prices should be compared to find the best quality for the best price available.

■ There are four basic sizes of letterhead stationery. Standard or letter stationery, which is most commonly used for business purposes, is $8\frac{1}{2} \times 11$ inches. Monarch or executive stationery is $8\frac{1}{4} \times 10\frac{1}{2}$ inches and is used for informal business correspondence. Baronial stationery is $5\frac{1}{2} \times 8\frac{1}{2}$ inches, whereas legal stationery is $8\frac{1}{2} \times 14$ inches.

■ The medical assistant should be familiar with the various parts of speech and the way to use them correctly in a sentence. Nouns name something, such as a person, place, or thing; pronouns are substitutes for nouns. Verbs are action words and express movement, a condition, or a state of being. Adjectives usually describe nouns, whereas adverbs usually describe verbs. Prepositions are connecting words, as are conjunctions. Interjections show strong feelings and are often followed by an exclamation point.

■ It is quite helpful to develop a personal tool collection that will assist the medical assistant with written communications in the medical office. An up-to-date dictionary, a medical dictionary, a composition handbook, an English-language reference manual, and a thesaurus will be valuable additions to the tool library.

■ Before any type of correspondence is answered, the piece should be read carefully. Often a highlighter is used for marking questions that must be answered, or notes may be written on the correspondence in pencil. A draft of the reply should be written first and then rewritten in its final draft.

■ Subsequent letters will be much easier to draft if the medical assistant develops a portfolio that contains sample letters and other types of communications. Once a letter is written, it can be saved on the computer hard drive or on a disk, or it can be printed and placed in a binder for easy viewing. If the letter is printed in a binder, it is wise to note on each example the file name as it is saved on the computer so that the document can be easily found again when needed. This is an excellent way to save time in the busy medical office.

■ Block is an efficient but less attractive letter style wherein all lines begin flush with the left margin of the paper. Modified block is similar, but some lines begin at the center of the page instead of the left margin. Modified block with indented paragraphs is identical to block style, with the exception of the indention of the paragraphs. Simplified letter style contains lines that begin flush at the left margin, but other items, such as the salutation and complimentary closing, are omitted.

■ The four standard parts of a business letter include the heading, the opening, the body, and the closing. The heading includes the letterhead and dateline, whereas the opening includes the inside address and any attention or salutation line. The body is the message of the document, and the closing is the signature, complimentary closing, reference initials, and special notations.

■ Money can be saved by consulting the post office when mailing, checking for better rates, and using ZIP codes. Consult a local post office when mailing in bulk to obtain the best rates.

INTERNET CONNECTIONS

- Airborne Express
  www.airborne.com
- DHL Worldwide Express
  www.dhl.com
- Emery Forwarding
  www.emeryworld.com
- Federal Express
  www.fedex.com
- Merriam-Webster Online Dictionary
  www.merriam-webster.com
- United Parcel Service
  www.ups.com
- United States Post Office
  www.usps.com

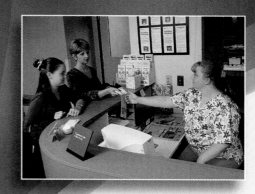

CHAPTER 13

Scenario

Susan Beezler has just begun her career in the medical assisting profession. She is attending medical assisting school in the morning hours and works part-time for a family practitioner in the afternoons as a clerical/records assistant. Susan is eager to learn about medicine and looks forward to taking on more responsibility at the office.

The practice is growing swiftly and recently added a new physician, Dr. Alex Thomas. Dr. Thomas has enjoyed working with Susan and feels that her energy will be just what his patients need. He has taken a special interest in Susan and often lets her assist him with patients when her other duties allow.

Susan knows that although she is a beginner in the office, she will gain trust from her supervisors and patients as long as she projects a teachable attitude. She cheerfully performs filing and often does transcription for Dr. Thomas. The other staff members are pleased with her willing attitude to perform even the most mundane tasks. Her warm personality and caring way with patients ensure that she has a great chance at a long career in this medical office.

Susan enjoys sharing her experiences with the other students in her class. She is the only person who is currently working in the medical field, so the other students ask many questions about what Susan has experienced in the real world of medicine. She is very careful not to breach patient confidentiality as she discusses situations in general, never mentioning any patient names.

Susan feels a great sense of pride that she is already a member of the healthcare team and able to make a positive contribution to the lives of her patients.

Medical Records Management

Learning Objectives

- Define and spell the terms listed in the vocabulary.
- List and discuss the basic equipment used in a filing system.
- Describe the steps in filing a document.
- List and discuss application of the basic filing systems.
- Explain how color coding of files can be useful in a medical facility.
- State several important reasons for keeping accurate medical records.
- Discuss the ownership of records.
- Explain the difference between a traditional medical record and a problem-oriented medical record.
- Illustrate the difference between subjective and objective information.
- Discuss changing an entry in the patient record and the importance of following correct procedures.
- Create a file for a new patient.
- Prepare an informed consent for treatment form.
- Add supplementary items to an established patient record.
- Prepare a record release form.
- Accurately transcribe a machine-dictated letter.
- File records using an alphabetical and numeric system.
- Accurately color code patient charts.

National Curriculum Competencies

ADMINISTRATIVE COMPETENCIES

1c. Perform medical transcription
1d. Organize a patient's medical record
1e. File medical records

CLINICAL COMPETENCIES

4c. Obtain and record patient history

TRANSDISCIPLINARY COMPETENCIES

1c. Establish and maintain the medical record
1d. Document appropriately

Vocabulary

alphabetical filing Any system that arranges names or topics according to the sequence of the letters in the alphabet.

alphanumeric Systems made up of combinations of letters and numbers.

audit A formal examination of an organization's or individual's accounts or financial situation; a methodical examination and review.

augment To make greater, more numerous, larger, or more intense.

caption A heading, title, or subtitle under which records are filed.

chronological order Of, relating to, or arranged in or according to the order of time.

continuity of care Care that continues smoothly from one provider to another, so that the patient receives the most benefit and no interruption in care.

dictation The act or manner of uttering words to be transcribed.

direct filing system A filing system in which materials can be located without consulting an intermediary source of reference.

gleaned Gathered bit by bit (e.g., information or material); picked over in search of relevant material.

indirect filing system A filing system in which an intermediary source of reference, such as a card file, must be consulted to locate specific files.

microfilm A film bearing a photographic record on a reduced scale of printed or other graphic matter.

numeric filing The filing of records, correspondence, or cards by number.

objective information Information that is gathered by watching or observation of a patient.

obliteration Act of making undecipherable or imperceptible by obscuring or wearing away.

OUTfolder A folder used to provide space for the temporary filing of materials.

OUTguide A heavy guide that is used to replace a folder that has been temporarily moved from the filing space.

power of attorney A legal instrument authorizing one to act as the attorney or agent of the grantor.

pressboard A strong, highly glazed composition board resembling vulcanized fiber; heavy card stock.

procrastination To put off intentionally the doing of something that should be done.

provisional diagnosis A temporary diagnosis made prior to receiving all test results.

quality control An aggregate of activities designed to ensure adequate quality, especially in manufactured products or in the service industries.

requisites Something considered essential or necessary.

retention schedule A method or plan for retaining or keeping medical records, and their movement from active, to inactive, to closed filing.

shelf filing A system that uses open shelves rather than cabinets for storing records.

shingling A method of filing whereby one report is laid on top of the older report, resembling the shingles of a roof.

subjective information Information that is gained by questioning the patient or taken from a form.

tickler file A chronological file used as a reminder that something must be taken care of on a certain date.

transcription To make a written copy of, either in longhand or by machine.

vested Granted or endowed with a particular authority, right, or property; to have a special interest in.

A medical records management system is only as good as the ease of retrieval of the data in the files. Since the pace of the medical office is usually quite rapid, patient charts must be found quickly and also be functional, so that the information inside is easily obtainable.

There are few phrases more frustrating to the patient than "we cannot locate your chart." Patients have every right to question the competence of the medical care they are receiving if the office has problems simply finding a chart. Organization and adherence to set routines will help to assure that charts are accessible when they are needed.

Ownership of the Medical Record

Who actually owns the medical record? Patients often assume that because the information contained in the medical record is about them, the ownership of the record rightfully belongs to the patient. However, the owner of the physical medical record is the physician or medical facility, often called the "maker," that initiated and developed the record. The patient has the right of access to the information within but does not own the physical chart or other document pertaining to the record. The patient has a **vested** interest and thus has the right to demand confidentiality of all of the information placed in the chart.

The actual patient chart should never leave the medical facility from which it originated. Even the physician should refrain from taking the chart from the office to the hospital or nursing facility. If information from the chart is needed, copies can be placed in a file, and progress notes written on-site and returned to the original chart later. Patient charts should be kept in a locked room or locked filing cabinets when the office is closed.

CRITICAL THINKING APPLICATION

On Susan's third day at work, a man comes to the office and demands to see his mother's medical chart. Susan pulls the chart and sees an entry stating that the mother does not wish the son to have any information about her. What should Susan do in this situation? Are there any viable reasons why the son should have access to the mother's medical information?

Why Medical Records Are Important

Medical records exist for four basic reasons. First, the medical record assists the physician in providing the best possible medical care for the patient. The physician examines the patient and enters the findings on the patient's medical record. These findings are the clues to diagnosis. The physician may order many types of tests to confirm or **augment** the clinical findings. As the reports of these tests come in, the findings fall into place like the pieces of a jigsaw puzzle. Then, with the confirmation data to support the diagnosis, the physician can prescribe treatment and form an opinion about the patient's chances of recovery, assured that every resource has been used to arrive at a correct judgment. The medical record provides a complete history of all of the care given to the patient.

The medical record also provides critical information for others. By reading through the chart and discovering the methods used to treat the patient, healthcare professionals can provide a **continuity of care**. Each person knows what the patient has experienced and can provide continued care, even from one facility to another. For example, when a patient is transferred from a hospital to a skilled nursing facility, the information from the patient's hospital chart will help the nursing facility to better care for the patient. When patients move from place to place or caregivers change, copies of the pertinent chart information should move with the patient to provide this continuity of care.

The second reason for keeping medical records is to offer legal protection for those who provided care to the patient. A documented medical chart is excellent proof that certain procedures were performed or medical advice was given. An accurate chart is the foundation for legal defense in cases of medical professional liability. This is one reason that it is critical to write legibly in the chart and document exactly what happens to the patient. As we have emphasized throughout the book: "If it isn't charted, it didn't happen."

Third, medical records provide statistical information that is helpful to researchers. The patient's chart provides information about medications taken and the reactions to them. Medical records may be used to evaluate the effectiveness of certain kinds of treatment or to determine the incidence of a given disease. Often, physicians take part in drug studies that track adverse reactions and side effects. The effects of various treatments and procedures can also be tracked and statistics **gleaned** from the information gathered from patient charts. Correlation of such statistical information may result in a new outlook on some phases of medicine and can lead to revised techniques and treatments. The statistical data from medical records are also valuable in the preparation of scientific papers, books, and lectures.

Fourth, medical records are vital for financial reimbursement. The information in the medical chart supports claims for reimbursement and is required by most third-party payors.

Creating an Efficient Medical Record Management System

The medical record management system used in the medical office should provide an easy method for retrieving information. The files should be organized in an orderly fashion, and all of the information within the chart must be completely legible to the average reader. The information must also be accurate, and corrections should be made and documented properly. The wording in the chart should be easily understood and grammatically correct. An efficient method of adding documents to the chart must be in place, so that the physician or other provider always has the most up-to-date information.

Above all, the medical record management system must be one that works for the individual facility. Attempting to adopt a method used by another facility may not always be best. The system should be adapted to the facility and provider's needs.

Types of Records

The two major types of patient records include the paper-based medical record and the computer-based medical record. As computer technology advances, the paper-based medical record seems more and more inefficient. It is difficult to use a paper-based record for multiple purposes. In most cases, only one person can use the paper-based record at any given time, and the record is not available to others who need it when it is in use by a single person. Misfiled information is common, and the entire record can be misfiled as well. Data cannot be accessed easily for research and **quality control**, and in facilities with multiple departments, the information is difficult to share. The paper-based record is a good evidence of patient care, but it not nearly as useful in other capacities.

The computer-based medical record (also called the electronic health record) is much more efficient than the paper-based record. The book *Electronic Health Records: Changing the Vision** offers the following definition:

> An electronic health record is any information relating to the past, present, or future physical/mental health, or condition of an individual which resides in electronic systems used to capture, transmit, receive, store, retrieve, link, and manipulate multimedia data for the primary purpose of providing healthcare and health related services.

The computer-based medical record is a great improvement over the paper-based record, but it is not without its disadvantages. Patient confidentiality is critical and sometimes difficult to maintain with computer-based records. Many providers worry about computer malfunctions that would inhibit access to the record in an emergency.

Still, the advantages of the computer-based record seem to far outweigh the disadvantages. Information can

---

*Murphy GF, Hanken MA, Waters K: *Electronic health records: changing the vision*, Philadelphia, 1999, WB Saunders.

be accessed in a variety of physical locations, and more than one person can see the record at any given time. The patient database usually allows various types of statistical information to be recalled, which is a valuable tool. Patient information is available quickly in an emergency, even when the patient is not in his or her hometown. All of these advantages mean that the computer-based record will continue to be a key tool in the future.

Organization of the Medical Record

Source-Oriented Records

The traditional patient record is source oriented; that is, observations and data are cataloged according to their source—physician, laboratory, radiology, nurse, technician—with no recording of a logical relationship between them. Forms and progress notes are filed in reverse **chronological order** (most recent on top) and filed in separate sections of the record by the type of form or service rendered—all laboratory reports together, all x-ray reports together, and so forth.

Problem-Oriented Medical Records

The problem-oriented medical record (POMR) is a radical departure from the traditional system of keeping patient records. It is sometimes referred to as the Weed system, because it was originated by Dr. Lawrence L. Weed, a professor of medicine at the University of Vermont's College of Medicine. The POMR is a record of clinical practice that divides medical action into four bases:

1. The *database* includes chief complaint, present illness, patient profile, review of systems, physical examination, and laboratory reports.
2. The *problem list* is a numbered and titled list of every problem the patient has that requires management or workup. This may include social and demographic troubles as well as strictly medical or surgical ones.
3. The *treatment plan* includes management, additional workups needed, and therapy. Each plan is titled and numbered with respect to the problem.
4. The *progress notes* include structured notes that are numbered to correspond with each problem number.

Several companies have developed file folders for the organization of patient data consistent with the problem-oriented medical record (Figure 13-1). The problem list is entered on the divider cover for laboratory reports. Special sections are provided for current major and chronic problems and for inactive major or chronic problems. The divider cover for progress notes is a chart for listing medications and other therapeutic modalities. Progress notes follow the SOAP approach. SOAP is an acronym for:

- Subjective impressions
- Objective clinical evidence
- Assessment or diagnosis
- Plans for further studies, treatment, or management

Some medical offices also used an "E" in the record, to represent "Evaluation." This section is used to record an assessment of the patient's understanding of and possible compliance with the treatment plan. As this is not used in every practice, the medical assistant may never see or use it to complete a patient record.

The POMR has the advantage of imposing order and organization on the information added to a patient's medical record. The records are more easily reviewed, and the likelihood of overlooking a problem is greatly reduced. The SOAP method essentially forces a rational approach to patient problems and assists in formulating a logical and orderly plan of patient care (Figure 13-2).

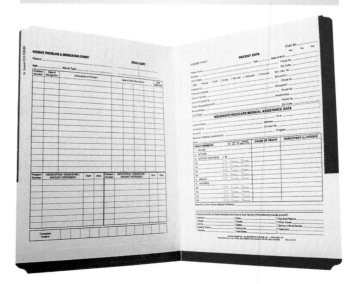

FIGURE 13-1 A chart designed for a problem-oriented medical record. Some charts are specifically adapted to the POMR. (Courtesy Bibbero Systems, Inc., Petaluma, Calif. 94954, (800) 242-2376, www.bibbero.com.)

OUTLINE FORMAT PROGRESS NOTES

Patient Name ___Fletcher, LeRoy_____

Prob. No. or Letter	DATE	**S** Subjective	**O** Objective	**A** Assess	**P** Plans		
2	01/26/00	Patient complains of two days of severe high epigastric pain and burning, radiating through to the back. Pain accentuated after eating.				Page 1	
			On examination there is extreme guarding and tenderness, high epigastric region. No rebound. Bowel sounds normal. BP 110/70				
				R/O gastric ulcer, pylorospasm.			
					To have upper gastrointestinal series. Start on Cimetidine, 300 mg. q.i.d. Eliminate coffee, alcohol, and aspirin. Return in two days.		

Start each Progress Note (Subjective, Objective, Assessment and Plans) at the appropriate margin of the page. Write through the intervening columns to the right shaded column to create an outline form.

ANDRUS/CLINI-REC® PRIMARY CARE CHARTING SYSTEM FORM NO. 26-7115, ©1976 BIBBERO SYSTEMS, INC., PETALUMA, CA.

FIGURE 13-2 SOAP progress notes. The SOAP method keeps information organized and in a logical sequence. An actual progress note would include the physician's signature or initials after this entry. (Courtesy Bibbero Systems, Inc., Petaluma, Calif. 94954, (800) 242-2376, www.bibbero.com.)

Popularity of the POMR has continued to grow since its introduction in the 1960s, and it is especially advantageous in clinics, group practices, and hospitals, where more than one person must be able to find essential information in the chart.

Contents of the Complete Case History

The medical case history is the most important record in a physician's practice. For completeness, each patient's record should contain **subjective information** provided by the patient and **objective information** provided by the physician. If all entries are completed, the case history will stand the test of time. No branch of medicine is exempt from the necessity of keeping patient history records.

Subjective Information

Personal Demographics. The patient's case history begins with routine personal data, which the patient usually supplies on the first visit (Procedure 13-1). Most patients are required to complete a patient information form (Figure 13-3). The basic facts needed are the following:

- Patient's full name, spelled correctly
- Names of parents if patient is a child
- Patient's sex
- Date of birth
- Marital status
- Name of spouse, if married
- Number of children, if any
- Home address and telephone number
- Occupation
- Name of employer
- Business address and telephone number
- Employment information for spouse
- Healthcare insurance information
- Source of referral
- Social Security number

Personal and Medical History. The personal and medical history, which is often obtained by having the patient complete a questionnaire, provides information about any past illnesses or surgical operations that the patient may have had and includes data about injuries or physical defects, whether congenital or acquired

---

PROCEDURE 13-1

Initiating a Medical File for a New Patient

GOAL: To initiate a medical file for a new patient that will contain all the personal data necessary for a complete record and any other information required by the facility.

EQUIPMENT AND SUPPLIES

- Computer or typewriter
- Clerical supplies (pen, clipboard)
- Information on the agency's filing system
- Registration form
- File folder
- Label for folder
- ID card if using numeric system
- Cross-reference card
- Financial card
- Routing slip
- Private conference area

PROCEDURAL STEPS

1 Determine that the patient is new to the office.

2 Obtain and record the required personal data.
Purpose: Complete information is necessary for credit and insurance claim processing.

3 Type the information onto the patient history form.

4 Review the entire form.
Purpose: To confirm that the information is complete and correct.

5 Select a label and folder for the record
Explanation: If color coding is used, a decision must be made regarding the appropriate color for the patient name.

6 Type the caption on the label and apply it to the folder.
Explanation: Use the patient's name for alphabetical filing or appropriate number for numeric filing.

7 For a numeric filing system, prepare a cross-reference card and a patient ID number.
Purpose: Numeric filing is an indirect system and requires a cross-reference to a patient's name for locating the chart. The patient will use the number of the ID card when arranging appointments or making inquiries.

8 Prepare the financial card, or place that patient's name in the computerized ledger.

9 Place the patient's history form and all other forms required by the agency into the prepared folder.

10 Clip an encounter form on the outside of the patient's folder.

Thank you for selecting our health care team!
To help us meet all your health care needs, please
fill out this form completely in ink. If you have any questions
or need assistance, please ask us - we will be happy to help.

Welcome

Patient #_____

Soc. Sec. #_____

Patient Information (CONFIDENTIAL)

Date_____

Name_____ Birth date _____ Home phone_____

Address_____ City_____ State_____ Zip_____

Check appropriate box: ☐ Minor   ☐ Single   ☐ Married   ☐ Divorced   ☐ Widowed   ☐ Separated

If student, name of school/college _____ City_____ State__ ☐ Full time ☐ Part time

Patient's or parent's employer_____ Work phone _____

Business address _____ City_____ State_____ Zip_____

Spouse or parent's name_____ Employer_____ Work phone _____

Whom may we thank for referring you?_____

Person to contact in case of emergency_____ Phone _____

Responsible Party

Name of person responsible for this account _____ Relationship to patient _____

Address _____ Home phone _____

Driver's license #_____ Birth date_____ Financial institution_____

Employer_____ Work phone_____ SSN#_____

Is this person currently a patient in our office?   ☐ Yes   ☐ No

Insurance Information

Name of insured _____ Relationship to patient _____

Birth date _____ Social Security #_____ Date employed_____

Name of employer_____ Union or local #_____ Work phone _____

Address of employer_____ City_____ State_____ Zip_____

Insurance company_____ Group #_____ Policy/ID #_____

Ins. co. address_____ City_____ State _____ Zip _____

How much is your deductible? _____How much have you used?_____ Max. annual benefit _____

| DO YOU HAVE ANY ADDITIONAL INSURANCE?   ☐ Yes   ☐ No   IF YES, COMPLETE THE FOLLOWING: |

Name of insured _____ Relationship to patient _____

Birth date _____ Social Security #_____ Date employed_____

Name of employer_____ Union or local #_____ Work phone _____

Address of employer_____ City_____ State_____ Zip_____

Insurance company_____ Group #_____ Policy/ID #_____

Ins. co. address_____ City_____ State _____ Zip _____

How much is your deductible? _____How much have you used?_____ Max. annual benefit _____

I authorize release of any information concerning my (or my child's) health care, advice and treatment provided for the purpose of
evaluating and administering claims for insurance benefits. I also hereby authorize payment of insurance benefits otherwise payable to me
directly to the doctor.

X _____   _____

Signature of patient or parent if minor   Date

FIGURE 13-3   The patient information form provides all of the information that the medical assistant needs to construct a patient chart.

(Figure 13-4). It also includes information about the patient's daily health habits.

The Patient's Family History. The family history comprises the physical condition of the various members of the patient's family, any past illnesses or diseases that individual members may have suffered, and a record of the causes of death. This information is important, because a hereditary pattern may be present in the case of certain diseases.

The Patient's Social History. The patient's social history includes information about the lifestyle the patient lives. If the patient drinks, how many drinks per day or

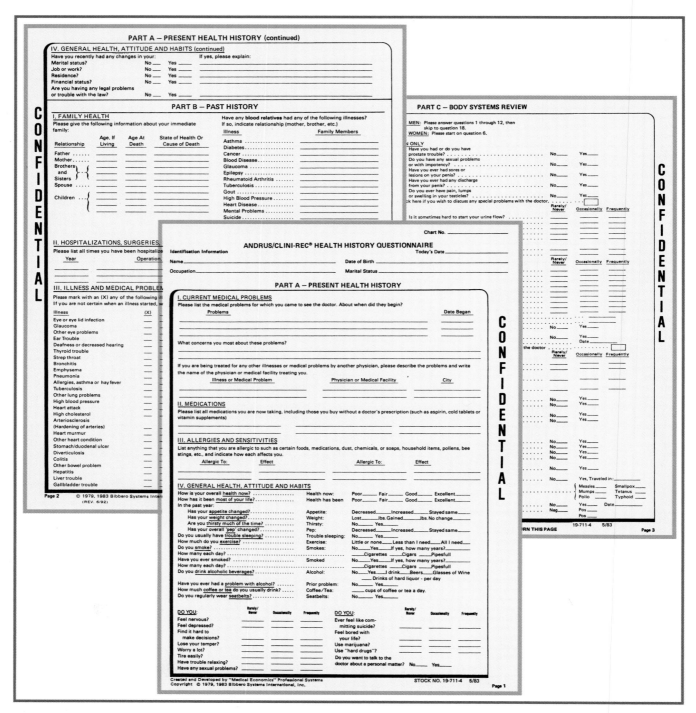

FIGURE 13-4 Database self-administered general health history questionnaire. Lengthy questionnaires should be completed by the patient before he or she is seen by the physician. Either mail the information to the patient in advance or ask the patient to come in early to complete the paperwork. (Courtesy Bibbero Systems, Inc., Petaluma, Calif. 94954, (800) 242-2376, www.bibbero.com.)

per week are consumed? If the patient uses cigarettes, how many packs a day are smoked? Drug use and even marital information can be considered the social history.

Patient's Chief Complaint. The patient's chief complaint is a concise account of the patient's symptoms, explained in the patient's own words. It should include the following:

- Nature and duration of pain, if any
- Time when the patient first noticed symptoms
- Patient's opinion as to the possible causes for the difficulties
- Remedies that the patient may have applied before seeing the physician
- Other medical treatment received for the same condition in the past

Objective Information

Objective findings, sometimes referred to as signs, become evident from the physician's examination of the patient.

Physical Examination and Findings and Laboratory and Radiology Reports. This section of the case history varies greatly with the specialty of the physician and the complaint of the patient. After the physician has examined the patient, the physical findings are recorded in the history (Figure 13-5). Results of other tests or requests for these tests are then recorded or, if they appear on separate sheets, attached to the history.

Diagnosis. The physician, on the basis of all evidence provided in the patient's past history, the physician's examination, and any supplementary tests, places the diagnosis of the patient's condition on the medical record. If there is some doubt, it may be termed **provisional diagnosis**.

Treatment Prescribed and Progress Notes. The physician's suggested treatment is listed after the diagnosis. Generally, instructions to the patient to return for follow-up treatment in a specific period of time are noted here as well (Procedure 13-2).

On each subsequent visit, the date must be entered on the chart and information about the patient's condition and the results of treatment added to the history, on the basis of the physician's observations. Notations of all medications prescribed or instructions given, as well as the patient's own progress report, should be placed in

the record. Any home visits are noted. If the patient is hospitalized, the name of the hospital, the reason for the admission, and the dates of admission and discharge are recorded. Much of this information may be obtained from the hospital discharge summary.

Condition at the Time of Termination of Treatment. When the treatment is terminated, the physician will record that information. For example:

August 18, 1999. Wound completely healed. Patient discharged.

Obtaining the History

The medical assistant usually secures the routine personal data. The personal and medical history and the patient's family history may be secured by asking the patient to complete a questionnaire, with the physician augmenting the information provided during the patient interview (see Appendix A).

The Medical Assistant's Role. When the medical assistant is responsible for recording the patient's history, care must be exercised to ensure that the patient's answers are not heard by others in the reception room. If privacy is not possible, it is better to give the patient a form to fill out and then transfer this information to permanent records later. When privacy is available, the medical assistant may ask the patient questions and at the same time write or type the answers directly on the record. This method offers an opportunity to become better acquainted with the patient while completing the necessary records. In facilities where lengthy questionnaires are to be completed by the new patient, the questionnaire may be mailed to the patient with a request that it be completed and returned to the physician before the appointment. If the record is to be computerized, requesting the information ahead of time gives the office staff the opportunity to transfer information to the computer before the new patient's visit.

The patient's chief complaint may have been indicated to the medical assistant, but the physician will question the patient in more detail. Many practitioners write their own entries on the chart in longhand. Some may keyboard the findings direct into the computer. Others may dictate the material, either directly to the medical assistant or by using a recording device. If the material is dictated and typed, the physician should check each entry and then initial the entry to verify accuracy. For a chart to be admissible as evidence in court, the person dictating or writing the entries must be able to attest that they were true and correct at the time they were written. The best indication of that is the physician's signature or initials on the typed entry.

Making Additions to the Patient Record

As long as the patient is under the physician's care, the medical history is building. Each laboratory report, radiology report, and progress note is added to the record with

PROCEDURE 13-2

Preparing an Informed Consent for Treatment Form

GOAL: To adequately and completely inform the patient regarding the treatment or procedure that he or she is to receive, and provide legal protection for the facility and the provider.

EQUIPMENT AND SUPPLIES
- Pen
- Consent form

PROCEDURAL STEPS

1 After the physician provides the details of the procedure to be done, prepare the consent form. Be sure that the form addresses the following:
- The nature of the procedure or treatment.
- The risks and/or benefits of the procedure or treatment.
- Any reasonable alternatives to the procedure or treatment.
- The risks and/or benefits of each alternative.
- The risks and/or benefits of not performing the procedure or treatment.

Purpose: To make certain that the patient is fully informed about the procedure or treatment and the risks and/or benefits of having or not having it performed.

2 Personalize the form with the patient's name and any other demographic information that the form lists.

Purpose: To correctly identify the patient and the procedure.

3 Deliver the form to the physician for use as the patient is counseled about the procedure.

Purpose: To avoid charges of practicing medicine without a license. The physician should explain procedures, risks, benefits, alternatives, and answer all of the patient's questions.

4 Witness the signature of the patient on the form, if necessary. The physician will usually sign the form as well.

5 Provide a copy of the consent form to the patient.

Purpose: To make certain that the patient is fully informed regarding the procedure and has a copy of the information for his or her personal records.

6 Place the consent form in the patient's chart. The facility where the procedure is to be performed may require a copy.

Purpose: To maintain a permanent copy of the signed consent form.

7 Ask the patient if he or she has any questions about the procedure. Refer questions that the medical assistant cannot or should not answer to the physician. Be sure that all of the questions expressed by the patient are answered.

Purpose: To make certain that the patient is fully informed.

8 Provide information regarding the date and time for the procedure to the patient.

the latest information always on top (Procedure 13-3). Although each item is important, the most recent is usually of greatest significance to the patient's care. Again, the physician should read and initial each of these reports before it is placed in the record.

Laboratory Reports

Different colors of paper are often used for reporting different procedures. For example, urinalysis report forms may be yellow, blood count forms pink, and so forth. When laboratory slips are smaller than the history form, they should be placed on a standard 8 1/2 ×11-inch sheet of colored paper. Type or print the patient's name in the upper right corner, and then, with transparent tape, fasten the first report even with the bottom of the page. The second laboratory report will be taped or glued in place on top of and about 1/2 inch above the first slip, allowing the date to show on the first report. By this method, called **shingling**, the latest report always appears on top (Figure 13-6). When checking previous reports, it

is necessary only to run a finger down the slips until the desired date is found; then flip up the slips above. Laboratory report carrier forms with adhesive strips may be purchased.

Radiology Reports

Radiology reports are usually typed on standard letter-size stationery. They are placed in the patient's history folder, with the most recent report on top. All radiology reports may be stapled together or kept behind a special divider in the chart.

Progress Notes

Reports on the patient's progress are continually being added to the case history. Each visit of the patient should be entered on the chart, with the date preceding any notations about the visit. The medical assistant can type or stamp the date on the chart when readying the charts for the patient's visits. Every instruction, pre-

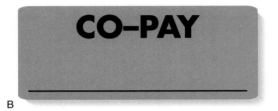

A

CO–PAY

_____

B

ADVANCE DIRECTIVES

_____ **Durable Power of Attorney for Healthcare**

_____ **Living Will**

_____ **Healthcare Surrogate**

C

FIGURE 13-5   A to C, Chart stickers. Information on stickers on the outside of the chart allows the physician and medical staff to quickly see important information about the patient. (Courtesy Bibbero Systems, Inc., Petaluma, Calif. 94954, (800) 242-2376, www.bibbero.com.)

PROCEDURE **13-3**

Adding Supplementary Items to Established Patient Files

GOAL: To add supplementary documents and progress notes to patient histories, observing standard steps in filing, while creating an orderly file that will facilitate ready reference to any item of information.

EQUIPMENT AND SUPPLIES

- Assorted correspondence, diagnostic reports, and progress notes
- Patient files
- Computer or typewriter
- Mending tape
- FILE stamp or pen
- Sorter
- Stapler

PROCEDURAL STEPS

1 Group all papers according to patients' names.
   Purpose: Some related papers may require stapling.

2 Remove any staples or paper clips.
   Purpose: Staples in the file folders are hazardous; paper clips are bulky and may become inadvertently attached to other materials.

4 Mend any damaged or torn records.

5 Attach any small items to standard-size paper.

Purpose: Small items are easily lost or misplaced in files.

6 Staple any related papers together.

7 Place your initials or FILE stamp in the upper left corner.
   Purpose: To indicate that the document is released for filing.

8 Code the document by underlining or writing the patient's name in the upper right corner.
   Purpose: To indicate where the document is to be filed.

9 Continue steps 2 through 7 until all documents have been conditioned, released, indexed, and coded.

10 Place all documents in the sorter in filing sequence.
   Explanation: Sorter can be taken to file cabinet or shelf for placing documents in patient folders.

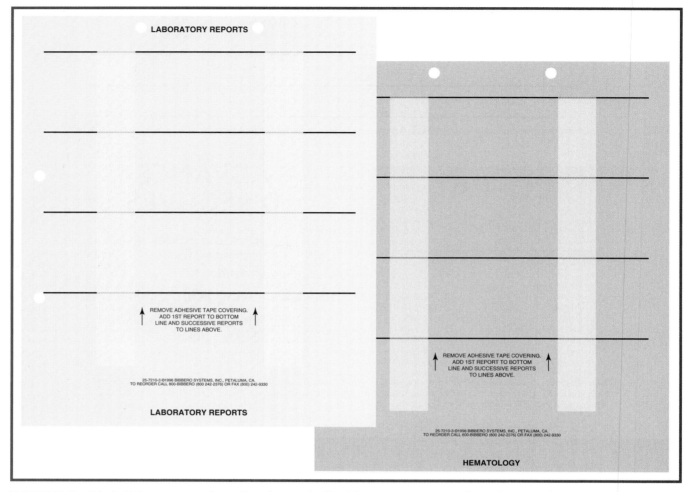

FIGURE 13-6 Shingled laboratory report forms. These forms make filing laboratory reports easy and provide a good adhesive so that the reports will not fall out of the chart if they are not standard size. (Courtesy Bibbero Systems, Inc., Petaluma, Calif. 94954, (800) 242-2376, www.bibbero.com.)

scription, or telephone call for advice should be entered with the correct date. It is always advisable to initial each entry, especially when several persons are handling and making entries on a patient's record. This aids in tracing entries about which there may be some question.

Making Corrections and Alteration of Medical Records

Sometimes it is necessary to make corrections on medical records. Erasing, correction fluid, or any other type of **obliteration** is never acceptable. To correct a handwritten entry, follow these three steps:
1. Draw a line through the error
2. Insert the correction above or immediately after the error.
3. In the margin, write correction or *Corr.*, the initial of the person correcting the entry, and the date.

Errors made while typing are corrected in the usual way. However, an error discovered in a typed entry at a later date is corrected in the same manner as described for a handwritten entry. Never attempt to alter medical

records without using this specific correction procedure, because this alteration of records may indicate a fraudulent attempt to cover up a mistake made by a staff member or the physician. Do not hide errors. If the error could in any way affect the health and well-being of the patient, it must immediately be brought to the attention of the physician.

CRITICAL THINKING APPLICATION

Susan has been using an incorrect abbreviation for several weeks and is having a difficult time remembering the right abbreviation. After taking a call from Mrs. Johnston, she remembers that she used the incorrect abbreviation in her chart last week. When Susan pulls the chart, she notices that entries have been made after the ones that Susan made on Mrs. Johnston's last visit. How does Susan correct her error?

Keeping Records Current

One of the greatest dangers to good record keeping is **procrastination**. The record must be methodically kept current. It is the medical assistant's responsibility to see that this is done.

Case histories and reports may accumulate on the physician's or the medical assistant's desk during the day. After the last patient has gone, check each history to make certain that all necessary information has been recorded and that each entry is sufficiently clear for future understanding. Give the physician all extra reports, such as laboratory and radiology reports, to read and initial so that they may be filed in the patient's case history folder.

While the physician is reviewing these reports, pull the histories of any patients seen outside the office that day, as well as those of patients who have been given special instructions by telephone or for whom prescriptions were ordered. These entries are made in the same manner as for an office visit, but the type of call is explained in parentheses after the date.

A prescription pad, printed on no-smear, carbonless paper, is available for a timesaving, write-it-once system. By placing the prescription blank over the patient's record, the prescription is automatically copied on the record as it is written. Prescription carriers with adhesive strips are also available for the physician who uses duplicate prescription blanks (Figure 13-7).

The patient record should not leave the office. A physician's pocket call record can be used for outside calls, and the information can be transferred to the chart in the office (Figure 13-8). Notations should be made of any missed appointments or of refusals to cooperate with instructions as they occur.

After all records have been reviewed for the day, they should be placed in a file tray and locked away for the night if there is insufficient time to file them. Do not leave histories out in view at night, especially if the facility has a night cleaning service. On arrival the next morning, the medical assistant can index the histories for filing. Attach extra reports and information sheets. Always attach material to the chart permanently—do not simply drop forms into the folders. When this has been done, the records are ready for filing.

The physician may prefer to dictate progress notes rather than write them in longhand. At appropriate times during the day, everything is dictated: patient histories, physical examination findings, medications prescribed, follow-up findings, and summaries of telephone conversations. At the end of the day, the recorded information is given to the medical assistant for transcribing onto the records.

A great deal of time may be saved in transcribing these notes by using a continuous roll or pages of self-adhesive strips. When the transcription has been completed, the physician may wish to check the notes, underline important points, and initial each entry before returning the notes to the medical assistant for insertion into the charts to verify that they are correct in the event

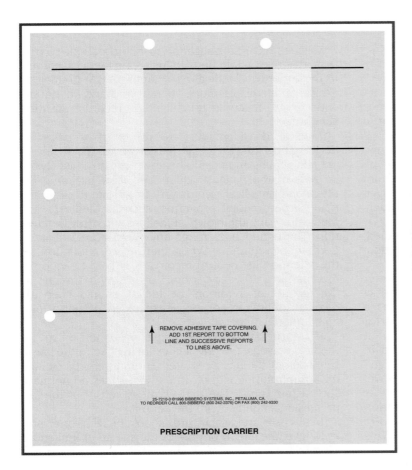

PRESCRIPTION CARRIER

FIGURE 13-7   Filing copies of prescriptions. The self-adhesive on this form allows a copy of the prescription to be filed inside the patient's chart, and saves time over handwriting the information a second time. (Courtesy Bibbero Systems, Inc., Petaluma, Calif. 94954, (800) 242-2376, www.bibbero.com.)

FIGURE 13-8 Physician pocket call record. The pocket call record may be used to record information about a patient seen away from the clinic, such as skilled nursing facility patients or hospital patients.

of **audit** or litigation. The use of self-adhesive strips saves removing the sheet from a chart that may be bound with metal fasteners, inserting the sheet into the typewriter, and putting the sheet back into the folder (Figure 13-9). It also simplifies the physician's part in checking and initialing the notes, because only the transcribed material is handled, not the bulky charts.

Transfer, Destruction, and Retention of Medical Records

Regular Transfer of Files

In most medical offices, records are filed according to three classifications:
- *Active files* are those of patients currently receiving treatment.
- *Inactive files* generally are those of patients whom the doctor has not seen for 6 months or longer. When such individuals return for care, their folders are replaced in the active file.
- *Closed files* are records of patients who have died, moved away, or otherwise terminated their relationship with the physician.

Some system must be established for regular transfer of files from active to inactive status or possibly destruction. The yearly expansion of charts and the file space available can influence the transfer period. Charts for patients who are currently hospitalized may be kept in a special section for quick reference, then placed in the regular active file when the patient is discharged from the hospital. In a surgical practice, there frequently is a specific date on which the patient is discharged from the physician's care and the notation made on the chart "Return prn" (for the Latin *pro re nata*, "as the occasion arises" or "when needed"). This record may safely be placed in the inactive file. In a general practice office, the outside of the folder may be stamped with the date of the visit each time the patient is seen. It will then be a simple matter to determine when the chart should be transferred to the inactive status. This is called the perpetual transfer method.

Retention and Destruction

Physicians have an obligation to retain patient records that may reasonably be of value to a patient, according to the American Medical Association (AMA) Council on Ethical and Judicial Affairs. There is no standard, nationwide rule to follow in establishing a records **retention schedule** at this time.

Medical considerations are the primary basis for deciding how long to retain medical records. For example, operative notes and chemotherapy records should always be part of the patient's chart. The laws regarding the retention of medical records vary from state to state, and many governmental programs, such as Medicare and Medicaid, have their own guidelines for records retention. These guidelines range anywhere from 3 years to permanent retention. When there is no restriction for the retention of medical records, it is best to keep the records for a 10-year period. However, when retaining the records of a minor, the facility should keep the records until the minor reaches the age of majority, plus an additional 3 years.

If a particular record no longer needs to be kept for medical reasons, the physician should check state law to see whether there is a requirement that records be kept for a minimum length of time (most states do not have such a provision). The time is measured from the last professional contact with the patient.

In all cases, medical records should be kept for at least as long as the length of time of the statute of limitations for medical malpractice claims, which may be 3 or more

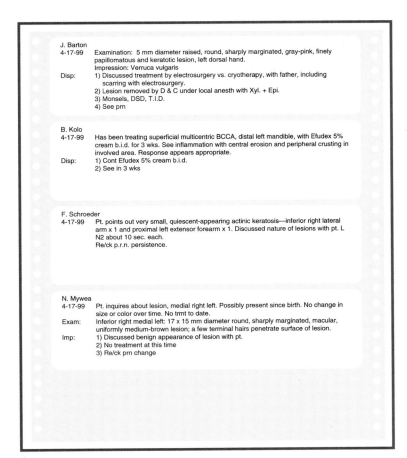

J. Barton
4-17-99   Examination: 5 mm diameter raised, round, sharply margined, gray-pink, finely
           papillomatous and keratotic lesion, left dorsal hand.
           Impression: Verruca vulgaris
Disp: 1) Discussed treatment by electrosurgery vs. cryotherapy, with father, including
              scarring with electrosurgery.
           2) Lesion removed by D & C under local anesth with Xyl. + Epi.
           3) Monsels, DSD, T.I.D.
           4) See prn

B. Kolo
4-17-99   Has been treating superficial multicentric BCCA, distal left mandible, with Efudex 5%
           cream b.i.d. for 3 wks. See inflammation with central erosion and peripheral crusting in
           involved area. Response appears appropriate.
Disp: 1) Cont Efudex 5% cream b.i.d.
           2) See in 3 wks

F. Schroeder
4-17-99   Pt. points out very small, quiescent-appearing actinic keratosis—inferior right lateral
           arm x 1 and proximal left extensor forearm x 1. Discussed nature of lesions with pt. L
           N2 about 10 sec. each.
           Re/ck p.r.n. persistence.

N. Mywea
4-17-99   Pt. inquires about lesion, medial right left. Possibly present since birth. No change in
           size or color over time. No trmt to date.
Exam: Inferior right medial left: 17 x 15 mm diameter round, sharply margined, macular,
           uniformly medium-brown lesion; a few terminal hairs penetrate surface of lesion.
Imp: 1) Discussed benign appearance of lesion with pt.
           2) No treatment at this time
           3) Re/ck prn change

A

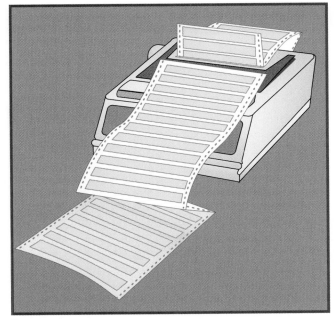

B

FIGURE 13-9 **A** and **B**, Self-adhesive progress notes. Progress notes can be quickly filed into the chart when self-adhesive forms are used.

years, depending on the state law. In the case of a minor, the statute of limitations may not apply until the patient reaches the age of majority.

The records of any patient covered by Medicare or Medicaid must be kept at least 6 years. HIPAA recom-mends that records for patients who have died should be kept for at least 2 years.

Before discarding old records, patients should be given an opportunity to claim a copy of the records or have them sent to another physician, if it is feasible to give the patient that opportunity. To preserve confidentiality when discarding old records, the documents should be destroyed by shredding or through a professional document destruction service.

Protection of Records

Releasing original case histories to anyone outside the healthcare facility should be avoided. Instead, prepare a summary or photocopy the materials needed for reference and retain the original in the physician's office. With the facsimile machine becoming standard equipment in business facilities, as well as in many of our homes, the transfer of information is simplified and the records remain in safekeeping. Often only certain aspects of the record are requested by colleagues or others, and these can easily be supplied by faxing the required pages, observing precautions for confidentiality.

Occasions may arise when records are temporarily out of the office. Some physicians release case histories to their colleagues, or an original record may be subpoenaed by the court. In such instances, a colored **OUTfolder** should be inserted in the file in place of the regular folder and a notation made of the name, date, and to whom the record was released. Interim papers may be placed in the OUTfolder until the original is returned.

Long-Term Storage

Large healthcare facilities may find it advisable to microfilm records for storage. Another option is the transfer of paper records by laser beam onto optical disks. *Microfilm* and optical disk technology are both expensive and probably are not practical for any but a very large group practice or health maintenance organization.

Facilities that have computerized the patient records will be able to keep those records indefinitely on disk. Scanners can convert a paper record into an image on the computer screen resulting in an electronic medical record. Records can be scanned and stored in electronic format on writeable CD- or DVD-ROMs. The bulky paper files can then be put in storage or eliminated. There is no longer a need to fill hundreds of square feet of storage space or search through stack upon stack of storage file boxes for an inactive or closed file.

Releasing Medical Record Information

The medical facility must be extremely careful when releasing any type of medical information. The patient must sign a release for information to be given to any third party (Procedure 13-4).

Often a family member will call to inquire about a patient, but without the patient's specific request or release, no information may be given. Some offices have a "code" system whereby the patient gives the facility a code word, which must be used by a family member to receive medical information about the patient.

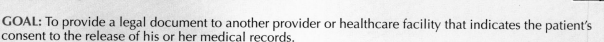

PROCEDURE 13-4

Preparing a Record Release Form

GOAL: To provide a legal document to another provider or healthcare facility that indicates the patient's consent to the release of his or her medical records.

EQUIPMENT AND SUPPLIES

- Medical record release form
- Pen
- Envelope

PROCEDURAL STEPS

1 Explain to the patient that a medical record release form will be necessary to obtain records from another provider. If the patient is having records sent to another provider, a release will also be required.

Purpose: To ensure the patient's understanding of the records release procedure and purposes.

2 Review the record release form with the patient and ask if the form is understood or if there are any questions about the form.

Purpose: To provide the opportunity for questions and to ensure the patient's understanding of the form.

3 Have the patient sign the form in the space indicated. If other demographic information is required, such as a social security number or other names used, complete that information as well.

Purpose: The patient must sign the form for records to be released by any medical facility.

4 Make a copy of the form for the file and then mail it to the appropriate facility. Note the date that the form was sent. Provide a copy to the patient if requested.

Purpose: To provide a record that the information or documents were actually requested on a certain date.

5 Follow-up to ensure that the requested records actually arrived.

Purpose: To make certain that the records needed by the physician to accurately and competently treat the patient are available in a timely manner.

RECORDS RELEASE AUTHORIZATION

TO _____
                              Doctor or Hospital

_____
                                  Address

I HEREBY AUTHORIZE AND REQUEST YOU TO RELEASE TO:

ALL RECORDS IN YOUR POSSESION CONCERNING _____

_____ILLNESS AND/OR

TREATMENT DURING THE PERIOD FROM _____TO _____.

NAME _____TEL. _____

ADDRESS_____

SIGNATURE _____DATE _____
                    (If relative, state relationship)

WITNESS_____DATE _____

25-8104 © 1973 BIBBERO SYSTEMS, INC., PETALUMA,, CA.

FIGURE 13-10   Medical record release authorization. All requests for medical records should be in writing and the request should be kept in the patient chart. (Courtesy Bibbero Systems, Inc., Petaluma, Calif. 94954, (800) 242-2376, www.bibbero.com.)

Requests for medical information should be made in writing (Figure 13-10). It is unwise to accept a faxed request for medical information or a faxed release of information from a patient. Even requests from the patient's attorney or third-party payors must be cleared by the patient to receive information. Some attorneys may present a legal document called a **power of attorney**, which authorizes them to see the records. Still, this document is signed by the patient, so it is a release in itself.

CRITICAL THINKING APPLICATION

Susan has never seen a power of attorney and is curious about this type of document. How might she investigate and learn more about them? Who should Susan approach first for this information? The physician has an attorney that Susan has met once. Should she call him and ask about the document without notifying the physician? Why or why not?

Sometimes, the patient will want to view his or her own record. They certainly have a right to see this information, but some patients may not understand the terminology used in the record. A staff member should always remain with the patient who is viewing his or her medical records. Remember, the original medical record should never leave the medical facility.

When a release is presented to the office, only copy the records requested in the release. Do not provide additional information that is not requested. It is acceptable to charge reasonable copying fees to the person requesting the information.

Dictation and Transcription

Administrative medical assistants may find that transcribing **dictation** is one of the job requirements they perform periodically. **Transcription** can be performed from handwritten notes, such as those in shorthand, or from machine dictation. In a healthcare facility, the medical transcriptionist is a part of the team. Smooth operation of the facility may depend on the timely and accurate performance of assigned responsibilities, such as record documentation and the preparation of special reports.

The transcriptionist will find that *accuracy* and *speed* are primary **requisites** (Figure 13-11). Income depends on the transcriptionist's productivity, which may be measured by the number of pages, characters, or lines typed. The person who intends to do transcribing exclusively would do well to take a special course in transcription techniques.

Machine Transcription

Three stages of activity are involved in the process of dictation and transcription:

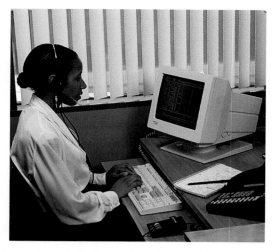

FIGURE 13-11 Medical transcriptionists must have excellent typing skills and good hearing. They must be accurate and use good grammatical skills while completing transcription duties.

- Dictating into a dictation unit
- Listening to what has been dictated
- Keyboarding the dictated text to a printed document using correct format and required punctuation

Dictation Unit

A dictation unit is used by the physician to record material to be typed. Dictation units vary in design and capabilities. A desktop dictation unit is common in an office setting. This may be a combination unit used for both dictation and transcription. Alternatively, a machine used only for dictation may remain at the physician's desk; a separate transcription unit, including headphones and a foot pedal, remains at the transcriptionist's station. A lightweight, portable, handheld dictation unit may be used for times when the physician wishes to dictate while traveling or attending meetings away from the office. Digital dictation machines are now available and are lightweight, portable, and hold more information than standard dictation recorders. Physicians in a larger setting may install transcribing equipment that they can access by telephone wherever they may be. Many hospitals have this arrangement. All produce a recording that the transcriptionist listens to while keyboarding the text.

CRITICAL THINKING APPLICATION

Susan would like to practice transcription skills at home, but she does not have a transcription unit. How could she do this without the proper equipment? Medical terminology is important to the medical assistant who does transcription. What are some ways Susan can improve her medical terminology skills?

Transcriber Unit

The unit operated by the transcriptionist may use magnetic tape, a cassette, or a disk. A desktop unit using mini-cassettes, microcassettes, or standard cassettes is typical in the physician's office.

There are many types and manufacturers of transcribing equipment, but most units contain certain standard features. Before using any equipment, the medical assistant should study the manufacturer's instruction manual. Most transcription units have a minimum of the following features:

- Stop and start control, with backup and fast-forward ability
- Speed control
- Volume control
- Tone control
- Indicator for locating special instructions and determining the document length

A beginning transcriptionist tends to listen to a few words, stop the machine, type those words, and then restart the transcriber unit. Through practice, the transcriptionist learns to coordinate keyboarding activity with listening skills and listen ahead, thereby retaining in memory more and more of the dictated material so that it becomes unnecessary to stop and start the machine for this purpose.

Keyboarding Unit

The most important piece of equipment for the transcriptionist is the typewriter or computer on which the printed text will be produced (Procedure 13-5). Many improvements have occurred within the past few years. Computers have attachable foot pedals and headphones that allow the medical assistant to perform transcription directly onto the unit. A variety of software programs are available to assist with transcription duties.

Filing Equipment

The vertical four-drawer steel filing cabinet, used with manila folders with the patient's name on the tab, was the traditional system of choice for years. The most popular system today is color coding on open shelves. There are also rotary, lateral, compactible, and automated files. Some records are kept in card or tray files. Regardless of the type or style of equipment, the best quality is always an economy. Some of the considerations in selecting filing equipment are as follows:

- Office space availability
- Structural considerations
- Cost of space and equipment
- Size, type, and volume of records
- Confidentiality requirements
- Retrieval speed
- Fire protection

Drawer Files

Drawer files should be full suspension; they should roll easily, close securely, and be equipped with a locking device. The best cabinets have a center trough at the bottom of each drawer with a rod for holding divider guides. Floor space of twice the depth of the drawer must

PROCEDURE 13-5

Transcribing a Machine-Dictated Letter Using a Computer or Word Processor

GOAL: To transcribe a machine-dictated letter into a mailable document without error or corrections, using a computer or word processor.

EQUIPMENT AND SUPPLIES

- Transcribing machine
- Word processor or computer with appropriate software
- Stationery
- Reference manual

PROCEDURAL STEPS

1 Assemble supplies.

2 Set up format for selected letter style.

3 Keyboard the text while listening to the dictated letter.

4 Edit the letter on the monitor.
   Purpose: The letter should be in mailable form before printing.

5 Execute a spell check.

6 Direct the letter to the printer.

---

be allowed so that the drawer can be pulled out to its full extent. A drawback of the vertical four-drawer files is that only one person can use a file cabinet at any given time. Filing is also slower because the drawer must be opened and closed each time a file is pulled or filed. Drawer files are relatively easy to move, but for safety reasons they should be bolted to the wall or to each other.

File drawers are heavy and can tip over, causing serious damage or injury unless reasonable care is observed. Open only one file drawer at a time and close it when the filing has been completed. A drawer left even slightly open can cause injury to a passerby.

Shelf Files

Shelf files should have doors to protect the contents. A popular type of shelf file has doors that slide back into the cabinet; the door from a lower shelf may be pulled out and used for work space. About 50% more material per square foot of floor space may be filed in shelf files when compared with the four-drawer file. Open shelf units hold files sideways and can go higher on the wall because there is no drawer to pull out (Figure 13-12). File retrieval is faster because several individuals can work simultaneously.

Open shelf units without doors are the most economical but offer little protection or confidentiality to the records. They are susceptible to water and fire damage. Shelf files are available in many attractive colors and can add a decorative note to the business office. Special storage or shelf space should be provided for x-ray films, if many films are stored.

Rotary Circular Files

Rotary circular files can hold a large volume of records. They save space and clerical motion. The files revolve

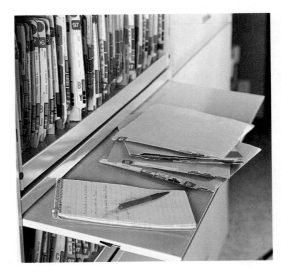

FIGURE 13-12   Open shelf filing is an efficient method, especially for color-coded filing systems. The shelf doors can often be used as workspace.

easily; some come with push-button controls. Several persons can work at one rotary file and use records at the same time. One disadvantage is that they afford less privacy and protection than files that can be closed and locked.

Lateral Files

Lateral files are good for personal files and are especially attractive for the physician's private office. They use more wall space than the vertical file but do not extend out into the room so far. The folders are filed sideways in the lateral file, left to right, instead of front to back as in a vertical file. Some have a pull-out drawer, as the vertical file does; others have doors that slide into the cabinet, exposing the filing space.

Compactible Files

The office with little space and a great volume of records might use compactible files, which are a variation of open shelf files. The files are mounted on tracks in the floor, and the units slide along the tracks so that access is gained to the needed records. They may be either automated or manual. One drawback is that not all records are available at the same time.

Automated Files

Automated files are very expensive initially and require more maintenance than do the other types of filing equipment. They will probably be found only in very large installations such as clinics or hospitals. These files bring the record to the operator instead of the operator going to the record. When the operator presses a button indicating the appropriate shelf, the shelf automatically moves into position in front of the operator for record retrieval. The automated or power file is fast and can store large amounts of records in a small amount of space. Only one person can use the unit at one time.

Card Files

Almost every office has some occasion to use a card file. This may be for patient ledgers, a patient index, library index, index of surgical tray setups, telephone numbers, or numerous other records. A good-quality steel box or tray is a sound investment.

Special Items

Metal framework is available that can convert a regular drawer file into suspension-folder equipment. The assistant with a great deal of filing may wish to purchase a portable filing shelf that fits on the side of an opened drawer and can be moved from place to place as needed. Another special filing item is a sorting file, which can be a great time saver. A portable file cart for the temporary filing of unbilled insurance claims may be quite useful. It may also be used for the preliminary sorting of charts to be refiled. This is sometimes called a *suspense file.*

Supplies

Divider Guides

Each file drawer or shelf should be equipped with plenty of dividers or guides. Some authorities recommend one guide for approximately each 1½ inches of material, or every eight to ten folders. Guides should be of good-quality **pressboard** or strong plastic. Economy guides will soon become bent and frayed and have to be replaced. Divider guides have a protruding tab, which may be either an integral part of the card or may be made of metal or plastic. The guides reduce the area of search and serve as supports for the folders. They are available in single, third, or fifth cut (one, three, or five different positions). The guide may have a projection at the bottom edge with a ring or hole through which a rod may go. This type of guide card is used in drawers that have a trough for the projection and a rod to hold the guides in place.

OUTguides

An **OUTguide** is a heavy guide that is used to replace a folder that has been temporarily removed (Figure 13-13). It should be of a distinctive color for quick detection. This makes refiling simpler and alerts the file clerk that a file is missing. Several colors may be used, each color designating the temporary location of the file. The OUTguide may have lines for recording information, or it may have a plastic pocket for inserting an information card.

Chart Covers of Folders

Most records to be filed are placed in covers or tabbed folders. The most commonly used is a general-purpose third-cut manila folder that may be expanded to ³/₄ inch. These are available with a double-thickness reinforced tab that will greatly lengthen the life of the folder. Folders kept in drawers have tabs at the top; those kept on shelves have tabs at the side. There are many variations of folder styles obtainable for special purposes.

The vertical pocket, which is heavier weight than the general purpose folder, has a front that folds down for easy access to contents and is available with up to 3½-inch expansion. These are used for bulky histories or correspondence.

Hanging or suspension folders are made of heavy stock and hang on metal rods from side to side of a drawer. They can be used only with files equipped with suspension equipment.

Binder folders have fasteners with which to bind papers within the folder. These offer some security for the papers but are time consuming in filing the materials.

The number of papers that will fit in one folder depends on the thickness of the papers. Near the bottom edge of most folders are one or more score marks, which should be used as the contents of the folders expand. If folders are refolded at these score marks, the danger of their bending and sliding under other folders is reduced, and a neater file results. Papers should never protrude from the folder edges, and they should always be inserted with their tops to the left. When papers start to ride up in any folder, the folder is overloaded.

Labels

The label is a necessary filing and finding device. Use labels to identify each shelf, drawer, divider guide, and folder. A label on the drawer or shelf identifies the nature of its contents. It should also indicate the range (alphabetical, numerical, or chronological) of the material filed in that space.

The label on the divider guide identifies the range of folder headings following that divider guide up to the next divider; for example, BaBo. The label on the folder

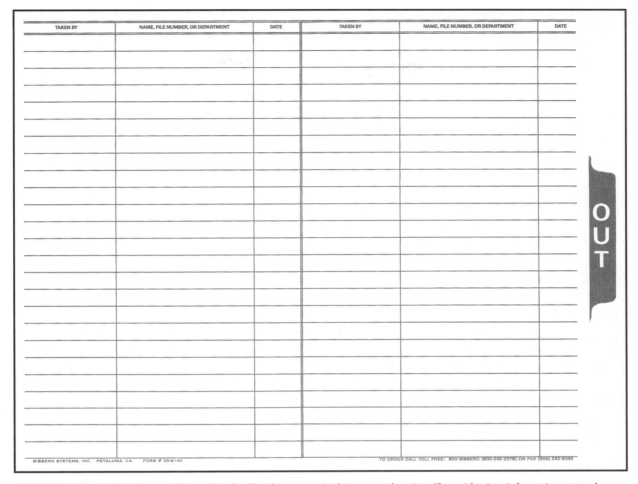

TAKEN BY	NAME, FILE NUMBER, OR DEPARTMENT	DATE	TAKEN BY	NAME, FILE NUMBER, OR DEPARTMENT	DATE

BIBBERO SYSTEMS, INC. PETALUMA, CA.   FORM # 33-8140   TO ORDER CALL TOLL FREE: 800-BIBBERO (800-242-2376) OR FAX (800) 242-9330

FIGURE 13-13   OUTguides provide tracking for files that are not in their proper location. The guide gives information as to where the file can be located. (Courtesy Bibbero Systems, Inc., Petaluma, Calif. 94954, (800) 242-2376, www.bibbero.com.)

identifies the content of that folder only. This may be the name of the patient, subject matter of correspondence, a business topic, or anything at all that needs to be filed. Label a folder when a new patient is seen or existing folders are full or when materials need to be transferred within the filing system.

Paper labels may be purchased in rolls of gummed tape; another type has adhesive backs that are peeled from a protective sheet. Labels are available in almost any size, shape, or color to meet the individual needs of any facility. Visit a stationer and study the catalogs to find the best product to meet the needs of the facility.

A narrow label applied to the front of the folder tab is the easiest to use and is satisfactory for folders kept in a drawer file. Labels for shelf filing should be identifiable from both front and back. Always type the label before separating it from the roll or protective sheet. Type the **caption** on the label in indexing order.

Filing Procedures

Filing of all materials involves five basic steps: conditioning, releasing, indexing and coding, sorting, and storing and filing.

Conditioning

Conditioning of papers involves (1) removing all pins, brads, and paper clips, (2) stapling related papers together, (3) attaching clippings or items smaller than page-size to a regular sheet of paper with rubber cement or tape, and (4) mending damaged records.

Releasing

The term *releasing* simply means that some mark is placed on the paper indicating that it is now ready for filing. This will usually be either the medical assistant's initials or a FILE stamp placed in the upper left corner.

Indexing and Coding

Indexing means deciding where to file the letter or paper, and coding means placing some indication of this decision on the paper (Table 13-1). This may be done by underlining the name or subject, if it appears on the paper, or writing the indexing subject or name in some conspicuous place. If there is more than one logical place to file the paper, the original is coded for the main location and a cross-reference sheet prepared, indicating this location and coded for the second

TABLE 13-1	Application of Indexing Rules			
Indexing Rule	Name	Unit 1	Unit 2	Unit 3
1	Robert F. Grinch	Grinch	Robert	F.
	R. Frank Grumman	Grumman	R.	Frank
2	J. Orville Smith	Smith	J.	Orville
	Jason O. Smith	Smith	Jason	O.
3	M. L. Saint-Vickery	Saint-Vickery	M.	L.
	Marie-Louise Taylor	Taylor	Marielouise	
4	Charles S. Anderson	Anderson	Charles	S.
	Anderson's Surgical Supply	Andersons	Surgical	Supply
5	Ah Hop Akee	Akee	Ah	Hop
6	Alice Delaney	Delaney	Alice	
	Chester K. DeLong	Delong	Chester	K.
7	Michael St. John	Stjohn	Michael	
8	Helen M. Maag	Maag	Helen	M.
	Frederick Mabry	Mabry	Frederick	
	James E. MacDonald	Macdonald	James	E.
9	Mrs. John L. Doe (Mary Jones)	Doe	Mary	Jones (Mrs John L.)
10	Prof. John J. Breck	Breck	John	J. (Prof.)
	Madame Sylvia	Madame	Sylvia	
	Sister Mary Catherine	Sister	Mary	Catherine
	Theodore Wilson, M.D.	Wilson	Theodore (M.D.)	
11	Lawrence W. Sloan, Jr.	Sloan	Lawrence	W. (Jr.)
	Lawrence W. Sloan, Sr.	Sloan	Lawrence	W. (Sr.)
12	The Moore Clinic	Moore	Clinic (The)	

location. Every paper placed in a patient's chart should have the date and name of the patient on it, usually in the upper right corner.

Sorting

Sorting is arranging the papers in filing sequence. Sort papers before going to the file cabinet or shelf. Do any necessary stapling of papers at the desk or filing table. Invest in a desktop sorter with a series of dividers between which papers are placed in filing sequence. One general-purpose sorter has six means of classification: alphabetical sections, numbers 1 to 31, days of the week, months of the year, numbers in groups of five, and space on the tabs for special captions to be taped when desired. In the preliminary sorting, place the papers in the appropriate division in the sorter. Then it is comparatively simple to arrange these groups into the proper sequence for filing.

Storing and Filing

In storing or filing papers in the folder, items should be placed face up, top edge to the left, with the most recent date to the front of the folder. Lift the folder 1 or 2 inches out of the drawer before inserting new material, so that the sheets can drop down completely into the folder. When refiling completed folders, arrange them in indexing order before going to the file cabinets.

Locating Misplaced Files

Unless files are promptly replaced after use, they may become lost. Papers may be misfiled, requiring a thor-

ough search to find them. After a methodical and complete search through the proper folder, there are several places one may look for a misplaced paper: (1) in the folder in front of and behind the correct folder; (2) between the folders; (3) on the bottom of the file under all the folders; (4) in a folder of a patient with a similar name; or (5) in the sorter.

Indexing Rules

Indexing rules are fairly well standardized, based on current business practices. The Association of Records Managers and Administrators takes an active part in updating the rules. Some establishments adopt variations of these basic rules to accommodate their needs. In any case the practices need to be consistent within the system.

1. Last names of persons are considered first in filing; given name (first name), second; and middle name or initial, third. Compare the names beginning with the first letter of the name. When there is a letter that is different in the two names, that letter determines the order of filing. For example:

abe
abi
abm
abx
acl
acm
ada
ade
adi

2. *Initials* precede a *name* beginning with the same letter. This illustrates the librarian's rule, "Nothing comes before something." For example:

> Smith, J.
> Smith, Jason

3. *Hyphenated personal names.* The hyphenated elements of a name, whether first name, middle name, or surname, are considered to be one unit. For example:

> Carlotta Freeman-Duque is filed as
> Freemanduque, Carlotta
> Cindy-Jean Green is filed as
> Green, Cindyjean

4. The apostrophe is disregarded in filing. For example:

> Andersons' Surgical Supply
> Andersons Surgical Supply

5. When indexing a foreign name and *cannot* distinguish the first and last name, index each part of the name in the order in which it is written:

> Cau Liu
> Talluri Devi

If you *can* make the distinction, you should use the last name as the first indexing unit:

> Liu, Jason

6. Names with prefixes are filed in the usual alphabetical order with the prefix being considered as part of the name. For example:

> von Schmidt is filed as Vonschmidt
> DeLong is filed as Delong
> LaFrance is filed as Lafrance

7. Abbreviated parts of a name are indexed as written if that is the form generally used by that person. For example:

> Ste. Marie is filed as Stemarie
> St. John is filed as Stjohn
> Wm. is filed as Wm
> Edw. is filed as Edw
> Jas. is filed as Jas

8. Mac and Mc are filed in their regular place in the alphabet:

> Maag
> Mabry
> *Mac*Donald
> Machado
> *Mac*Hale
> Maville
> *Mc*Aulay
> *Mc*Williams
> Meacham

If the files contain a great many names beginning with Mac or Mc, some offices file them as a separate letter of the alphabet for convenience.

9. The name of a married woman is indexed by her legal name (her husband's surname, her given name, and her middle name or maiden surname). For example:

> Doe, Mary Jones (Mrs. John L.)
> *not* Doe, Mrs. John L. (unless first name is unknown)

10. Titles, when followed by a complete name, may be used as the *last* filing unit if needed to distinguish from another identical name. For example:

> Mr. James D. Conley
> Conley James D Mr.
> Dr. James D. Conley
> Conley James D Dr.

Titles without complete names are considered the *first* indexing unit:

> Madame Sylvia
> Sister Theresa

11. Terms of seniority, or professional or academic degree, are used only to distinguish from an identical name. For example:

> Theodore Wilson, PhD
> Theodore Wilson, Sr.
> Theodore Wilson, Jr.
> Theodore Wilson, MD

These examples would be filed in the following order:

> Theodore Wilson, Jr.
> Theodore Wilson, MD
> Theodore Wilson, PhD
> Theodore Wilson, Sr.

12. Articles such as *The* or *A* are disregarded in indexing:

Moore Clinic (The)	

Filing Methods

The three basic methods of filing used in healthcare facilities are these:
- Alphabetical by name
- Numeric
- Subject

Patient charts are filed either alphabetically by name or by one of several numeric methods. Subject filing is used for business records, correspondence, and topical materials.

Alphabetical Filing

Alphabetical filing by name is the oldest, simplest, and most commonly used system. It is the system of choice for filing patient records in the majority of physicians' offices. If the medical assistant can find a word in the dictionary or a name in the telephone directory, then he or she already knows some of the rules.

The alphabetical system of filing is traditional and simple to set up, requiring only a file cabinet or shelf, folders, and some divider guides (Procedure 13-6). It is a **direct filing system**, in that the person filing need only know the name in order to find the desired file. Alphabetical filing does have some drawbacks:
- The correct spelling of the name must be known.
- As the number of files increases, more space is needed for each section of the alphabet. This results in periodic shifting of folders from drawer to drawer or shelf to shelf to allow for expansion.
- As the files expand, more time is required for filing or retrieving each folder because of the greater number of folders involved in the search. The time can be greatly reduced by color coding.

Numeric Filing

Some form of **numeric filing** combined with color and **shelf filing** is used by practically every large clinic or hospital. Management consultants differ in their recommendations; some recommend numeric filing only if there are more than 5000 charts, more than 10,000 charts, or in some cases more than 15,000 charts. Others recommend nothing but numeric filing. Numeric filing is an **indirect filing system**, requiring the use of an alphabetical cross-reference to find a given file. Some people object to this added step and overlook the advantages, which are that it:
- Allows unlimited expansion without periodic shifting of folders, and shelves are usually filled evenly.
- Provides additional confidentiality to the chart.

PROCEDURE **13-6**

Filing Medical Records and Documents Using the Alphabetical System

GOAL: To file records efficiently using an alphabetical system and ensure that the records can be easily and quickly retrieved.

EQUIPMENT AND SUPPLIES
- Medical records
- Physical filing equipment
- Cart to carry records, if needed
- Alphabetical file guide
- Staple remover
- Stapler

PROCEDURAL STEPS

1 Using alphabetical guidelines, place the records to be filed in alphabetical order. If a stack of documents is to be filed, place them in alphabetical order inside an alphabetical file guide or sorter. Use rules for filing documents alphabetically.

Purpose: To organize the filing process and file the record or document quickly without retracing steps and skipping from letter to letter.

2 Go to the filing storage equipment (shelves, cabinets, or drawers) and locate the spot in the alphabet for the first file.

3 Place the file in the cabinet or drawer in correct alphabetical order.

4 If adding a document to a file, place it on top so that the most recent information is seen first. This puts the information in the file in reverse chronological order.

Purpose: To provide access to the most pertinent and recent information.

5 Securely fasten documents to the chart. Do not just drop the documents inside the chart.

Purpose: To keep vital information from falling out of the chart and being lost.

6 Refile the chart in its proper place.

- Saves time in retrieving and refiling records quickly. One knows immediately that the number 978 falls between 977 and 979. By contrast, an alphabetical system, even with color coding, requires a longer search for the exact spot.

There are several types of numeric filing systems. In the straight or consecutive numeric system, patients are given consecutive numbers as they visit the practice. This is the simplest of the numeric systems and works well for files of up to 10,000 records. It is time consuming, and there is a greater chance for error when filing documents with five or more digits. Filing activity is greatest at the end of the numeric series.

In the terminal digit system, patients are also assigned consecutive numbers, but the digits in the number are usually separated into groups of twos or threes and are read in groups from right to left instead of from left to right. The records are filed backward in groups. For example, all files ending in 00 are grouped together first, then those ending in 01, etc. Next the files are grouped by their middle digits so that the 00 22s come before the 01 22s. Finally the files are arranged by their first digits, so that 01 00 22 precedes 02 00 22.

Middle-digit filing begins with the middle digits, followed by the first digit and finally by the terminal digits.

Some practices use the last four digits of each patient's Social Security number to file patient records. However, there is no legal requirement that every United States resident have a Social Security number, in which case a "pseudo number" would have to be issued.

Numeric filing requires more training, but once the system is mastered, fewer errors occur than with alphabetical filing (Procedure 13-7).

CRITICAL THINKING APPLICATION

Susan is unsure whether alphabetical or numeric filing is best in the medical office. What are some advantages and disadvantages of each method?

Subject Filing

Subject filing can be either alphabetical or **alphanumeric** (A 1-3, B 1-1, B1-2, and so on) and is used for general correspondence. The main difficulty with subject filing is indexing, or classifying—deciding where to file a document. Many papers require cross-referencing. All correspondence dealing with a particular subject is filed together. The papers within the folders are filed chronologically, the most recent on top. The subject headings are placed on the tabs of the folders and filed alphabetically.

Color Coding

When a color coding system is used, both filing and finding are easier, and misfiled folders are kept to a minimum (Procedure 13-8). The use of color visually

---

PROCEDURE 13-7

Filing Medical Records and Documents Using the Numeric System

GOAL: To file records efficiently using a numeric system and ensure that the records can be easily and quickly retrieved.

EQUIPMENT AND SUPPLIES

- Medical records
- Physical filing equipment
- Cart to carry records, if needed
- Numeric file guide
- Staple remover
- Stapler
- Paper clips

PROCEDURAL STEPS

1 Using numeric guidelines, place the records to be filed in numeric order. If a stack of documents is to be filed, write the chart number on the document. Use rules for filing documents alphabetically.

Purpose: To organize the filing process and file the record or documents quickly without retracing steps and skipping from letter to letter.

2 Go to the filing storage equipment (shelves, cabinets, or drawers) and locate the numeric spot for the first file.

3 Place the file in the cabinet or drawer in correct numeric order.

4 If adding a document to a file, place it on top so that the most recent information is seen first. This puts the information in the file in reverse chronological order.

Purpose: To provide access to the most pertinent and recent information.

5 Securely fasten documents to the chart. Do not just drop the documents inside the chart.

Purpose: To keep vital information from falling out of the chart and being lost.

6 Refile the chart in its proper place.

restricts the area of search for a specific record. A misfiled chart is easily spotted even from a distance of several feet. In color coding, a specific color is selected to identify each letter of the alphabet. The application of the principle may be through using colored folders, adhesive colored identification labels, or various combinations of these. Any selection of colors may be used, and the division of the alphabet is determined by one's own needs. However, studies have shown that there is wide variation in the frequency with which different letters occur.

Alphabetical Color Coding. There are several ways of color coding files. One alphabetical system utilizes five different colored folders, with each color representing a segment of the alphabet. The *second* letter of the patient's last name determines the color.

As medicine continues to consolidate into larger facilities, with more patients under one management, the filing of patient charts becomes more complicated and color coding becomes more useful. Several color-coding systems use two sets of 13 colors—one set for letters A–M, and a second set of the same colors on a different background for the letters N–Z.

There are many ready-made systems available (e.g., Bibbero, Colwell, Kardex, Remington Rand, Smead, TAB, VisiRecord). Self-adhesive colored letter blocks with either two or three letters in the specific colors are supplied in rolls. The color blocks with the appropriate letter are placed on the index tab of the folder, along with the patient's full name. The letters are in pairs so that they can be seen from either side of the chart. Strong, easily differentiated colors are used, creating a band of color in the files that makes it easy to spot out-of-place folders (Figure 13-14).

Numeric Color Coding. Color coding is also used in numeric filing. Numbers 0 through 9 are each assigned a different color. In a terminal digit filing system, the colors for the last two numbers would be affixed to the tab. If the number 1 is red and 5 is yellow, all files with numbers ending in 15 form a red and yellow band. Usually a predetermined section of the number is color coded.

Other Color Coding Applications. There are many other ways to make color work for the efficient medical office. Small pressure-sensitive tabs in a variety of colors may be used to identify certain types of insured patients and other specific information. For example, a red tab over the edge of the folder may identify a patient on Medicaid, a blue tab may identify a CHAMPUS patient; a green tab may identify a workers' compensation patient; matching tabs may be attached to the insured's ledger card; research cases may be identified by a special color tab; and brightly colored labels on the outside of a patient chart can indicate certain health conditions, such as drug allergies. In a partnership practice, a different color folder or label may identify each physician's patients. Color can also be used to differentiate dates—one color for each month or year.

Business records may also utilize color coding. Main divider guide headings may be of one color, subheadings in a second color, and subdivisions in a third color. A fourth color might be used for personal items.

The use of color in filing is limited only by the imagination. One word of caution: Every person in the facility who uses the files must know the key to the coding, and the key should also be written in the facility's procedures manual.

PROCEDURE **13-8**

Color Coding Patient Charts

GOAL: To color code patient charts using the agency's established coding system to effectively facilitate filing and finding.

EQUIPMENT AND SUPPLIES

- List of patient charts to code
- File folders
- Information on agency's coding system
- Full range of color tabs

PROCEDURAL STEPS

1 Assemble patient charts.

2 Arrange charts in indexing order.
Purpose: When charts have been color coded, they will be in filing order.

3 Pick up the first chart and note the second letter of the patient's surname.

Explanation: For purpose of activity, the color coding system in the text will be used.

4 Choose a folder and/or caption label of the appropriate color.

5 Type patient's name on label in indexing order and apply to folder tab.
Purpose: To identify sequence of folder in filing system.

6 Repeat steps 4 and 5 until all charts have been coded.

7 Check entire group for any isolated color.
Purpose: If the order and color of the folders is correct, all charts of the same color within each letter of the alphabet will be grouped together.

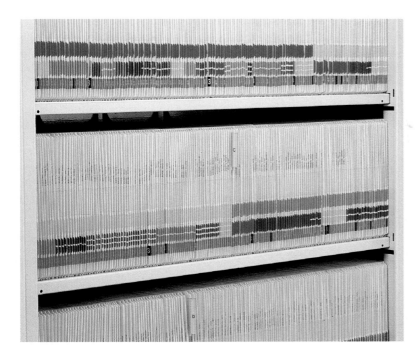

FIGURE 13-14   Color coding patient charts makes it easy to see a file that is misplaced. (Courtesy Bibbero Systems, Inc., Petaluma, Calif. 94954, (800) 242-2376, www.bibbero.com.)

Organization of Files

It is very difficult for a physician to study a disorganized history. Some systematic method must be followed in placing items in the patient folder. The content of the patient record has already been discussed. From the filing standpoint, it should be emphasized that when a patient record is not in actual use, there is only one place it should be—in the filing cabinet or shelf. Many precious hours can be lost in searching for misplaced or lost records that were carelessly left unfiled.

The patient's full name, in indexing order, should be typed on a label and attached to the folder tab. A strip of transparent tape can be placed on the label to prevent smudging if this is a problem. The patient's full name should also be typed on each sheet within the folder.

Health-Related Correspondence

Correspondence pertaining to patients' medical records should be filed with the case history. Other medical correspondence should probably be filed in a subject file.

General Correspondence

The physician's office operates as a business as well as a professional service. There will be correspondence of a general nature pertaining to the operation of the office. In all likelihood, a special drawer or shelf will be set aside for the general correspondence. The correspondence is indexed according to subject matter or names of correspondents. The guides in a subject file may appear in one, two, or three positions, depending on the number of headings, subheadings, and subdivisions.

Practice Management Files

The most active financial record is, of course, the patient ledger. In facilities that still use a manual system, this will be a card or vertical tray file, and the accounts will be arranged alphabetically by name. There will be at least two divisions:

- Active accounts
- Paid accounts

Miscellaneous Folder

Papers that do not warrant an individual folder are placed in a miscellaneous folder. Within the folder, all papers relating to one subject, or with one correspondent, are kept together in chronological order, the most recent on top, and then filed alphabetically with other miscellaneous material. Related materials may be stapled together. Never use paper clips for this purpose. When as many as five papers accumulate with one correspondent or subject, a separate folder should be prepared. Other business files include records of income and expense, financial statements, income and payroll tax records, canceled checks, and insurance policies. These papers may be filed chronologically.

Tickler or Follow-Up Files

The most frequently used follow-up method is that of a **tickler file**, so called because it tickles the memory that something needs to be done or followed up on a particular date. The tickler file is always a chronological arrangement. In its simplest form, it consists of notations on the daily calendar. If information, such as an x-ray report or laboratory report, is expected concerning a patient who has an appointment to come in, the medical assistant might make a note on the calendar or tickler file a day ahead to check on whether the report has arrived.

The tickler file is often a card file with 12 guides for the names of the months and 31 guides printed with numbers 1 through 31 for the days of the month. The guide for the current month, followed by the 31-day guides, is placed at the front of the file. Notations of actions to be taken are placed behind the guides for specific days of the current month. Notations for future months are placed behind the guide for that month. To be effective, the tickler file must be checked the first thing each day.

CRITICAL THINKING APPLICATION

Susan is responsible for checking the tickler file on a daily basis. What types of documents and duties might she find inside these files?

There are many ways to use the tickler file. It is a useful reminder for recurring events such as payments, meetings, and so forth. On the last day in each month, all the notations from behind the next month's guide are distributed among the daily numbered guides, and the guide for the month just completed is placed at the back of the file.

Transitory or Temporary File

Many papers are kept longer than necessary because no provision is made for segregating those that have a limited usefulness. This situation is avoided by having a *transitory* or *temporary* file. For example, if a medical assistant writes a letter requesting a reprint, the file copy is placed in the transitory folder. When the reprint is received, the file copy is destroyed. The transitory file is used for materials having no permanent value. The paper may be marked with a *T* and destroyed when the action is completed.

Closing Comments

Just like every aspect of the medical profession, advances in medical records management are occurring rapidly, allowing physicians and other caregivers to perform their duties in a more efficient and accurate way. A medical assistant must constantly be willing to learn and adapt to changes that result from legislation and technological strides. Because patients are fast becoming more computer literate, computers will become more generally accepted as a viable means of recording medical information. This is a positive change, because many patients and providers were not in favor of computer-based medical records when the concept was first presented to the general public.

Patient Education

The medical assistant should always explain any paperwork to the patient that he or she may be required to

complete. Patients do not like to be told to simply "sign here." Take the time to explain any form that needs completion or a signature, so that the patient will understand the reason for collecting the information and the necessity of the information being available to the medical facility.

Many forms are similar, and patients may complain about answering the same questions on multiple forms. It can be frustrating for patients when they must list their address and phone numbers on each of several forms. Review and revise the forms used in the office often so that they are user-friendly for the office and patient alike.

Patients may need reassurance that each staff member in the physician's office is committed to complete patient confidentiality. Always be open to answering questions regarding the patient medical record.

Legal and Ethical Issues

The authority to release information from the medical record lies solely with the patient unless required by law by subpoena. Ownership of the record is often a subject of controversy. The record belongs to the physician; the information belongs to the patient.

When a medical record is used as evidence in a court case, the person who entered information in the chart must be able to read it, no matter how much time has lapsed since the entry was created. When a chart is corrected, the proper method must be followed and the record should never be obliterated.

Be sure to understand the laws concerning records retention. Records should be kept through the period of the statute of limitations, and possibly longer in certain situations. Take care with the medical chart, as it is the lifeline of patient care in the medical facility.

SUMMARY OF SCENARIO

Susan looks forward to attending her medical assisting classes each day and works diligently to perform to the best of her ability in the classroom. She strives to do well on each procedure check-off and each examination that she completes. Her instructors provide excellent feedback and appreciate her contributions to the classroom experience.

Susan has the attitude that everything she is allowed to do in the medical office is a learning tool. She regularly asks for additional responsibilities and is always ready to assist a co-worker. Dr. Thomas has recognized that she has the desire to learn, and he gives her many opportunities to glean more knowledge through the everyday activities in the office.

Although she is new to the medical profession, Susan learns quickly and thinks logically. She knows the rules and regulations regarding patient confidentiality and is always careful about the information she provides to those who request it. She is never hesitant about asking her office manager for guidance if she is unsure about any aspect of her duties. Susan is understanding and respectful when patients are concerned about their privacy. Her confidence and warm personality play a role in the trust that she earns from the patients at the clinic.

Susan is willing to admit when she has made an error and has sought advice from Dr. Thomas and her office manager when an error needed correction. Although filing is not one of her favorite duties, she can be counted on to give her best while completing this important task. She takes pride in her work and is efficient and accurate where medical records are concerned. When she is faced with a task that is new to her, she considers it a learning experience and seeks help when she is not completely certain about the way to handle a given situation.

Susan's co-workers are supportive and always willing to assist her as she learns to be the best medical assistant that she can possibly be. Her future as a professional medical assistant will certainly be laden with opportunity and advancement.

SUMMARY OF LEARNING OBJECTIVES

■ Several types of equipment and supplies are necessary when managing patient records. A variety of shelving units and filing containers are available. Open shelving allows the maximized use of color coded charts, which make finding misfiles quick and easy. Many file folder styles are available, and there are several types of forms to use within the patient charts. The preference of the physician and staff members who use these tools is important, as well as concerns such as cost and availability. A medical assistant should be conservative when ordering supplies and purchasing equipment, only ordering the number needed to save on office supply costs.

■ Five basic steps are involved in filing documents. The papers are conditioned, which is the preparatory stage for filing. Releasing the documents means that they are ready to be filed because they have been reviewed or read, and some type of mark is placed on the document to indicate this. Indexing involves the decision as to where the document should be filed, and coding is placing some type of mark on the paper relative to that decision. Sorting is placing the files in filing sequence. The last step is the actual filing and storing of the document.

■ Alphabetical filing is a simple and traditional filing system, whereby documents are filed in alphabetical order. Numeric filing systems use a number code to give order to the files. An alphanumeric system is a combination of the two.

■ Color coding is an excellent way to keep patient charts in order and swiftly locate those charts that have been misfiled. The medical assistant can tell at a glance when a chart is out of place. Color coding also makes retrieval of and refiling files quick and easy.

■ Medical records must be accurate primarily so that the right care can be given to the patient. The record also helps to provide continuity of care between providers, so that there is no lapse in treatment to the patient. The record serves as indication and proof in court that certain treatments and procedures were performed on the patient, so it can be excellent legal support if it is well maintained and accurate. Medical records also aid researchers with statistical information.

■ The physician owns the physical medical record, whereas the patient owns the information contained within.

■ The problem-oriented medical record categorizes each problem that a patient has and elaborates on the findings and treatment plan for all concerns. Detailed progress notes are kept for every individual problem. This method separates each of the patient's concerns and addresses them separately, whereas a traditional record may address all problems and concerns at one time. The problem-oriented medical record helps to assure that all individual problems are addressed.

■ Very simply, subjective information is provided by the patient, whereas objective information is provided by the physician or provider. Subjective information includes items such as the patient address, social security number, insurance information, and the patient's explanation of the condition he or she is experiencing. Objective information is obtained through the questions the physician asks and the observations made during the examination.

■ Correct procedures must be followed when making corrections to a patient chart. A single line should be drawn through the incorrect information, then initialed and dated. Some offices require a notation of "Corr." or "correction" on the chart as well. A medical assistant should never try to alter the medical record or cover up an error in charting.

INTERNET CONNECTIONS

- American Health Information Management Association http://www.ahima.org
- The Health Insurance Portability and Accountability Act http://www.cms.hhs.gov/hipaa
- The Informatics Review http://www.informatics-review.com
- Professional Standards Review Council of America http://www.psrc-of-america.org

UNIT three

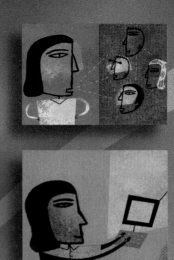

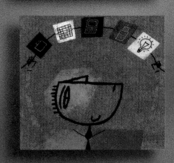

Financial Management

CHAPTER 14

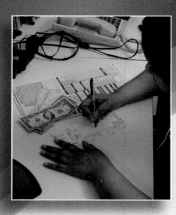

Scenario

Myra Morrison has worked for Dr. Jerry Wallace, an endocrinologist, for 3 years. She began as a receptionist, but she always had a knack for mathematics. This led Dr. Wallace to place her in charge of the accounting functions for the practice. When patients are ready to leave the clinic, Myra totals their bill and enters the charges and payments into the computerized ledger system. She also schedules their return appointments. Myra has learned quite a bit about medical insurance as well, so she can answer many of the patients' questions about their coverage and the benefits or exclusions of their insurance policies. There have been many cases in which she was able to decipher a confusing insurance claim and explain the reimbursement to the patient. Myra has a great attitude about assisting patients with insurance questions and does not hesitate to call the insurance company to ask questions on behalf of the patient. She provides the patients with exceptional customer service.

Myra knows that care must be taken when dealing with numerical transactions. Her handwriting is clear and legible, and she writes numbers the same way each time to avoid confusion and errors. She is able to use a manual pegboard but prefers the computer programs that do most of the work for her. Myra has some basic accounting background, so she can find errors easily and correct them. She even enjoys balancing the accounts on a daily basis to be sure all transactions were entered correctly.

Myra provides a valuable service to the patients that visit Dr. Wallace. She can always be counted on to follow up on any detail that needs attention. When patients call her for assistance, she takes no more than 24 hours to respond with the answers to their questions. She is a great patient advocate in the office. Some patients even tease her and ask her to balance their checkbooks! Myra is also willing to help any staff member with other duties whenever necessary. She is an enthusiastic team player who puts the patients first.

Professional Fees, Billing, and Collecting

Learning Objectives

- Define and spell the terms listed in the vocabulary.
- List three values that are considered in determining professional fees.
- Distinguish among the terms *usual*, *customary*, and *reasonable*.
- Discuss the value of estimates for patient treatment.
- Explain the concept of professional courtesy.
- Name the ways by which payment for medical services is accomplished.
- Explain why itemizing statements is important.
- Discuss why patients fail to pay accounts.
- Explain how to handle a "skip."
- Briefly explain some of the guidelines of telephone collecting.
- Explain professional fees to patients.
- Effectively use a pegboard system.
- Establish credit arrangements for patient payment.
- Prepare accurate monthly statements.
- Evaluate patient accounts for necessary collection procedures.

National Curriculum Competencies

2c. Post entries on a day sheet
2f. Perform billing and collecting procedures
3b. Post adjustments
3c. Process a credit balance

3d. Process refunds
3e. Post nonsufficient fund checks
3f. Post collection agency payments

Vocabulary

account A statement of transactions during a fiscal period and the resulting balance.

account balance The amount owed on an account.

accounts receivable ledger A record of the charges and payments posted on an account.

credit An entry on an account constituting an addition to a revenue, net worth, or liability account; the balance in a person's favor in an account.

debit An entry on an account constituting an addition to an expense or asset account or a deduction from a revenue, a net worth, or a liability account.

debit cards A card that looks like a credit card and by which money may be withdrawn or the cost of purchases paid directly from the holder's bank account without the payment of interest.

disbursements Funds paid out.

fee profile A compilation or average of physician fees over a given period of time.

fee schedule A compilation of preestablished fee allowances for given services or procedures.

fiscal agent An organization under contract to the government as well as some private plans to act as financial representatives in handling insurance claims from providers of health care; also referred to as fiscal intermediary.

guarantor A person who makes or gives a guarantee of payment for a bill.

instigate To goad or urge forward; to provoke.

medically indigent Able to take care of ordinary living expenses but not able to afford medical care.

payables The balance due to a creditor on an account.

pegboard system Also called the write-it-once system; a method of tracking patient accounts that allows the figures to be proved accurate through mathematical formulas.

posting Transferring or carrying from a book of original entry to a ledger; entering figures in an accounting system.

premium The consideration paid for a contract of insurance.

preponderance A superiority or excess in number or quantity; a majority.

professional courtesy Reduction or absence of fees to professional associates.

receipts Amounts paid on patient accounts.

receivables Total monies received on accounts.

third party payor Someone other than the patient, spouse, or parent who is responsible for paying all or part of the patient's medical costs.

transaction An exchange or transfer of goods, services, or funds.

The practice of medicine is a business as well as a profession, and the details of conducting the business aspects are often the responsibility of the medical assistant. Although service to the patient is the primary concern of the medical profession, a physician must charge and collect a fee for such services to continue providing medical care. The physician is one of many contributors in determining the amount of the fees. The medical assistant usually has the responsibility of informing the patient about financial matters, collecting the payment, and in some cases, making arrangements for deferred payment.

Why Patients Do Not Pay

Most patients truly want to pay the bills that they owe. However, there may be times that the patient experiences difficulties in meeting his or her obligations. The patient may have lost a job or insurance coverage. An emergency could arise that depletes finances. When patients are in a position in which they must choose between paying their medical bills or having electricity, the physician is often forced to wait for reimbursement for the services rendered. Although a few patients will absolutely refuse to pay for medical care they have received, most are honest and willing to pay but may need help with a payment plan. Terms can be arranged for collecting payment in full when both the office and the patient cooperate with each other. The medical assistant should attempt to work out a plan that the patient can abide by, and the patient should be expected to make promised payments.

How Fees Are Determined

Setting fees is no simple matter. The physician has three commodities to sell—time, judgment, and services. Yet the value of these commodities is never exactly the same to any two individuals. Medical care has little value except to the patient, and the value may not be consistent with his or her ability to pay. In every case, the physician must place an estimate on the value of the services. Such an arrangement is known as *fee for service*. This value may then be modified by other considerations.

Impact of Managed Care

An important consideration in today's atmosphere of managed care is the **preponderance** of patients who are enrolled in health maintenance organization (HMO) insurance contracts. Under managed care, the physician agrees to accept predetermined fees for specific procedures and services instead of the fee-for-service arrangement described in the preceding paragraph. The patient may be subject to a co-payment that is determined by the insurance contract and is collected at the time of service. A base capitation plan pays the provider a set amount for each patient enrolled that is meant to cover all of the person's healthcare expenses. Usually, capitation plans cover a group of individuals.

Prevailing Rate in the Community

One of the bases for determining charges on the fee-for-service basis is the economic level of the community. Different communities have different living scales, and this situation is reflected in medical fees as well. Consequently, the prevailing rate in the community—the average composite fee—must be taken into consideration by each physician. Strangely enough, fees that are too low drive patients away just as quickly as fees that are too high because the average person tends to judge worth of a product on its cost—low cost translates as low value.

Usual, Customary, and Reasonable Fees

Most insurance plans base their payments on what has become known as a *usual, customary, and reasonable (UCR) fee* for a given procedure.

- *Usual*—The physician's usual fee for a given service is the fee that an individual physician most frequently charges for the service.
- *Customary*—The customary fee is a range of the usual fees charged for the same service by physicians with similar training and experience practicing in the same geographical and socioeconomic area. There is now a growing tendency for fees to be determined by national trends rather than by local custom.
- *Reasonable*—The term *reasonable* usually applies to a service or procedure that is exceptionally difficult or complicated, requiring extraordinary time or effort on the part of the physician.

To illustrate, let us suppose that Dr. Wallace usually charges patients $100 for a first office visit. The usual fees charged for a first visit by other physicians in the same community with similar training and experience range from $75 to $125. Dr. Wallace's fee of $100 is within the customary range and would therefore be paid by an insurance plan that pays on a usual and customary basis. If, on the other hand, the range of usual fees in the community is from $60 to $85, the insurance plan would allow only the maximum within the range, or $85, to Dr. Wallace.

CRITICAL THINKING APPLICATION

Myra realizes that many of Dr. Wallace's patients are confused about insurance policies and are easily frustrated when payments are not as high as the patient thinks they should be. How can Myra help patients understand their policies better?

UCR rates were developed many years ago when indemnity plans were the most common type of health insurance coverage. However, since the majority of insurance plans today are some type of managed care, the UCR rates now are based on the prevailing managed care rate of payment in a region.

Fee Setting by Third Party Payors

The physician does not act alone in determining fees. A third party payor may provide the physician with a predetermined fee schedule that it will approve for payment. Some require preapproval of the fee before service is rendered. A third party payor may require precertification before it will pay for a specific service. Government programs such as Medicare and Medicaid have strict guidelines regarding reimbursement for fees and the raising of fees.

Physician's Fee Profile

The **fiscal agent**, or fiscal intermediary, for government-sponsored insurance programs as well as some private plans keeps a continuous record of the usual charges submitted for specific services by each physician. When these fees have been compiled and averaged over a given period, usually a year, the physician's **fee profile** is established. This fee profile is then used in determining the amount of third party liability for services under the program. One of the objections voiced by physicians is the lag between the time of a private fee increase and the time it is reflected in payments by an insurance carrier. It may be as long as 2 to 3 years.

Insurance Allowance

In some individual cases, the physician may not wish to charge the patient in addition to what will be allowed by the patient's insurance. This is often a professional courtesy for other healthcare professionals. The full fee should be quoted to the patient and charged to the account, with the understanding that after the insurance allowance has been received, the balance may be discounted. If a smaller fee is quoted and charged, the following problems may arise:

- The lower fee will alter the physician's fee profile.
- If it becomes necessary to bring suit for payment of the fee, only the reduced fee can be recovered.
- If the insurance allowance is paid on the basis of a certain percentage of the physician's fee and a lower fee is charged, the insurance allowance will be correspondingly lower.
- If the physician does this with many patients, the insurance company may take the position that the reduced fee is the physician's usual fee and base its payments accordingly. It may even be considered fraudulent in some instances.

Explaining Costs to Patients

It is natural for the patient, particularly one new to the practice, to wonder, "How much is this going to cost?" However, some patients may be reluctant to voice this concern. Do not wait for the patient to ask about the fees. It is the responsibility of the physician or the medical assistant to approach the subject if the patient does not do so (Procedure 14-1). Be prepared to discuss costs with any patient who is interested, and ask all patients if they have questions about the fees. A good way to open the discussion would be to ask the following:

"Mr. Willardson, do you have any questions about the costs of your operation? If you do, I'll be glad to review them."

In this preliminary discussion of fees, the physician or medical assistant must not sidestep the issue by saying,

PROCEDURE **14-1**

Explaining Professional Fees

GOAL: To explain the physician's fees so that the patient understands his or her obligations and rights for privacy.

EQUIPMENT AND SUPPLIES

- Patient's statement
- Copy of physician's fee schedule
- Quiet, private area where the patient feels free to ask questions

PROCEDURAL STEPS

1 Determine that the patient has the correct bill.
Purpose: To make certain that the bill belongs to this patient and that the insurance numbers, the address, and the telephone number are correct.

2 Examine the bill for possible errors.
Purpose: To demonstrate that the patient's concerns are important and that you are willing to make any necessary adjustments.

3 Refer to the fee schedule for services rendered.
Purpose: To explain how physicians determine their fees. If an error has occurred, correct it immediately with a sincere apology.

4 Explain itemized billing:
- Date of each service
- Type of service rendered
- Fee
Purpose: To make certain that the patient realizes the number and extent of the services rendered.

5 Display a professional attitude toward the patient.
Purpose: To reassure the patient that you have a thorough understanding of the fee schedule and show willingness to answer questions politely and completely.

6 Determine whether the patient has specific concerns that may hinder payment.
Purpose: To provide an opportunity for making special arrangements if needed.

7 Make appropriate arrangements for a discussion between the physician and patient if further explanation is necessary for resolution of the problem.

"*Don't worry about the bill; let's just get you well first.*" The patient may later complain about the bill because he or she misunderstood the complexity of the service.

Even in cases in which the physician quotes a fee, the medical assistant often has the responsibility of explaining the physician's fees to the patient. The medical assistant must know how fees are determined and why charges vary, as well as have a thorough knowledge of the physician's practice and policies to handle perplexing situations involving fees.

CRITICAL THINKING APPLICATION

Mr. Reynolds, one of Dr. Wallace's long-standing patients, continually complains about his insurance policies and the small payments made on his medical claims. He frequents the office at least twice a month for checkups and goes into a long speech about the problems with his insurance each time he stops to pay his bill at Myra's desk. He will continue complaining even when other patients come to pay their bills. How can Myra tactfully handle Mr. Reynolds and stop his complaints?

As the medical assistant's understanding of the practice increases, he or she can build respect for the physician's

services by educating patients that money spent for medical care is an excellent investment in the future. It is a rare patient who understands the intricate procedures involved in diagnosis and treatment, especially when third party payors are involved. Be patient and understanding when questions arise in this area.

Advance Discussion of Fees

Advance fee discussions help the patient plan ahead for medical expenditures (Figure 14-1). Most patients want to pay their financial obligations but rightly insist on an accurate estimate of those obligations before they contract for purchase of goods or services. When a physician frankly discusses fees in advance with patients, even to the point of describing how a fee is established, misconceptions and complaints about overcharging and fee discrepancies are usually eliminated.

Explanation of Additional Costs

Explanations of medical costs should extend beyond the physician's own charges. For example, if a patient is to undergo surgery, the physician should also explain the costs of the operation, the anesthesiologist's and radiologist's charges, the laboratory fees, and the approximate hospital bill. The importance of calling in another physician for consultation should be explained to patients when consultation becomes necessary. It should be made

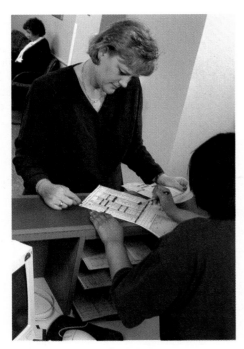

FIGURE 14-1 Taking a short amount of time to explain fees will often result in prompt payment for services.

clear, in advance, that there will be a separate bill submitted by the consulting physician. Patients do not always understand that the consultation is for the benefit of the patient, not the physician.

Estimates on Costs

Some physicians give patients an estimate of medical expenses before hospitalization. A few medical societies cooperatively develop estimate sheets or forms with local hospitals. Individual physicians occasionally work up their own estimate forms when a patient is embarking on long-term treatment. The physician should, however, emphasize that it is an estimate only and that the actual cost may vary somewhat.

Estimate slips should be prepared in duplicate so that the patient may have a copy and the original is retained in the patient's file. Duplicate estimate slips may help in the following ways:

- It may help to avoid forgetting that a fee was quoted.
- It may help eliminate the possibility of later misquoting the fee.
- It may help simplify collection by preventing misunderstanding and confusion over charges.

Guarantor's Ultimate Responsibility: The Bill

Patients must understand that the **guarantor** is the person ultimately responsible for the entire bill. The insurance policy is a contract between the policy holder and the insurance company or between a group of people (such as an employer) and a managed care organization. The actual physician is not a party to that contract. Therefore it is not the responsibility of the physician or staff to

pursue insurance payment for the benefit of the patient. However, it is in the best interest of the staff to actively assist the patient if there are problems in securing payment for several reasons.

First, the staff is almost always more knowledgeable about the insurance business than the patient. Many patients have never even read their insurance policies and have no idea as to what is or is not covered. Some patients expect the insurance to pay all costs simply because they are paying a high **premium**. The medical assistant may need to educate these patients about their policies and offer advice as to how the patients can effectively work with the insurance company to get answers to questions and make certain that they are receiving all of the benefits to which they are entitled.

Second, it is in the best interest of the staff to assist the patient in collecting from the insurance company so that the physician will be compensated for services rendered. Helping the patient in this area will usually result in the bill for care being paid. Another reason to actively assist the patient is that the medical assistant will gain knowledge about the insurance industry. The more experience the medical assistant has in working with third party payors, the more helpful he or she can be to the patients of the clinic. It is a good idea to keep a notebook with specific information about each type of policy that the office handles. This reference notebook will provide excellent guidance and suggestions for the medical assistant when working with a particular payor.

Always be sure to secure guarantors in writing. Most patient information sheets have a section that refers to the guarantor. There may be a statement that the guarantor signs indicating an agreement to pay the costs of medical care. States have varying statutes that deal with guarantors, so be sure that the office policies reflect compliance with those laws. It is especially important to secure a written agreement to pay for services when the care will be long term or when a costly treatment or surgical procedure must be done.

Encounter Forms

Encounter forms are the slips that are attached to charts while the patient is in the office; they are used for billing purposes. The encounter form provides information about the patient, such as the name, account number, and previous balance. Current charges and payments for the visit are added after the physician sees the patient. The physician can indicate on the encounter form when the patient should return to the clinic (Figure 14-2). The medical assistant then schedules an appointment and can even use the patient's copy of the encounter form to note the next appointment date and time.

The encounter form normally consists of three parts, with a white top sheet, a yellow sheet, and a pink sheet. The colors can vary, but usually the white copy is kept as a permanent record by the office, and the yellow and pink copies are given to the patient. The yellow copy is

FIGURE 14-2   An encounter form. The encounter form is used by the physician and staff to document what was done to the patient during an office visit and indicate when the physician wishes the patient to return. The copies of the form may be used to bill third party payors. (Courtesy Bibbero Systems, Inc., Petaluma, Calif. 94954, (800) 242-2376, www.bibbero.com.)

used by the patient for insurance billing (if not done by the office), and the pink copy is a receipt for the patient.

Encounter forms are sometimes designed to work with a **pegboard system** or may be available in continuous forms that can be placed in the printer for computer use. Encounter forms have been known by many aliases throughout the years; these include *superbills*, *charge slips*, and *multipurpose billing forms*.

Patient Account Transactions

A business **transaction** is the occurrence of an event or of a condition that must be recorded. For example, when a service is performed for which a charge is made, when a debtor makes a payment on account, when a piece of equipment is purchased, or when the monthly rent is paid, a business transaction has been completed.

Each of these examples is a transaction that must be recorded within the accounting system. The medical assistant will very likely encounter various other business transactions as he or she becomes more familiar with the individual needs of the employer's practice.

A patient's financial record is called an **account**. All of the patients' accounts together constitute the **accounts receivable ledger**. Account cards vary in design, but all will have at least three columns for entering figures. In the manual system these columns are as follows:

- *Debit column*—It is on the left, is used for entering charges, and is sometimes called the *charge column*.
- *Credit column*—It is to the right, is sometimes headed *Paid*, and is used for entering payments received.
- *Balance column*—It is on the far right and is used for recording the difference between the debit and the credit columns.

An *adjustment column* is available in some systems and is used for entering professional discounts, write-offs, disallowances by insurance companies, and any other adjustments. In a computer system, when a patient is called up by name or identification number, the patient's balance will appear. This is the individual patient's ledger.

Posting means the transfer of information from one record to another. Transactions are posted from the journal to the ledger; this is accomplished in one writing on the pegboard system. The **account balance** is normally a debit balance, which means that the charges exceed the payments on the account. A **debit** balance is entered by simply writing the correct figure in the balance column. A **credit** balance exists when payments exceed charges (e.g., when a patient pays in advance). This is common in obstetric practices.

Discounts are also credit entries and are entered in the adjustment column, or if there is no adjustment column, the discount is entered in the debit column and enclosed in parentheses. When the entry is made this way, it is recognized as a subtraction from the charges. When columns are totaled, any figure in red or in parentheses is always subtracted. **Receipts** are cash and checks taken in payment for professional services. **Receivables** are charges for which payment has not been received—amounts that are owing. **Disbursements** are cash amounts paid out. **Payables** are amounts owed to others but not yet paid.

Manual Posting

All charges and payments for professional services are posted to the ledger daily. The ledger then becomes a reliable source of information for answering all inquiries from patients about their accounts.

A separate account card or page is prepared for each patient at the time of the first visit or service. The heading of the account should include all information pertinent to collecting the account, such as the following:

- Name and address of person responsible for payment (the guarantor)
- Insurance identification
- Social Security number
- Home and business telephone numbers
- Name of employer
- Any special instructions for billing

Billing statements to the patient and the patient's insurance carrier are prepared from the ledger.

Computer Posting

The patient's name, date, diagnosis, and procedures are posted when the patient leaves the office. The database will retrieve the correct charges and post the charges on the computerized patient record and the accounts receivable ledger.

Write-It-Once, or Pegboard, System

The initial cost of materials for the pegboard system is slightly more than that for other accounting systems but is still moderate. The system is simple to operate, and training is included in most medical assisting programs.

The system gets its name from the lightweight aluminum or Masonite board with a row of pegs along the side or top that holds the forms in place. The accounting forms are perforated for alignment on the pegs. All of the forms used in any system must be compatible so that they may be aligned perfectly on the board. The pegboard system generates all the necessary financial records for each transaction with one writing, as follows:

- Encounter form
- Receipt
- Ledger card
- Journal entry

It may also include a statement and bank deposit slip.

The system provides current accounts receivable totals and a daily record of bank deposits and cash on hand, in addition to the record of income and expenses. The need for separate posting to patient accounts is eliminated, and the chance for error is decreased.

Using the Pegboard System

The pegboard system provides positive control over cash, collections, and receivables and ensures that every cent is accounted for and properly entered. It provides a record of every patient, every charge, and every payment, plus a daily recap of earnings—a running record of receivables and an audited summary of cash. The system requires a minimum of time. One writing allows a medical assistant to do the following:

- Enter a transaction on the day sheet.
- Give the patient a receipt for payment.
- Bring the patient's account up to date.
- Provide a current statement of account for the patient.
- Give the patient a notation of the next appointment.

All of these features communicate the money message to patients effectively and courteously and generate good financial records.

Gathering Required Materials. The pegboard may be of inexpensive Masonite construction with pegs down the left side, or it may be a more sophisticated aluminum sliding board that allows flexible positioning of materials. The basic pegboard forms follow:

- Day sheet (Figure 14-3)
- Patient ledger
- Encounter form

All of the forms must be compatible and are available from medical office supply companies. They may be customized to the practice, incorporating the usual services and procedure codes of the practice.

Preparing the Board. At the beginning of each day, place a new day sheet on the accounting board. Some systems have a sheet of clean carbon attached to the day sheet, others use special carbon with holes for the pegs, and some use NCR (no carbon required) paper. The carbon goes on top of the day sheet. Over the carbon, place the encounter form. The receipt has a carbonized writing line that should align with the first open writing line on the day sheet. If the slips are shingled, lay the entire bank of receipts over the pegs, with the top one aligned as mentioned. The remainder will be automatically in place. Receipts should be used in numerical order.

Pulling the Ledger Cards. If a great many patients are to be seen in a day, pull the ledger cards for all scheduled patients in the morning to save time (Figure 14-4). Keep the cards in the order in which the patients are scheduled to be seen.

Entering and Posting Transactions. As each patient arrives, insert the patient's ledger card under the first receipt, aligning the first available writing line of the card with the carbonized strip on the receipt. Enter the receipt number and date, the account balance in the space labeled *previous balance*, and the patient's name.

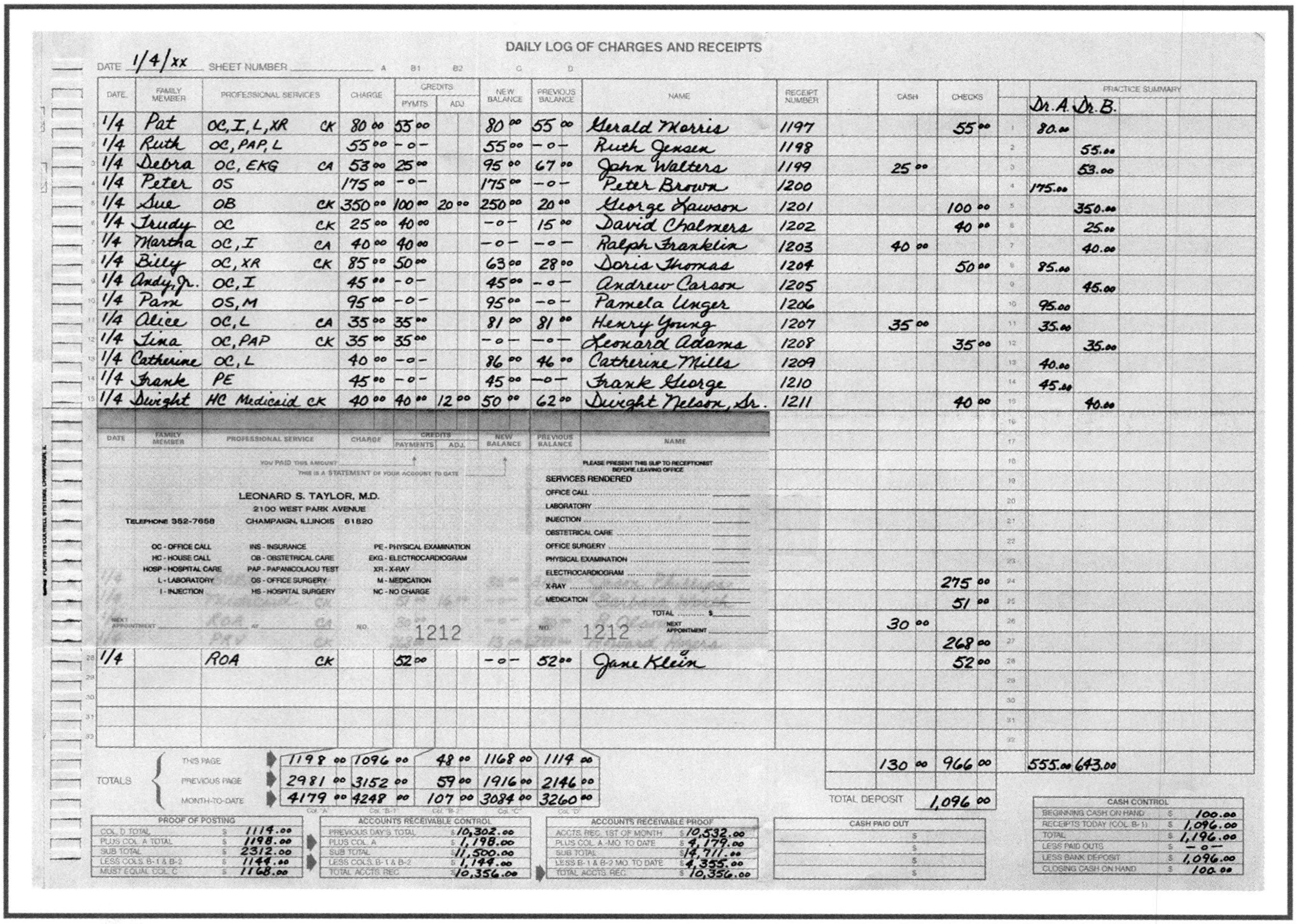
DAILY LOG OF CHARGES AND RECEIPTS

DATE 1/4/xx SHEET NUMBER

DATE	FAMILY MEMBER	PROFESSIONAL SERVICES	CHARGE	CREDITS PYMTS	CREDITS ADJ	NEW BALANCE	PREVIOUS BALANCE	NAME	RECEIPT NUMBER	CASH	CHECKS		Dr. A.	Dr. B.
1/4	Pat	OC, I, L, XR CK	80.00	55.00		80.00	55.00	Gerald Morris	1197		55.00	1	80.00	
1/4	Ruth	OC, PAP, L	55.00	-0-		55.00	-0-	Ruth Jensen	1198			2		55.00
1/4	Debra	OC, EKG CA	53.00	25.00		95.00	67.00	John Walters	1199	25.00		3		53.00
1/4	Peter	OS	175.00	-0-		175.00	-0-	Peter Brown	1200			4	175.00	
1/4	Sue	OB CK	350.00	100.00	20.00	250.00	20.00	George Lawson	1201		100.00	5		350.00
1/4	Trudy	OC CK	25.00	40.00		-0-	15.00	David Chalmers	1202		40.00	6		25.00
1/4	Martha	OC, I CA	40.00	40.00		-0-	-0-	Ralph Franklin	1203	40.00		7		40.00
1/4	Billy	OC, XR CK	85.00	50.00		63.00	28.00	Doris Thomas	1204		50.00	8	85.00	
1/4	Andy, Jr.	OC, I	45.00	-0-		45.00	-0-	Andrew Carson	1205			9		45.00
1/4	Pam	OS, M	95.00	-0-		95.00	-0-	Pamela Unger	1206			10	95.00	
1/4	Alice	OC, L CA	35.00	35.00		81.00	81.00	Henry Young	1207	35.00		11	35.00	
1/4	Tina	OC, PAP CK	35.00	35.00		-0-	-0-	Leonard Adams	1208		35.00	12		35.00
1/4	Catherine	OC, L	40.00	-0-		86.00	46.00	Catherine Mills	1209			13	40.00	
1/4	Frank	PE	45.00	-0-		45.00	-0-	Frank George	1210			14	45.00	
1/4	Dwight	HC Medicaid CK	40.00	40.00	12.00	50.00	62.00	Dwight Nelson, Sr.	1211		40.00	15		40.00
											275.00	24		
											51.00	25		
										30.00		26		
											268.00	27		
1/4		ROA CK	52.00			-0-	52.00	Jane Klein			52.00	28		

LEONARD S. TAYLOR, M.D.
2100 WEST PARK AVENUE
CHAMPAIGN, ILLINOIS 61820
TELEPHONE 352-7658
NO. 1212

TOTALS	CHARGE	PYMTS	ADJ	NEW BALANCE	PREVIOUS BALANCE	CASH	CHECKS	Dr. A.	Dr. B.
THIS PAGE	1198.00	1096.00	48.00	1168.00	1114.00	130.00	966.00	555.00	643.00
PREVIOUS PAGE	2981.00	3152.00	59.00	1916.00	2146.00				
MONTH-TO-DATE	4179.00	4248.00	107.00	3084.00	3260.00				

TOTAL DEPOSIT 1,096.00

PROOF OF POSTING	
COL. D TOTAL	$ 1114.00
PLUS COL. A TOTAL	$ 1198.00
SUB TOTAL	$ 2312.00
LESS COLS. B-1 & B-2	$ 1144.00
MUST EQUAL COL. C	$ 1168.00

ACCOUNTS RECEIVABLE CONTROL	
PREVIOUS DAY'S TOTAL	$ 10,302.00
PLUS COL. A	$ 1,198.00
SUB TOTAL	$ 11,500.00
LESS COLS. B-1 & B-2	$ 1,144.00
TOTAL ACCTS. REC.	$ 10,356.00

ACCOUNTS RECEIVABLE PROOF	
ACCTS. REC. 1ST OF MONTH	$ 10,532.00
PLUS COL. A -MO. TO DATE	$ 4,179.00
SUB TOTAL	$ 14,711.00
LESS B-1 & B-2 MO. TO DATE	$ 4,355.00
TOTAL ACCTS. REC.	$ 10,356.00

CASH CONTROL	
BEGINNING CASH ON HAND	$ 100.00
RECEIPTS TODAY (COL. B-1)	$ 1,096.00
TOTAL	$ 1,196.00
LESS PAID OUTS	$ -0-
LESS BANK DEPOSIT	$ 1,096.00
CLOSING CASH ON HAND	$ 100.00

FIGURE 14-3 Sample day sheet for use with a pegboard bookkeeping system. The pegboard system allows the user to write bookkeeping entries once, prepare deposit slips, and perform business analysis functions. (Courtesy Colwell Systems, Inc., Champaign, Illinois.)

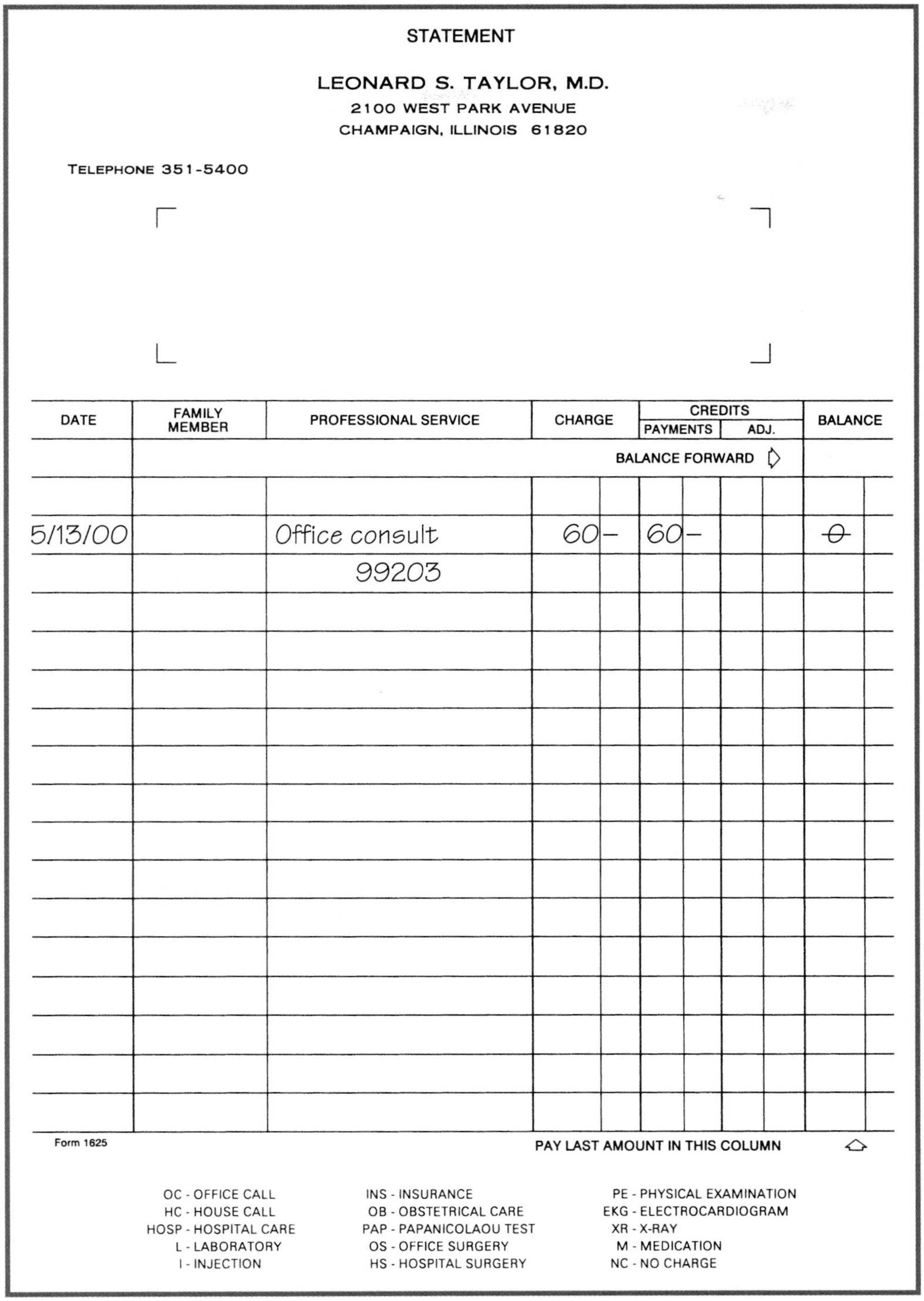

FIGURE 14-4 Patient ledger card. A ledger card showing the charge and payment for an office consultation. (Courtesy Colwell Systems, Inc., Champaign, Illinois.)

The information recorded on the receipt is automatically posted to the ledger and the day sheet (Figure 14-5). The charge slip is then detached and clipped to the patient chart to be routed to the physician, who now has an opportunity to see how much the patient owes and can discuss the account in privacy, if desired.

After the service has been performed, the physician enters the service on the encounter form and asks the patient or the nurse to return it to the medical assistant. The assistant then has an opportunity to ask the patient whether this is to be a charge or cash transaction before completing the posting. Again, insert the ledger card under the proper receipt, checking the number that was previously entered to make sure the correct card is being used. Record the service by procedure code, post the charge from the fee schedule, enter any payment made, and write in the current balance (Procedure 14-2). If there is no balance, place a zero or a straight line in the balance column. If another appointment is required, enter the date and time at the bottom of the receipt.

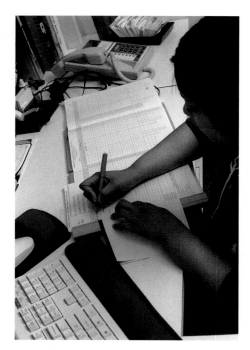

FIGURE 14-5 The pegboard system saves time by allowing several entries to be made at one time.

The transaction has now been posted to the journal and the ledger, and if payment was made by the patient, a receipt has been generated. The service receipt is given to the patient; no other receipt is necessary. The ledger card is ready for refiling.

File the encounter forms in numerical order for any internal audit. At the end of the month, the total of the encounter forms should equal the total of the charges recorded on the day sheets for the month (Figure 14-6).

Recording Other Payments and Charges. Payments will be received in the mail and may be brought in by patients some time after a service was performed. These payments are entered on the day sheet and the ledger card in the same manner as previously explained. Payments by mail do not require a receipt.

The physician may have daily charges for visits to patients in a hospital or convalescent facility. Enter these charges on the day sheet and ledger card only. Surgery fees are usually recorded as one entry that includes the surgery and aftercare.

CRITICAL THINKING APPLICATION

- Dr. Wallace sometimes forgets to write down information for billing when he goes to the hospital to check on his patients. Myra has a difficult time entering the charges for hospital visits because Dr. Wallace's records are not reliable in this area. How might Myra rectify this situation?
- How can Myra help Dr. Wallace to be more accurate in this area?

Summarizing Accounting Transactions. At the end of the day, all columns must be totaled and proved. Although all bookkeeping is done in ink, it is a good idea to write the totals in pencil until they have been proved. If an error is discovered, correct the entry in which it occurred. Do not attempt to erase or write over the incorrect entry. Simply draw one line through it and make a new entry on the first open writing line. Remember to reinsert the ledger card for these corrections. Also, if the entry included a receipt for the patient, make a new receipt and notify the patient of the correction.

Special Bookkeeping Entries

The following special entries are necessary occasionally and may be used with a pegboard or any other accounting system:
- Adjustments
- Credit balances
- Refunds
- Nonsufficient fund checks

Adjustments

At times, it is necessary to enter a credit adjustment. These could be for professional discounts, insurance disallowances, account write-offs, or payments that come to the office after the account has been placed for collections. If a patient or guarantor files bankruptcy, the charge will usually have to be adjusted off the books.

If the system has an adjustment column, enter them there. Otherwise, because the adjustment is actually a subtraction from the charge, enter it in the charge column with the figure enclosed in parentheses or circled and an explanation of the entry in the description column. When the column of figures is totaled, the circled figure is subtracted rather than added. The learner has a tendency to ignore the circled figures. This is incorrect—they must be subtracted.

Credit Balances

A credit balance occurs when a patient has paid in advance or there has been an overpayment or duplicate payment. For example, an overpayment occurs if the patient made a partial payment and later the insurance allowance was more than the remaining balance. The difference between the total amount of money received and the amount owed must be entered in the balance column and enclosed within parentheses or circled. This indicates a credit balance. Some credit balances are created when there has been an error in posting.

The credit balance is money owed to the patient. If the patient has paid in advance or wishes to leave the overpayment in the account in anticipation of future charges, care must be taken in figuring the balance on future transactions. Whereas normally a charge increases the balance, it will decrease a credit balance.

PROCEDURE 14-2

Posting Service Charges and Payments Using a Pegboard

GOAL: To post 1 day's charges and payments and compute the daily bookkeeping cycle using a pegboard.

EQUIPMENT AND SUPPLIES

- Pegboard
- Calculator
- Pen
- Day sheet
- Receipts
- Ledger cards
- Balances from previous day

PROCEDURAL STEPS

1 Prepare the board:
- Place a new day sheet on the board.
- Place a bank of receipts over the pegs, aligning the top receipt with the first open writing line on the day sheet.

2 Carry forward balances from the previous day.
Purpose: To keep all totals current.

3 Pull ledger cards for patient being seen that day.

4 Insert the ledger card under the first receipt, aligning the first available writing line of the card with the carbonized strip on the receipt.
Purpose: To ensure that one writing will correctly post the entry to receipt, ledger, and day sheet.

5 Enter the patient's name, the date, the receipt number, and any existing balance from the ledger card.

6 Detach the charge slip from the receipt and clip it to the patient's chart.
Purpose: The physician will indicate the service performed on the charge slip and return it to you.

7 Accept the returned charge slip at the end of the visit.

8 Enter the appropriate fee from the fee schedule.

9 Locate the receipt on the board with a number matching the charge slip.
Purpose: To make certain it is the correct receipt.

10 Reinsert the patient's ledger card under the receipt.

11 Write the service code number and fee on the receipt.

12 Accept the patient's payment and record the amount of payment and the new balance.
Purpose: To bring the patient's account up to date and provide a current statement for the patient.

13 Give the completed receipt to the patient.

14 Follow your agency's procedure for refilling the ledger card.

15 Repeat Steps 4 to 14 for each service of the day.

16 Total all columns of the day sheet at the end of the day.
Purpose: To determine total amount of the charges, receipts, and resulting balances for the day.

17 Write preliminary totals in pencil.
Purpose: To facilitate any necessary changes.

18 Complete proof of totals and enter totals in ink.

19 Enter figures for accounts receivable control.
Purpose: To complete daily accounting cycle.

Refunds

If a patient wishes to have an overpayment refunded, write a check for the amount due and enter the transaction on the day sheet. In most cases, the refund will result in a patient balance of zero.

CRITICAL THINKING APPLICATION

- Myra receives a phone call from a patient who says that she is due a refund, since her insurance company sent her an explanation of benefits for $654.00, and her balance was only $436. She demands an immediate refund, but Myra has not yet received the check. What should she do?
- Myra suspects that the check sent to pay on the account was an error. What should she do in this situation?

Nonsufficient Fund Checks

Sometimes, a patient sends in a check without having sufficient funds to cover it; this check is later deposited to the physician's account. The bank will return the check to

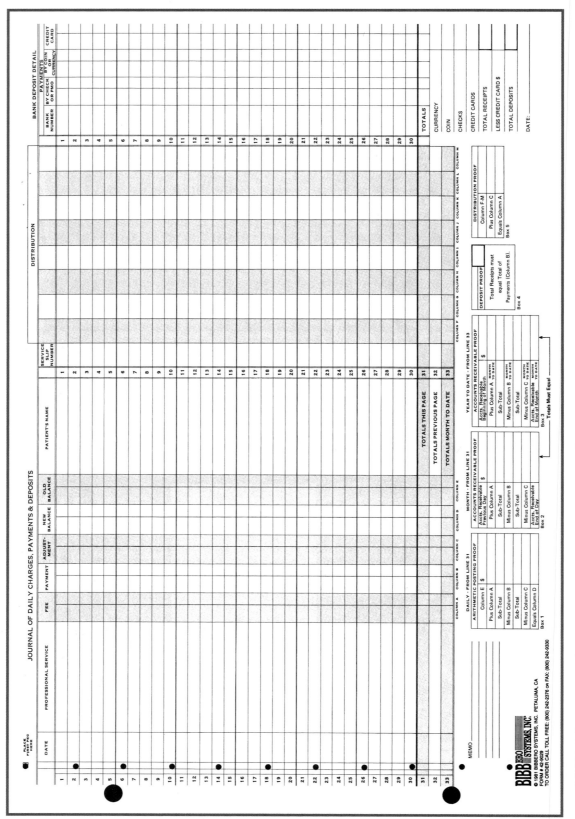

FIGURE 14-6 Sample day sheet used to log patient charges and receipts. (Courtesy Bibbero Systems, Inc., Petaluma, Calif. 94954, (800) 242-2376, www.bibbero.com.)

you marked NSF (*nonsufficient funds*). Two accounting functions must be performed. First, deduct the amount from the practice's checking account balance. Then add the amount back into the patient's account balance by entering the amount in the paid column in parentheses and increasing the balance by the same amount. Write a brief explanation of the transaction in the description column.

Balancing the Accounts Receivables and Accounts Receivables Control

The accounts receivable control is a daily summary of what remains unpaid on the accounts. Most offices also complete an end-of-day summary. These are integral parts of the office accounting system and are discussed in Chapter 23.

Paying for Medical Services and Treatment

The payment for medical services is accomplished in the following four ways:
1. Payment at the time of service
2. Internal billing when extension of credit is necessary
3. Internal insurance or other third party billing
4. Outside billing and collection assistance

Payment at the Time of Service

A large percentage of patients will have some type of health insurance for at least major items. Every practice in which there are patient visits should encourage time-of-service collection. It is especially important to collect co-payments and payment for office visits not covered by insurance. If patients get into the habit of paying their current charges before they leave the office, there are no further billing and bookkeeping expenses. If patients are informed when making an appointment that payment is expected at the time of service, they are not surprised when asked for payment at the end if the visit. Use a phrase, such as the following:

> "Your charge for today is $25.00. Will that be cash, check, or credit card?"

Many patients are hesitant to ask about charges and are unsure whether to offer to pay or to wait until asked. Make it easier for the patients by offering to accept their payments, because most people are prepared to pay small bills on a cash basis. If a patient requests to be billed, the medical assistant may say:

> "Our normal procedure is to pay at the time of service, unless other arrangements are made in advance."

Many offices accept credit cards for the convenience of their patients. **Debit cards** are now widely accepted for payment as well. Computers have made the electronic transfer of funds easy and convenient.

The medical assistant must believe that the physician and the facility have a right to charge for the services provided. Do not be embarrassed to ask for payment for the value of the service. When tact and good judgment are used in billing and collecting, patients appreciate the service they receive and the help the medical assistant provides. Give individual attention and personal consideration to each patient, and be courteous, showing a sincere desire to help the patient who has financial problems.

Billing After Extension of Credit

In some types of practice, particularly those involving large fees for surgery or long-term care, it becomes necessary to extend credit and establish a regular system of billing. This requires informing the patient of what the charges will be, what professional services these charges cover, and what the credit policy of the office is (Procedure 14-3).

Many practices do not have a true credit policy; thus each account continues to be evaluated individually. It is almost impossible to judge accounts objectively and equitably under such circumstances.

The physician and the staff should think through their situation, decide what they expect of patients with respect to payments, and how they will inform the patient. Although there will always be exceptions to any rule, there must be a rule, which should be in writing and conveyed to the patient at the outset of the relationship.

Some medical practices prepare an information booklet that includes the payment policy. New patients are given a copy of the booklet. Any patient who needs special consideration can be counseled by the medical assistant. The medical assistant who has the guidance and support of an established credit policy can perform with confidence when handling patient accounts. The credit policy must be fair and must address the following issues:
- Time when payment is due from patients
- Payment at the time of service
- Times when or if assignment of insurance benefits is accepted
- Completion of insurance forms by the office staff (or not)
- Billing procedures
- Collection protocol
- Length of time an account will be carried without payment
- Telephone collection protocol
- Use of a collection agency

PROCEDURE **14-3**

Making Credit Arrangements With a Patient

GOAL: To assist the patient in paying for services by making mutually beneficial credit arrangements according to established office policy.

EQUIPMENT AND SUPPLIES

- Patient's ledger
- Calendar
- Truth in Lending form
- Assignment of benefits form
- Patient's insurance form
- Private area for interview

PROCEDURAL STEPS

1 Answer all questions about credit thoroughly and kindly.

2 Inform the patient of the office policy regarding credit:

3 Payment at the time of first visit

4 Payment by bank card

5 Credit application
Purpose: To ensure complete understanding of mutual responsibilities.

6 Have the patient complete the credit application.
Purpose: To comply with office practices on the extension of credit.

7 Check the completed credit application.
Purpose: To confirm that all the necessary information is included.

8 Discuss with the patient the possible arrangements and ask the patient to decide which of those arrangements is most suitable.
Purpose: To ensure better compliance, which can be expected when the patient makes the choice.

9 Prepare the Truth in Lending form and have the patient sign it if the agreement requires more than four installments.
Purpose: To comply with Regulation Z.

10 Have the patient execute an assignment of insurance benefits.
Purpose: To comply with credit policy.

11 Make a copy of the patient's insurance card and have the patient sign a consent for release of the information to the insurance company.
Purpose: To ensure that a claim can be processed because consent for the release of information is necessary on most insurance forms.

12 Keep credit information confidential.

Installment Buying of Medical Services. Because installment buying is so much a part of our economic system today, the physician's office must be prepared to help patients budget for their medical care. Patients expect to use their credit resources and appreciate business-like assistance in establishing a payment plan. The medical profession has too long suffered a poor collection record because of its fear of appearing too commercial. The physician should be ready to arrange credit when medical bills will be high or when a patient for some reason is unable to pay at the time of service. In general, fees for routine office calls and small medical bills should be kept on a pay-as-you-go basis.

In recent years, companies have begun to offer credit or loans specifically for medical procedures. This is very popular for cosmetic surgeries. Offices that offer these types of procedures may wish to investigate these alternative financing services.

Truth in Lending Act. Regulation Z of the Truth in Lending Act, which is enforced by the Federal Trade Commission, requires that when there is a bilateral agreement between physician and patient to accept payment in more than four installments, the physician is required to provide disclosure of information regarding finance charges (Figure 14-7). Even if there are no finance charges

involved, the form must be completed stating this fact. The physician retains a copy of the form, and the original is given to the patient. Specific wording is required in the disclosure. Have the patient sign the agreement in your presence, because you must have proof of signing. The disclosure statement must be kept on file for 2 years. Although the disclosure statement is designed as protection for the debtor, it can be a good collection tool for the creditor.

It is recognized that physicians generally permit their patients to pay in installments, and as long as there is no specific agreement on the part of the physician for payment to be made in more than four installments and no finance charge is made, the account is not subject to the regulation. If the patient chooses to pay in installments instead of the full amount, this is considered a unilateral action. The physician, in accepting such payments, probably would not be subject to the provisions of the regulation. The physician's office, however, must be certain to bill for the full balance each time. If the statement is for only a partial payment, it then becomes a bilateral agreement and as such is subject to Regulation Z.

Helping patients budget their medical expenses is a rather new aspect of the business side of medical practice. However, it is a real service to patients and demonstrates

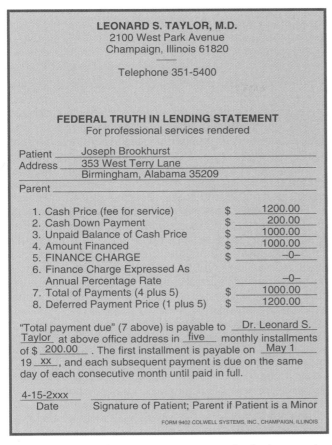

LEONARD S. TAYLOR, M.D.
2100 West Park Avenue
Champaign, Illinois 61820

Telephone 351-5400

FEDERAL TRUTH IN LENDING STATEMENT
For professional services rendered

Patient _____ Joseph Brookhurst
Address _____ 353 West Terry Lane
_____ Birmingham, Alabama 35209
Parent _____

1. Cash Price (fee for service)	$	1200.00
2. Cash Down Payment	$	200.00
3. Unpaid Balance of Cash Price	$	1000.00
4. Amount Financed	$	1000.00
5. FINANCE CHARGE	$	–0–
6. Finance Charge Expressed As Annual Percentage Rate		–0–
7. Total of Payments (4 plus 5)	$	1000.00
8. Deferred Payment Price (1 plus 5)	$	1200.00

"Total payment due" (7 above) is payable to __Dr. Leonard S.__
__Taylor__ at above office address in __five__ monthly installments
of $ __200.00__ . The first installment is payable on __May 1__
19 __XX__ , and each subsequent payment is due on the same
day of each consecutive month until paid in full.

__4-15-2xxx__
Date   Signature of Patient; Parent if Patient is a Minor

FORM 9402 COLWELL SYSTEMS, INC., CHAMPAIGN, ILLINOIS

FIGURE 14-7   Disclosure statement. An example of a document for compliance with the Federal Truth in Lending Act. (Courtesy Colwell Systems, Inc., Champaign, Illinois.)

that the physician and the office staff are sincerely anxious to help patients pay their own way. It may also prevent many collection problems.

Confidentiality

Obtaining Credit Information. Credit information is confidential. It should be guarded as carefully as a confidential medical history and should be disclosed to no one. When asking for credit information from patients in the office, do so in a private area where others cannot overhear the conversation. A desk or table away from the reception area where a patient can sit in total privacy and complete a credit application is a great asset. Credit information is personal—it should be kept that way.

Credit Bureaus. Some physicians join a credit bureau, particularly in large cities where it is more difficult to gauge informally the patients' ability to pay. Credit bureaus gather credit information from many sources, pool it, and make it available to dues-paying bureau members. If the office receives a request for credit information about a patient, it is permissible to furnish it because the debtor, by giving the physician's name as a reference, has given implied consent; otherwise, the credit bureau would not have contacted the office. According to the Fair Credit Practices Act Amendments of 1975, the following information only can be given:

- When the account was opened
- How much the patient now owes

- What the highest amount of the account is at any time

You should avoid any reference to the following:
- Character
- Paying habits
- Credit rating

Billing Insurance or Other Third Parties

Insurance billing in the medical office is a courtesy to patients. Often, patients do not understand the policies and appreciate the assistance given by the medical office. Information on completing insurance forms and diagnostic and procedure coding is found in Chapters 15 through 18.

Independent Billing and Collection Services

Many healthcare facilities find it advantageous to refer their billing and collections to an independent billing service. The information related to services and fees is sent to the billing service on a daily or weekly basis. The servicing agent then handles all billing and collections, as well as any telephone inquiries. This system frees the regular office staff for more patient-oriented duties. An added advantage is that a person who is not connected with the patient care on a personal basis handles any dispute that may arise.

Internal Billing by the Account Manager

Billing Methods

In a practice with only a moderate number of accounts, the medical assistant handles the preparation and mailing of statements. This may be accomplished by using the following:
- A computer-generated statement
- An encounter form
- A typewritten statement
- A photocopied statement

The appearance of the statement carries a visual impact just as a letter does, so the statement heads should be carefully chosen and the typing clean and accurate. Statement heads are usually imprinted with the same information as the physician's letterhead. They should be of good quality and large enough to allow itemization of charges. Envelopes should be imprinted with *Address Correction Requested* under the return address to maintain up-to-date mailing lists. A self-addressed return envelope included with the statement encourages prompt payment. This is mainly for the convenience of patients who do not always have stationery available for sending a return payment or who are less likely to return a payment immediately if they must address an envelope.

Computer-Generated Statement. Patient accounts are generated and stored in the computer, and a statement can be produced whenever needed. The statement can show the service rendered on each date, the charge for each service, the date on which a claim was submitted to the insurance company, the date of payment, and the balance due from the patient. The computer may also be programmed to print messages on the statement, such as *Balance now 30 days past due* or a selection of other messages.

Encounter Form as a Bill. There are variations in style, but encounter forms are usually personalized for the practice. The form has space for all the elements required in submitting medical insurance claims, such as the following:

- Name and address of the patient
- Name of the insurance carrier
- Insurance identification number
- Brief description of each service by code number
- Fee for each service
- Place and date of service
- Diagnosis
- Physician's name and address
- Physician's signature

The encounter form can be used as a charge slip for office treatments if the physician checks the services performed at the completion of the visit and asks the patient to hand it to the medical assistant when leaving. Either the physician or the medical assistant may write in the amount of the fee. If a payment is made, it can be so indicated. Instructions to the patient for filing insurance claims are on the bottom left.

Statements. Statements must be correct and must include the patient's name and address as well as the balance owed. If statements are photocopied or microfilmed, special care must be taken that the ledger card is correct because it will be duplicated in the billing process.

Typewritten Statements. The use of continuous-form billing statements is a timesaver. The statements are printed in a roll with perforated edges for separation. The roll is fed into the typewriter for the first statement and remains until the last statement is typed, eliminating the time and energy necessary for inserting and removing each statement form from the typewriter.

Photocopied Statements. Coordinated ledger cards and copy paper are used in preparing photocopied statements. A perfect statement is ready for mailing in minimal time. Extra care must be used in posting the ledgers. A black pen should be used in making entries on the ledger card, because other ink colors do not reproduce well. Writing must be clear and legible. No personal notes should be made on the ledger cards unless there is something you wish conveyed to the patient. (It is possible to buy pencils with nonreproducible lead if you believe this is necessary for making collection entries.) Usually, a window envelope is used for mailing, which means that the name and address on the ledger must be neat, correct, and positioned correctly for the envelope window.

Internal Billing Procedures

Itemizing the First Statement. If the medical fee has been explained in advance, the monthly statement is merely a confirmation of what is owed, and there should be no misunderstanding. However, it is good business practice—and a courtesy to the patient—to

itemize the charges. This is essential if the statement is to be used for billing the patient's insurance. Patients are entitled to an understanding of the physician's statement for medical services.

Itemizing statements is not difficult, and computerized statements usually automatically itemize the first statement. The simplest method is merely to allow space on the original statement, below the *For Professional Services* line, on which to list the separate charges for office visits, hospital calls, or treatments or tests performed in the medical facility.

Many physicians have devised their own itemized encounter forms, which are given to the patient when payment is made at the time of service or later mailed in a combination statement-reply envelope. The use of such charge slips simplifies the itemization procedure, because filling out the slips is usually just a matter of checking the procedures listed. Although the itemization of bills may seem tedious, the medical assistant will spend less time in explaining services provided, clearing up misunderstandings with patients, and following up on delinquent accounts by itemizing.

CRITICAL THINKING APPLICATION

Mrs. Deaton is frustrated because she claims she was never sent an itemized statement and now refuses to pay her account. Myra feels that this is a delay tactic, because she specifically recalls sending an itemized statement to the patient. How can this situation be remedied?

Time and Frequency of Billing

A regular system of mailing statements should be put into operation. Most people expect to receive statements from their creditors, and they plan their budgets around first-of-the-month bills received. Punctuality in billing encourages prompt payment.

Statements should be sent at least once each month. Some offices send bills immediately after treatment; others bill all patients on the same day each month. Mailing statements twice a month (e.g., half of the accounts on the tenth and the remaining half on the twenty-fifth) is also a common practice.

Once-a-Month Billing. If a monthly pattern is followed, bills should leave the office in time to reach the patient no later than the last day of each month and preferably before the twenty-fifth of the month. Planning ahead for the preparation of statements can lighten the burden of once-a-month billing (Procedure 14-4). The statement can be prepared at the time of service, postdated, and mailed at the end of the month.

Cycle Billing. Many physicians prefer to use the cycle billing system, which calls for the billing of certain portions of the accounts receivable at given times during the month instead of preparing all statements at the end of each month. Cycle billing is used in large businesses such as department stores, banks, and utility companies. Its many advantages include avoiding once-a-

PROCEDURE 14-4

Preparing Monthly Billing Statements

GOAL: To process monthly statements and evaluate accounts for collection procedures in accordance with the agency's credit policy.

EQUIPMENT AND SUPPLIES

- Typewriter or computer
- Patient accounts
- Agency's credit policy
- Statement forms

PROCEDURAL STEPS

1 Assemble all accounts that have outstanding balances.

2 Separate accounts that need special attention in accordance with the agency's credit policy.
  Explanation: Routine statements should be prepared first, after which special attention can be given to delinquent accounts.

3 Prepare routine statements, including the following:

- Date the statement is prepared
- Name and address of the person responsible for payment
- Name of the patient, if different from the person responsible for payment
- Itemization of dates, services, and charges for the month
- Any unpaid balance carried forward (may or may not be itemized, depending on office policy)

4 Determine the action to be taken on accounts separated in Step 2.

5 Make a note of the necessary action on the ledger card (telephone call, collection letter series, small claims court, or assignment of collection agency).
  Purpose: To be used for guidance in executing an action and for later follow-up when necessary.

---

month peak workloads and stabilizing the cash flow. In a small office in which billing is done only once a month, the unexpected illness or absence of the medical assistant for any emergency can leave the physician in a financial bind if the statements do not go out.

The accounts are separated into fairly equal divisions, the number of divisions depending on how many times billing will be done during a month. For example, if the office expects to bill twice per month, divide the accounts into 2 equal groups; for weekly billing, divide into 4 groups, and for daily billing, divide into 20 groups.

Small alphabetical groups can be combined to keep the divisions nearly equal in the number of statements to prepare on each billing day. If the files are color coded, the medical assistant may wish to use the same alphabetical breakdown in billing. Regardless of constant changes in the individual accounts, the mailing dates for accounts in each section remain the same. A schedule for processing and mailing is thus established, and the workload is apportioned throughout the entire month.

Cycle billing allows the medical assistant to continue all routine duties each day, handling the statements on a day-to-day or weekly schedule rather than in one intensive period at the end of the month. This means that whole days need not be sacrificed from other duties to get statements in the mail. When the billing is spaced throughout the month, more time and consideration can be given to each statement, the itemization of bills is less burdensome, and the likelihood of error is decreased.

Patients generally accept the cycle billing system quickly, often with enthusiasm. However, if your office decides to change from a once-a-month billing system to a cycle billing system, patients should be notified in advance, and the new plan should be explained to them. To explain the new system to established patients, enclose a notice in each statement for 2 months before the transfer, describing the plan and indicating the future dates on which each patient will receive the bill.

Before a physician adopts the cycle billing system, particularly in a small community, several factors should be taken into consideration, such as the following:

- What is the general income level of the community, and how and when does the average patient get paid?
- Do local companies pay employees at various times during the month, or are most paychecks handed out at the beginning of the month?
- Would cycle billing benefit patients as well as the overall operation of the office?

Billing Third Party Payors. Collection problems may arise if the medical assistant fails to get the necessary insurance information, particularly Medicare and Medicaid information. In some instances, if the insurance forms are not completed correctly, the claim may be denied because of minor infractions such as failing to name the responsible party or omitting Social Security information, the policy number, or the group number.

Time limits must also be observed in billing third party payors. In cases of Medicare patients with a terminal illness, it may be best to accept assignment of benefits. If the physician does not take assignment, he or she may receive nothing because the family is not obligated to pay, and Medicare will not pay after a certain time or if the claim has not been correctly filed.

Billing Minors. Minors cannot be held responsible for payment of a bill unless they are emancipated. Bills for minors must be addressed to a parent or legal guardian. If a bill is addressed to a minor, the parent or parents could take the attitude that they are not responsible because they never received the bill.

If the parents are separated or divorced, the parent who brings the child in for treatment is responsible for payment. Whatever financial agreement exists between the parents is strictly their personal business and should not concern the medical office. The responsible parent should be so informed from the beginning.

If a minor appears in the office and requests treatment and you can ascertain that the person is legally emancipated, the minor is responsible for the bill. It may be wise to make a determination either with the business manager or with the physician as to whether your office wishes to treat this emancipated minor.

Care for Those Who Cannot Pay

The medical profession has traditionally accepted the responsibility of providing medical care for individuals unable to pay for these services. In spite of the increased scope of government-sponsored care for the **medically indigent**, physicians still donate thousands of dollars' worth of such medical services each year.

In many instances, medical care of the indigent is available through social service agencies. The medical assistant should learn about any local organizations and agencies that can aid the patient in obtaining the necessary assistance. The physician can provide only medical services. Other agencies must provide hospitalization, for example, or arrange for paying the costs of special therapy, rehabilitation, or medications. Unfortunately, there is still another segment of the population that consists of uninsured employees who are not eligible for public assistance, are not covered under a group policy, and cannot afford the high premiums for private medical insurance. Special attention must be given to helping these people arrange to pay their medical bills.

If a physician accepts a case for which a fee will not be paid, complete records must still be kept on the patient. The only deviation in procedure is that the financial record indicates no charge (n/c) in the debit column.

Fees in Hardship Cases

Sometimes a physician is faced with the problem of deciding whether to reduce or cancel a fee in a hardship case. Before adjusting or canceling a fee, the physician or the medical assistant should engage in a frank discussion of the patient's financial situation. Find out whether the patient is entitled to an insurance settlement of some kind. For instance, if the patient's injuries are the result of a car accident, there may be insurance through the automobile policy. Circumstances may qualify the patient for local or state public assistance, such as crime victim

assistance. If so, the assistant may direct the patient to the appropriate agency.

If the circumstances of hardship are known before the services are rendered, thorough discussion of what the fee will be and how it will be paid should take place at that time. The physician may suggest that a medically indigent patient seek care at a county hospital with public assistance. A physician should be free to choose his or her form of charity and not feel obligated to substantially reduce or cancel a fee when the circumstances are known in advance.

After the physician and patient have agreed on a fee, special circumstances may arise that create a hardship. If the physician then agrees to reduce the fee, the patient should be told that the reduction will be effective only after the adjusted amount is paid in full. For instance, if a fee of $500 is reduced to $350, the full amount of the $500 charge should appear on the ledger and when $350 has been received the remainder can be written off as an adjustment.

Pitfalls of Fee Adjustments

When a physician begins to reduce his or her fees, problems can arise. Patients may begin to expect that fees will be reduced in all circumstances. Patients may even doubt the competency of a physician who habitually reduces fees.

Great care should be taken in reducing the fee for care of a patient who dies. The physician's sympathy is with the family in such instances, but the physician's generosity in reducing a fee could be misinterpreted and result in a suit for malpractice. The family may suspect that the fee was reduced because the physician knows he or she made an error.

If the physician agrees to settle for a reduced fee in a situation in which the patient is disputing the fee, care should be taken to make certain the negotiations are without prejudice. By taking this precaution, the physician protects the right to collect the original sum should the patient refuse to pay the lowered fee. The offer of a discount therefore should be made in writing, with the insertion of the words "without prejudice" and a definite time limit for making payment stated. Prepare two copies of the agreement and have the signatures witnessed. Keep the original for the physician and give a copy to the patient.

A fee should never be reduced on the basis of a poor result or as a means of obtaining payment to avoid the use of a collection agency. A reduction for these reasons degrades the physician and the practice of medicine.

Professional Courtesy

Traditionally, physicians do not charge professional colleagues or their immediate dependents for medical care. Although the concept of **professional courtesy** is often attributed to Hippocrates, the foundations of professional courtesy today are derived from Thomas Percival's Code of 1803.

In some cases, giving professional courtesy represents the loss of a large amount of potential income. If there is a substantial outlay in the cost of materials, the professional colleague will probably wish to reimburse the physician for the materials used. Most physicians today subscribe to a health insurance plan. If the care they receive is covered by insurance, it is entirely ethical for the attending physician to accept the insurance benefits in payment for services.

If the services are frequent enough to involve a significant portion of the physician's professional time or if they extend over a long time, the physician may wish to charge on an adjusted basis. When professional courtesy has been offered and the recipient still insists on paying, the physician need not hesitate on ethical grounds to accept a fee for service.

Professional courtesy is often extended beyond fellow physicians and their dependents. Most physicians treat their own medical assistants, and often their families, without charge and grant discounts to nurses and medical assistants not in their direct employ. Student externs should never expect to be treated while serving in an externship capacity. Professional courtesy is sometimes extended to others in the healthcare field (e.g., pharmacists and dentists).

CRITICAL THINKING APPLICATION

Dr. Franklin has just finished seeing Dr. Wallace as a patient and insists to Myra that Dr. Wallace always extends him professional courtesy. This is not indicated on the ledger card, since several payments are shown on the record. Dr. Wallace has just left the office and is in an important meeting at the hospital. What should Myra do?

Collection Techniques

Sometimes, it becomes necessary to aggressively attempt to collect the balances that patients owe the physician (Procedure 14-5). Persuasive collection procedures include telephone calls, collection reminders and letters, and personal interviews.

Telephone Collection Calls

A telephone call at the right time, in the right manner, will be more successful than notes, a statement, or a collection letter. The personal contact of a telephone call will bring in more money than if a call is not made. In the absence of time to make calls, the collection letter is the next best avenue. If collections are a serious problem, it may pay to hire an extra person to do the telephoning. Written notification is a must before making a final demand for payment indicating that legal or collection proceedings will be started. There are no hard and fast rules for pursuing collections by telephone. Each case should be handled individually on the basis of the experience with the person involved.

GENERAL RULES TO FOLLOW IN TELEPHONE COLLECTIONS

What To Do

- Call the patient when it can be done with privacy.
- Call between 8 AM and 9 PM.
- Determine the identity of the persons with whom you are speaking. If you ask, "Is this Mrs. Noble?" and she answers, "Yes," it could be the patient's mother-in-law or daughter-in-law, who is also "Mrs. Noble." Use the person's full name.
- Be dignified and respectful. One can be friendly and formal at the same time.
- Ask the patient if it is a convenient time to talk. Unless you have the attention of the called party, there is little to be gained by continuing. If told that it is an inopportune time, ask for a specific time to call back, or get a promise for the patient to call the office at a specified time.
- After a brief greeting, state the purpose of the call. Make no apology for calling, but state the reason in a friendly, business-like way. The physician expects payment and the medical assistant is interested in helping the patient meet the financial obligation. Open the call with a phrase such as, "This is Alice, Dr. Wallace's financial secretary. I'm calling about your account." A well-placed pause at this point in the call sometimes gets an immediate response from the debtor in regard to the nonpayment.
- Assume a positive attitude. For example, convey the impression that the patient intended to pay and it is only a matter of working out some suitable arrangements.
- Keep the conversation brief and to the point, and avoid threats of any kind.
- Try to get a definite commitment—payment of a certain amount by a certain date.
- Follow up on promises. This is best accomplished by a tickler file or a note on the calendar. If the payment does not arrive by the promised date, remind the patient with another call. If the medical assistant fails to do this, the whole effort has been wasted.

What Not To Do

- Do not call between 9 PM and 8 AM. To do so may be considered harassment.
- Do not make repeated telephone calls.
- Do not call the debtor's place of work if the employer prohibits personal calls.
- If a call is placed to the debtor at work and the person cannot take the call, leave a

---

GENERAL RULES TO FOLLOW IN TELEPHONE COLLECTIONS—Cont'd

message asking the debtor to "call Mrs. Black at 727-9238" without revealing the nature of the call; that is, do not state that the call is from "Dr. Wallace's office" or "Dr. Jones's medical assistant."

• Do not show hostility. An angry patient is a poor-paying patient. Insulted patients often do not pay at all.

Collection Letters or Reminders

Some consultants believe that a printed collection letter or reminder enclosed with a statement is more effective than a personal letter. Their attitude is that a patient may be embarrassed by a personal letter and feel that he or she has been singled out for attention. An impersonal printed message will probably encourage the debtor to send a payment. The printed form is a time saver and is recommended if a lack of time is contributing to poor collection follow-up. Standard printed forms are readily available, and the medical assistant can also design original forms.

Letters that are friendly requests for an explanation of why payment has not been made are still effective in

---

PROCEDURE 14-5

Aging Accounts Receivables

GOAL: To determine the age of accounts and decide what collection activity is needed.

EQUIPMENT AND SUPPLIES

• Patient ledger cards with a balance due
• Pen
• Computer
• Calculator

PROCEDURAL STEPS

1 Prompt the computer to compile a report on the age of accounts receivable. Many programs will have this report option that can be easily accessed.
Purpose: To determine which accounts have a balance due.

2 Divide the accounts into categories as listed below:
• 0–30 days old
• 30–60 days old
• 60–90 days old
• 90–120 days old
• Over 120 days old
Purpose: To determine how old the various accounts are and place the accounts into categories as to when the last payment was made.

3 If the computer program does not perform this function, manually pull all ledger cards that have a balance due and divide them into the categories listed above.

4 Examine the accounts to see which are awaiting an insurance payment. Action need not be taken if an insurance payment is expected and is not long overdue. Return those ledgers to the ledger tray.
Purpose: To avoid collection activity on accounts for which a payment is expected.

5 Follow the office procedure for collections on the accounts left. Collection reminder stickers may

be placed on the statements sent to the patient, or a collection letter may be sent. Be sure that the stickers are inside the envelope, not on the outside.
Purpose: To prompt the patient to make a payment by pointing out the age of the account.

6 Call patients whose accounts are over 90 days old. Attempt to make payment arrangements with the patient.
Purpose: To attempt to collect from the patient or determine why the patient has not yet paid the account.

7 Send a collection letter to patients whose accounts are over 120 days old, if indicated, to encourage the patient to pay the account. If it is the office policy, mention that the account is in danger of being sent to a collection agency.
Purpose: To reach patients who are not available by telephone.

8 Add the total accounts receivable for each category and arrive at a figure outstanding for each. The physician may wish to have a report weekly or monthly on these figures.
Purpose: To have a current accounting of the amounts owed to the physician, and to double check the amount outstanding according to the pegboard system or computer software system.

9 Note any arrangements made with patients regarding payment of the accounts in the chart and/or on the ledger. Send a follow-up letter to remind the patients of their payment agreements.
Purpose: To document arrangements made and remind the patients of their obligation and promise to pay.

many cases. These letters should indicate that the physician is sincerely interested in the patient and wishes to help straighten out the financial obligations. The patient should be invited to visit the office to explain the reasons for nonpayment so that, if possible, special arrangements can be worked out. To give the patient an opportunity to save face, these letters can suggest that the patient may have overlooked previous statements.

On receipt of such a letter, most patients make some effort to explain their failure to make payment. If a patient really is having financial difficulties, the physician may be able to get public assistance for him or her. If it is a temporary financial embarrassment, the physician and the patient may together be able to work out a satisfactory installment plan for payment.

The medical assistant often is given a free hand in designing collection patterns and composing collection letters. Many medical assistants compose a series of collection letters, using model letters that they have found to be effective (Figure 14-8). Such a series usually includes at least five letters in varying degrees of forcefulness.

Sometimes, even the person with poor paying habits will pay the bill if treated with respect and consideration. The medical assistant should never go beyond the authority granted by the physician in pursuing collections. If there are questions about special collection problems, always check with the physician before proceeding. This is particularly important with patients whom you do not know personally (e.g., patients who the physician has seen in the hospital or at home and patients with no credit history). It is difficult to say whether pressing collections too hard loses more good will of patients than not pursuing collections diligently enough. The physician and the medical assistant together should agree on general collection policies as outlined earlier in this chapter, and then the policies should be followed. In all cases in which an account is to be assigned to a collection agency, be certain that the physician is aware of it.

Signing Collection Letters. In most medical offices, the medical assistant signs collection letters with the identification "Assistant to Dr. Brown" or "Financial Secretary" below the typewritten signature. Some physi-

---

1. Your account has always been paid promptly in the past, so this must be an oversight. Please accept this note as a friendly reminder of your account due in the amount of $ _____ .

2. Since your care in this office in March, we have had no word from you in regard to how you are feeling or your account due. If it is impossible for you to pay the full amount of $ _____ at this time, please call this office before June 15 so that satisfactory arrangements can be worked out.

3. Medical bills are payable at the time of service unless special credit arrangements are made. Please send your check in full or call this office before June 30.

4. If you have some question about your statement, we will be happy to answer it for you. If not, may we have a payment before the end of this month?

5. Unless some definite arrangement is made to reduce your balance of $ _____ , we can no longer carry your account on our books. Delinquent accounts are turned over to our collection agency on the 25th of the month.

6. **When a payment plan has been established, it can be reinforced by recognizing the first remittance with a letter of acknowledgment:**

   Thank you for the recent payment of $ _____ on your account. We are glad to cooperate with you in this arrangement for clearing your account. We will look for your next check at about the same time next month, and your final payment the following month.

7. **When a payment schedule has been arranged by a telephone call, it can be confirmed by letter.**

   As agreed upon in our telephone conversation today, we will expect you to mail a payment of $50 on February 10; $50 on March 10; and the balance on April 10. If some emergency should prevent your making one of these payments on time, please notify us immediately by telephone.

DO'S AND DON'TS

DO:

1. Individualize letters to suit the situation.

2. Design your early letters as mere reminders of debt.

3. Always imply that the patient has good intentions to pay, until lack of response over a period of time proves otherwise.

4. Send letters with a firmer tone only after you have sent one or two friendly reminders.

DON'T

1. Use the same collection letter for a patient with good paying habits as for one who is known to neglect financial obligations.

2. Place an overdue notice of any kind on a postcard or on the outside of an envelope. This is an **invasion of privacy.**

FIGURE 14-8 Suggestions for composing collection letters. Brief collection letters that ask patients to explain the lack of payment are often effective.

cians may wish to personally sign these communications, but generally the medical assistant who handles the accounts also signs the collection letters.

Personal Interviews

Personal interviews with patients can sometimes be more effective than a whole series of collection letters. By talking to a patient face to face, the medical assistant can come to an understanding of the problem more quickly and reach an agreement about future payment plans.

Occasionally, a patient may undergo a long course of treatment and yet make no attempt to pay anything on account. Perhaps such a patient is only waiting for the physician or the medical assistant to suggest that a payment be made. When there is advance knowledge that the patient will require extensive treatment, the matter of payment should be discussed early in the course of treatment, the credit policy explained, and some agreement reached as to a payment plan.

Because the fee for medical services is far more intangible than that of any commercial account, collection efforts must not be delayed too long. Any responsible, sincere patient will call or write the physician's office after receiving a second statement and explain the delay in payment or ask for a payment plan.

If it becomes necessary to refer the account to a collector, a good agency should have a 35% to 40% recovery rate with an account that is assigned within 4 or 5 months. This may drop to 25% if the account is held only a few more months. If recovery by the agency is greater than 40%, it may indicate that the collection effort by the medical assistant needs to be intensified.

The value of medical accounts diminishes in direct proportion to the length of time that has elapsed since service was rendered. Do not fight the law of diminishing returns. All collection activity is costly. Know when to stop and call on the services of a professional agency.

Special Collection Situations

Tracing "Skips." When a statement is returned marked *Moved—no forwarding address*, you may consider this account as a "skip." This generally is accepted as an indication that the patient is attempting to avoid liability for debts. Some so-called skips are innocent errors. The person may have been careless in not leaving a forwarding address, or the mistake may have occurred in the physician's office; the wrong name or address may have been placed on the statement. However, immediate action should be taken in regard to returned statements. Do not wait until the next billing time to attempt to trace the debtor.

SUGGESTIONS FOR TRACING SKIPS

- Examine the patient's original office registration card.
- Call the telephone number listed on the card. Occasionally a patient may move without leaving a forwarding address but will transfer the old telephone number. The new telephone number may be given when you call the old number.
- If you are unable to contact the individual by telephone, make a few discreet calls to the references listed on the registration card to get leads.
- Check the Internet to secure the names and telephone numbers of neighbors or the landlord, and contact these people to secure information about the debtor's whereabouts.
- Do not inform a third party that the person owes you money. Simply state that you are trying to locate or verify the location of the individual.
- Check the debtor's place of employment for information. If the person is a specialist in his or her field of work, the local union or similar organizations may be contacted. Although they may not give you the person's current address, they will relay the message that you are seeking to contact him or her. Often, people will be stirred into paying a bill if they think that their employer may learn of their payment failure.
- Do not communicate with a third party more than once. This is specifically forbidden by law (Public Law 95-109, Sec. 804) unless the third party requests the collector to do so.

The tracing of skips is a challenge to any medical assistant. A certified letter can be sent; by paying additional fees, you can ask the Postal Service to obtain a receipt including the address where the letter was delivered. The certified letter may be sent in a plain envelope so that the patient will not refuse to accept the letter because of the return address.

If all attempts fail, turn the account over to a collection agency without delay. Do not keep a skip account too long, because the trail may become so cold as time elapses that even collection experts will be unable to follow it.

Claims Against Estates. A bill owed by a deceased patient may be handled a little differently than regular bills. Courtesy dictates that a bill not be sent during the initial period of bereavement, but do not delay more than 30 days. The person responsible for settling the affairs of the estate will be assembling outstanding accounts and will expect to receive the medical bills along with all others. Address the statement using the following:

Estate of (name of patient)
c/o (spouse or next of kin, if known)
Patient's last known address

Do not address the statement to a relative unless you have a signed agreement that that person will be responsible. If for some reason the statement cannot be addressed as just suggested (e.g., if the patient was in a convalescent home and there is no name of a relative), seek information from the county seat in the county in which the estate is being settled.

A will is generally filed within 30 days of a death. A request to the Probate Department of the Superior Court, County Recorder's Office, will usually provide the name of the executor or administrator. The time limits for filing an estate claim are determined by the state in which the decedent resided.

After the name of the administrator or executor of the estate has been obtained, a duplicate itemized statement of the account should be sent to that person by certified mail, return receipt requested. If no response is received in 10 days, contact the executor or the county clerk where the estate is being settled and obtain forms for filing a claim against the estate. (Some states do not have special claim forms but will accept simple itemized statements.) This claim against the estate must be made within a certain length of time, varying from 2 to 36 months, depending on the state in which it is filed.

The executor of the estate will either accept or reject the claim and if it is accepted, will send an acknowledgment of the debt. Payment is often delayed because of the legal complications in settling an estate, but if the claim has been accepted, you will receive your money in due time. If the claim is rejected and there is full justification for claiming the bill, file a claim against the executor within a limited time, according to state laws. The time limit in such cases starts with the date on the letter of rejection that was sent in response to the original claim.

Because states have different time limits and statutes in regard to such matters, it is advisable for the medical assistant to contact the physician's attorney or the local court for the exact procedure to follow.

Bankruptcy. Bankruptcy laws were passed to secure equal distribution of the assets of an individual among the individual's creditors. Bankruptcy laws are federal and are applicable in all states. When notified that a patient has declared bankruptcy, do not send statements or make any attempt to collect on the account from the patient.

Chapter VII bankruptcy is usually a "no asset" situation. Because the physician's fee is an unsecured debt, there is little purpose in pursuing collection. Chapter XIII is known as *wage-earner bankruptcy*. Under Chapter XIII, the patient/debtor pays a fixed amount (agreed on by the court) to the trustee in bankruptcy. This is then passed on to the creditors. During this period, none of the creditors can attach the debtor's wages or otherwise attempt to collect the debt. It is sometimes beneficial to file a claim under Chapter XIII because small payments will be made by the debtor under the supervision of the court over a period of 3 years.

Using Outside Collection Assistance

When everything possible has been done internally to follow up on an outstanding account and the office has not received payment, the question arises as to what step to take next, as follows:

- Should the facility sue for the payment?
- Should the account be sent to a collection agency?
- Should the account be written off as a bad debt?

Before forcing an account, first consider the time element: Has the patient been given a fair chance to pay this bill? Have statements been sent regularly and used a systematic method of following the account? Ask if there might be a misunderstanding about the fee charged. Was the first statement fully itemized? A large unexplained bill may frighten a patient into making no payments at all because the whole balance looks too large.

If the correct registration forms to secure advance credit information were used, the medical assistant should know the financial abilities of the patient to pay. However, illness may have caused a loss of salary and resulted in temporary inability to pay. Try to thoroughly analyze the situation.

Could the patient have been dissatisfied with the care received? For some unknown reason, a patient may feel that he or she was not treated correctly. Perhaps the patient expected a complete cure too soon. Only an explanation of the condition, prognosis, and care can enlighten such patients, and this is best handled by the physician. If payment of a bill is pressed too hard and the patient is dissatisfied for some reason, a malpractice suit may be filed by the patient to seek retribution against the physician. The court can approve a period longer than 3 years in special cases, but cannot approve a period longer than 5 years.

Collecting Through the Court System

Making the Decision to Sue. Will a physician lose more good will by suing for a bill than by writing it off as a loss? One management official has related that, strangely enough, when a physician-client sued two patients for large amounts, the patients lost the cases, paid up, and were back in the office for treatment very shortly! However, most physicians believe it is unwise to resort to the court to collect medical bills unless there are extraordinary circumstances.

An account must be considered a 100% loss to the physician before legal proceedings are started. Remember to never threaten to **instigate** legal proceedings unless prepared to carry out the threat and have the physician's consent to issue such a warning. If the physician decides in favor of a lawsuit, investigate thoroughly before taking action. Litigation to collect a bill is generally in order when the following occur:

- The patient can afford to pay without hardship.
- The physician can produce office records that support the bill.
- The physician can justify the amount of the bill by comparing it with fee practices in the community.
- The patient's general condition after treatment is satisfactory.
- The persuasive powers of an ethical collection agency have been exhausted and the agency advises suing.
- The patient can be given ample warning of the physician's intention to sue.

- The defendant (whether a patient or a parent or legal guardian) is legally liable for the services rendered to the patient.
- The statute of limitations has ruled out any possible malpractice action.
- The physician is not bubbling over with indignation and is not in a negative frame of mind.

Small Claims Court. Many medical practices find the small claims court a satisfactory and inexpensive way to collect delinquent accounts. The law places a limit on the amount of debt for which relief may be sought in the small claims court. Because this varies from state to state (from $300 to $5000) and in some instances even within a state, this limit should be checked locally before seeking recovery in this manner.

Parties to small claims actions cannot be represented by an attorney at the trial but may send another person to court in their behalf to produce records supporting the claim. Physicians often send their bookkeeper or medical assistant with records of unpaid accounts to show the judge.

If the court awards a judgment for the amount owed, the plaintiff in small claims court may also recover the costs of the suit. For a very small investment in time and money, the physician who uses this method has done the following:

- Saved the time of a regular court action
- Had no attorney's fee to pay
- Not sacrificed the commission charged by a collection agency

After being awarded a judgment, the medical assistant must still collect the money. The only person in a small claims action who has the right of appeal is the defendant. An appeal by the defendant may have the judgment set aside. The plaintiff cannot file an appeal in a small claims action; the decision of the court is final.

The necessary papers for filing action and full instructions on the course to follow may be obtained from the clerk of the small claims court. The medical assistant who has never appeared in the court would probably be wise to attend once as a spectator to preview the procedure and feel more at ease when appearing for the physician.

A collection agency to which an account may have been assigned may not file or handle a small claims action. It must either sue in the regular municipal or justice court or attempt to collect the debt in some other manner.

Using a Collection Agency

The medical assistant should try every means possible to collect accounts before they become delinquent. As soon as the account is determined *uncollectible* through the office (i.e., the patient has failed to respond to the final letter or has failed to fulfill a second promise on payment), send the account to the collector without delay. Skips should be assigned immediately.

Even though collection by an agency will mean sacrificing from 40% to 60% of the amount owed, further delay will only reduce the chances of recovery by the professional collector. If the agency finds that the case

deserves special consideration, it will seek the physician's advice before proceeding further.

Selecting a Collection Agency. There are a number of agencies either owned and operated as an integral part of the county medical society or operated separately from the medical society but supervised by the medical profession. These bureaus provide specialized medical collection services.

Another type of collection agency is a division of the local credit association, recognized by the National Retail Credit Association. If the local credit association does not maintain a collection department, it will be able to recommend a reputable one. A nationally recognized credit association has considerable responsibility and a high standard to maintain. These factors serve as monitors to its reliability.

The most common type of collection agency throughout the United States is the privately owned and operated agency. Many of these work with the local professional societies and strive to keep their work on a high ethical standard. Because a few bureaus are unethical and unscrupulous in their tactics, care should be taken to be sure that the one chosen is reliable and ethical. For the sake of comparison, many healthcare facilities use two or three agencies.

Responsibilities to the Collection Agency. When a reputable agency is selected, the medical assistant must be prepared to provide the agency with all the necessary data to enable it to begin prompt collection procedures on overdue accounts. The agency should receive the following:

- Full name of the debtor
- Name of the spouse
- Last known address
- Full amount of the debt
- Date of the last entry on account (debit or credit)
- Occupation of the debtor
- Business address
- Any other pertinent data

After an account has been released to a collection agency, the office makes no further collection attempts. Once the agency has begun its work, adhere to the following guidelines and procedures:

1. Send no more statements.
2. Mark the patient's ledger or stamp it so that everyone will know it is now in the hands of the collector.

3. Refer the patient to the collection agency if he or she contacts the office in regard to the account.

4. Promptly report any payments made directly to your office (a percentage of this payment is due the agency).

5. Call the agency if any information is obtained that will be of value in tracing or collecting the account.

6. Do not push the agency with frequent calls. The representatives of the agency will report regularly and will keep the office posted on collection progress.

Collection Agency Payments. If a patient sends a payment after the account has been turned over to a collection agency, the amount will need to be adjusted on the patient ledger. The collection agency will be due a percentage of the payment.

Closing Comments

Billing and collecting are critical duties in the medical office, and a responsible medical assistant is a great asset in this important area. Always maintain a positive attitude with the patients and guarantors. Remember that those who are ill or facing challenges are not always at their best and may not respond in a positive way to calls regarding their accounts. Make every attempt to work with each patient to develop a workable plan to clear their accounts.

Patient Education

Most patients are unaware of the actual coverage they have through their insurance policies. The medical assistant should encourage patients to read the entire policy so that they become familiar with its limitations and exclusions. Tell patients that when calling the company with questions, they should always write down the date, time, and name of the person with whom they spoke. Using email is helpful, because a record of the correspondence can be easily saved or printed. It is well worth the effort to make sure that patients have a general understanding of their health insurance coverage.

Often, patients do not dispute or question the company when a claim is rejected or not paid in the expected amount. Encourage them to call the company and question rejections if they do not understand why the claim was denied. Patients are paying for coverage and they should receive all of the benefits to which they are entitled.

Patients appreciate receiving an office-policy brochure or booklet that informs them about payment and credit options. The patient can use the printed booklet as a reference whenever questions arise, and its regular use by most patients will reduce the number of calls made to the office. Encourage patients to use the booklet. Helpful phone numbers or extensions, as well as instructions as to whom the patient should call for answers to questions at the medical facility, should be included.

Legal and Ethical Issues

A patient who has filed bankruptcy cannot be contacted or billed further. A threat to take collection action must be fulfilled or the creditor is in violation of the federal Fair Debt Collection Practices Act. Never say that the physician intends to take action if he or she does not plan to follow through.

The Federal Equal Credit Opportunity Act of 1977 bars discrimination in all areas of credit. If the physician agrees to extend credit to one credit-worthy patient, then the same arrangement must be offered to any other patient who requests it, as long as the patient is also credit worthy.

Since laws vary greatly from state to state, the medical assistant should review the statutes pertaining to billing and collecting in the area in which he or she lives. Develop a good understanding of what is required of the small business, such as a physician's office, in collecting fees and billing for amounts due. Remember that laws change often, and constantly update policies to reflect current statutes.

SUMMARY OF SCENARIO

Myra is a well-respected member of Dr. Wallace's office team. Her friendly attitude and flexibility make her a pleasure to interact with in the facility. She knows that there are only a few patients for whom she cannot work out some type of payment arrangements. She is professional in her dealings with those whom she contacts about outstanding accounts.

Dr. Wallace has noticed that more and more patients pay their accounts, and he attributes this to the care that Myra shows when working with them. She is never hesitant to ask for payment from the patient but is sensitive to their needs and struggles at the same time. She urges her patients to cooperate and make a good attempt to pay their accounts, and in return, Myra arranges a payment schedule that the patient can meet.

Myra's flexibility as an employee has paid off for Dr. Wallace several times. During a week-long period when the computer bookkeeping system was malfunctioning, Myra was able to retrieve information from her backup disks and use a pegboard system until the system was repaired. Her preparation allowed the office to continue operations without skipping a beat. Most patients did not even notice that the computer was not in use for the week.

Myra has also been able to fill in for other employees because of the versatility she gained from her medical assistant training. She has scheduled appointments and even assisted Dr. Wallace with minor office surgery. Myra feels that performing other duties is a nice change periodically, and she keeps her skills sharp. She has proved herself to be a valuable and efficient employee.

SUMMARY OF LEARNING OBJECTIVES

- Medical services are valuable to the patient who receives them. The physician sets fees based on three commodities. The physician offers the patient his *time* and makes the most accurate *judgments* possible about the patient's medical condition. The *services* provided to the patient also figure into the fees that are set for various procedures.

- Many third party payors use the UCR method of determining fees for procedures. The *usual* fee is what the physician normally charges for a given service. The *customary* fee is the range of fees charged by physicians who have similar experience in the same geographic area. Services or procedures that are exceptionally complicated and that require extra time deserve a *reasonable* fee and may be higher than the usual fee.

- Providing estimates for medical care helps patients plan their finances when an illness or injury occurs. When estimates are provided, the possibility of later misquoting the fee is avoided. The office staff should keep a copy of the estimate in the patient's chart, which will help to avoid misunderstandings and confusion over charges.

- Some physicians choose to extend professional courtesy to other physicians, medical professionals, and medical staff employees. This means that the physician either discounts or eliminates the charges for all or part of the services provided. The decision to offer professional courtesy should remain with the physician.

- Payment for medical services is accomplished in several ways. Most physicians prefer that payment be received at the time of service. When the extension of credit is offered, internal billing is necessary. Some offices contract with external billing services. Often, patients have some type of insurance or managed care policy that pays at least a portion of the bill. When patients fail to meet their obligations, outside collection services may be used.

- The first statement should always be itemized. This provides the patient and the guarantor with a record of each procedure and each charge. Insurance companies require itemized bills to reimburse the charges.

- Rarely do patients not wish to meet their obligations by paying bills. Some do not have the money to pay for medical services, and if they do not have health insurance, it could be even more difficult to obtain medical care. The financial problem that the patient faces may be temporary, or it may be a long-standing situation. Only a few patients are actually unwilling to pay, so the medical assistant should work with the patient to develop a payment plan that the patient can meet.

- Immediate action should be taken when the office classifies a patient as a "skip." Search the patient chart for all possible telephone numbers and call those that the patient has given. Do not reveal that the patient owes money. If it is necessary to leave a message, do not indicate that the call is from a physician's office. The employer may be called if the patient has not given specific permission not to call the place of business. Never communicate with a third party more than once unless invited to call back. A certified letter may be sent, and when address corrections are requested, the new address is often obtainable. Unless the skip is found quickly, the account is generally turned over to a collection agency.

■ When making collection calls to patients or guarantors, be sure to call within accepted calling hours, which are 8 AM to 9 PM. Be sure to correctly identify the person speaking, and always be respectful and courteous. State the purpose for the call, and keep the conversation business-like and professional. Keep a positive attitude, and convey to the patient that the call is to help devise a way that his or her obligations to the physician can be met. Never threaten the patient, and make every effort to get a commitment as to when payment can be expected. Most important, follow up on collection calls to ensure that patients send in the payment as promised.

INTERNET CONNECTIONS

- Fair Credit Billing
  http://www.ftc.gov/bcp/conline/pubs/credit/fcb.htm
- Fair Credit Reporting Act
  www.fair-credit-reporting-act.com
- Federal Trade Commission
  www.ftc.gov
- Truth In Lending Act
- http://www.uslaw.com/library/article/bbktilact.html?
  area_id = 11

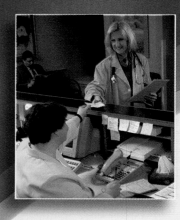

CHAPTER 15

Scenario

Kay James has been an administrative assistant for Shuman & Taylor, MD, a gastroenterology practice, for 2 years. She simultaneously has been enrolled in the medical assistant program at her local college. As she has become quite knowledgeable, it is an appropriate decision for Kay to become more involved in ICD-9-CM and CPT coding.

When it comes to reimbursement, Kay is very aware of the legalities and importance of proper billing. Now she will use her experience and advance her position within the office. She knows that the practice is committed to compliance and feels assured that the patient charts are well documented so that her new task will be easier to carry out. Kay is hard working and looks forward to excelling in her new role as she is exposed to more aspects of becoming a medical assistant.

Basics of Diagnostic Coding

Brenda K. Burton
Carol A. Turiello

Learning Objectives

- Define and spell the terms listed in the vocabulary.
- Identify three purposes of ICD-9-CM.
- Explain the proper utilization of the ICD-9-CM.
- Understand and apply the basic coding rules in the use of the ICD-9-CM.
- Realize the Tabular List contains the most specific coding information.
- Comprehend and utilize instructional terms and symbols as defined in ICD-9-CM.
- Understand the use of V and E codes.
- Properly perform basic diagnostic coding.

National Curriculum Competencies

ADMINISTRATIVE COMPETENCIES

4e. Perform diagnostic coding

Vocabulary

ancillary diagnostic services Services that support patient diagnoses (e.g., laboratory or radiology services).

ancillary therapeutic services Services that support patient treatment (specialists or surgery).

"and" In the context of ICD-9-CM, the word "and" should be interpreted as "and/or."

"code also" When more than one code is necessary to fully identify a given condition, "code also" or "use additional code" is used.

"code if applicable" Notation meaning that the designated code may be principal if no casual condition is applicable or known.

coding Converting verbal or written descriptions into numerical and alphanumerical designations.

comorbidities Preexisting conditions that will, because of their presence with a specific principal diagnosis, cause an increase in length of an inpatient hospital stay by at least 1 day in approximately 75% of cases.

complications Conditions that arise during a hospital stay that prolong the length of stay by at least 1 day in approximately 75% of cases.

"diagnosis" The determination of the nature of a disease, injury, or congenital defect.

etiology The cause of the disorder; a claim may be classified according to etiology.

"excludes" Exclusion terms are always written in italics, and the word "excludes" is often enclosed in a box to draw particular attention to these instructions. Exclusion terms may apply to a chapter, a section, a category, or subcategory. The applicable code number usually follows the exclusion term.

"includes" This term appearing under a subdivision, such as a category (three-digit code) or two-digit procedure code, indicates that the code and title include these terms. Other terms also classified to that particular code and title are listed in the Alphabetic Indexes.

***International Classification of Diseases, Ninth Revision, Clinical Modification* (ICD-9-CM)** System for classifying disease to facilitate collection of uniform and comparable health information, for statistical purposes and indexing medical records for data storage and retrieval.

***International Classification of Diseases, Tenth Revision* (ICD-10)** System containing the greatest number of changes in ICD's history. To allow more specific reporting of disease and newly recognized conditions, the ICD-10 contains approximately 5500 more codes than ICD-9.

mandated Required by an authority or law.

"note" Notes are found in both the Alphabetic Index and the Tabular List as instructions or guides in classification assignments, defining category content or the use of subdivision codes.

"omit code" Term used primarily in Volume 3 of the ICD-9-CM when the procedure is the method of approach for an operation.

preexisting condition Physical condition of an insured person that existed before the issuance of the insurance policy.

principal diagnosis That condition that after study is determined to be chiefly responsible for the patient's admission to the hospital.

"see" A direction given to the coder to look in another place. This term must always be followed and is found in the Alphabetic Index, Volumes 2 and 3.

"see also" A direction given to the coder to look elsewhere if the main term or subterm (or subterms) for that entry are not sufficient for coding the information. If a code number follows, "see also" is enclosed in parentheses. If there is no code number, "see also" is preceded by a dash.

"see category" A direction given to the coder to see a specific category (three-digit code). This must always be followed.

superbill A form on which to list procedures and ICD-9-CM codes most frequently used in a specific practice. The encounter is marked off on this form at the time of patient check out and utilized for billing purposes. This is usually called an encounter form.

"use additional code" This term appears only in volume 1 in those subdivisions in which the user should add further information by means of an additional code to give a more complete picture of the diagnosis. In some cases you will find "if desired" following the term. For the purpose of coding, the "if desired" phrase will not be used. When the term "use additional code...if desired" appears, you will disregard "if desired" and assign the appropriate additional code.

"with" In the context of ICD-9-CM, the terms "with," "with mention of," and "associated with" in a title dictate that both parts of the title be present in the statement of the diagnosis order to assign the particular code.

To facilitate accurate medical record-keeping and the processing of claims, it is essential to identify appropriate services and descriptions of diseases, injuries, and procedures. *The International Classification of Diseases, Ninth Revision, Clinical Modification* (ICD-9-CM) statistically classifies elements of a subject according to diseases, injuries, and operations.

For **coding** and reporting clinical information, the ICD-9-CM is used by healthcare providers, as required for participation in Medicare and Medicaid programs, in addition to its uses for tracking healthcare statistics. Practice management software and third party payers also recognize these codes.

Medical assistants are expected to adhere to ethical standards, only assigning and reporting codes that are clearly supported by concise documentation in the patient chart. When in doubt, a medical assistant should consult the attending healthcare provider for clarification. Maintaining and continually enhancing coding skills and keeping informed of changes in codes, guidelines, and regulations are necessary responsibilities for a coding professional.

The medical assistant, because of his or her involvement in both clinical and administrative aspects of the healthcare setting, is a key person in transitioning the verbal and written reasons for an encounter into the universally accepted numerical codes (ICD-9-CM).

Getting to Know ICD-9-CM

The Evolution of ICD Coding

The systematic classification of disease dates back to seventeenth century England. The classification of disease has progressed from the *International List of Causes of Death* in 1937, changing over the years to the *International Classification of Causes of Death*. In 1948, the list was revised yet again to become the first *International Classification of Disease* (ICD), published by the World Health Organization (WHO).

In 1979, the ICD-9-CM was published by the Department of Health and Human Services in the United States. The intention was to describe the clinical picture of the patient more precisely. Rather than just basic health statistical analysis, the term *clinical* emphasizes the modification's intent to better define morbidity data for indexing medical records, medical and ambulatory care, and review.

Since the passage of the Medicare Catastrophic Coverage Act of 1988, physicians have been required by law to submit **diagnosis** codes for Medicare reimbursement. The appropriate diagnosis is required when billing for services to Medicare beneficiaries.

Centers for Medicare and Medicaid Services (CMS), formerly known as the Health Care Financing Administration (HCFA), designated the coding system ICD-9-CM to be used by physicians.

Updates to the ICD-9-CM

The new ICD-9-CM numbers are published yearly; the responsibility for maintenance of the classification system is shared between the National Center for Health Statistics (NCHS) and CMS. The ICD-9-CM Coordination and Maintenance Committee is co-chaired by these organizations. The committee, meeting twice a year, was formed in 1985 to provide a public forum to discuss possible updates and revisions. The committee plays an advisory role, addressing suggestions. The public is welcome and encouraged to share their comments both before and at the meetings. The Director of NCHS and the Administrator for CMS make the final decisions after the December meeting, and the resultant revisions become effective October 1 of the following year.

Each year, before the October 1 effective date, the official code revisions (referred to as addenda) are published and made available to the public (Figure 15-1). The new codes and code extensions are published in the *Federal Register*.

ICD-10-CM. *The International Statistical Classification of Diseases and Related Health Problems, Tenth Revision* **(ICD-10)**, used to code and classify mortality data from death certificates, replaced the ICD-9-CM in 1999. The NCHS is the federal agency responsible for use of the ICD-10 in the United States. The NCHS has developed a clinical modification of the classification for

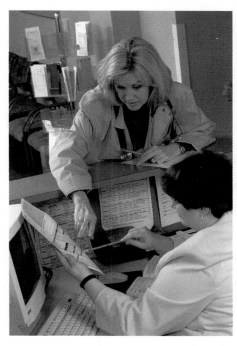

FIGURE 15-1   The team depends on the medical assistant to help keep them updated on coding changes.

morbidity purposes. The current draft of ICD-10-CM contains a significant increase in codes over those in ICD-9-CM.

The Health Insurance Portability and Accountability Act of 1996 (HIPAA), also known as the Kennedy-Kassebaum Act, includes "Standards for Electronic Transactions and Code Sets." HIPAA Transactions and Code Sets regulations were implemented to improve efficiency in healthcare delivery by standardizing electronic data interchange (EDI). Although there is currently no indication of when it will be released, ICD-10-CM is planned as the replacement for ICD-9-CM, Volumes 1 and 2. According to the Centers for Disease Control and Prevention (CDC):

> "There is not yet an anticipated implementation date for the ICD-10-CM. Implementation will be based on the process for adoption of standards under the Health Insurance Portability and Accountability Act of 1996. There will be a two year implementation window once the final notice to implement has been published in the Federal Register."

Additionally, of note, the draft version of ICD-CM-10 is now available for public viewing at: http://www.cdc.gov/nchs/about/otheract/icd9/icd10cm.htm.

CRITICAL THINKING APPLICATION

If Kay wanted to be prepared on behalf of the office by researching proposed changes or address concerns about ICD-9-CM coding issues, how would she best go about it?

Why Use ICD Codes?

In addition to the logistical layout of a standard system used in billing, some pertinent reasoning behind the utilization of ICD-9-CM codes would include the following:

- For data storage and retrieval
- To maximize reimbursement by accurate coding
- To shorten claims processing time
- To facilitate measurement of compliance with clinical guidelines

Compiling healthcare data also helps to measure the appropriateness and timeliness of medical care, enabling third party payers and providers to analyze payments for health services.

Format and Conventions of ICD-9-CM

The ICD-9-CM is published in various media, including book, CD, and downloadable file. It is ideal to have a printed book because of the limitations that an electronic format may present. This set comprises Volumes 1, 2, and 3.

Volume 1, Tabular List

Volume 1, containing 5 appendices and 17 chapters, is referred to as the Tabular List. This Volume classifies diseases and injuries according to **etiology** and organ system, dividing them into groups:

- Anatomical system type of condition
- Related groups of codes
- Three-digit codes (category codes)
- Fourth digit (subcategory codes)
- Fifth digit (subclassification codes)

Classifications of Sections and Structure of Chapters 1 Through 17. Each of the 17 chapters in Volume 1 is subdivided as follows:

- *Section:* A group of three-digit code numbers describing a general disease category
- *Category:* A three-digit code representing a specific disease within the section
- *Subcategory:* A further breakdown of the category, assigning a fourth digit
- *Subclassification:* Five-digit code giving the highest level of specificity to the disease state

---

EXAMPLE OF THE CHAPTER STRUCTURE

Chapter: Diseases of the Circulatory System
  Chapter Seven (390-459)
Section: Hypertensive Disease (401-405)
Category: Hypertensive Heart Disease (402)
Subcategory: Malignant (402.0)
Subclassification: Without heart failure (402.00)

Volume 2, Alphabetic Index

Volume 2 contains an Alphabetic Index of disease and injury. This Volume contains more information than is contained in the Tabular List and is divided into three sections:

- Index of diseases
- Poison and external causes of adverse affects of drugs and other chemical substances
- Alphabetic Index of external cause of injury and poisoning

Volume 3, Procedures: Tabular List and Alphabetic Index

Volume 3 contains a tabular and alphabetic index of procedures. Unlike Volumes 1 and 2, it is not used in a physician's office but is primarily used in hospitals and other facilities to code the procedures performed in those settings. The procedure codes are two digits followed by a decimal and one or two additional digits.

Symbols, Abbreviations, Punctuations, and Notations

Symbols, abbreviations, punctuations, and notations appear in the listings to serve as instructional notes. Understanding their meaning and using their guidance is crucial to accurate coding. Many different publishers offer the ICD-9-CM, and there may be some differences in the symbols, notations, colors, or other reference marks used for convenience or to convey specific meaning. The medical assistant should be familiar with the manual in use in his or her office. Several examples are listed below.

Symbols

□	The lozenge symbol precedes a disease code when indicating that the content of a four-digit category has been moved or modified.
§	The section mark symbol is only used in the Tabular List of diseases and precedes a code denoting a footnote on the page.
•	The bullet symbol indicates a new entry.
▲	The triangle symbol indicates a revision in the Tabular List and a code change in the Alphabetic Index.
►◄	These symbols mark both the beginning and ending of new or revised text.
♀	Female diagnosis only.
♂	Male diagnosis only.
√4th	Code requires a fourth digit.
√5th	Code requires a fifth digit.

Abbreviations

NEC	Not elsewhere classifiable. The category number for the term including NEC is to be used only when the coder lacks the information necessary to code the term to a more specific category.
NOS	Not otherwise specified. This abbreviation is the equivalent of "unspecified."

Punctuation

[ ]	Brackets are used to enclose synonyms, alternative wordings, or explanatory phrases.
( )	Parentheses are used to enclose supplementary words, which may be present or absent in the statement of a disease or procedure without affecting the code number to which it is assigned.

:   Colons are used in the Tabular List after an incomplete term that needs one or more of the modifiers that follow to make it assignable to a given category.

{ }   Braces enclose a series of terms, each of which is modified by the statement appearing to the right of the brace.

Bold   Bold type is used for all codes and titles in the Tabular List.

Italics   Italic type is used for exclusion notes and to identify diagnosis that cannot be used as primary.

Notations

DEF   Appearing in blue indicates a definition of disease or a procedure term.

MSP   Identifies a specific trauma code that will alert the carrier that another carrier should be billed first. Medicare is to be billed second if payment from the first payer is not equal to or greater than what Medicare would reimburse.

PDx   Indicates a V code that can only be used as a primary diagnosis.

SDx   Indicates a V code that can only be used as a secondary diagnosis.

CRITICAL THINKING APPLICATION

It is Kay's responsibility to make sure the superbill and the practice management software contain valid, updated ICD-9-CM codes. How can she begin to prepare for the upcoming fiscal year during the last quarter of this fiscal year?

Steps in ICD Coding

As in other administrative duties, developing good coding habits starts in the beginning. Practicing coding as outlined below will assist the medical assistant to develop good coding habits and become an asset to the physician.

The following steps are always necessary to assign the appropriate ICD-9-CM code (Procedure 15-1):

1. Identify the key terms in the diagnostic statement, determining the main reason for the encounter (Figure 15-2). Keep in mind that the definitive diagnosis should be coded first. Some important points to remember:
   - Check documentation regarding a preexisting condition. Be sure this condition is currently being treated and not part of the past medical history.
   - *Never code conditions described as "rule out," "suspected," "probable," or "questionable."* (You do not want to give a patient a disease he or she does not have!)
   - If a patient requests that a different diagnosis be used that is not the correct or appropriate diagnosis for the visit, stating that his or her insurance company will not reimburse, you have a legal and ethical responsibility to code the diagnosis as documented in the patient's medical record.

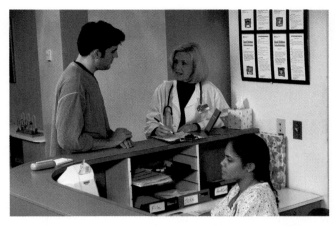

FIGURE 15-2 Coding begins with proper documentation of the patient's reason for visiting the physician.

   - If no definitive diagnosis is made, code the reason for the encounter.
2. Locate the diagnosis in the Alphabetic Index (Volume 2).
3. Read and understand any footnotes, symbols or instructions, following any cross-references, such as "**code also.**"
4. Locate the diagnosis in the Tabular List.
5. Read and understand the inclusions and exclusions.
6. Make certain you include fourth and fifth digits when available, assigning to the highest level of specificity.
7. Assign the code, until all diagnosis elements are identified.
8. After assigning the code, double check to ensure accurate transfer from the book to the patient form and subsequent data entry.
9. Use the same process for secondary diagnoses and other conditions *addressed* during the encounter.

CODING EXAMPLE

A patient comes to the office with dehydration, nausea, and vomiting.
- Dehydration is the definitive diagnosis; the Alphabetic Index refers you to 276.5 in the tabular list
- 276.5—Volume depletion includes dehydration; it excludes hypovolemic shock
- Next code the signs and symptoms
- Nausea (see also Vomiting) with vomiting refers you to 787.01. This is a perfect example of why you need to read all the exclusions. If this patient were an infant, the code would be different.

The code for this adult patient would be:
- Dehydration 276.5
- Nausea and vomiting 787.01

Special Codes

In addition to the 17 chapters in Volume 1, two supplementary classifications are provided in ICD-9-CM. When

PROCEDURE **15-1**

ICD-9-CM Coding

GOAL: To assign the proper ICD-9-CM code based on a medical documentation for auditing and billing purposes.

EQUIPMENT AND SUPPLIES

- Patient medical record
- Current ICD-9-CM code book
- Medical dictionary

Case Study:

Follow Up Visit

Name: Ms. Patient   ID: 3456

Date: 10/8/XX   DOB: 6/10/XX

This 82-year-old female was seen in the office 3 days ago with new onset CHF. She states she feels much better. She does note some small amount of leg edema but she feels this is significantly less than 3 days ago. She denies any chest pain in the last 3 days.

There has been no change in her History as noted in my note of 3 days ago.

On examination, her blood pressure is 150/70. Pulse is 72 and irregularly irregular. Her weight is 158 pounds, down 7 pounds in 3 days. HEENT examination reveals pupils to be equal, round, and reactive. Extraocular movements are intact. Conjunctiva pink. Neck is supple. No JVD. Carotids are 2 + bilaterally without bruits. Lungs are clear to auscultation and percussion. Cardiac examination reveals no heaves or thrills. There is a normal S1 and S2 with an irregularly irregular rhythm. There is a grade 2/6 systolic ejection murmur at the left sternal border and apex. The abdomen is soft, nontender, bowel sounds are present. The liver and spleen do not appear enlarged. Examination of her extremities reveals no edema, clubbing, or cyanosis. She is alert, oriented, with no focal motor deficits.

Impression: This pleasant 82-year-old woman has experienced a dramatic improvement in her CHF symptoms in the last 3 days. Her physical examination and CXR today reflect this improvement. At this time she is reluctant to undergo any further testing.

I will have her continue with the same medication, weigh herself daily, and return for follow-up in 2 weeks. Before she returns I will have her obtain a chemistry profile. She is instructed to call with any weight gain or chest pain.

PROCEDURAL STEPS

1 Identify the key term in the diagnostic statement.
Purpose: To determine the definite diagnosis.

2 Locate the diagnosis in the Alphabetic Index.

3 Read and understand footnotes.
Note: This includes any symbols, instructions, or cross-references.

4 Locate the diagnosis in the Tabular List.

5 Read and understand the inclusions and exclusions.

6 Make certain you include fourth and fifth digits where available.

7 Assign the code.
Note: All diagnosis elements need to be identified. Double-check the code to ensure an accurate transfer to the patient form.

recording a code from these classifications, always write the alpha character first to distinguish the V or E code from a diagnosis code that has the same number of digits but no alphabetical character.

CRITICAL THINKING APPLICATION

Dr. Taylor has inadvertently circled the diagnosis for dysphagia on the patient's superbill. Kay assisted with the examination and knows the patient came in for rectal bleeding. What is the proper approach in correcting this code?

V Codes

The V code is used on occasions when the patient is not currently ill or to explain problems that influence his or her current illness or injury. The Supplementary Classification of Factors Influencing Health Status and Contact with Health Service (V Code, V01-V82) is used in cases such as preventive vaccination or chronic disease states such as dialysis for renal disease.

Example: Exposure to rabies by rabid skunk
Code as: Rabies V01.5

CRITICAL THINKING APPLICATION

Mr. Smith has been a patient for several years and presents for a routine physical examination. Mr. Smith has Medicare as his primary insurance and asks Kay to list his long-standing hypertension as the reason for his visit, knowing that Medicare does not cover routine physicals. How should Kay handle this?

E Codes

The E code is used to classify environmental causes of injury, poisoning, or other adverse effects on the body. Supplemental Classification of External Causes of Injuries and Poisoning (E Code, E800-E999).

Example: Injury from butane explosion
Code as: Accident caused by explosive material, explosive gases, Butane E923.2

Symptoms, Signs, and Ill-Defined Conditions (Chapter 16, 780-799)

Unlike the other chapters that contain diagnoses in Volume 1, Chapter 16 comprises symptoms, signs, and ill-defined conditions. If the terms "suspected," "suspicious," or "rule out" are used within the diagnosis, code the reason for the encounter. This could be the symptoms, signs, abnormal test results, or any other reason that the patient sought medical care (Figure 15-3). If there is any question about the reason for the encounter, check with the physician.

Example: Rule out myocardial infarction
Code as: Chief complaint: "chest pain"(central) 786.50

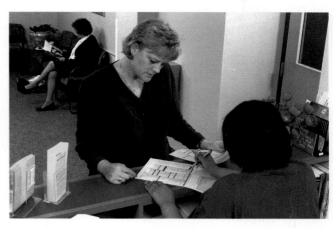

FIGURE 15-3 The encounter form is an important tool in gathering the diagnosis and symptoms needed for coding.

CRITICAL THINKING APPLICATION

If a patient presented with right lower quadrant pain and the physician simply wrote "R/O appendicitis" on the encounter form, how would Kay go about coding this?

Appendices

The five appendices included in Volume 1, Tabular List, serve as a reference to the coder to provide additional information to futher define a diagnosis, classifying new drugs and to provide a quick reference for three-digit categories. The five appendices are as follows:

- *Morphology of Neoplasms:* The WHO established an adaptation of the ICD for Oncology (ICD-O). The morphology code numbers consist of five digits. The first four digits identify the histological type of neoplasm and the fifth digit indicates its behavior. M codes are used for statistical data only and are not used in physician billing. This section of the appendix is usually utilized by inpatient coders.
- *Glossary of Mental Disorders:* This glossary is an alphabetical listing of the psychiatric terminology that appears in Chapter 5, "Mental Disorders."
- *Classification of Drugs by AHFS List:* The adverse effect of drugs is coded according to the American Hospital Formulary Service (AHFS) list. The list is continuously revised and published under the direction of the American Society of Hospital Pharmacists (ASHP). This section is usually used by pharmacies.
- *Classification of Industrial Accidents According to Agency:* This appendix concerns the Statistics of Employment Injuries categorized by industrial agency. This section is usually used by government organizations, such as OSHA.
- *List of Three-Digit Categories:* This appendix is a breakdown of the chapters' categories; includes V and E codes.

Maximizing Third Party Reimbursement

The most important aspect to remember with ICD-9-CM is to code the diagnosis to the highest level of specificity, linking the ICD-9-CM code to the Current Procedural Terminology (CPT) code. The CPT coding is further explained in Chapter 16.

Obtaining the correct reimbursement is important to the practice cash flow and depends on proper coding and billing techniques. Some other crucial points to remember when submitting diagnostic codes for claims are as follows:

- Use the current ICD-9-CM manual, staying informed of changes.
- Code accurately from documented information (Figure 15-4).
- Be sure diagnosis corresponds with symptoms and treatment.
- Review data entry to ensure no transposition of digits.
- Know insurance carriers' rules for submitting claims; for example, some insurance carriers allow only one or two codes per claim.
- Incomplete or inaccurate codes may result in insurance denial because of a lack of medical necessity.

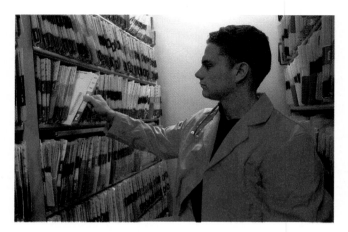

FIGURE 15-4 The patient's chart is used to support the diagnosis and can be accessed by authorized personnel should any questions arise.

the medical assistant realizes these codes are updated yearly, this makes them an asset in coding compliance.

Legal and Ethical Issues

Medical assistants are entrusted by the physician and practice that employs them. To this extent, a medical assistant must be responsible and knowledgeable to ensure that no fraud takes place in the coding and claims submission process.

The coding professional should not change codes or narratives in patient chart documentation to accommodate insurance reimbursement or policy coverage requirements. Deliberate misrepresentation may carry criminal and/or civil penalties.

CODING TIPS AND HINTS

- Always have a good medical dictionary.
- Use the most recent ICD manual and have your own copy.
- Make notes in your books.
- Do not code from the Alphabetic Index alone.
- Diagnoses are listed by first word, by a key word in a phrase, or by anatomical site involved.
- Avoid nonspecific codes.
- Be very careful when coding preexisting conditions.
- Make certain the documentation supports the diagnosis.
- Remember, inaccurate coding can lead to accusations of fraud and abuse.

SUMMARY OF SCENARIO

Kay has been very enthusiastic throughout her learning experiences at the practice. She knows that as time continues and she earns her certificate, she will enjoy being a medical assistant. As Kay progresses with diagnostic coding, she will also be able to help the physicians and nursing staff be attentive to details in documentation of the patient chart.

Although using the superbill to enter the codes for billing is an easy tool, knowing how to use the ICD-9-CM volumes is a necessary asset to ensure accurate coding when there is a question at checkout. Also, if additional information is requested by the insurance company to support a given diagnosis code, Kay can pull the patient's chart for research and documentation. Keeping in mind the aspect of maximum reimbursement, Kay will be knowledgeable in coding to the highest level of specificity.

Having access to the Internet will help Kay to be ready for new codes and to revise the superbill when needed. This will also be advantageous in an expedient revenue cycle.

Closing Comments

The medical assistant's knowledge of accurate diagnostic coding contributes to the legal and financial health of the practice. In most cases, ICD-9-CM codes are found on the provider's encounter form (or **superbill**) and/or in the practice management software. However, with literally thousands of current diagnostic codes, it may be necessary to code from the ICD-9-CM manual. Because

SUMMARY OF LEARNING OBJECTIVES

■ The medical assistant will become very comfortable with diagnostic coding with practice and patience. The ICD-9-CM is used to track healthcare statistics, as well as to facilitate accurate medical record keeping and ease in processing claims. Use of the ICD-9-CM is mandatory for participation in many federal, state, and private insurance programs.

■ Each of the three Volumes has a specific use. Start with the alphabetic list and then proceed to the tabular list when assigning a code. Only the inpatient coder uses Volume 3 of the ICD-9-CM.

■ Several basic coding rules exist that will assist the medical assistant in coding. Be sure that the most recent ICD-9-CM manual is being used, and keep a medical dictionary handy. As difficult codes are assigned, keep notes in the book for future reference. Proofread the claim and be sure that it makes good sense. Avoid nonspecific codes and use care when coding preexisting conditions.

■ Never code directly from the index. The tabular list contains the most specific information. Check and recheck the codes, making certain that the documentation supports the codes that are used on the claim.

■ The medical assistant should become familiar with all of the symbols used in the ICD-9-CM. Instructional codes should be read thoroughly and all directions followed while coding a claim.

■ E or V codes may help to clarify a code or explain the code further. V codes are used when the patient is not currently ill, but is being seen by health service professionals. This would include preventative visits to the physician or visits for vaccinations. E codes are used to explain that some external cause contributed to an adverse effect within the body.

INTERNET CONNECTIONS

• American Academy of Professional Coders
http://www.aapc.com/
• American Medical Association
www.ama-assn.org
• Centers for Medicare and Medicaid Services
http://www.cms.gov/
• National Center for Health Statistics
http://www.cdc.gov/nchs/
• US Government Printing Office (to access *Federal Register*)
http://www.access.gpo.gov/

REFERENCES

Fordney M: *Insurance handbook for the medical office*, ed 6. Philadelphia, 2002, WB Saunders.
ICD-9-CM easy coder, Montgomery, Ala, 2002, UnicorMed.
International classification of diseases, ninth revision, clinical modification (ICD-9-CM), volumes 1 and 2. Chicago, 2002, American Medical Association.

PROCEDURE 15-1

ANSWERS TO PROCEDURE 15-1

1 CHF

2 Congestion (heart) 428.0

3 None

4 428

5 Excludes:
Following cardiac surgery (429.4)
Rheumatic (398.91)
That complicating:
Abortion (634-638 with .7, 639.8)
Ectopic or molar pregnancy (639.8)
Labor or delivery (668.1, 669.4)

6 Code, if applicable, heart failure due to hypertension first (402.0-402.9, with fifth digit 1 or 404.0-404.9 with fifth digit 1 or 3).

7 428.9 Hearth failure, unspecified
Cardiac failure NOS
Heart failure NOS
Myocardial failure NOS
Weak heart

CHAPTER 16

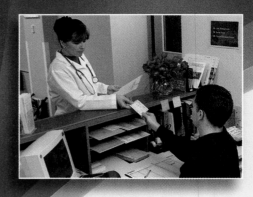

Scenario

As Kay James progresses in her education and continues as administrative assistant for Drs. Shuman and Taylor, she has enjoyed the challenges and has excelled on her diagnostic coding exams. She looks forward to being equally competent with procedural coding. Now, she is ready to move on to procedural coding. As with ICD-9-CM, Kay can rely on accurate record keeping within the practice to perform this task.

As she prepares to graduate from her medical assisting educational program, Kay is excited to receive her degree and continue to be an asset to the practice. She anticipates gaining more responsibility as her knowledge becomes more well rounded.

Basics of Procedural Coding

Brenda K. Burton
Carol A. Turiello

Learning Objectives

- Define and spell the terms listed in the vocabulary.
- Identify three purposes of the CPT.
- List the classifications of sections in the CPT.
- Explain the use of guidelines and where they are located.
- Discuss the importance of modifiers.
- Briefly explain the importance of correctly assigning evaluation and management codes.
- Define *upcoding* and explain why it must be avoided.
- Accurately assign a CPT code based on medical documentation.
- Explain the basic rules for CPT coding.

National Curriculum Competencies

4d. Perform procedural coding

Vocabulary

bundled codes Procedures or services that are grouped together and paid as one.

component A constituent part; a part of a larger group.

downcoding A change in code done by the insurance company that receives a claim resulting in a lesser reimbursement. The change will usually be the code closest to the one submitted on the claim, because the code does not match in some way to the specifications of the insurance company.

modifiers Code additions that explain circumstances that alter a service that has been provided and clarify exactly what was done to the patient.

morbidity The relative incidence of disease.

mortality The number of deaths in a given time or place.

revenue The total income produced by a given source.

unbundled codes Separating the components of a procedure and reporting them separately.

upcoding A deliberate increase in a CPT code to receive higher reimbursements.

utilization Related to the process of reviewing procedures and services for medical necessity.

As with diagnostic coding, accurate use of the CPT-4 is essential. The medical assistant facilitates accurate medical record keeping and the efficient processing of claims by using the CPT-4, which identifies appropriate procedures and services common to the physician's office. CPT-4 is used in the claims submission process to receive reimbursement from payors as well as to track physician productivity.

Medical assistants are expected to adhere to ethical standards when involved in all aspects of coding. Again, as with diagnostic coding, the medical assistant should consult the attending healthcare provider for clarification when a question arises. CPT codes must be maintained, following the changes in guidelines and regulations. Medical assistants, because of their involvement in both clinical and administrative aspects of the healthcare setting, are key persons in converting the verbal and written reasons for an encounter into the universally accepted numeric and alphanumeric codes of CPT-4.

Getting to Know the CPT-4

The Evolution of CPT Coding

Current Procedural Terminology was first published in 1966 by the American Medical Association. It was based on the California Relative Value Study, developed by the California Medical Society. Its primary purpose was to simplify the reporting of procedures and/or services provided by physicians. In 1992 the most significant change was made to CPT with the replacement of the office and hospital visit codes with the Evaluation and Management (E&M) codes, identifying key elements to be documented in the medical record. CPT has been revised three times; the edition in current use is CPT-4.

Updates to the CPT

CPT is updated every October by the AMA and published for the next calendar year. The CPT is available as a printed manual or as an electronic file. As with the ICD-9-CM, it is ideal to purchase the printed version to be certain you have the entire contents for easy reference. Because the practice of medicine is constantly changing and new procedures are being developed, the AMA encourages suggestions from physicians, medical societies, and organizations. Forms are available from the AMA CPT Editorial Research and Development Department and on the AMA website (given at the end of the chapter). These changes are found in Appendix B of the CPT manual.

Why Use the CPT?

Medicare and most commercial insurance companies use CPT to identify and classify claims for payment. Although its use is standard in physicians' practices, CPT is not recognized in some facility settings or under special guidelines within an insurance company.

Physicians' practices use CPT to:
- Submit claims for services and procedures
- Track **utilization** of services and procedures
- Measure physician productivity

CRITICAL THINKING APPLICATION

As Kay learns more about CPT codes, what will she find similar to what she learned with ICD-9-CM?

Format of the CPT

There are three levels of CPT:
- Level I codes are developed by the AMA and contained in the current CPT Manual. They are five-digit codes and two-digit modifiers.
- Level II codes, known as HCPCS, are national codes developed by CMS to describe medical services and supplies not covered in the CPT. They consist of alphabetic characters (A through V) and four digits. Modifiers are either alphanumerical or two letters (AA to VP).
- Level III codes are local codes. Unlike Level I and II, these codes are not common to all carriers. They are assigned by local Medicare carriers to describe new procedures that are not yet in Levels I and II. These codes start with a letter (W through Z) followed by four digits. Note: when the HIPAA standards for electronic transactions are implemented, Level III codes will no longer be recognized for reimbursement reporting.

Symbols

Symbols appear in the listings to serve as instructional notes. Understanding their meaning and using their guidance is crucial to accurate coding.

- New code
- ▲ Code revision
- + CPT add-on codes
- Ø Exempt from the use of modifier –51
- ▶◀ Revised guidelines, cross-references, and explanations
- → With a circle around it refers to *CPT Assistant*
- * Surgical procedure only

Sections

Evaluation and Management (E&M). The E&M section appears in the front of the CPT Manual and must be thoroughly understood. There is the most room for error when coding in this section. Since all specialties bill these services and these codes constitute 65% of the total Medicare part B payments to physicians, it is extremely important to understand this section. A full section devoted to understanding E&M coding appears later in this chapter.

Anesthesia Codes. This section contains anesthesia and modifier codes plus the very specific physical status modifiers developed by the American Society of Anesthesiologists to rank patients by level of complexity. The modifiers range from P1 (normal healthy) through P6 (brain dead) patients whose organs are being removed for transplantation. There are also add-on codes (+) that explain difficult circumstances. These are located in the Anesthesia Guidelines found at the beginning of the section and also in the medicine section of the CPT-4.

Surgery. The surgery section is further divided into 18 subsections by specific type of surgery. General guidelines are found at the beginning of the section and apply to all subsections. The subsections have specific guidelines that apply to that particular area. The subsections are further divided into subheadings. One of the most important explanations in the general guidelines is the definition of the surgical package; it is essential to know exactly what is and is not included in the package. All surgeries have *global periods*. These range from 0 (the actual calendar day of the procedure) up to 90 days (starting the day before the surgery and continues for 90 days). These global periods cover normal "routine" care during that time. Complications, new problems, or other injuries are reported using modifiers.

Radiology. In addition to radiology (x-ray diagnostic procedures), this section includes nuclear medicine and diagnostic ultrasound. This section requires a written report from the radiologist to the physician that ordered the test.

Pathology and Laboratory. Codes in the pathology and laboratory section cover laboratory tests and services of pathologists. It is important to understand that some tests are grouped into panels. These panels give a clearer picture of problems with an organ or disease.

Medicine. The medicine section covers a multitude of services provided to patients ranging from immunization through testing that is not included in other sections to services provided by a psychiatrist or a physical therapist, and osteopathic manipulation to home healthcare.

Classifications of Sections

- *Section* is a general grouping of codes, such as surgery, medicine, laboratory or radiology. It is the largest grouping within CPT.
- *Subsection* better defines the section.
- *Subheading* further defines the subsection.
- *Category* directs you to the specific procedures in which you will find the correct code.

CLASSIFICATIONS OF SECTIONS

Example

Section: Surgery
  Subsection: Integumentary
    Subheading: Skin; subcutaneous and accessory structures
      Category: Incision and drainage of abscess, CPT code 10060*

The * symbol indicates surgical procedure only.

Guidelines at the beginning of each section of the CPT manual refer to the whole section; guidelines specific to the subsections are listed as Notes at the beginning of the subsection. A medical assistant needs to read and understand these guidelines. Each section is unique and has very specific requirements. Attempting to code services without a working knowledge of the guidelines can lead to improper coding and possibly loss of **revenue**.

Steps in CPT Coding

The following is a brief outline of the considerations you will use in CPT coding. (To assign a CPT code, see Procedure 16-1.)

1. Know the CPT code book; there are changes each year, so even if you have been coding for years, you need to read the *introduction, guidelines, and notes* (Figure 16-1).
2. Review all services and procedures performed on the day of the encounter. Include all medications administered and trays and equipment used.
3. Find the procedures and/or services in the index in the back of the CPT book. This will direct you to a code (not a page number!). The code you are looking for may be listed as a procedure, body system, service, or abbreviation (this will usually refer you to the full spelling).
4. Read the description in the code and also any related descriptions that follow a semicolon; this will lead you to the most accurate code.
5. If the service is an E&M code, identify and perform the following:
   - Whether this is a new or established patient
   - Whether this is a consultation
   - Where the service was performed

PROCEDURE **16-1**

Assigning a CPT Code

GOAL: To assign the proper CPT codes based on medical documentation for auditing and billing purposes.

EQUIPMENT AND SUPPLIES

- Patient medical record
- Current CPT code book
- Medical dictionary

Case Study:

Initial Office Visit

Name: Mr. Patient   ID: 2345
Date: 3/28/XX   DOB: 9/12/XX

Mr. Patient is a 52-year-old white male who for the last 2 months has experienced moderate chest discomfort, radiating to his jaw when he shovels snow. The pain generally lasts about 5 minutes and is relieved with rest. He states he becomes short of breath when he experiences the chest discomfort.

The patient denies any chest pain or pressure at the present time. He is a diabetic and has been on insulin for the past 10 years. He has no known allergies.

His mother is living and well. His father was a diabetic and died when he was 40. The patient is not sure, but he thinks his father had a stroke. He has no brothers or sisters.

Mr. Patient is an electrical engineer and lives at home with his wife and two teenage children. He does not smoke and drinks an occasional beer.

Present medications: NPH insulin, multiple vitamins.

On physical examination: B/P 160/90. Pulse 90 and regular. Respiratory rate 20. Height 5'8". Weight 250 lbs. Face is somewhat flushed. Neck is supple. Carotid upstroke 2 + without bruits. No JVD. The lungs are clear. Heart sounds somewhat distant; S1, S2 regular; no systolic murmur appreciated. The abdomen is soft and nontender. The abdominal aorta is not palpable. Femoral and pedal pulses are strong. There is no lower extremity edema, no clubbing or cyanosis. No lymphadenopathy or scars noted. Heme negative brown stool. Prostate not enlarged.

ECG done today in my office shows NSR, rate 90. No ST-T abnormalities. The tracing is within normal limits. CXR—negative. Normal cardiac silhouette.

Given Mr. Patient's symptoms, diabetes, obesity, and probable family history, further work-up will include a fasting lipid profile and a nuclear stress test. After these tests, we can further discuss the possible need for a left heart catheterization.

- Review the documentation to determine the level of service
- Check to determine whether there is a reason to use a modifier

- Assign the five-digit CPT code

_____

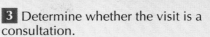

PROCEDURE 16-1—Cont'd

PROCEDURAL STEPS

1 Identify if the patient is new or established.
   Note: Using the case described, assume that the key components for Mr. Patient's encounter with regard to evaluation and management are:
   - A detailed history
   - A detailed examination
   - Medical decision making of low complexity

2 Indicate where the patient is being seen.

3 Determine whether the visit is a consultation.

4 Determine whether the visit is due to illness or is a preventive medical service.

5 Determine the level of history.

6 Determine the level of examination.

7 Determine the level of medical decision making.

8 Assign the most accurate CPT code.

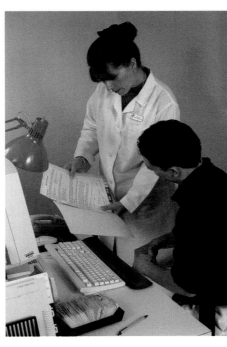

FIGURE 16-1   A medical assistant should always check with the healthcare provider when there is a question about which CPT code to use.

Modifiers

When used, **modifiers** explain circumstances that alter a service that has been provided. These circumstances do not change the basic meaning of the code but help clarify exactly what was done. It may be that the professional or technical component is being billed, more than one physician was involved in providing the service, a procedure had to be discontinued, and other circumstances. Modifiers can now be found in Appendix A of the CPT codebook.

Multiple Modifiers

Sometimes more than one modifier is needed. When this happens, the first modifier used is –99. This signals the person reviewing the claim that more than one modifier is being used.

Understanding Evaluation and Management

Factors Considered in E&M Coding

Type of Service. Services covered in the E&M section include, but are not limited to, physician encounters in all locations for "well" or "sick" visits, patient transport, case management services, preventative medicine services and prolonged services.

Place of Service. For payment purposes the place of service needs to match the type of service. The places of service are as follows:
- Office (11)
- Patient's home (12)
- Inpatient hospital (21)
- Outpatient hospital (22)
- Emergency department (ED) hospital (23)
- Ambulatory surgery center (ASC) (24)
- Birthing center (25)
- Skilled nursing facility (SNF) (31)
- Nursing facility (32)
- Custodial care facility (33)
- Hospice (34)
- Federally qualified health center (50)
- Inpatient psychiatric facility (51)
- Partial hospitalization, psychiatric facility (52)
- Community mental health center (53)
- Psychiatric residential treatment center (56)
- Comprehensive inpatient rehabilitation facility (61)
- Comprehensive outpatient rehabilitation facility (62)
- End-stage renal disease treatment facility (65)
- State or local public health clinic (71)
- Rural health clinic (72)
- Other unlisted facility (99)

Patient Status. Many of the CPT codes are classified by whether a patient is a new or established patient. A *new patient* is new to the practice or has not been seen by the specialty in group practice for more than 3 years. An *established patient* is one who has a continuing relationship with the practice and has been seen within the last 3 years.

CRITICAL THINKING APPLICATION

Dr. Shuman performed a colonoscopy at the hospital on a patient, Cecil Matthews, who has been Dr. Shuman's patient for several years. Mr. Matthews presented to the office with left lower quadrant pain and a history of colon cancer. What other factors or information would Kay need to know to properly code this encounter?

Levels of E&M Services

Determining Factors. To understand the levels of history it is important to know the definition and components of the patient's history. The history relates to the patient's clinical picture and depends on the patient for answers to specific questions. The history is composed of the chief complaint, or reason the patient is being seen. This is usually in the patient's own words.

The *history of present illness* identifies the location, severity, timing, modifying factors, quality, duration, context and associated signs and symptoms relating to the chief complaint.

The *review of systems* has the patient answer questions about the following systems: constitutional, eyes, ear/nose /throat (ENT) and mouth, cardiac, gastrointestinal, musculoskeletal, endocrine, neurological, integumentary, psychiatric, genitourinary, allergic/immunologic, respiratory, and hematological/lymphatic.

The *past medical, family, and social history* is important, because patients' experiences with illness and surgery, whether they smoke, use illicit drugs and/or alcohol, if they are married, have children, where they live, and what diseases their blood relatives have had play an extremely important part in determining their risk factors for illness (Figure 16-2).

Now that it is understood what makes up the history, the various levels can be discussed.

- *Problem focused:* A problem-focused history concentrates on the chief complaint; it looks at the symptoms, severity, and duration of the problem. It usually does not include a review of systems (ROS) or family and social history.
- *Expanded problem focused:* The physician proceeds the same as for the problem-focused history but includes a review of the systems that relate to the chief complaint. Usually past, family, and social histories are not included.
- *Detailed:* The physician will document a more extensive history, ROS, and will document pertinent past, family, and social histories.
- *Comprehensive:* The physician will document responses to *all* of the components listed previously. A comprehensive history is usually taken during an initial visit with patients who have a significant history of illness.

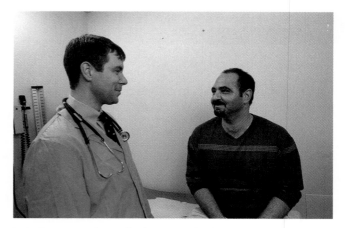

FIGURE 16-2   The medical assistant should document any history obtained from the patient.

Medical Decision Making. When a physician makes medical decisions, the decisions are based on many years of education and experience. To understand what goes into these decisions, the following guidelines have been developed.

NUMBER OF DIAGNOSES/MANAGEMENT OPTIONS. When we read the note the physician writes, we should be able to tell whether the patient's problem is minor or an established problem that is stable or getting worse or whether the patient has a new problem that the physician wants to watch or perhaps to order or perform more tests on.

AMOUNT AND COMPLEXITY OF DATA REVIEWED. The physician's note should tell us what laboratory tests, x-ray diagnostic procedures, and other tests have been ordered or reviewed.

RISK OF COMPLICATIONS AND MORBIDITY OR MORTALITY. There is often risk involved in medical care, either from the treatment given to the patient or from the lack of treatment and professional care. **Morbidity,** the relative incidence of disease, and **mortality,** which relates to the number of deaths from a given disease, are part of the assessment of risks made by the physician.

These three elements play a role in the complexity of the decision-making process used when treating a patient. The physician determines the level of care given to a patient, but must consider these three factors when choosing the E&M levels assigned to a patient on a given encounter. The physician cannot base the choice of E&M levels solely on the time spent with the patient. All elements must be considered when assigning the code. Usually, the physician circles this service code and other procedure codes on the encounter form as or just after the patient is seen in the office. Although a physician may allow the medical assistant to make notations on the encounter form, only the physician makes the decision as to which services and procedures are performed.

MEDICAL DECISION–MAKING COMPLEXITY LEVELS
- *Straightforward:* Minimal diagnosis/management options, minimal/none for the amount and complexity

---

of data to be reviewed, and minimal risk to the patient of complications or death if untreated.

- *Low-complexity:* Limited number of diagnoses/management options, limited data to be reviewed, and low risk to the patient of complications or death if untreated.
- *Moderate-complexity:* Multiple diagnoses/management options, moderate amount and complexity of data to be reviewed, and moderate risk to the patient of complications or death if untreated.
- *High-complexity:* Extensive diagnoses/management options, extensive amount and complexity of data to be reviewed, and high risk to the patient for complications and/or death if the problem is untreated.

Examination. The examination is the objective part of the patient's visit (Figure 16-3). The physician examines the patient and makes notes referring to body areas and/or organ systems:

- *Body areas:* Head including face and neck, chest, including breasts and axillas, abdomen, genitourinary (GU), back, including spine and extremities.
- *Organ systems:* Constitutional, eyes, ears/nose/throat and mouth, cardiovascular, respiratory, gastrointestinal (GI), GU, musculoskeletal, skin, neurological, psychiatric, and hematological/lymphatic/immunologic.

The examination is divided into the following levels:

- *Problem-focused:* The examination is limited to the single body area or single system mentioned in the chief complaint.
- *Expanded problem-focused:* In addition to the limited body area or system, related body areas or organ systems are examined.
- *Detailed:* An extended examination is performed on the related body areas or organ systems.

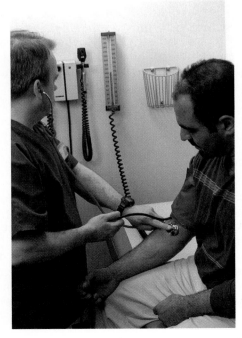

FIGURE 16-3 Examinations conducted by all members of the team are part of the documentation requirements for CPT coding.

- *Comprehensive:* A "complete" multisystem examination is performed.

Contributing Factors

Although the determining factors just discussed are the basis for E&M coding, there are circumstances in which other factors contribute to determining the level of service.

Counseling. Almost all E&M services contain a degree of counseling with the patient and/or the family. This is factored into the E&M code, and as long as this factor does not exceed 50% of the time spent with the patient, it is included in the E&M code.

Coordination of Care. Some patients need assistance in arranging for care beyond the visit or hospitalization. Some will need care in a skilled nursing facility or home health care. Others will need hospice care. The primary physician usually coordinates this care.

Nature of the Presenting Problem. The presenting problem is usually explained in the chief complaint. It can range from something as simple as a cold in an otherwise healthy patient to a life-threatening problem.

Time. CPT has provided assigned times for each of the CPT E&M codes. Time should not be the determining factor, *with one exception:* if more than 50% of the visit is spent counseling, *only time* determines the level of complexity.

PUTTING IT ALL TOGETHER TO DETERMINE THE CODE

- Determine whether the patient is new or established.
- Where is the patient being seen—office, hospital, or other setting?
- Is this a patient of the practice, or is someone requesting a consultation?
- Is the patient "sick" or here for preventative medicine services?
- Is the history problem-focused, expanded problem-focused, detailed, or comprehensive?
- Is the examination problem-focused, expanded problem-focused, detailed, or comprehensive?
- Is medical decision making straightforward, low, moderate, or high?
- Pick the code.

CPT Coding Definitions

- **Bundled codes** describe procedures or services that are grouped together and paid as one. An example would be code 90700 Diphtheria, tetanus

<oids, and acellular pertussis vaccine for intramuscular use.

- **Unbundled codes** describe separating the components of a procedure and reporting them separately. To use the diphtheria example, if someone reports the three vaccines separately, it gives the impression that three injections rather than one were given.
- **Upcoding** is a deliberate increase in a CPT code to receive higher reimbursements. This is a target of CMS investigations and should never be done.
- **Downcoding** is usually done by the insurance companies if, on review, the examiner feels the documentation does not match the code description.

CRITICAL THINKING APPLICATION

If a patient was referred for epigastric pain and Dr. Shuman performed an ultrasound examination of the gallbladder, what would Kay need to consider to properly code this encounter?

CODING TIPS AND HINTS

- Always have the latest edition of CPT and HCPCS.
- Follow the CCI information quarterly.
- Never code something because it is "close" to the description; research it further.
- Review the guidelines and refer to them as part of your routine. It would be extremely difficult for any one person to know all the specific guidelines.
- Keep the lines of communication open with the physician and never hesitate to ask for clarification.
- Develop and use an audit sheet that you are comfortable with and do periodic code reviews. This may not be your responsibility, but understanding how a chart audit is done can help you in your coding responsibilities.
- Know the modifiers and use them when appropriate.
- Know abbreviations, especially for laboratory procedures.

Legal and Ethical Issues

Medical assistants must be responsible and remain knowledgeable about CPT to ensure that no fraud takes place in the coding and claims submission process. Medical assistants should also ensure that proper precautions are taken to avoid incorrect coding, data entry errors, and false claims submissions.

Codes or narratives should not be altered in patient chart documentation to increase insurance reimbursement or to accommodate policy coverage requirements. Deliberate misrepresentation may carry criminal and/or civil penalties.

SUMMARY OF SCENARIO

Kay enjoys working toward becoming a medical assistant. As Kay progresses with learning procedural coding, she envisions herself as becoming more well rounded in her knowledge of the practice's administrative operations.

The encounter form is a common document used to enter the procedure when a patient checks out, but knowing how to use the CPT manual is essential when notes must be coded from outpatient procedures performed by Dr. Shuman or Dr. Taylor. As with diagnostic coding, Kay can pull the patient chart for research and documentation if any questions arise about a claim. Kay knows that coding to the highest level of specificity will help in accuracy and obtaining maximum reimbursement.

Kay continues to use the Internet to network and research. She stays informed of the changes in procedural coding by ordering the CPT Manual each year.

SUMMARY OF LEARNING OBJECTIVES

■ The CPT serves three basic purposes. First, it is used to submit claims to third-party payors for reimbursement. Second, the CPT is used to track utilization and ensure that the procedures performed relate to the patient diagnosis. Third, the CPT is a method of measuring physician productivity.

■ The CPT contains several sections, including general groupings of codes; subsections, which better define the sections; subheadings, which make the subsection even more specific; and categories, where the actual code can be found.

■ Guidelines are provided at the beginning of each section of the CPT and offer information about the codes in that particular section and specific coding instructions. Special circumstances for coding may be included. These should be read thoroughly and clearly understood before a medical assistant attempts any coding in that section.

■ Modifiers are important, because they further clarify and explain a service that may have been difficult to perform or a complicated procedure. The modifier offers the payor a logical explanation for extra charges that were incurred because of the special circumstances. If these are not used, the provider may be paid a reduced amount of money.

The payor must be completely convinced that the amount charged is a fair amount for the procedure performed.

■ Most claims for services in a physician's office include an evaluation and management code. This code indicates how much time, decision making, and evaluation were employed by the physician as he or she examined the patient. Not all patient encounters take the same amount of time or use the same amount of decision-making ability. Therefore no physician should charge for 1 hour of time with the patient when only 15 minutes was spent. The evaluation and management codes clarify exactly what was needed to provide quality care to the patient.

■ Upcoding is assigning a code for a procedure that is deliberately "higher" than the actual code to increase the amount of reimbursement to the provider. Physicians sometimes upcode because they feel the amount of reimbursement is too low, but this practice can constitute fraud and must be avoided at all times.

INTERNET CONNECTIONS

- American Academy of Professional Coders
  http://www.aapc.com/
- American Medical Association
  http://www.ama-assn.org
- Centers for Medicare and Medicaid Services
  http://www.cms.gov/
- National Center for Health Statistics
  http://www.cdc.gov/nchs/
- US Government Printing Office (to access *Federal Register*)
  http://www.access.gpo.gov/

REFERENCES

Fordney M: *Insurance handbook for the medical office*, ed 6. Philadelphia, 2002, WB Saunders.

Buck C: *Step-by-step medical coding*, ed 4. Philadelphia, 2002, WB Saunders.

CHAPTER 17

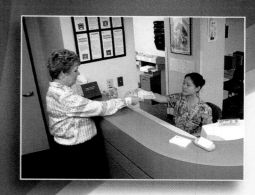

Scenario

The school where Kalene Umber receives her medical assistant training offers an optional job-shadowing module. For her assignment, she chose a nearby health center, where she observed the administrative responsibilities of the medical assistants employed in this multispecialty practice. Kalene found that some of the offices were organized and efficient, whereas others lacked a structured routine, especially in the insurance department. Kalene, a detail-oriented person who enjoyed her studies related to billing and coding, heard numerous comments from employees in the administrative area related to the volumes of work in the billing offices. Her office manager explained that the mountainous paperwork was created as a result of managed care requirements, rejected claims needing further research, and inconsistencies in the demands of the various insurance companies. Kalene agreed that keeping up with the requirements and regulations of the many third-party payors and government entitlement programs must be an overwhelming task. She concluded that billing and reimbursement are at the heart of the medical facility, and the correct completion of insurance claim forms is central to the success of the practice. She realized that becoming familiar with the complexities of the insurance claims process would be challenging, but through education, organization, and dedication, she was convinced that she could become a valuable employee and an advocate for the patients that needed her assistance in resolving issues related to their claims for reimbursement.

The Health Insurance Claim Form

Janet Beik
Alexandra P. Young

Learning Objectives

- Define and spell the terms listed in the vocabulary.
- Discuss the differences between paper claims and electronic claims.
- Differentiate between "clean" and "dirty" claims.
- Understand the guidelines for completing the CMS-1500 claim form.
- Explain how to complete each of the 33 blocks of the CMS-1500 claim form.
- List the OCR guidelines.
- Discuss methods of preventing claim rejections.
- Describe ways of checking the status of claims.

National Curriculum Competencies

ADMINISTRATIVE COMPETENCIES

4a. Apply managed care policies and procedures
4b. Apply third-party guidelines
4f. Complete insurance claim forms

TRANSDISCIPLINARY COMPETENCIES

1b. Recognize and respond to verbal communication
2a. Identify and respond to issues of confidentiality
2b. Perform within legal and ethical boundaries
2d. Document appropriately
3a. Explain general office policies
4c. Utilize computer software to maintain office systems

Vocabulary

assignment of benefits The transfer of the patient's legal right to collect benefits for medical expenses to the provider of those services, authorizing the payment to be sent directly to the provider.

audit trail The path left by a transaction when it has been completed, often referred to when tracking medical services used by patients or researching claims.

beneficiary Individual entitled to receive benefits from an insurance policy or program, or a governmental entitlement program offering healthcare benefits. Also called a *participant, subscriber, dependent, enrollee,* or *member.*

carrier As related to insurance, a company that assumes the risk of an insurance policy.

carrier-direct system A system for electronic data submission in which the medical facility has a computer system designed to transmit claims to a specific carrier directly, without first passing through a clearinghouse.

clean claim An insurance claim form that has been completed correctly (no errors or omissions) and can be processed and paid promptly if the claim meets the restrictions on covered services and items.

clearinghouse A centralized facility, sometimes called a *third-party administrator* (TPA), to whom insurance claims are transmitted. Clearinghouses separate, check, and redistribute claims electronically to various insurance carriers, and may offer additional services to the physician.

commercial insurance Plans (sometimes called *private insurance*) that reimburse the insured for expenses resulting from illness or injury according to a specific fee schedule as outlined in the insurance policy and on a fee-for-service basis.

digital signature A signature used for electronic claims; it consists of lines of text or a text box and is attached through a software application.

dingy claim A claim that is delayed because it cannot be processed, usually because the software used to transfer the claim or system changes make it incompatible with the receiving system.

dirty claim Claims that contain errors or omissions that cannot be processed or must be processed by hand because of OCR scanner rejection.

electronic claims Claims that are submitted to insurance processing facilities using a computerized medium, such as direct data entry, direct wire, dial-in telephone digital fax, or personal computer download/upload.

electronic data interchange The transfer of data back and forth between two or more entities using an electronic medium.

electronic signature A scanned signature or other such mark that is accepted as proof of approval and/or responsibility for the content of an electronic document.

employer identification number (EIN) The number used by the Internal Revenue Service that identifies a business or individual functioning as a business entity for income tax reporting.

fiscal intermediary An organization that contracts with the government to handle and mediate insurance claims from medical facilities, home health agencies, or providers of medical services or supplies.

incomplete claim A claim that is missing information and is returned to the provider for correction and resubmission.

insured An individual or organization who is covered by an insurance policy according to the policy terms, usually the individual or group who pays the premiums. Blue Cross/Blue Shield refers to this person or group as the *subscriber*.

invalid claim A claim that is incorrect in some manner or does not present a logical picture of the patient's situation.

Medigap A term sometimes applied to private insurance products that supplement Medicare insurance benefits.

national provider identifier (NPI) A lifetime number consisting of 10 digits that Medicare will use to replace the provider identification number (PIN) and the unique physician identification number (UPIN).

optical character recognition (OCR) The electronic scanning of printed items as images and use of special software to recognize these images (or characters) as ASCII text.

paper claims Hard copies of insurance claims that have been completed and sent by surface mail.

policyholder A person who pays a premium to an insurance company and in whose name the policy is written in exchange for the insurance protection provided by a policy of insurance, usually applicable to an automobile policy.

provider The company, individual, or group that provides medical services to a patient.

provider identification number (PIN) A number assigned to providers by carriers for use in submission of claims.

rejected claim A claim returned to the provider for clarification of any question and that must be corrected prior to resubmission.

third-party administrator An organization that processes claims and performs other business-related functions for a health plan.

third-party payor An entity that makes a payment on an obligation or debt but is not a party of the contract that created the debt.

unique provider identification number (UPIN) A number assigned by fiscal intermediaries to identify providers on claims for services.

universal claim form The form developed by the Health Care Financing Administration (HCFA) (now known as the Centers for Medicare and Medicaid Services [CMS]) and approved by the AMA for use in submitting all government-sponsored claims.

Medical insurance can be many things to many people. To some, it is a mound of paperwork. To others, it is a mass of confusion and regulations that seem to constantly change. But to a patient, medical insurance can quite literally be the difference between life and death. The lack of adequate and affordable healthcare is one of the most challenging issues faced by the government and the citizens of the United States. This makes health insurance a valuable benefit to most Americans. The enormous healthcare industry is the source of billions of dollars spent in this country each year. The leaders of the healthcare industry are constantly looking for ways to reduce costs and simplify the processes related to healthcare expense reimbursement.

The **universal claim form** (Figure 17-1), now called the CMS-1500 (formerly the HCFA-1500), was first developed in 1988 by the Health Care Financing Administration and approved by the American Medical Association Council on Medical Service for use in submitting Medicare claims. The CMS-1500 claim form answers the needs of healthcare insurers and can be downloaded along with detailed instructions on the CMS website.

The CMS-1500 form was renamed since HCFA became the Centers for Medicare and Medicaid Service on July 1, 2001. This governmental agency divides the former responsibilities of the Health Care Financing Administration into three entities, which are the Center for Medicare Management, the Center for Medicaid and State Operations, and the Center for Beneficiary Choices.

Because many changes will take place over the next several years, as healthcare facilities move into compliance with HIPAA regulations and more claims are submitted through **electronic data interchange**, medical assistants will need to stay abreast of the guidelines as they are released and implement those that are applicable to their individual facilities. Each facility should designate a person or persons to be responsible for implementation and continuous compliance with HIPAA.

Audit Trails

Electronic transactions leave behind a path or trail as they are processed, and this trail can be tracked or audited to provide a record. This record, called an **audit trail**, can be used to verify that information was processed correctly or to locate the source of an error. If an office uses a computerized accounting program and submits claims electronically, the task of keeping track of claims is simple, because the software is capable of printing out an "insurance aging report" by date, by patient name, or by carrier name. If **paper claims** are used, however, the medical assistant should establish a follow-up procedure for tracking insurance claims. This can be accomplished by using an insurance claims register or log (Figure 17-2). This document can be developed and updated with little effort using a spreadsheet software program.

Another method of tracking claims is a tickler file, also called a *suspense* or *follow-up file*. With this method, a copy of each insurance claim is filed chronologically, and the file is checked periodically for unprocessed (delinquent) claims. When the claim is paid, the copy is removed, and the information is posted on the patient's ledger card.

Delinquent claims remaining in the file after the normal contract time limits are pulled and then traced. If the claim has been denied, a letter may be sent to the insurance carrier's appeals department with a copy to the patient. (For more information on this topic, see Tracking Insurance Claims later in this chapter.)

Types of Claims

A medical assistant may submit insurance claims to a **third-party payor** or an insurance **carrier** either by hard copy (paper) or electronically. Most of today's computer software programs generate claims internally from the information that is entered into the database.

It is estimated that more than 6 billion insurance claims are filed every year—about 500 million per month. Of those claims, less than half are filed electronically. The remaining claims are still filed manually on a paper claim form. However, as the government and private insurers continue the migration toward time-saving electronic submissions, more claims will be submitted by electronic means. If a patient furnishes a different form from a **commercial insurance** company, it is usually acceptable to complete the CMS-1500 form and attach it to the commercial form for submission.

Paper

Paper claims often contain errors, which significantly lengthens payment turnaround time. About 30% to 35% of all paper claims are rejected because of typographical errors and errors of omission. Paper claims have advantages and disadvantages.

Advantages
- Documentation explaining unusual circumstances can be readily attached, if necessary and allowed.
- Start-up cost is minimal.
- Forms are readily available.
- Accepted by most third-party payors.

Disadvantages
- Completing forms is labor intensive.
- Costs of mailing, follow-up, and resubmission can become excessive.
- Greater chance for rejection.
- Cash flow is delayed because of slower reimbursements.
- Require a lot of storage space.

Electronic

Electronic claims processing reduces payment turnaround time by shortening the payment cycle and can reduce average error rates to less than 1% or 2%. Some insurance companies even waive the attachment requirements for many procedures when claims are submitted electronically. Some facilities use a **carrier-direct system**, in which claims are submitted directly to the specific carrier without first passing through a **clearinghouse**. There are also advantages and disadvantages to using electronic claims.

PLEASE
DO NOT
STAPLE
IN THIS
AREA

CARRIER

[ ] PICA

HEALTH INSURANCE CLAIM FORM

PICA [ ]

1. MEDICARE   MEDICAID   CHAMPUS   CHAMPVA   GROUP HEALTH PLAN   FECA BLK LUNG   OTHER
[ ] (Medicare #)   [ ] (Medicaid #)   [ ] (Sponsor's SSN)   [ ] (VA File #)   [ ] (SSN or ID)   [ ] (SSN)   [ ] (ID)

1a. INSURED'S I.D. NUMBER   (FOR PROGRAM IN ITEM 1)

2. PATIENT'S NAME (Last Name, First Name, Middle Initial)

3. PATIENT'S BIRTH DATE   MM | DD | YY   SEX   M [ ]   F [ ]

4. INSURED'S NAME (Last Name, First Name, Middle Initial)

5. PATIENT'S ADDRESS (No., Street)

6. PATIENT RELATIONSHIP TO INSURED
Self [ ]   Spouse [ ]   Child [ ]   Other [ ]

7. INSURED'S ADDRESS (No., Street)

CITY   STATE

8. PATIENT STATUS
Single [ ]   Married [ ]   Other [ ]

CITY   STATE

ZIP CODE   TELEPHONE (Include Area Code) ( )

Employed [ ]   Full-Time Student [ ]   Part-Time Student [ ]

ZIP CODE   TELEPHONE (INCLUDE AREA CODE) ( )

9. OTHER INSURED'S NAME (Last Name, First Name, Middle Initial)

10. IS PATIENT'S CONDITION RELATED TO:

11. INSURED'S POLICY GROUP OR FECA NUMBER

a. OTHER INSURED'S POLICY OR GROUP NUMBER

a. EMPLOYMENT? (CURRENT OR PREVIOUS)
[ ] YES   [ ] NO

a. INSURED'S DATE OF BIRTH   MM | DD | YY   SEX   M [ ]   F [ ]

b. OTHER INSURED'S DATE OF BIRTH   MM | DD | YY   SEX   M [ ]   F [ ]

b. AUTO ACCIDENT?   PLACE (State)
[ ] YES   [ ] NO

b. EMPLOYER'S NAME OR SCHOOL NAME

c. EMPLOYER'S NAME OR SCHOOL NAME

c. OTHER ACCIDENT?
[ ] YES   [ ] NO

c. INSURANCE PLAN NAME OR PROGRAM NAME

d. INSURANCE PLAN NAME OR PROGRAM NAME

10d. RESERVED FOR LOCAL USE

d. IS THERE ANOTHER HEALTH BENEFIT PLAN?
[ ] YES   [ ] NO   *If yes,* return to and complete item 9 a-d.

READ BACK OF FORM BEFORE COMPLETING & SIGNING THIS FORM.

12. PATIENT'S OR AUTHORIZED PERSON'S SIGNATURE I authorize the release of any medical or other information necessary to process this claim. I also request payment of government benefits either to myself or to the party who accepts assignment below.

SIGNED _____ DATE _____

13. INSURED'S OR AUTHORIZED PERSON'S SIGNATURE I authorize payment of medical benefits to the undersigned physician or supplier for services described below.

SIGNED _____

14. DATE OF CURRENT: MM | DD | YY   ◀ ILLNESS (First symptom) OR INJURY (Accident) OR PREGNANCY(LMP)

15. IF PATIENT HAS HAD SAME OR SIMILAR ILLNESS. GIVE FIRST DATE   MM | DD | YY

16. DATES PATIENT UNABLE TO WORK IN CURRENT OCCUPATION   FROM MM | DD | YY   TO MM | DD | YY

17. NAME OF REFERRING PHYSICIAN OR OTHER SOURCE

17a. I.D. NUMBER OF REFERRING PHYSICIAN

18. HOSPITALIZATION DATES RELATED TO CURRENT SERVICES   FROM MM | DD | YY   TO MM | DD | YY

19. RESERVED FOR LOCAL USE

20. OUTSIDE LAB? $ CHARGES
[ ] YES   [ ] NO

21. DIAGNOSIS OR NATURE OF ILLNESS OR INJURY. (RELATE ITEMS 1,2,3 OR 4 TO ITEM 24E BY LINE)

1. L___ . ___   3. L___ . ___

2. L___ . ___   4. L___ . ___

22. MEDICAID RESUBMISSION CODE   ORIGINAL REF. NO.

23. PRIOR AUTHORIZATION NUMBER

24. A DATE(S) OF SERVICE			B Place of Service	C Type of Service	D PROCEDURES, SERVICES, OR SUPPLIES (Explain Unusual Circumstances) CPT/HCPCS	MODIFIER	E DIAGNOSIS CODE	F $ CHARGES	G DAYS OR UNITS	H EPSDT Family Plan	I EMG	J COB	K RESERVED FOR LOCAL USE
From MM DD YY	To MM DD YY												
1													
2													
3													
4													
5													
6													

25. FEDERAL TAX I.D. NUMBER   SSN EIN [ ] [ ]

26. PATIENT'S ACCOUNT NO.

27. ACCEPT ASSIGNMENT? (For govt. claims, see back) [ ] YES   [ ] NO

28. TOTAL CHARGE $

29. AMOUNT PAID $

30. BALANCE DUE $

31. SIGNATURE OF PHYSICIAN OR SUPPLIER INCLUDING DEGREES OR CREDENTIALS (I certify that the statements on the reverse apply to this bill and are made a part thereof.)

SIGNED _____ DATE _____

32. NAME AND ADDRESS OF FACILITY WHERE SERVICES WERE RENDERED (If other than home or office)

33. PHYSICIAN'S, SUPPLIER'S BILLING NAME, ADDRESS, ZIP CODE & PHONE #

PIN# _____   GRP# _____

(APPROVED BY AMA COUNCIL ON MEDICAL SERVICE 8/88)   **PLEASE PRINT OR TYPE**   APPROVED OMB-0938-0008 FORM CMS-1500 (12-90), FORM RRB-1500, APPROVED OMB-1215-0055 FORM OWCP-1500, APPROVED OMB-0720-0001 (CHAMPUS)

PATIENT AND INSURED INFORMATION

PHYSICIAN OR SUPPLIER INFORMATION

FIGURE 17-1   The CMS-1500 claim form.

Patient's Name Group/policy No.	Name of Insurance Company	Claim Submitted		Follow-Up		Claim Paid		Difference
		Date	Amount	Date	Date	Date	Amt	
Jones, Bob	BC/BS	1-7-03	319.37			2/28/03	294.82	24.55
Carson, David	BC	1-8-03	268.08	2-10-03	3-10-03			
Linden, Jan	Medicaid	1-9-03	146.15	2-10-03				
Paul, Emma	Medicare	1-10-03	96.28	2-10-03				
Cortez, Jose	Unicare	1-10-03	647.09	2-10-03				
Dimico, Joe	Tricare	2-1-03	134.78	3-10-03				
Coldman, Billy	Aetna	2-4-03	607.67	3-10-03				
Fritz, Renee	Travelers	2-10-03	564.55	3-10-03				
Wong, Chang	Prudential	2-15-03	1515.79					
Billings, Harry	Allstate	2-21-03	121.21					
Green, James	BC	2-24-03	124.99					

INSURANCE CLAIMS REGISTER   Page No. _____

FIGURE 17-2   Insurance claims register.

Advantages

- Cost savings as a result of shortened preparation time.
- Cost savings in postage.
- Reduced claim rejection.
- Quicker payment turnaround time.
- Generation of claim status reports.

Disadvantages

- Computer hardware/software glitches and/or power outages that delay preparation or transmission.
- Issue of creating electronic attachments.
- Initial start-up is expensive.

Electronic claims can be submitted either directly to the carrier via modem, after being validated by the computer software program, or through a claims clearinghouse. A clearinghouse (also called a *third-party administrator*, or *TPA*) is a company that offers the healthcare **provider** (for a fee) the service of receiving claim transmissions, checking and preparing the claims for processing, consolidating claims so that one transmission can be sent to each carrier, and submitting claims in correct data format to the applicable insurance payor. Clearinghouses provide the following additional services:

- Audit claims to make sure all required fields are completed and data are correct.
- Report the number of claims submitted and the number of errors and their specifics.
- Forward claims to insurance carriers that accept electronic claims (Medicare, Medicaid, Blue Cross/Blue Shield, and others) or to another clearinghouse that may hold the contracts with specific payors.
- Keep provider offices updated as new carriers are added to the database,
- Generate informative statistical reports.

Typically with electronic claims processing, payments are received in half the time when compared with turnaround time for paper claims. Very soon after claims are transmitted, reports will be sent from the clearinghouse for tracking purposes, and the medical assistant will know in a very short time which claims have been rejected and which ones need additional information.

Whether the medical facility chooses to submit claims directly to the carrier or use the services of a clearinghouse, there is usually an "enrollment" process. Most government and many commercial carriers require enrollment so they can set up information about the medical office on their computer system. Some require a signed contract. The biggest obstacle in getting set up for electronic claims processing is the time it takes for approval from state, federal, and in some cases, commercial/HMO carriers. The only equipment requirements for electronic claims submission besides a computer are a modem and a working phone line. Clearinghouse services are not free, however. In addition to the set-up cost, many charge a nominal fee (usually less than a dollar) on a per-claim basis.

CRITICAL THINKING APPLICATION

Kalene is interested in learning more about filing claims electronically. In the medical facility where she is doing her externship, she has asked to work with Mrs. Leonard, who performs this procedure in the office. How can working closely with Mrs. Leonard benefit Kalene on this subject?

Claim Status

Obtaining timely and correct payment from third-party payors is a concern for many medical practices. Lost claims, delayed claims, and dirty claims result in healthcare providers waiting months for payment of professional services rendered. Most providers will agree that claim processing payment issues are at the heart of most provider-payor conflicts.

Clean Claims

A **clean claim** is one that has been filled out correctly, contains no missing data or errors, and has been submitted for payment within the time allowed by the insurer. Additionally, it has passed all claim edits and audits and can be processed and paid on the first submission.

Dirty Claims

If there are errors or omissions on claim forms, if they are improperly filled out, or if they are submitted after the time allowed by the third-party payor, claims are subsequently denied. Claims like these are known as **dirty claims**. The two main reasons for denial are (1) technical errors and (2) insurance policy coverage issues. Technical errors include typographical or mathematical errors and incorrect or incomplete information. Coverage issues are usually more complex and are not as readily resolved as technical errors. A common reason for rejection in this category is that a procedure listed on the claim is not a covered service or is involved with a preexisting condition.

Dingy Claims

A **dingy claim** results when the fiscal intermediary for Medicare cannot process a claim for a particular service or bill type, and the claim is put on hold until the necessary system changes are implemented and the claim can be paid correctly.

Incomplete Claims

An **incomplete claim** is missing some type of information.

Invalid Claims

An **invalid claim** is complete, but does not make logical sense or is incorrect in some way.

Rejected Claims

A *rejected claim* is one that has missing or incorrect information. **Rejected claims** subsequently require investigation, need further clarification, and/or possibly require answers or documentation for specific questions.

Denied Claims

Claims can be denied as the result of a technical error but are usually not paid because the medical service submitted is not covered under the policy, is an ineligible service, or must be applied to the deductible in accordance with the policy.

Rules for Completing the Health Insurance Claim Form

When the first appointment is made, the medical assistant should ask the patient for all pertinent insurance information. Much of this information is on the patient information form that is completed when the patient comes to the medical office for the initial visit and is inserted into the medical chart as well as entered into the computer's patient database. Additional information will have to be abstracted from the patient record for processing the insurance claim. Remember that the patient may not be the **beneficiary** of insurance reimbursement.

Patients should be asked during each visit whether their insurance information is complete and current. Many offices use a form that allows the patient to provide address and phone updates, as well as new insurance information. The use of sign-in sheets is now questionable, because such logs usually list all of the patients who visited the facility by name, and this violates privacy guidelines.

Health Insurance Claim Form Guidelines

A medical assistant can use the following general guidelines for completing a health insurance claim form:
- Photocopy the back and front of the patient's insurance card and place it in the medical record.
- If a patient has more than one insurance policy, it is important to get the name, address, group, and policy number for each company.
- Record the name of the subscriber if it is someone other than the patient.
- Obtain a signed authorization form for releasing information to the insurance carrier; for Medicare, obtain authorization to pay benefits directly to the physician (Figure 17-3).
- Complete all required blocks of the CMS-1500 claim form (Procedure 17-1).
- Proofread the form carefully.
- Make certain any necessary attachments are included with the completed form.
- Follow office policies and guidelines for claim review and signatures.
- Forward the original (red print) claim to the proper insurance carrier either by mail or electronically.
- If creating a paper claim, make a copy of the completed and signed claim form for the office records.
- Enter the appropriate information in the insurance log and record the insurance submission information on the patient's ledger (Figure 17-4).

Optical Scanning (OCR) Guidelines

Because many insurance carriers are using **optical character recognition (OCR)** scanners to transfer the information on claim forms to their computers' memories, the CMS-1500 claim form is printed in red ink. The reason for this is that the OCR process uses a red-bulb scanner, which causes the preprinted portion of the form to disappear or "drop out." The resulting image allows for "clean" recognition of the data inserted without the characters being obstructed by the lines and text of the form.

A medical assistant should use OCR scanning rules for completing the CMS-1500 form. Entries should be clear and sharp; carbon copies are not acceptable. A proportionally spaced 12-point font such as Courier works best. The following are additional guidelines:

ASSIGNMENT OF INSURANCE BENEFITS

I, the undersigned, represent that I have insurance coverage with and do hereby authorize
_____ to pay and assign directly to _____
  (NAME OF COMPANY)   (NAME OF DOCTOR)

all surgical and/or medical benefits, if any, otherwise payable to me for services as described on the attached forms hereof, but not to exceed the charges for those services. I understand that I am financially responsible for all charges whether or not paid by said insurance. I hereby authorize said assignee to release all information necessary to secure the payment of said benefits.

Date _____   Signed _____

FIGURE 17-3   Assignment of benefits form.

PROCEDURE **17-1**

Complete an Insurance Claim Form

GOAL: Accurately complete a CMS-1500 (formerly HCFA-1500) claim form.

EQUIPMENT AND SUPPLIES

- Patient information form
- Photocopy of patient's insurance ID card
- Encounter form
- Patient record
- Patient's ledger
- CMS-1500 form
- Typewriter or computer

PROCEDURAL STEPS

Patient/Insured Section

Block 1　Check the type of health insurance coverage applicable to the claim.

Block 1a　Enter the patient's insurance identification number or Medicare ID number exactly as it appears on his or her insurance card.

Block 2　Enter the patient's last name, first name, and middle initial following OCR guidelines.

Block 3　Enter the patient's birth date in MM DD YYYY format, and enter an "X" in the appropriate box for sex.

Block 4　For commercial and Blue Cross/Blue Shield claims, enter "SAME" if patient and insured (policyholder) are the same person. If the insured's name is different from the patient, enter the last name, first name, and middle initial in this block. If there is insurance primary to Medicare, list the name of the insured here. If Medicare is primary, leave blank. For CHAMPUS/TRICARE, enter the "sponsor's" name

Block 5　Enter the patient's street address on the first line, city and state on the second line, and the ZIP code and telephone number on the third line. Remember to use all capital letters and no punctuation.

Block 6　Check the appropriate box for the patient's relationship to insured. If Medicare is primary, leave blank.

Block 7　Enter the insured's address and telephone number, unless the insured and the patient are the same, in which case enter "SAME." Complete this item only when blocks 4 and 11 are completed. For Medicare and Medicaid, leave blank.

Block 8　Check the appropriate box for the patient's marital status and whether employed or a student.

Block 9　(Required if 11d is marked "yes.") If the patient has other medical insurance coverage, and he or she is not the insured, enter the insured's name, and complete boxes 9a through 9d. If there is no other insurance, leave 9a through 9d blank and proceed to block 10.

Block 9a　Enter the policy or group number of the insured's secondary insurance coverage. If the secondary policy is Medigap, enter the policy and/or group number preceded by MEDIGAP.

Block 9b　Enter the insured's birth date in MM DD YYYY format, and enter an "X" in the appropriate sex box.

Block 9c　Enter the name of the insured's employer or school, if applicable. Leave blank if a Medigap PayerID is entered in item 9d. Otherwise, enter the claims processing address of the Medigap insurer.

Block 9d　Enter the name of the secondary insurance plan or program. If the secondary insurer is a Medigap policy, enter the nine-digit PayerID number of the Medigap insurer. If there is no PayerID number, enter the Medigap insurance program or plan name.

Continued

Block 10 Check the appropriate boxes in this section to identify whether the patient's condition was related to either his or her employment, auto accident, or other accident.

Block 10a Check "no" unless the illness, accident, or injury was the result of employment or occurred on the job or in the process of performing one's job.

Block 10b Check "no" unless the claim is related to an injury resulting from an automobile accident. In the case of an auto accident, enter the two-letter state code where the accident occurred.

Block 10c Enter an "X" in the appropriate box.

Block 10d This block is usually reserved for Medicaid as secondary payor claims. In some states, this block is used only if the patient is entitled to Medicaid. If this is the case, enter the patient's Medicaid number, preceded by MCD. For Medicare, leave blank. Some third-party payors want the word "ATTACHMENT(S)" entered into this field if there are attachments included with the claim.

Block 11 For commercial carriers, enter the group policy name/number from the patient's card. For BC/BS and Medicaid, leave blank. For insurance primary to Medicare, enter the insured's policy or group number. If Medicare is primary, the word "NONE" must appear in this block. By doing so indicates that Medicare is primary. NOTE: For a claim to be considered for Medicare Secondary Payer, a copy of the primary payor's explanation of benefits (EOB) must be included with the claim form.

Block 11a Enter the insured's birth date and sex if different from block 3. For Medicare and Medicaid, leave blank.

Block 11b Enter the employer's name if applicable. On Medicare claims, if there is a second policy and the insured's status is retired, enter the date of retirement preceded by the word "RETIRED."

Block 11c Enter the nine-digit PayerID number of the primary insurer. If no such number exists, enter the complete name of the primary payor's program or plan name.

Block 11d Check "no" if patient is covered by only one insurance policy. If the answer is "yes," give the name of the company and any other information available in block 9. For Medicare and Medicaid, leave blank.

Block 12 The patient or authorized person must sign and date this item unless a signature is on file. If this is the case, the words "SIGNATURE ON FILE" should be entered here. Leave blank on Medicaid claims.

Block 13 The patient or authorized person should sign and date this item if he or she agrees that benefits are to be paid directly to the provider. For Medicare supplements and cross-over claims, "SIGNATURE ON FILE" must also appear in this block. For Medicaid, leave blank.

Physician/Supplier Information

Block 14 Enter the date of the first symptom of the current illness, injury, or pregnancy in this block if one is documented in the chart notes or the date of the last menstrual cycle if the claim is related to pregnancy.

Block 15 Enter the date the patient was first treated for this condition. Leave blank for Medicare claims.

Block 16 Enter date(s) patient is unable to work in current occupation if it is a workers' compensation claim. Not required for most other carriers.

Block 17 Enter the name of the referring (or ordering) physician, if applicable.

Block 17a Enter the UPIN/NPI number of the referring/ordering physician listed in block 17.

Block 18 If the claim is for a related hospital stay, enter the dates of hospital admission and discharge. If the patient has not been discharged, leave the "to" box blank.

Block 19 This block is usually left blank. Some private payors insert the word "ATTACHMENT(S)" when specific documentation accompanies the claim.

Block 20 If laboratory procedures are listed on the claim in block 24, and these services were performed in the provider's facility, the "no" box is checked with an "X" or left blank. If lab work shown on the claim was done by an outside lab and billed to the provider, check the "yes" box, and enter the total amount of the charges. Leave this block blank if no lab tests were done.

Block 21 Enter the patient's diagnosis or diagnoses using ICD-9-CM code number(s), listing the primary diagnosis first. Up to four codes (in priority order) can be entered in block 21.

PROCEDURE 17-1—cont'd

Block 22   Required only for replacement claims for Medicaid. Enter the appropriate 3-digit replacement code followed by the 17-digit transaction control number of the most current incorrectly paid claim.

Block 23   For private and commercial carriers and Medicaid, enter the 10-digit prior authorization number for those procedures requiring prior approval assigned by the peer review organization (PRO). Consult the specific guidelines for the payor to whom the claim is being submitted.

Block 24a   The first date of service for the charge on this line should be placed in the "From" column. When a claim is for more than one day of the same service on a line item, the days must be in consecutive order. The last date of service is required in the "To" column. Enter the month, day, and year (in the MM DD YYYY format) for each procedure, service, or supply. When "from" and "to" dates are shown for a series of identical services, enter the number of days or units in 24G.

Block 24b   Enter the appropriate place of service code.

Block 24c   Enter the appropriate type of service code. NOTE: For private payors and Medicare, leave blank. All others, refer to specific guidelines.

Block 24d   Enter the procedure, service, or supply code using appropriate five-digit CPT or HCPCS procedure code. Enter a two-position modifier when applicable.

Block 24e   Link the procedure/service code back to the diagnosis code in block 21 by indicating the applicable number of the diagnosis code (1, 2, 3 or 4) to that line's procedure code.

Block 24f   Enter the charge for each listed procedure, supply, and/or service.

Block 24g   Enter the number of days or units. If only one service is performed, enter the number 1.

Block 24h   Leave blank for all claims with the exception of certain Medicaid claims.

Block 24i   For certain carriers, enter an "X" or "E" as appropriate if documentation indicates a medical emergency existed. Leave blank for Medicare claims.

Block 24j   For commercial claims, BC/BS, Medicare, Medicaid, and TRICARE, leave blank. (Refer to specific third-party payor guidelines.)

Block 24k   Enter the five-digit number that has been assigned when the provider was approved by the third-party payor. For Medicare, it is referred to as the "billing number." Blue Cross-Blue Shield and Medicaid have their own numbers. This is not the same as the UPIN number.

Block 25   Enter the provider's nine-digit Federal tax identification number and check the appropriate box in this field; or, in the case of an unincorporated practice or sole proprietorship, enter the provider's Social Security number.

Block 26   Enter the patient's account number as assigned by the provider's accounting system, if available. If you are submitting the claim electronically, you are required to provide a patient account number.

Block 27   Check the appropriate block to indicate whether the provider accepts assignment of benefits. If the supplier is a participating provider (PAR), assignment must be accepted for all covered charges. For nonPAR providers, this can be left blank. For Medicaid, check "yes."

Block 28   Total column 24f and enter the total charges in this field.

Block 29   Enter the total amount, if any, that has been paid by the patient. Leave blank if no payment has been made.

Block 30   Used when there is a secondary insurance. Enter the balance owing as indicated on the explanation of benefits (EOB).

Block 31   Enter the signature of the provider, or his or her representative and his or her initials, and the date the form was signed. The signature may be typed, stamped, or handwritten; however, the characters should not fall outside of the block.

Block 32   Enter the name and address of the facility where the services were performed if other than patient's home or physician's office. For Medicare, enter the name and address of the facility regardless of where services were provided.

Block 33   Enter the provider's billing name, address, zip code, and telephone number. Also, enter the billing number (from block 24k). Enter the Group NPI number, if the provider is a member of a group practice. Refer to specific third-party payor guidelines.

INSURANCE CLAIM REGISTER					
PATIENT	INSURANCE COMPANY	DATE FILED	AMOUNT BILLED	AMOUNT PAID	DIFFERENCE

FIGURE 17-4 Insurance log showing the date each claim was filed, the amount billed, the amount paid, and the difference that must be either discounted or billed to the patient.

- Use all uppercase letters.
- Omit all punctuation.
- Use the MM DD YYYY format (with a space between each set of digits) for all birth dates.
- Keep all entries within their respective boxes. "X's" must fall completely within the designated box. NOTE: If a computer software program is being used to generate forms, print a test pattern before printing the final form to ensure proper alignment. If a typewriter is being used, use the test strips on the right and left margins. To check horizontal alignment, type "X's" in both the left and right test patterns.
- For the following, substitute a blank space:
  - Dollar signs and decimal points in charges and ICD codes
  - Dashes preceding procedure code modifiers
  - Parentheses around telephone area codes
  - Hyphens in Social Security numbers
- Omit titles and other designations, such as Sr., Jr., II, or III, unless they appear on the ID card.
- When the charge is expressed in whole dollars, use two zeros in the "cents" column.
- If using a typewriter, do not use lift-off tape, correction tape, or correction fluid.
- Since photocopies of claims cannot be scanned, all resubmissions must be prepared using the original (red print) claim form.
- Do not include any handwritten data (other than signatures) on the forms.

- Do not staple anything to the form.
- Insert the name and address of the insurance company in the proper area in the top margin of the claim form.

Signatures on Health Insurance Claim Forms

A signature verifies that a person agrees with the statements in a document. On a health insurance claim form, there are spaces for the patient and/or **insured** to sign, as well as the provider. As with any document that is verified by signature, the text should be read thoroughly for accuracy prior to signing. The provider is ultimately responsible for the accuracy of the claim, but this does not release the individual who billed the claim from any liability.

Patient Signatures. The patient must sign the release of medical information authorization so that the provider can submit the claim for reimbursement. A signed authorization for a specific period of time may be used, in which case future claims during that time period can be noted "signature on file." Some patients may also sign a lifetime signature authorization, such as persons who are in a skilled nursing facility.

The patient may also sign the **assignment of benefits** block if he or she wants the payment to go directly to the provider. When the patient has already paid the provider, he or she may not sign this block so that the payment will come directly to the patient for reimbursement.

Provider Signatures. Providers may sign the insurance claim form by original signature or by signature stamp. They may also authorize an employee to sign the form, use a signature stamp, or use an **electronic signature** or **digital signature**. Providers who use billing services may offer this same type of authorization to the billing company that files claims on their behalf. Providers may also complete a certification letter for electronic claims once which serves the same purpose as an actual signature, when allowed by third-party payors and governmental entities.

The Health Insurance Claim Form

The CMS-1500 form is divided into two parts (see Figure 17-1). The top part of the form is the patient/insured section; the bottom half is the physician/supplier section. The name and address of the insurance company or government agency should appear in the upper right portion in the margin of the form. This information must be restricted to a 2-inch area just right of the bar code at the top (Figure 17-5).

When completing the CMS-1500 form, follow the guidelines that begin below. NOTE: Comments on filling out each individual block on the CMS-1500 form apply primarily to commercial, Medicare/Medicaid, and Blue Cross/Blue Shield claims.

CHAMPUS/TRICARE claims are similar to commercial claims, except where noted. To become proficient in completing forms for all major payors, a medical assistant should prepare a guidelines manual with detailed instructions on how each of the 33 blocks should be completed for each payor. Usually, claims guidelines can be obtained from the third-party payor. This manual should be updated periodically so that it remains current.

The following are general guidelines for completing the CMS-1500 claims forms.

Patient/Insured Section

Block 1 **Type of Insurance (required).** Check the type of health insurance coverage applicable to the claim. EXAMPLE: If the claim is primary for Medicare, check the Medicare box. If Medicare is secondary, check the "Other" box.

1. MEDICARE (Medicare #) | MEDICAID (Medicaid #) | CHAMPUS (Sponsor's SSN) | CHAMPVA (VA File #) | GROUP HEALTH PLAN (SSN or ID) | FECA BLK LUNG (SSN) | OTHER (ID)

Block 1a **Insured's ID Number (required).** Enter the patient's insurance identification number or Medicare ID number exactly as it appears on his or her insurance card. For CHAMPUS/TRICARE, the sponsor's Social Security number is used.

1a. INSURED'S I.D. NUMBER (FOR PROGRAM IN ITEM 1)

Block 2 **Patient's Name (required).** Enter the patient's last name, first name, and middle initial following OCR guidelines.

2. PATIENT'S NAME (Last Name, First Name, Middle Initial)

Block 3 **Patient's Birth Date (required).** Enter the patient's birth date in MM DD YYYY format, and enter an "X" in the appropriate box for gender.

3. PATIENT'S BIRTH DATE MM DD YY — SEX M F

Block 4 **Insured's Name.** For commercial and Blue Cross/Blue Shield claims, enter "SAME" if patient and insured **(policyholder)** are the same person. If the insured's name is different from the patient, enter the last name, first name, and middle initial in this block. If there is insurance primary to Medicare, either through the patient or spouse's employment or any other source, list the name of the insured here. If Medicare is primary, leave blank. For CHAMPUS/TRICARE, enter the "sponsor's" name.

4. INSURED'S NAME (Last Name, First Name, Middle Initial)

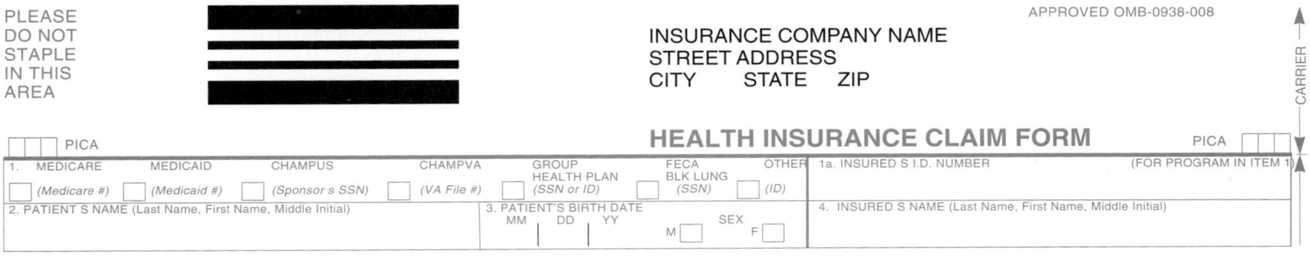
PLEASE DO NOT STAPLE IN THIS AREA

APPROVED OMB-0938-008

INSURANCE COMPANY NAME
STREET ADDRESS
CITY STATE ZIP

CARRIER

PICA HEALTH INSURANCE CLAIM FORM PICA

1. MEDICARE (Medicare #) MEDICAID (Medicaid #) CHAMPUS (Sponsor s SSN) CHAMPVA (VA File #) GROUP HEALTH PLAN (SSN or ID) FECA BLK LUNG (SSN) OTHER (ID)
1a. INSURED S I.D. NUMBER (FOR PROGRAM IN ITEM 1)
2. PATIENT S NAME (Last Name, First Name, Middle Initial)
3. PATIENT'S BIRTH DATE MM DD YY SEX M F
4. INSURED S NAME (Last Name, First Name, Middle Initial)

FIGURE 17-5 Correct placement of insurance company's address.

Block 5   **Patient's Address.** Enter the patient's street address on the first line, the city and state on the second line, and the ZIP code and telephone number on the third line. Remember to use all capital letters and no punctuation.

```
5. PATIENT'S ADDRESS (No., Street)

CITY                                          STATE

ZIP CODE              TELEPHONE (Include Area Code)
                        (    )
```

Block 6   **Patient's Relationship to Insured.** Check the appropriate box for the patient's relationship to the insured. If Medicare is primary, leave blank.

```
6. PATIENT RELATIONSHIP TO INSURED
  Self □   Spouse □   Child □   Other □
```

Block 7   **Insured's Address.** Enter the insured's address and telephone number, unless the insured and the patient are one and the same, in which case enter "SAME." Complete this item only when blocks 4 and 11 are completed. For Medicare and Medicaid, leave this blank.

```
7. INSURED'S ADDRESS (No., Street)

CITY                                          STATE

ZIP CODE              TELEPHONE (INCLUDE AREA CODE)
                        (    )
```

Block 8   **Patient Status.** Check the appropriate box for the patient's marital status and whether he or she is employed or a student.

```
8. PATIENT STATUS
   Single □   Married □      Other □

   Employed □   Full-Time □   Part-Time □
                Student        Student
```

Block 9   **Other Insured's Name (required if 11d is marked "yes").** If the patient has other medical insurance coverage, and he or she is not the insured, enter the insured's name and complete boxes 9a through 9d. If there is no other insurance, leave 9a through 9d blank and proceed to block 10.

Block 9a   **Other Insured's Policy or Group Number.** Enter the policy or group number of the insured's secondary insurance coverage. If the secondary policy is **Medigap**, enter the policy and/or group number preceded by "MEDIGAP."

Block 9b   **Other Insured's Date of Birth.** Enter the insured's birth date in MM DD YYYY format and enter an "X" in the appropriate sex box.

Block 9c   **Employer's Name or School Name (optional).** Enter the name of the insured's employer or school, if applicable. Leave blank if a Medigap Payer ID is entered in box 9d. Otherwise, enter the claims processing address of the Medigap insurer.

Block 9d   **Insurance Plan Name or Program Name.** Enter the name of the secondary insurance plan or program. If the secondary insurer is a Medigap policy, enter the nine-digit Payer ID number of the Medigap insurer. If there is no Payer ID number, enter the Medigap insurance program or plan name. (Medigap policies are identifiable by the numbers "99" in the seventh and eighth digits of the Payer ID.)

```
9. OTHER INSURED'S NAME (Last Name, First Name, Middle Initial)

a. OTHER INSURED'S POLICY OR GROUP NUMBER

b. OTHER INSURED'S DATE OF BIRTH          SEX
   MM   DD   YY                    M □      F □

c. EMPLOYER'S NAME OR SCHOOL NAME

d. INSURANCE PLAN NAME OR PROGRAM NAME
```

Block 10   **Is Patient's Condition Related to (required).** Check the appropriate boxes in this section to identify whether the patient's condition was related to his or her employment, an auto accident, or another accident. If any of the boxes in this block are checked "Yes," this may indicate that the patient's health insurance is not primary and that other insurance, such as workers' compensation or an automobile insurance policy, may be primary.

Block 10a   Check "No" unless the illness, accident, or injury was the result of employment or occurred on the job or in the process of performing one's job.

Block 10b   Check "No" unless the claim is for an injury resulting from an automobile accident. In the case of an auto accident, enter the two-letter state code where the accident occurred.

Block 10c   Enter an "X" in the appropriate box.

```
10. IS PATIENT'S CONDITION RELATED TO:

a. EMPLOYMENT? (CURRENT OR PREVIOUS)
       □ YES          □ NO
b. AUTO ACCIDENT?           PLACE (State)
       □ YES          □ NO ____
c. OTHER ACCIDENT?
       □ YES          □ NO
```

Block 10d **Reserved for Local Use (optional).** This block is usually reserved for Medicaid as secondary payor claims. In some states, this block is used only if the patient is entitled to Medicaid. If this is the case, enter the patient's Medicaid number, preceded by "MCD." For Medicare, leave this blank. Some third-party payors want the word "Attachment(s)" entered into this field if there are attachments included with the claim.

```
10d. RESERVED FOR LOCAL USE
```

Block 11 **Insured's Policy or Group Number.** For commercial carriers, enter the group policy name/number from the patient's card. For Blue Cross/Blue Shield and Medicaid, leave this blank. For insurance primary to Medicare, enter the insured's policy or group number. If Medicare is primary, the word "NONE" must appear in this block. Doing so indicates that Medicare is primary. NOTE: For a claim to be considered for Medicare Secondary Payer, a copy of the primary payor's explanation of benefits (EOB) must be included with the claim form.

Block 11a **Date of Birth.** Enter the insured's birth date and sex if different from block 3. For Medicare and Medicaid, leave this blank.

Block 11b **Employer's Name.** Enter the employer's name if applicable. On Medicare claims, if there is a second policy and the insured's status is retired, enter the date of retirement, preceded by the word "RETIRED."

Block 11c **Insurance Plan Name or Program Name (conditionally required).** Enter the nine-digit Payer ID number of the primary insurer. If no such number exists, enter the complete name of the primary payor's program or plan name.

Block 11d **Is There Another Health Benefit Plan (required).** Check "No" if covered by only one insurance policy. If the answer is "Yes," give the name of the company and any other information available in block 9. For Medicare and Medicaid, leave this blank.

```
11. INSURED'S POLICY GROUP OR FECA NUMBER

a. INSURED'S DATE OF BIRTH        SEX
   MM   DD   YY            M        F

b. EMPLOYER'S NAME OR SCHOOL NAME

c. INSURANCE PLAN NAME OR PROGRAM NAME

d. IS THERE ANOTHER HEALTH BENEFIT PLAN?
     YES      NO   If yes, return to and complete item 9 a-d.
```

Block 12 **Patient's or Authorized Person's Signature (conditionally required).** The patient or authorized person must sign and date this item unless a signature is on file. If this is the case, the words "SIGNATURE ON FILE" or "SOF" should be entered here. Leave this blank on Medicaid claims.

```
READ BACK OF FORM BEFORE COMPLETING & SIGNING THIS FORM.
12. PATIENT'S OR AUTHORIZED PERSON'S SIGNATURE I authorize the release of any medical or other information necessary
to process this claim. I also request payment of government benefits either to myself or to the party who accepts assignment
below.

SIGNED _____                DATE _____
```

Block 13 **Insured's or Authorized Person's Signature.** As in block 12, the patient or authorized person should sign and date this item if he or she agrees that benefits are to be paid directly to the provider. For Medicare supplements and crossover claims, "SIGNATURE ON FILE" or "SOF" must also appear in this block. For Medicaid, leave this blank.

```
13. INSURED'S OR AUTHORIZED PERSON'S SIGNATURE I authorize
    payment of medical benefits to the undersigned physician or supplier for
    services described below.

    SIGNED _____
```

CRITICAL THINKING APPLICATION

It is office policy to request that patients assign benefits when the patient does not pay for services immediately. One of the patients, Mr. Jones, seems hesitant to sign block 13 of the CMS-1500 form. How should Kalene explain the office policy to Mr. Jones?

Physician/Supplier Information

Block 14 **Date of Current Illness Injury (required on accident or medical emergency claims).** Enter the date of the first symptom of the current illness, injury, or pregnancy in this block if one is documented in the chart notes, or the date of the last menstrual cycle if the claim is related to pregnancy. Use caution here, because an incorrect date may indicate a preexisting condition, and the claim will be rejected.

```
14. DATE OF CURRENT:    ILLNESS (First symptom) OR
    MM   DD   YY         INJURY (Accident) OR
                         PREGNANCY(LMP)
```

Block 15 **Same or Similar Illness (optional).** Enter the date the patient was first treated for this condition. Leave this blank for Medicare claims.

15. IF PATIENT HAS HAD SAME OR SIMILAR ILLNESS.
GIVE FIRST DATE   MM   DD   YY

Block 16 Patient Unable to Work (optional).
Enter date(s) the patient is unable to work in his or her current occupation if it is a workers' compensation claim. Not required for most other carriers.

16. DATES PATIENT UNABLE TO WORK IN CURRENT OCCUPATION
          MM   DD   YY   MM   DD   YY
FROM   TO

Block 17 Name of Referring Physician or Other Source (conditionally required). Enter the name of the referring (or ordering) physician, if applicable. If the physician orders a test or procedure that is performed by an ancillary healthcare giver but the physician/source interprets the results, his or her **unique provider identification number (UPIN)** or **national provider identifier (NPI)** must be entered here, and the UPIN number entered in block 17a. EXAMPLE: If Dr. Smith orders an ECG, which is performed by the medical assistant but is interpreted by Dr. Smith, his name is entered into block 17 and his UPIN/NPI number in block 17a. This block is also required if billing for a consultation.

17. NAME OF REFERRING PHYSICIAN OR OTHER SOURCE

Block 17a ID Number of Referring Physician (required if a referring physician is listed in block 17). Enter the UPIN/NPI number of the referring/ordering physician listed in block 17.

17a. I.D. NUMBER OF REFERRING PHYSICIAN

Block 18 Hospitalization Dates Related to Current Services (conditionally required). If the claim is for a related hospital stay, enter the dates of hospital admission and discharge. If the patient has not been discharged, leave the "To" box blank.

18. HOSPITALIZATION DATES RELATED TO CURRENT SERVICES
          MM   DD   YY   MM   DD   YY
FROM   TO

Block 19 Reserved for Local Use (not required). This block is usually left blank. Some private payors insert the word

"Attachment(s)" when specific documentation accompanies the claim. There are circumstances on Medicare and/or Medicaid claims when information might be entered here. Check with the local fiscal intermediary or the guidelines of the individual third-party payor for details.

19. RESERVED FOR LOCAL USE

Block 20 Outside Lab? (conditionally required). If laboratory procedures are listed on the claim in block 24, and these services were performed in the provider's facility, the "NO" box in block 20 is checked with an "X" or left blank. If laboratory work shown on the claim was done by an outside laboratory and billed to the provider, check the "YES" box, and enter the total amount of the charges. Leave this block blank if no laboratory tests were performed.

20. OUTSIDE LAB? $ CHARGES
    ☐ YES   ☐ NO

Block 21 Diagnosis or Nature of Illness/Injury (required). Enter the patient's diagnosis or diagnoses using ICD-9-CM codes, listing the primary diagnosis first, and code to the highest level of specificity. Up to four codes (in priority order) can be entered in block 21.

21. DIAGNOSIS OR NATURE OF ILLNESS OR INJURY. (RELATE ITEMS 1,2,3 OR 4 TO ITEM 24E BY LINE)
1. ⌊___.___   3. ⌊___.___
2. ⌊___.___   4. ⌊___.___

Block 22 Medicaid Resubmission. Required only for replacement claims for Medicaid. Enter the appropriate three-digit replacement code followed by the 17-digit transaction control number of the most current incorrectly paid claim.

22. MEDICAID RESUBMISSION
    CODE   ORIGINAL REF. NO.

Block 23 Prior Authorization Number. This block can be completed in various ways. For private and commercial carriers and Medicaid, enter the 10-digit prior authorization number for those procedures requiring prior approval assigned by the peer review organization

(PRO). Consult the specific guidelines for the payor to whom the claim is being submitted.

23. PRIOR AUTHORIZATION NUMBER

Block 24a Date(s) of Service (required). The first date of service for the charge on this line should be placed in the "From" column. When a claim is for more than one day of the same service on a line item, the days must be in consecutive order. The last date of service is required in the "To" column. Enter the month, day, and year (in the MM DD YYYY format) for each procedure, service, or supply. When "From" and "To" dates are shown for a series of identical services, enter the number of days or units in block 24g.

Block 24b Place of Service (required). Enter the appropriate place of service code for the payor to which the claim is being submitted (Figure 17-6).

Block 24c Type of Service (if required). Enter the appropriate type of service code if required (Figure 17-7). NOTE: For private payors and Medicare, leave blank. For all others, refer to specific guidelines.

Block 24d Procedure Codes/Modifiers (required). Enter the procedure, service, or supply code using the appropriate five-digit CPT or HCPCS procedure code. Enter a two-position modifier when applicable. NOTE: If an unlisted procedure code is used (codes ending in –99), a complete description of the procedure must be given. Use a separate attachment to do this, if the carrier allows attachments.

Block 24e Diagnosis Code (required for multiple diagnoses). Link the procedure/service code back to the diagnosis code in block 21 by indicating the applicable number of diagnosis codes (1, 2, 3, or 4) to that line's procedure code.

Block 24f Charges (required). Enter the charge for each listed procedure, supply, and /or service.

Block 24g Days or Units (required). Enter the number of days or units. This field is normally used for multiple visits, units of supplies, anesthesia minutes, or oxygen volume. If only one service is performed, enter the number "1."

Block 24h EPSDT/Family Plan. Leave blank for all claims with the exception of certain Medicaid claims. (EPSDT is an acronym for "early and periodic screening diagnosis and treatment.") If this is applicable, enter the appropriate alpha referral code.

BLOCK 24B
PLACE OF SERVICE CODES

11 Doctor's office
12 Patient's home
21 Inpatient hospital
22 Outpatient hospital
23 Emergency department—hospital
24 Ambulatory surgical center
25 Birthing center
26 Military treatment facility/ uniformed service treatment facility
31 Skilled nursing facility (swing bed visits)
32 Nursing facility (intermediate/long-term care facilities)
33 Custodial care facility (domiciliary or rest home services)
34 Hospice (domiciliary or rest home services)
35 Adult living care facilities (residential care facility)
41 Ambulance–land
42 Ambulance–air or water
50 Federally qualified health center
51 Inpatient psychiatric facility
52 Psychiatric facility–partial hospitalization
53 Community mental health care (outpatient, twenty-four-hours-a-day services, admission screening, consultation, and educational services)
54 Intermediate care facility/mentally retarded
55 Residential substance abuse treatment facility
56 Psychiatric residential treatment center
60 Mass immunization center
61 Comprehensive inpatient rehabilitation facility
62 Comprehensive outpatient rehabilitation facility
65 End-stage renal disease treatment facility
71 State or local public health clinic
72 Rural health clinic
81 Independent laboratory
99 Other unlisted facility

FIGURE 17-6

Block 24i EMG (if applicable). For certain carriers, enter an "X" as appropriate if documentation indicates a medical emergency existed. Leave this blank for Medicare claims.

Block 24j Coordination of Benefits (COB) (if applicable). For commercial claims, Blue Cross/Blue Shield, Medicare, Medicaid, and TRICARE, leave blank. In some instances, the first two digits of the NPI number are entered in block 24j, with the remaining eight digits of the NPI in block 24k, including the two-digit location identifier. (Refer to specific third-party payor guidelines.)

Block 24k Reserved for Local Use. Enter the five-digit number assigned when the provider was approved by the third-party payor. For Medicare, it is referred to as the *billing number.* Blue Cross/Blue Shield and Medicaid have their own numbers. This is not the same as the UPIN number.

BLOCK 24C TYPE OF SERVICE CODES FOR MEDICAID, TRICARE, AND WORKERS' COMPENSATION

These codes should be selected depending on the procedure code used on each line. Codes may vary according to regions and claim administrators.

1 Medical care (e.g., evaluation and management services)
2 Surgery
3 Consultation
4 Diagnostic x-ray (e.g., ultrasound and nuclear testing)
5 Diagnostic laboratory
6 Radiation therapy
7 Anesthesia
8 Assistant at surgery
9 Other medical service (e.g., laboratory, venipuncture, handling of specimen)
0 Blood or packed red cells
A DME rental/purchase
B Drugs
C Ambulatory surgery
D Hospice
E Second opinion on elective surgery
F Maternity
G Dental
H Mental health care
I Ambulance
J Program for persons with disabilities
L Renal supply in home
M Alternate payment for maintenance
N Kidney donor
V Pneumococcal vaccine
Z Third opinion on elective surgery

FIGURE 17-7

Block 25 **Federal Tax ID Number (required).** Enter the provider's nine-digit federal tax identification number and check the appropriate box in this field; or, in the case of an unincorporated practice, enter the provider's Social Security number.

Block 26 **Patient's Account No. (conditionally optional).** Enter the patient's account number as assigned by the provider's accounting system. If you are submitting the claim electronically, you are required to provide a patient account number.

Block 27 **Accept Assignment.** Check the appropriate box to indicate whether the provider accepts assignment of benefits. If the supplier is a *participating provider* (PAR), assignment must be accepted for all covered charges. For nonPAR providers, this can be left blank. For Medicaid, check "YES."

Block 28 Total Charge (required). Total column 24f and enter the total charges in this field.

```
28. TOTAL CHARGE
$
```

Block 29 Amount Paid. Enter the total amount, if any, that has been paid by the patient. Leave this blank if no payment has been made.

```
29. AMOUNT PAID
$
```

Block 30 Balance Due. Used when there is secondary insurance. Enter the balance owing as indicated on the explanation of benefits (EOB).

```
30. BALANCE DUE
$
```

Block 31 Signature of Physician or Supplier Including Degrees or Credentials. Enter the signature of the provider or representative, his or her initials, and the date the form was signed. The signature may be typed, stamped, or handwritten; however, the characters should not fall outside the block.

```
31. SIGNATURE OF PHYSICIAN OR SUPPLIER
INCLUDING DEGREES OR CREDENTIALS
(I certify that the statements on the reverse
apply to this bill and are made a part thereof.)
SIGNED                        DATE
```

Block 32 Name and Address of Facility Where Services Were Rendered. Enter the name and address of the facility where the services were performed if other than the patient's home or physician's office.

```
32. NAME AND ADDRESS OF FACILITY WHERE SERVICES WERE
RENDERED (If other than home or office)
```

Block 33 Physician's, Supplier's Billing Name, Address, Phone Number (required). Enter the provider's billing name, address, ZIP code, and telephone number. (NOTE: A missing phone number may be cause for rejection.) Also enter the billing number

(from block 24k). Enter the group NPI number, including the two-digit location identifier, if the provider is a member of a group practice (although this is not required in most cases). (Refer to specific third-party payor guidelines.)

```
33. PHYSICIAN'S, SUPPLIER'S BILLING NAME, ADDRESS, ZIP CODE
& PHONE #
PIN#                          GRP#
```

Appendix C lists and compares HCFA form requirements for each type of payor.

Preventing Claim Rejection

If a claim form is not sufficiently detailed, complete, and accurate, the insurance company may reject it.

Common Problems Areas

The following is a troubleshooting list of problem areas to check when proofreading claims:

- The patient's name, address, and ID number should be identical to the information printed on the insurance card.
- Patient's birth date and sex should correspond with the medical record.
- The word "NONE" should appear in block 11 if Medicare is the primary payor.
- The referring, consulting, or ordering provider's name and number should be entered in block 17 and 17a, if applicable.
- The physician's correct billing number should be entered in block 24k and again to the right of "PIN #" in block 33.
- The federal **employer identification number (EIN)** should be correct. (Often these numbers contain transpositions.)
- If services were rendered in a location other than the provider's office or the patient's home, the name and address of the facility should be entered in block 32.
- Accept assignment should be checked "Yes" if the physician is PAR.
- Be sure the diagnosis is not missing or incomplete.
- The diagnosis must be coded accurately and must correspond with the treatment.
- The patient must have authorized the release of information and the patient section completed accurately.
- Fees for each charge must be listed.
- The physician signature must be on the form in an accepted manner.

A medical assistant should be proactive rather than reactive when working with claim forms. He or she should make every effort possible to produce clean claims, rather than try to "fix" them after the fact.

The best way to avoid repeated claim rejections is to identify the reason for the rejection or denial. Everyone who has worked with medical insurance knows the process can be frustrating, because there are so many insurance companies, and each has its own requirements as to how the claim form should be completed. One way that a medical assistant might approach this challenge is by creating a "comparison chart" for the major payors. Keeping this chart handy for easy reference can minimize claim problems.

If a service is not covered because it is deemed medically unnecessary or unreasonable, but the Medicare patient still wishes to have the service, the patient should be required to sign an Advance Beneficiary Notice (ABN). This document means that the service cannot be claimed to Medicare, and if the notice is not signed in advance of the service taking place, the charges cannot be collected from the patient.

Medical assistants might consider the following items when creating a work-friendly routine for completing insurance claims:

- If possible, set aside a definite time for completing insurance claims.
- Have a central location for all insurance forms.
- Have readily available the necessary manuals, code books, and other references needed.
- Create a master list of codes most often used by the practice, including fourth and fifth digits, if appropriate. The list should be updated annually and never be considered a replacement for the coding manuals.
- Make it a practice to complete the forms as soon as possible after service is rendered, usually at the end of the day.
- Complete the forms by category (e.g., all Blue Cross, all Medicare)
- If using a computer billing program to print insurance forms, the computer will store insurance information on outstanding claims that can be printed in batches using the CMS-1500 forms. Adjust the printer so that the information prints correctly on the form.
- Transmit claims electronically whenever possible.

At times, a denied claim may involve policy issues beyond the control of the medical assistant. When this happens, he or she should contact the patient and discuss the problem. Normally, it is the patient's responsibility to resolve disputes regarding payment with the payor. The insurance policy is a contract between the company and the insured. However, the provider and those involved with the billing process in the medical facility should have a strong grasp for the types of claims and various insurers handled most often in the facility. If the medical assistant knows that the payor will deny the claims for any reason or that the benefits will not cover a service, the patient should be informed in advance and payment arrangements made.

It is often necessary to send a "tracer" to an insurance company to determine the status of a delinquent insurance claim (Figure 17-8). The accepted practice is to submit the tracer a day or two after the usual turnaround time of the payor.

Checking Claim Status

As mentioned earlier in this chapter, a duplicate copy of all submitted claims should be retained, and the medical assistant should establish some sort of structured routine for following up on pending claims. The Insurance Claim Register (see Figure 17-4), tickler files, and reports from the insurance database all help to keep track of paid and pending claims. The database can also generate an insurance aging report, which is useful in the follow-up of claims that have yet to be paid.

If claims are being submitted electronically either directly or through a clearinghouse, the medical assistant might allow 2 to 3 weeks before reimbursement is expected. For paper claims, allow an additional week or two to allow for necessary manual processing and mailing time. Time lengths between when a claim is submitted and when it is paid varies from payor to payor; however, an experienced medical assistant will soon become familiar with individual payment patterns of third-party payors and their claim turnaround times.

Complementary to a follow-up file, it is also a good idea to create an insurance log (Figure 17-9). An insurance log can be designed to track the status of each claim. By using this kind of tool, the medical assistant can easily see at a glance which claims are becoming delinquent and need follow-up. Any software with spreadsheet capabilities can easily accommodate this task.

Patient Education

The medical assistant needs to be well versed in completing CMS-1500 claim forms, and he or she should be able to explain confusing technical issues to patients in simple, understandable terms. Patients, especially

INSURANCE CLAIM TRACER

INSURANCE COMPANY NAME _____ DATE _____

ADDRESS: _____

PATIENT NAME _____ INSURED: _____

POLICY/CERTIFICATE NUMBER _____ GROUP NAME/NUMBER _____

EMPLOYER NAME AND ADDRESS: _____

DATE OF INITIAL CLAIM SUBMISSION _____ AMOUNT: _____

An inordinate amount of time has passed since submission of our original claim as described above. We have not received a request for additional information and still await payment of this assigned claim. Please review the attached duplicate and process for payment within seven (7) days.

If there is any difficulty with this claim, please check one of these below and return this letter to our office.

Claim pending because: _____
Payment of claim in process: _____
Payment made on claim: Date: _____ To whom: _____
Claim denied: (Reason) _____
Patient notified: Yes _____ No _____
Remarks: _____

Thank you for your assistance in this important matter. Please contact _____ in our office if you have any questions regarding this claim.

Office of: _____ M.D.

Address: _____

_____ TELEPHONE NUMBER: _____

FIGURE 17-8 Example of an insurance claim tracer. (Modified from Fordney M: *Insurance handbook for the medical office,* ed 7. Philadelphia, 2002, WB Saunders, p 266.)

General Physicians, Inc.
5515 Lake Dr.
Chicago, IL 00000

INSURANCE LOG

Patient's Name	Date of Service	Fee	Amt. Paid	Insurance Reimbursements Date	Amount	Amt. Due from Patient	Date	Amt. Reimbursed to Patient	Date	Current Balance
Terry Holmes	2/5/03	$85	Ø	3/15/03	$75	$10	3/15			
	2/17/03	$30	30	3/30/03	$25	$5	3/30			
	3/24/03	$65	40	4/15/03	$32			$22	5/25/03	Ø

FIGURE 17-9 Example of an insurance log.

elderly ones, quickly become confused and frustrated over insurance issues—especially Medicare rules and regulations, which change nearly every year.

The medical assistant should attempt to keep patients fully informed of changes in insurance guidelines and patiently explain why some procedures and services are paid and others are not. It is the medical assistant's responsibility to become well acquainted with the various insurance plans used by the patients in their medical facility. When a claim is delayed or rejected, the medical assistant should make every effort to assist the patient or the insured to come to an acceptable resolution.

Whenever possible, the medical assistant must be able to explain insurance submission policies and patient financial responsibilities before the patient receives care. Signatures to authorize insurance billing, supplying information to insurance companies, and accepting assignments of benefits (if appropriate) should be obtained from all new patients.

Legal and Ethical Issues

The practice of medicine and the responsibilities of the medical assistant are greatly affected by the legislative process. It is extremely important to stay current on the laws that affect medicine, and in particular, the completion of the CMS-1500 claim form.

CRITICAL THINKING APPLICATION

An irate patient comes to the office and insists that his insurance claim was not filled out properly, because it was rejected by his insurance company. When she investigates, Kalene discovers that the reason for the rejection was that the insurance company considered the procedure "not medically necessary." What should she do? How can Kalene explain this situation to the patient?

The Health Insurance Portability and Accountability Act of 1996 (HIPAA), developed by the Centers for Medicare and Medicaid Services (CMS), is responsible for the implementation of various acts that protect individuals' health insurance and privacy standards. Medical assistants should familiarize themselves with this important insurance act.

Because of the emphasis on compliance in medical practices today, every medical office must create and implement a plan to identify potential compliance problems and correct them before a liability risk is incurred. It is mandated that all providers avoid fraud and abuse charges by following the regulations and guidelines provided by governmental entities and third-party payors.

SUMMARY OF SCENARIO

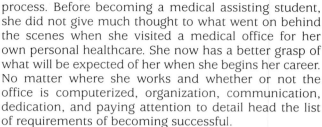

Kalene feels that she now has a better understanding of the insurance claims process. Before becoming a medical assisting student, she did not give much thought to what went on behind the scenes when she visited a medical office for her own personal healthcare. She now has a better grasp of what will be expected of her when she begins her career. No matter where she works and whether or not the office is computerized, organization, communication, dedication, and paying attention to detail head the list of requirements of becoming successful.

Kalene has asked for her instructor's help in developing a reference manual for the various third-party payors common to her area. She is looking forward to more hands-on experience in the medical office where she is doing her externship so she can gain as much knowledge as possible in every facet of medical assisting. She is also establishing positive relationships with the staff at her externship site. She feels the knowledge and expertise they share with her will do much to round out her education in the medical field in preparation for her career.

SUMMARY OF LEARNING OBJECTIVES

- For a better understanding of the medical insurance claims process, a medical assistant should familiarize himself or herself with the language and terms used in this area of administrative work.

- Insurance claims can be submitted in two forms: paper and electronic. There are advantages and disadvantages for both; however, electronic claims normally have fewer errors and historically are paid faster.

- Clean claims are those that can be processed and paid quickly; dirty claims contain errors and/or omissions that often result in rejection, thus greatly slowing down the reimbursement process.

- The insurance claim cycle begins when the patient first makes an appointment. The medical assistant should follow an established list of guidelines for CMS-1500 form completion, including obtaining a signed authorization to release information, and assign benefits, if applicable.

- There are 33 blocks in the CMS-1500 claim form and, except for a few blocks that ask for standard information, completion requirements vary from payor to payor. The medical assistant should familiarize himself or herself with each major payor's unique requirements in order to maximize reimbursement.

■ Optical character recognition (OCR) scanning is the electronic transfer of information to data banks that simplify and speed up the claims process. Specific guidelines should be followed when completing claims to facilitate OCR scanning. A medical assistant should know and follow these guidelines precisely.

■ Claim rejection and delay cost the medical facility time and money. Proven methods of preventing claim rejections should be established and adhered to.

■ It is important to track claims once they are submitted. An insurance claim register, or log, can be created and used as one method of tracking claims. A routine should be established for claims follow-up.

INTERNET CONNECTIONS

- American Association of Medical Assistants
  http://www.aama-ntl.org/
- Centers for Medicare and Medicaid Services
  http://www.cms.gov
- Electronic Claims Processing Facts
  http://www.webcom.com/medical/elec_clm.htm
- Health Insurance Portability and Accountability Act
  http://www.cms.hhs.gov/hipaa
- Sunrise Services: electronic claims clearinghouse
  http://www.sunrize.com/clearinghouses.htm

REFERENCES

Fordney M: *Insurance handbook for the medical office*, ed 7. Philadelphia, 2002, WB Saunders.

CHAPTER 18

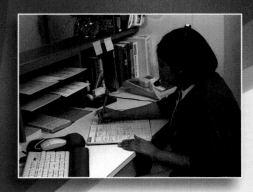

Scenario

The instructor in Beverly Studevant's administrative medical assistant class, Sandra Dickson, realizes that today's medical insurance can be challenging to understand. She asks Teresa Ward, a 25-year veteran in medical insurance billing and collecting, for assistance. Ms. Dickson knows that working with medical insurance can be quite rewarding, and experienced billers find the field financially rewarding as well. Ms. Ward agrees to come to class twice a week to work with Beverly and her classmates, answering their questions and helping them to see that medical insurance is not as complicated as it seems.

Ms. Ward shares her on-the-job experiences with Beverly and her classmates. Through a series of role-playing events, Ms. Ward acquaints the students with the guidelines of the various third-party payors. Beginning with simple case studies, Ms. Ward walks the students through the various stages of third-party reimbursement.

Beverly soon realizes that when insurance billing is broken down into manageable segments of information and applied to real life situations, it becomes an interesting task. Beverly feels almost like a detective as she follows up on claims and checks to ensure that the correct codes are used for diagnoses and procedures. She decides to investigate medical billing as a career and talks with Ms. Dickson about the possibility of performing her externship in a billing office.

Third-Party Reimbursement

Janet Beik
Alexandra P. Young

Learning Objectives

- Define and spell the terms listed in the vocabulary.
- Discuss the purpose of health insurance.
- Differentiate among the various types of insurance policies.
- Explain the numerous classifications of insurance benefits available.
- Demonstrate how insurance benefits are determined.
- Understand the healthcare reform efforts.
- Describe managed care, its history, and its effect on modern medicine.
- Differentiate among the different types of managed care options.
- List and discuss other major third-party payors.
- Interpret the procedure for verifying insurance benefits.
- Discuss the different types of fee schedules.
- Explain the procedure for tracking insurance claims.
- Obtain managed care referrals and precertifications.

National Curriculum Competencies

ADMINISTRATIVE COMPETENCIES

4a. Apply managed care policies and procedures
4b. Apply third-party guidelines
4c. Obtain managed care referrals and precertifications

TRANSDISCIPLINARY COMPETENCIES

1b. Recognize and respond to verbal communication
1c. Recognize and respond to nonverbal communication
2a. Identify and respond to issues of confidentiality
2b. Perform within legal and ethical boundaries
3a. Explain general office policies

Vocabulary

allowed charge The maximum amount of money that many third-party payors allow for a specific procedure or service.

authorization A term used in managed care for an approved referral.

benefits The amount payable by an insurance company for a monetary loss to an individual insured by that company, under each coverage.

birthday rule Under law, when an individual is covered under two insurance policies, the insurance plan of the policyholder whose birthday comes first in the calendar year (month and day—not year) becomes the primary insurance.

capitation Payment method used by many managed care organizations wherein a fixed amount of money is reimbursed to the provider for patients enrolled during a specific period of time, no matter what services received or number of visits made.

Civilian Health and Medical Program of the Uniformed Services (CHAMPUS) A government-sponsored program wherein authorized dependents of military personnel receive medical care. This program is now referred to as TRICARE.

Civilian Health and Medical Program of the Veterans Administration (CHAMPVA) A health benefits program run by the Department of Veterans Affairs (VA) that helps eligible beneficiaries pay the cost of specific healthcare services/supplies.

coinsurance A policy provision frequently found in medical insurance whereby the policyholder and the insurance company share the cost of *covered* losses in a specified ratio (i.e., 80/20 means 80% is covered by the insurer and 20% by the insured).

coordination of benefits (COB) The mechanism used in group health insurance to designate the order in which multiple carriers are to pay benefits to prevent duplicate payments.

copayment A sum of money that is paid at the time of medical service; a form of coinsurance.

deductible A specific amount of money a patient must pay out-of-pocket before the insurance carrier begins paying. Usually this amount ranges from $100 to $500. This deductible amount is met on a yearly or per-incident basis.

dependents The spouse, children, and sometimes domestic partner or other individuals designated by the insured who are covered under a healthcare plan.

disability income insurance Insurance that provides periodic payments to replace income when an insured person is unable to work as a result of illness, injury, or disease.

effective date The date on which an insurance policy or plan takes effect so that benefits are payable.

exclusions Limitations on an insurance contract for which benefits are not payable.

fee for service An established schedule of fees set for services performed by providers and paid by the patient.

government plan An entitlement program or healthcare plan that is sponsored and/or subsidized by the state or federal government, such as Medicaid and Medicare.

group policy Insurance written under a policy that covers a number of people under a single master contract issued to their employer or to an association with which they are affiliated.

guarantor The person who is responsible for paying a medical bill.

health insurance Protection in return for periodic *premium* payments, which provides reimbursement of expenses resulting from illness or injury. Includes these forms of insurance: accident, disability income, medical expense, and accidental death and dismemberment. Also known as *accident and health insurance* or *disability income insurance*.

Health Insurance Portability and Accountability Act (HIPAA) The Kassebaum-Kennedy Act designed to improve portability and continuity of health insurance coverage; to combat waste, fraud, and abuse in health insurance and healthcare delivery; to promote the use of medical savings accounts; to improve access to long-term care services and coverage; to simplify the administration of health insurance; and for other purposes.

health maintenance organization (HMO) An organization that provides a wide range of comprehensive healthcare services for a specified group at a fixed periodic payment. HMOs can be sponsored by the government, medical schools, hospitals, employers, labor unions, consumer groups, insurance companies, and hospital-medical plans.

indemnity plan Traditional health insurance plan that pays for all or a share of the cost of covered services, regardless of which physician, hospital, or other licensed healthcare provider is used. Policyholders of indemnity plans and their dependents choose when and where to get healthcare services.

individual policy An insurance policy designed specifically for the use of one person (and his or her dependents), not associated with the amenities of a group policy, namely higher premiums. Often called *personal insurance*.

managed care plans An umbrella term for all healthcare plans that provide healthcare in return for preset monthly payments and coordinated care through a defined network of primary care physicians and hospitals.

medical savings account A tax-deferred bank or savings account combined with a low-premium/high-deductible insurance policy, designed for individuals or families who choose to fund their own healthcare expenses and medical insurance.

medically indigent An individual who may be able to afford to pay for his or her normal daily living expenses but cannot afford adequate healthcare.

medically necessary Phrase indicating that the patient's symptoms and diagnosis justify or support specific medical services or procedures, as determined through a decision-making process used by third-party payors. Also known as *medical necessity*.

participating provider (PAR) A physician or other healthcare provider who enters into a contract with a specific insurance company or program, and by doing so, agrees to abide by certain rules and regulations set forth by that particular third-party payor.

policyholder The individual in whose name an insurance policy is written and who pays the premium; thus the "holder" of the policy.

premium The periodic (monthly, quarterly, or annual) payment of a specific sum of money to an insurance company for which the insurer, in return, agrees to provide certain benefits.

primary diagnosis The condition or chief complaint for which a patient is treated in an outpatient (physician's office or clinic) medical care setting.

principal diagnosis A condition established after study that is chiefly responsible for the admission of a patient to the hospital. Used in coding inpatient hospital insurance claims.

resource-based relative value system (RBRVS) A fee schedule designed to provide national uniform payment of Medicare benefits after being adjusted to reflect the differences in practice costs across geographic areas.

rider A special provision or group of provisions that may be added to a policy to expand or limit the benefits otherwise payable. It may increase or decrease benefits, waive a condition or coverage, or in any other way amend the original contract.

self-insured plan An insurance plan funded by an organization having a large enough employee base that they can afford to fund their own insurance program.

self-referral The act of a patient or insured individual who refers himself or herself to a specialist without requesting the referral to the primary provider, such as a woman seeking an annual gynecological examination. Managed care guidelines may require the patient to report the self-referral.

service benefit plan Plan that provides its benefits in the form of certain surgical and medical services rendered, rather than cash. A service benefit plan is not restricted to a fee schedule.

TRICARE See CHAMPUS.

utilization review A review of individual cases by a committee to make sure that services are medically necessary and to study how providers use medical care resources.

workers' compensation Insurance against liability imposed on certain employers to pay benefits and furnish care to employees who are injured and to pay benefits to dependents of employees killed in the course of or arising out of their employment.

The Purpose of Health Insurance

The purpose of **health insurance** is to help individuals and families offset the costs of medical care. Health insurance is defined as projection against financial losses resulting from sickness or accidental bodily injury. This protection provides payment of **benefits** for covered

sickness or injury. There are various types of health insurance, such as accident insurance, disability income insurance, medical expense insurance, and accidental death and dismemberment insurance.

Increasingly, the trend has been for health insurance policies to cover services that prevent illness or lead to early diagnosis. Health insurance normally covers **medically necessary** services and procedures; elective procedures (such as certain cosmetic surgeries) are usually not included under health insurance policies.

Cost of Coverage

In light of the rising costs of healthcare, to keep **premiums** in check, most insurance policies and programs do not pay all expenses resulting from accident or illness. A premium is the periodic (monthly, quarterly, or annual) payment of a specific sum of money to an insurance company for which the insurer agrees to provide certain benefits. Most policies do not begin to pay medical expenses immediately. The real cost to the individual at the time of treatment includes the following:

- Deductibles
- Copayment or coinsurance
- Costs for noncovered services

A **deductible** is an amount a **policyholder** agrees to pay out-of-pocket, per claim or per accident, toward the total amount of an insured loss before insurance coverage is effective. A deductible amount is stated in the insurance contract and normally ranges from $100 to $500. The higher the deductible, the lower the premium cost. Remember that the patient may not be the **guarantor** for the medical account. Be sure to verify who the guarantor is and obtain written documentation, if necessary, that this person agrees to be responsible for the account.

Coinsurance is a policy provision frequently found in medical insurance whereby the policyholder and the insurance company share the cost of *covered* losses in a specified ratio, such as 80/20 (80% by the insurer and 20% by the insured). Many plans now require a **copayment**, which is a type of coinsurance that is collected at the time of service. Copayments usually range from $10 to $25 for office visits but can vary according to the services rendered.

CRITICAL THINKING APPLICATION

Beverly notes that a patient, Mrs. Brent, underwent a covered procedure that cost $1000, which was the *allowable charge* of the insurance carrier. Mrs. Brent has a policy that provides coverage with a $250 deductible and an 80/20 coinsurance ratio. Mrs. Brent inquires how much of the total bill is her responsibility. How can Beverly calculate this? What would her response be to the patient? How can Beverly help the patient understand this complex information?

Under most circumstances, the deductible must only be paid one time per calendar year; however, some policies have a deductible per occurrence. The medical assistant should always verify the **effective date** on the patient's insurance card. It may be necessary to call the company to verify coverage and **exclusions**.

Some **managed care plans** require a copayment, which is a flat fee per office visit—from $5 to $20 or greater, depending on the charges. Any services or procedures that are not covered under the terms of the policy are the responsibility of the policyholder.

Coordination of Benefits (COB)

Coordination of benefits is a mechanism used in group health insurance to designate the order in which multiple carriers are to pay benefits and prevent duplicate payments. The purpose of COB provisions is to limit benefits to no more than 100% of the cost. If a plan does not have COB provisions, it becomes the primary payor and pays benefits first.

Laws establishing which payor is primary, including the **birthday rule**, were enacted in many states in January 1987. In the case of an employed person who is eligible for Medicare benefits, the employer's group plan is the primary carrier, and Medicare is secondary. However, because of the tremendous increase in health-care premiums in the last few years, a medical assistant might not encounter this phenomenon as much as in the past, because most couples and families are covered by only one policy. Still, some seniors work full-time and are also covered by Medicare benefits, so the medical assistant must be familiar with COB restrictions.

COB follows the rules of the plan that is the primary payor. If both plans have COB provisions, then:
- The policyholder's own plan is primary for that individual. There are some exceptions; for instance, the policyholder may have more than one policy or may be covered by another entity that is required to pay first, such as car insurance in the event of a motor vehicle accident. The primary coverage for **dependents** of the policyholder is determined by the birthday rule. The insurance plan of the policyholder whose birthday comes first in the calendar year (month and day—not year) provides primary coverage for each dependent.

The primary plan for dependents of legally separated or divorced parents is more complicated:
- The birthday rule is in effect if the parent who has custody of the dependent has not remarried. If the custodial parent has remarried, that parent's plan is primary for that dependent.
- If one parent has been decreed by the court to be the responsible party, that parent's policy is primary. This is not always the parent with legal custody of the child.
- If one of the plans originated in a state not having the COB law, the plan that did originate in a state having a COB law will determine the order of benefits.

All of this emphasizes the need to determine whether there is a birthday rule in the state in which the medical assistant is employed. To avoid complications and confusion later, it is important to establish primary and secondary payors before the patient is treated.

The Availability of Health Insurance

Health insurance is available to the majority of persons in this country through group, individual, or prepaid plans. In addition, many people are covered by government plans or entitlement programs. However, although health insurance might be available, it is not always affordable. A recent survey revealed that more than 46 million Americans—roughly 18% of the population—have no regular source for obtaining medical care, and lack of health insurance was a major obstacle.

Group Policies

Insurance written under a group policy covers a number of people under a single master contract issued to their employer or to an association with which they are affiliated. Group coverage usually provides greater benefits at lower premiums because of the large pool of people from whom premiums are collected. Physical examinations are normally not required and preexisting conditions are often waived. Often the employee shares the cost of coverage through payroll deductions.

Recently some smaller companies are finding themselves hard pressed to provide group coverage to their employees because of increasing premiums. Many have found it necessary to circumvent this problem by increasing deductibles and limiting eligibility to full-time workers only (over 30 hours per week). Congressional efforts have increased to find available and affordable health insurance for uninsured individuals, families, and people who lose their coverage as a result of job changes.

Individual Policies

Individuals who do not qualify for inclusion in a group or government-sponsored plan may apply to companies that offer individual policies—often called *personal insurance*. The applicant is normally required to fill out an extended health questionnaire and undergo a physical examination before acceptance. Unlike group policies, there is a risk that coverage may be denied, or the individual may have to accept a **rider**, or limitation, on benefits the policy will cover. Premiums are almost always higher with individual policies and often the benefits are less.

Government Plans

The federal government first became responsible for insuring a large group of people in 1956 with passage of Public Law 569. This law authorized dependents of military personnel to receive treatment by civilian physicians at the expense of the government. The program administering these benefits became the **Civilian Health and Medical Program of the Uniformed Services (CHAMPUS)**, which today is known as TRICARE (discussed in detail later in this chapter).

In 1965 the federal government provided for another group—the **medically indigent**—through a program that is still known as Medicaid. Title XIX of Public Law 89-97, under the Social Security Amendments of 1965, provided for agreements with states for assistance from the federal government to provide medical care for people meeting specific eligibility criteria.

On July 1, 1966, Medicare was established under the Social Security Administration as a national health insurance program for persons age 65 and older. The scope of coverage increased in 1973 to include Medicare coverage for disabled persons younger than age 65 receiving Social Security benefits, railroad retirees, and civil service retirees. This also included disabled workers of any age, disabled widows, disabled dependent widowers, adults disabled before age 18 whose parents are eligible or are retired on Social Security benefits, children and adults with end-stage renal disease, and living kidney donors (including all expenses related to the kidney transplant).

The passage of the Health Maintenance Organization Act in 1973 provided for federal aid to health insurance prepayment plans that met certain criteria. This brought about a rapid growth of the **health maintenance organization (HMO)**, which is an organization that provides comprehensive healthcare to an enrolled group for a fixed periodic payment. Some of these plans pay by **capitation**, which means that the provider is paid a fixed amount for each individual enrolled in the plan during a specified time period, regardless of the number of services provided to the patient. The provider still only collects the contracted rate, even if expenses cost much more than that rate for the time period.

Title VI of the Social Security Amendments Act of 1983 contained the prospective payment system (PPS) for hospitals, which was the beginning of the radical restructuring of the payment system to hospitals for Medicare inpatient services.

The most fundamental change in determining physicians' fees under Medicare since its inception was the **resource-based relative value scale (RBRVS)** reimbursement system put into effect in 1992.

Many large groups of people are covered by government plans or entitlement programs. A patient who is older than age 65 is covered by Part B of Medicare. A medically indigent patient may be eligible for Medicaid with or without Medicare. Dependents of military personnel are covered by **TRICARE** (formerly known as CHAMPUS); surviving spouses and dependent children of veterans who died as a result of service-related disabilities are covered by the **Civilian Health and Medical Program of the Veterans Administration (CHAMPVA)**.

Some wage earners are protected against the loss of wages and the cost of medical care resulting from an occupational accident, disease, or disability through **workers' compensation** insurance. An individual may collect benefits for health expenses from an automobile policy if the injury is related to a car accident or other such loss.

Self-Insured Plans

Many large companies or organizations have a big enough employee base that they choose to fund their own insurance program. This is called a **self-insured plan**. Technically, a self-funded plan is not insurance by true definition. The employer pays employee healthcare costs from the firm's own coffers. Recent surveys indicate about 40% of workers with employment-based health insurance are enrolled in plans that their employers self-insure. Usually benefits and premium costs under self-insured plans are similar to group plans. Self-funded plans tend to work best for companies that are large enough to offer good coverage, reasonable premium rates, and are able to pay large claims for expensive medical services. Often a third-party administrator (TPA) handles paperwork and claim payments for a self-insured group.

Medical Savings Account

In 1996 Congress made tax-free Medical Savings Accounts (MSAs) available to 750,000 American workers and their families. This is a type of self-insurance. Under a provision of the Kassebaum-Kennedy health insurance reform bill, small companies (with 50 or fewer employees), self-employed persons, and the uninsured can purchase health insurance policies and make tax-free deposits to an MSA. They can use their MSA money to pay small and routine healthcare expenses, reserving a high-deductible medical insurance policy to pay large, catastrophic expenses. Money that remains in the account at year's end earns tax-free interest. People can also elect to use MSA money to pay their health insurance premiums during a job change, which should reduce *job lock*, a situation in which people do not change jobs for fear of losing their health insurance.

There are both advantages and disadvantages to an MSA, and it is wise to investigate it thoroughly to learn its values and limitations.

Types of Insurance Benefits

An insurance package is tailored to the needs of each individual or group policy, and the combinations of benefits are limitless. A policy may contain one or any combination of the following benefits.

Hospitalization

Hospital coverage pays the cost of all or part of the insured person's hospital room and board and specific hospital services, such as the costs involved in having surgery in a hospital. Hospital insurance policies frequently set a maximum amount payable per day and a maximum number of days of hospital care. Some insurance companies require that the hospital be an accredited or a licensed hospital. Most hospital plans exclude admission for diagnostic studies.

Surgical

Surgical coverage pays all or part of a surgeon's fee; some plans also pay for an assistant surgeon. Surgery includes any incision or excision, removal of foreign bodies, aspiration, suturing, and reduction of fractures. Surgery may be accomplished in a hospital, physician's office, or elsewhere. The insurer frequently provides the subscriber with a surgical fee schedule that establishes the amount the insurer will pay for commonly performed procedures.

Basic Medical

Basic medical coverage pays all or part of a physician's fee for nonsurgical services, including hospital, home, and office visits. Usually there is a deductible amount payable by the patient as well as a copayment or coinsurance each time service is received. The insurance plan may include a provision for diagnostic laboratory, radiology, and pathology fees. Some medical plans do not cover routine physical examinations when the patient does not have a specific complaint or illness.

Major Medical

Major medical insurance (formerly called *catastrophic coverage*) provides protection against especially large medical bills resulting from catastrophic or prolonged illnesses. It may be a supplement to basic medical coverage or a comprehensive integrated program providing both basic and major medical protection. (For additional information on this topic, see the section on Disability Programs.)

Disability (Loss of Income) Protection

Weekly or monthly cash benefits are provided to employed policyholders who become unable to work as a result of an accident or illness. Many disability policies do not start payment until after a specified number of days or until a certain number of sick leave days have been used. Payment is made directly to the individual and is intended to replace lost income resulting from an illness or other disability. It is not intended for payment of specific medical bills, and it should not be confused with a regular insurance plan, entitlement program, or workers' compensation, in which compensation is provided for an employee who is injured on the job or cannot work as a result of a job-related illness or other disability.

Dental Care

Dental coverage is included in many *fringe benefit* packages. Some policies are based on a copayment and incentive program, in which preventive dental care (such as cleaning and x-ray films) is covered 100%, with most other coverage paid at 50%.

Vision Care

Vision care insurance may include reimbursement for all or a percentage of the cost for refraction, lenses, and frames.

Medicare Supplement

Many Medicare beneficiaries purchase a supplemental health insurance policy to help defray medical costs not covered, or only partially covered, by Medicare. Federal regulations now require that Medicare supplement contracts must be uniform in benefits to avoid confusion for the purchaser.

Special Risk Insurance

Special risk insurance protects a person in the event of a certain type of accident, such as an automobile or airplane crash, or for certain diseases, such as tuberculosis or cancer. There is usually a maximum benefit.

Liability Insurance

There are many types of liability insurance, including automobile, business, and homeowners' policies. Liability policies often include benefits for medical expenses payable to individuals who are injured in the insured person's home or car, without regard to the insured person's actual legal liability for the accident.

Life Insurance

Life insurance provides payment of a specified amount on an insured's death, either to his or her estate or to a designated beneficiary, or in the case of an endowment policy, to the policyholder at a specified date. Life insurance policies sometimes provide monthly cash benefits if the policyholder becomes permanently and totally disabled. Sometimes the proceeds from life insurance are used to meet the expenses of the insured person's last illness.

Long-Term Care Insurance

Long-term care insurance is a relatively new type that covers a continuum of broad-ranged maintenance and health services to chronically ill, disabled, or mentally retarded persons. Services may be provided on an inpatient (rehabilitation facility, nursing home, or mental hospital), outpatient, or at-home basis. The **Health Insurance Portability and Accountability Act (HIPAA)** of 1996 gives some federal income tax advantages to people who buy certain long-term care insurance policies.

How Benefits Are Determined

Insurance benefits may be determined and paid in one of several ways:
- By indemnity schedules
- By service benefit plans
- By determination of the usual, customary, and reasonable fee
- By relative value studies

Indemnity Schedules

Indemnity plans are traditional health insurance plans that pay for all or a share of the cost of covered services, regardless of which physician, hospital, or other licensed healthcare provider is used. Policyholders of indemnity plans and their dependents choose when and where to get healthcare services. In exchange for premiums that members pay, the indemnity plan reimburses members or the provider when claims are filed. The subscriber is often given a schedule of indemnities (fee schedule) when the policy is purchased, which explains the benefit payment amounts of the policy.

Indemnity plans typically have an annual deductible before the plan pays anything. Usually members also must pay a percentage of each charge—coinsurance. Most indemnity plans have an annual "out-of-pocket limit" on the amount members must pay for coinsurance payments. Because physicians and other providers are paid for each office visit, test, procedure, or other service they deliver, indemnity plans are often called **fee-for-service** plans.

This type of plan takes the major expense out of medical bills and helps keep premium costs down. The amount of premiums often determines the schedule of benefits. Indemnity benefits are usually paid to the person insured unless that person has authorized payment directly to the provider.

Service Benefit Plans

In a **service benefit plan** the insuring company agrees to pay for certain surgical or medical services without additional cost to the person insured. There is no set fee schedule.

In a service benefit plan, surgery with complications would warrant a higher fee than an uncomplicated procedure would. Premiums are sometimes higher for this type of coverage, but often payments are larger. Frequently payment of benefits is sent directly to the physician and is considered full payment for services rendered.

Usual, Customary, and Reasonable (UCR) Fee

Some insurance companies agree to pay on the basis of all or a percentage of the physician's usual, customary, and reasonable fee. Charges for a specific service are compared to a database of charges for the same service to other patients by the same type of physician, and to patients by other physicians performing same or similar services in the same geographic area. The insurance company determines whether the charge is usual, customary, and reasonable, and any amount over this **allowed charge** will not be paid.

Resource-Based Relative Value Scale

The RBRVS is one of the outcomes of the Medicare Physician Payment Reform that was enacted in the Omnibus Budget Reconciliation Act of 1989 (usually called *OBRA '89*). Since the beginning of Medicare, Part B of the program has paid physicians using a fee-for-service system based on customary, prevailing, and reasonable charges. The RBRVS, effective in 1992, changed this. The RBRVS consists of three parts:

1. Physician work
2. Charge-based professional liability expenses
3. Charge-based overhead

The physician work component includes the degree of effort invested by a physician in a particular service or procedure and the time it consumed. The professional liability and overhead components are computed by the Centers for Medicare and Medicaid Services (CMS).

The fee schedule is designed to provide national uniform payments after being adjusted to reflect the differences in practice costs across geographic areas. The fee schedule includes a conversion factor, which is a single national number applied to all services paid under the fee schedule. Conversion factors change according to Congressional enactment. (For more information on RBRVS, see the section on RBRVS under Fee Schedules.)

Healthcare Reform Efforts

Healthcare reform is not a new concept. It has recently been thrust to the forefront of the news since the advent of managed care. Changes in the way people in this country pay for healthcare began in the early 1900s, when Theodore Roosevelt made national health insurance one of the major issues during his 1912 presidential campaign.

In the middle of the twentieth century, it became apparent that some kind of taxpayer-funded healthcare program was needed for the growing elderly population. During President Lyndon Johnson's term in office, federal legislation in the form of Medicare for the aged and Medicaid for the indigent was enacted.

A variety of national health insurance plans were debated in Congress in the 1960s and 1970s. In 1973 Congress passed the Health Maintenance Organization (HMO) Act, which provided grants to employers who set up HMOs.

In the 1980s and 1990s politicians again proposed a variety of national health insurance plans. One such plan was known as "pay or play," because it would have forced employers to provide health insurance or pay into a national fund that would cover uninsured workers. A second plan, championed by President George Bush in 1991, would have provided tax breaks, vouchers, and other incentives to employers to extend health insurance benefits. A third proposal was based on the Canadian model of nationalized healthcare, which was opposed by most doctors and the insurance industry.

When President Bill Clinton took office in 1993, healthcare reform was a major issue on his platform. His proposals included a national health insurance program that would have ultimately provided coverage for most U.S. citizens, but the program was opposed by many insurance companies, medical entities, and small businesses.

In 1999 President Clinton and Congress struggled over the development of a "patient bill of rights" to protect people from service denials and other HMO limitations. Now many individual states have developed their own health insurance alternatives by using managed healthcare systems that monitor the type of services offered, setting fees for each service.

Efforts of healthcare reform continue today. Much activity is alive at the state level, where legislatures are gradually making changes in healthcare costs and delivery. A few states are enacting price control reform on prescription drugs, and many have granted patients greater rights relating to their health maintenance organizations—in some cases, the right to sue. Efforts are underway, and dedicated individuals and groups will make the difference in tomorrow's healthcare delivery methods.

The Advent of Managed Care

What is managed care? **Managed care** is an umbrella term for all healthcare plans that provide healthcare in return for preset scheduled payments and coordinated care through a defined network of physicians and hospitals. *Managed care* refers to healthcare plans that provide healthcare in return for scheduled payments and coordinate healthcare through a defined network of primary care physicians, hospitals, and other providers.

Under managed care, a medical group, such as an HMO or an independent practice association (IPA), is contracted to assume some of the responsibilities of the insurance company, such as claims processing, provider relations, member services, utilization review, and eligibility. A primary care physician (PCP) is usually selected by the patient (although not all managed care plans force the patient to choose a primary provider), and that physician manages all patient services. Managed care is essentially an attempt to lower healthcare costs in this country.

The History of Managed Care

Managed healthcare evolved in the 1970s in response to rising healthcare costs and national interest in new, cost-effective ways for providing access to quality healthcare. Membership in managed care plans is growing rapidly and is expanding into areas of the nation that previously did not have these types of healthcare delivery system models. An estimated 58 million Americans are enrolled in HMOs, and another 81 million are enrolled in other types of managed care plans. Managed healthcare plans may take many forms, ranging from staff/group model HMOs, to loose IPAs, to preferred provider organizations (PPOs).

The phenomenon of managed healthcare, however, is not new. The organization that is now Kaiser Permanente, one of the largest and best-known managed care systems in the nation, began during the Great Depression when an inventive young surgeon named Sidney R. Garfield looked at the thousands of men involved in building the Los Angeles Aqueduct and saw an opportunity. He borrowed money to build Contractors General Hospital, a 12-bed hospital in the middle of the Mojave Desert, 6

miles from a tiny town called Desert Center, and began treating sick and injured workers. But financing was difficult, and Dr. Garfield was having trouble getting insurance companies to pay his bills in a timely fashion. To compound matters, not all of the men had insurance.

Dr. Garfield refused to turn away any sick or injured worker, so he often was left with no payment at all for his services. In no time, the hospital's expenses far exceeded its income. This is when Harold Hatch entered the picture. He suggested that the insurance companies pay Dr. Garfield a fixed amount per day, per covered worker, up front. This "prepayment" idea solved the hospital's immediate money problems. Dr. Garfield also began emphasizing maintaining health and safety as opposed to merely treating injuries and sickness, which gave birth to "preventive" healthcare. For an additional nickel a day, workers could also receive coverage for non–job-related medical problems. Thousands of workers enrolled, and Dr. Garfield's hospital became a financial success.

Hearing of Dr. Garfield's success with the Southern California desert project, Henry Kaiser persuaded him to set up a similar plan for the workers on the Grand Coulee Dam and later for workers and their families at the shipyards in San Francisco and other Kaiser-managed facilities. At the peak of World War II, there were about 200,000 members in the plans. Health plans continued to grow and new ones opened across the country. Today the organization known as Kaiser Permanente serves nearly 9 million members.

The Health Maintenance Organization Act of 1973

Although managed care organizations have been in existence since the 1920s, it was not until the early 1970s that the federal government began to regulate managed care as a model of healthcare delivery. In 1973 Congress passed legislation creating federal standards and encouraging the expansion of HMOs. The Health Maintenance Organization Act of 1973 defined the characteristics of an HMO to include the following:

- An organized system for providing healthcare
- An agreed set of basic and supplemental health maintenance and treatment services
- A voluntary group of enrollees.

In 1976 Congress established the first specific federal requirement for Medicare contracts with HMOs and other managed care organizations. However, it was not until the 1980s that corporate America began to move its work force out of fee-for-service plans and into managed care arrangements. Corporate payments for health insurance benefits began to decline in the early 1990s.

The Effects of Managed Care on Modern Medicine

What impact has managed care had on healthcare costs? Managed care payors attempt to contain costs by limiting where patients can obtain services, from whom they receive these services, and what particular kinds of services they receive. Some managed care plans limit a patient's access to specialty care and simultaneously negotiate reduced payments to providers for services.

Managed care has been met with considerable controversy, and there are pros and cons that must be considered. It is important that medical assistants be well versed in the various types of managed care plans to fully understand their impact on healthcare costs.

Advantages of managed care include the following:
- Healthcare costs are usually contained.
- There are established fee schedules.
- Authorized services are usually paid.
- Most preventive medical treatment is covered.
- Patients' out-of-pocket expenses tend to be smaller than traditional insurance.

Disadvantages of managed care include the following:
- Access to specialized care and referrals can be limited.
- Physician choices in treatment of patients can be limited.
- The amount of paperwork may be increased.
- Treatment may be delayed because of preauthorization requirements.
- Reimbursement is historically less than that through traditional insurance.

Models of Managed Care

Health Maintenance Organizations

An HMO is an organization that provides healthcare in return for preset payments over a specified time period from its members. HMOs contract with healthcare providers (physicians, hospitals, and other health professionals), to provide services to plan members through a network of doctors, hospitals, and other healthcare professionals. HMO members must use these specific providers in order for their healthcare needs to be covered. Several types of HMOs are as follows:

- A *prepaid group practice model*, in which physicians form a group and contract with an HMO. These physicians' group practices are not owned by the HMO, but operate independently and contract with an HMO to provide medical treatment to enrolled members. Although the physicians work for a salary, it is paid by their own independent group, not by the administrators of the health plan.
- A *staff model*, in which the facility is owned by the HMO, and the health plan hires physicians directly and pays their salaries. Routine medical care is given by, or authorized by, the patient's PCP.
- An *independent practice association* is a closed-panel HMO. Instead of maintaining its own staff and clinic buildings, an IPA contracts with independently practicing physicians who continue to practice in their own offices. The IPA may pay each doctor a set amount per patient in advance (*capitation*), or fees charged for services to group members may be billed directly to the IPA rather than to the patient. Fees for services to nonmember patients are handled the same as any other fee for service. The physician may be contracted with several IPAs.

- An *exclusive provider organization* (EPO) combines features of HMOs (e.g., enrolled population, limited provider panel, gatekeepers, utilization management, capitated provider reimbursement, and authorization system) and PPOs (e.g., flexible benefit design, negotiated fees, and fee-for-service payments). It is referred to as "exclusive" because employers agree not to contract with any other plan. Members must choose medical care from network providers, with certain exceptions for emergency or out-of-area services. If a patient decides to seek care outside the network, he or she generally will not be reimbursed for the cost of treatment. Technically, many HMOs can be considered EPOs; however, EPOs are regulated under insurance statutes rather than federal and state HMO regulations.

Preferred Provider Organizations

The PPO model of managed healthcare preserves the fee-for-service concept that many physicians prefer. An insurer representing its clients contracts with a group of providers (physicians) who agree on a predetermined list of charges for all services including those for complex and usual procedures.

The care is not prepaid. Usually there are deductibles or coinsurance payments of 20% to 25% of the predetermined charge that the patient pays; the insurer pays the balance. A provider who joins a PPO does not need to alter the manner of providing care and continues to treat and bill the patients on a fee-for-service basis. When a patient covered under a PPO plan comes for treatment, the physician treats the patient and bills the PPO.

Technically, PPOs are not HMOs, but they do have more patient care management than regular indemnity insurance plans. PPOs furnish their subscribers with a list of member-providers from which subscribers can receive healthcare at PPO rates. Rates are quite often lower than those charged to non-PPO patients. If a patient goes to a physician who is not in the PPO network, the out-of-pocket cost is higher.

CRITICAL THINKING APPLICATION

The physicians in the practice in which Beverly is doing her externship are not members of a PPO that is well known in that geographic area. Many patients are confused when they have to pay a larger out-of-pocket fee for their medical services. How can Beverly explain the reason for larger out-of-pocket fees to nonmember patients?

More Third-Party Payors

Blue Cross and Blue Shield

Blue Cross and Blue Shield (BC/BS) is America's oldest and largest system of independent health insurers. It began in 1929 when an executive at Baylor University in Dallas came up with a plan for teachers to budget for their future hospital bills. The teachers paid $6 a year into a fund and were, in turn, guaranteed 21 days of free hospital care. Within 10 years the American Hospital Association officially embraced the concept of prepaid hospital care and symbolized their new program with a blue cross.

At the same time, workers in lumber camps in the Northwest developed a similar approach to deal with frequent logging accidents. Camp owners provided medical care for workers by paying physicians monthly fees for which a doctor would provide all the care the workers needed. Physicians formed groups, or medical service bureaus, which were linked to specific employers. The bureaus were identified with a blue shield, and they too quickly expanded in popularity.

Originally, Blue Cross plans were formed to cover the cost of hospital care, whereas Blue Shield plans were established to cover physicians' services. Today both brands represent the full spectrum of healthcare coverage. Now there are local Blue Cross plans operating in all 50 states, the District of Columbia, Canada, Puerto Rico, and Jamaica.

BC/BS no longer operates at the national level; plans are locally based, and they maintain their commitment to serving community needs. Each plan operates independently in its own service area, where it has the flexibility to respond to local healthcare needs. Plans can be organized as not-for-profit corporations or as for-profit companies, depending on the general business climate, their capital needs, and the regulatory environment.

BC/BS offers incentive contracts to healthcare providers. If the provider chooses to sign a member contract, he or she becomes a **participating provider (PAR)**. The healthcare provider then agrees to accept BC/BS reimbursement as payment in full for covered services. In turn, BC/BS agrees to reimburse providers directly and in a shorter time.

BC/BS identification cards carry the subscriber's name and identification number with a three-character alphabetical prefix. The letters are an important part of the number and must be included on the claim form.

MEDICAID

Title XIX of Public Law 89–97 under the Social Security Amendments of 1965 provides for agreements with states for assistance from the federal government in providing healthcare for the medically indigent. All states and the District of Columbia have Medicaid programs, but wide variations may exist among these programs.

The federal government provides basic funding to the state, after which the states individually elect whether to provide funds for extension of benefits. The state determines the type and extent of medical care that will be covered within the minimum requirements established by the federal government. Some local areas and states are developing HMOs that serve only patients who qualify for Medicaid.

A physician may accept or decline to treat Medicaid patients. The physician who does accept Medicaid

patients automatically agrees to accept Medicaid payment as payment in full for covered services. The patient cannot be billed for the difference between the Medicaid fee and the physician's normal fee. The patient can be billed for any services that are not covered by Medicaid. Eligibility for benefits is determined by the respective states.

Examples of individuals who qualify for benefits include the following:
- Persons receiving certain types of federal and state aid
- Persons who are medically needy
- Recipients of Aid to Families with Dependent Children
- Persons who receive Supplemental Security Income (SSI)
- For Qualified Medicare Beneficiaries (QMBs), Medicaid pays for Medicare Part B premiums, deductibles, and coinsurance for qualified low-income elderly
- Persons in institutions or other long-term care in nursing facilities and intermediate care facilities
- Medicaid purchase of COBRA coverage (low income persons who lose employer health insurance coverage)

A benefits identification card (BIC), which looks like a white credit card, or a sticker or label showing proof of eligibility is usually issued to the beneficiary. The BIC is verified by a point of service (POS) device similar to a credit card verification machine. The medical assistant must verify coverage each time the patient comes into the office before being seen if the state uses a BIC.

MEDICARE

Medicare is a federal health insurance program for:
- People 65 years of age and older
- People who are permanently disabled or blind
- People receiving dialysis for permanent kidney failure or who have had a kidney transplant

Medicare was developed in 1966 as a national health insurance program for the elderly. Before Medicare, only 50% of the nation's elderly had any health insurance. Today Medicare is the world's largest insurance program. It serves more than 38 million older and disabled Americans.

Medicare is administered by the CMS (formerly HCFA), a division of the Department of Health and Human Services (DHHS), and is based on laws enacted by Congress. Medicare has two parts, Part A and Part B.

Part A: Hospital Insurance. Retired people 65 years of age and older and people who receive monthly Social Security or railroad retirement checks are automatically enrolled for hospital insurance benefits and pay no premiums for this insurance. Part A covers:
- Inpatient hospital
- Skilled nursing facilities
- Home healthcare
- Hospice services

Part A is financed with special contributions deducted from employed individuals' salaries with matching contributions from their employers. These sums are collected, along with regular Social Security contributions, from wages and self-employment income earned during a person's working years. There is a deductible that a hospitalized patient must pay toward hospital expenses.

Medicare health insurance cards (Figure 18-1) identify whether a person has Part A alone or has both Part A and Part B insurance. A patient whose Medicare claim number ends in the letter *A* will have the same Social Security number and Medicare number. If a person has different Social Security numbers and Medicare numbers, the Medicare number ends in a *B* or a *D*. The letters after the Social Security number denote the patient's status, such as wage earner (A), widow (D), or other designations.

Part B: Medical Insurance. Persons who are eligible for Part A are also eligible for Part B, but they must apply for this coverage and pay a monthly premium. Some federal employees and former federal employees who are not eligible for Social Security benefits and Part A may still enroll in Part B. Certain disabled persons younger than age 65 years are also eligible. Part B covers:

- Outpatient hospital care
- Durable medical equipment
- Physicians' services
- Other medical services

A patient with Medicare Part B must meet an annual deductible before benefits become available, after which Medicare pays 80% of the *covered* benefits. Usually the physician *accepts assignment* of benefits for Medicare patients and is paid directly. In these cases the physician must accept the payment that Medicare allows and bills the patient for 20% of the charge allowed by Medicare. If the physician does not accept assignment, the patient must pay the entire bill (which cannot be greater than the limit set by Medicare for nonparticipating physicians), and the patient will receive a reimbursement check directly from Medicare.

Many Medicare enrollees also carry private supplemental insurance that pays the deductible and the 20% copayment not covered by Medicare.

TRICARE/CHAMPUS

TRICARE is the Department of Defense and military's comprehensive healthcare program for family members of active duty personnel, military retirees and their eligible family members under the age of 65, and survivors of all uniformed services. Before January 1994, this program was known as CHAMPUS, which stood for **Civilian Health and Medical Program of the Uniformed Services**, created in 1966 under Public Law 89-614.

The TRICARE program is managed by the military in partnership with civilian hospitals and clinics. It is designed to expand access to healthcare, ensure high-quality care, and promote medical readiness. All military hospitals and clinics are part of the TRICARE program and offer high-quality healthcare at low costs to plan users.

To be eligible for TRICARE, an individual must be a TRICARE/CHAMPVA recipient and entitled to retired, retainer, or equivalent pay and listed in the Defense Department's Defense Enrollment Eligible Reporting System (DEERS), which is a computerized data bank that lists all active and retired service members. Coverage is also available for a TRICARE-eligible spouse under age 65, and dependent, unmarried children under age 21 (23 if in college). Eligible spouses and children of active-duty service members may enroll as well as TRICARE-eligible widows, widowers, and ex-spouses (who have not remarried).

There are three choices under TRICARE:

- TRICARE Prime: The Department of Defense's managed care option, similar to a civilian HMO
- TRICARE Extra: A preferred provider network option
- TRICARE Standard: A traditional fee-for-service option formerly known as CHAMPUS

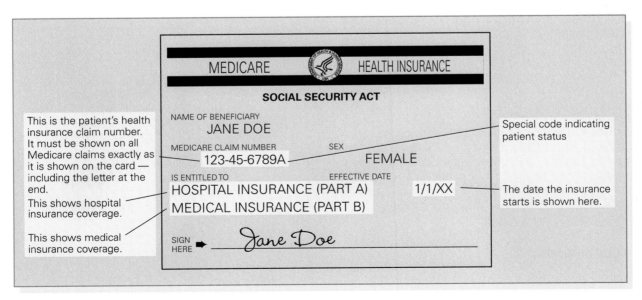

This is the patient's health insurance claim number. It must be shown on all Medicare claims exactly as it is shown on the card — including the letter at the end.

This shows hospital insurance coverage.

This shows medical insurance coverage.

MEDICARE   HEALTH INSURANCE

SOCIAL SECURITY ACT

NAME OF BENEFICIARY
JANE DOE

MEDICARE CLAIM NUMBER   SEX
123-45-6789A   FEMALE

IS ENTITLED TO   EFFECTIVE DATE
HOSPITAL INSURANCE (PART A)   1/1/XX
MEDICAL INSURANCE (PART B)

SIGN HERE ➤ _Jane Doe_

Special code indicating patient status

The date the insurance starts is shown here.

FIGURE 18-1 Medicare health insurance identification card. (From Fordney M: *Insurance handbook for the medical office,* ed 7. Philadelphia, 2002, WB Saunders, p 354.)

CHAMPVA

In 1973 a program similar to TRICARE/CHAMPUS was established for the spouses and dependent children of veterans suffering total, permanent, service-connected disabilities, and for surviving spouses and dependent children of veterans who had died as a result of service-related disabilities. This program, the **Civilian Health and Medical Program of the Veterans Administration (CHAMPVA)**, is a health benefits program in which the Department of Veterans Affairs (VA) shares with eligible beneficiaries the cost of certain healthcare services and supplies. The administration of CHAMPVA is centralized to VA's Health Administration Center (HAC) in Denver, Colorado.

After eligibility for CHAMPVA has been determined and identification cards are issued, the insured persons may obtain covered services and supplies from any provider who is appropriately licensed or certified to perform the services offered. Exceptions include certain mental health categories and free-standing ambulatory surgical centers.

Workers' Compensation

All state legislatures have passed workers' compensation laws to protect wage earners against the loss of wages and the cost of medical care resulting from occupational accident or disease. State laws differ as to the classes of employees included and the benefits provided.

No state's workers' compensation laws cover all employees. However, if a patient says that he or she was injured in the workplace or is suffering from a work-associated illness, the medical assistant should check with the patient's employer to verify the insurance coverage.

Compensation benefits include medical care benefits, weekly income replacement benefits for temporary disability, permanent disability settlements, and survivor benefits when applicable. The provider of service (e.g., doctor, hospital, therapist) accepts the workers' compensation payment as payment in full and does not bill the patient. Time limitations are set for the prompt reporting of workers' compensation cases. The employee is obligated to promptly notify the employer; the employer, in turn, must notify the insurance company and must refer the employee to a source of medical care.

In some states the employer and insurance company have the right to select the physician treating the patient. In essence, the purpose of workers' compensation laws is to provide prompt medical care to an injured or ill worker so that the person may be restored to health and return to full earning capacity in as short a time as possible.

Disability Programs

Disability income insurance is a form of health insurance that provides periodic payments to an individual to replace income (actual or presumed) when a sickness, injury, or disability (which is not a work-related condition) results in the insured being unable to work. A disability insurance policy can be obtained through employer-sponsored and/or government-funded programs, or private policies can be purchased through a commercial insurance company.

Mandated Programs. Several states require that employees be covered by nonindustrial disability (time loss) insurance. A small percentage (ranging from 0.3% to 1.2%) of the employee's salary may be deducted to cover the cost of this insurance. All regular employees, part-time or full-time, are covered until they retire.

Weekly benefits are based on the employee's salary and calculated using a predetermined formula. There is a waiting period before benefits begin (usually 7 days) and a time limit ranging from 26 to 52 weeks for benefits to continue.

Voluntary Programs. In states that do not have mandated disability insurance, employees or groups may solicit coverage from a commercial carrier.

Commercial Insurance

Many people are covered by health insurance issued by private (commercial) insurance companies. Physicians and medical societies control neither the premiums paid nor the benefits received from such policies. For traditional types of policies, payment is normally made to the subscriber unless the subscriber has authorized that payment be made directly to the physician.

Precertification and Preauthorization

Most insurance companies require precertification or preauthorization, usually within 24 hours, when a patient is going to be hospitalized or undergo certain procedures. Additionally, most managed care systems require preauthorization for a patient to be referred to a specialist or even for certain laboratory tests or other procedures.

It is necessary when a new patient makes an appointment to ask what type of insurance the patient has. If the patient belongs to an HMO, the medical assistant should check that plan contract for precertification or preauthorization requirements (Procedure 18-1). If you are not sure of the requirements, call the plan's contact number and keep a record of the requirements on a reference guide that you prepare with the following information:

- Plan name
- Address
- Telephone number (or numbers)
- Name and phone number of contact person
- Copayment amount or deductible
- Hospital benefits for inpatient and outpatient surgery
- Second opinion, preauthorization requirements, telephone number, and assistant surgeon with percentage
- Participating hospitals, radiology service providers, laboratories, and physicians

PROCEDURE **18-1**

Obtaining Precertification

GOAL: Using the information in the case study, obtain precertification from a patient's HMO for requested services/procedures.

EQUIPMENT AND SUPPLIES

- Patient record
- Precertification form
- Patient's insurance information
- Telephone/FAX machine
- Pen/pencil

CASE STUDY

PATIENT NAME: Kasandra J. Schaffer 4444 Morning Glory Drive Creston, IL xxxxx	PATIENT NO. 54398 SS# XXX-22-3333
DATE OF VISIT: 9/22/XX	DATE OF BIRTH 11/21/XX

S. This elementary school teacher returns to the office today for follow-up of the course of treatment prescribed and testing from her initial visit one month ago. (See detailed H&P from 10/16/xx.) She reports no improvement. Her symptoms, including constant exhaustion, ringing in the ears, sinus problems, pain in the joints, sore throat, gastrointestinal "problems," and decreased libido persist. She reports she is keeping to her prescribed diet.

O. Vitals are within normal limits. HEENT: Negative; Heart RRR, Lungs CTA. Abdomen: Soft, nontender. Bowel sounds are normal. Initial testing, including blood, urine, stool and a mental status exam were all within normal limits. Results of these tests were reviewed with the patient.

A. The fact that all tests were negative and the fact that Kasandra has been suffering from the above symptoms for more than 6 months leads me to the diagnosis of chronic fatigue syndrome.

P. 1. Continue with lorazepam, 0.5 mg as needed for insomnia.
    2. Refer to Physical Therapy for strength/endurance training.
    3. Follow up in one month.

Ralph Lopez, MD/xx

FACT SHEET:

Insurance Carrier: John Deere HMO 1345 John Deere Road Moline, IL xxxxx	Phone/Fax: 555-222-3321 Group # 54JD Patient's ID No. 22-3333HMO

Patient's Employer: Creston School District

PCP: Ralph Lopez, MD (NPI#345 543 876)

Name of Health Care Provider to whom patient is being referred: Anton Moss, PT

Reason for request: 12 1-hour physical therapy sessions

Diagnosis Code: 780.71

Continued

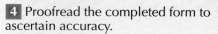

PROCEDURE 18-1—cont'd

PROCEDURAL STEPS

1 Assemble the necessary documents and equipment.

2 Examine the patient record, and determine the service/procedure for which preauthorization is being requested, including the specialist's name and phone number, and the reason for the request.

Purpose: To correctly complete the required form for gaining authorization from the patient's insurance carrier for the specified treatment.

3 Complete the referral form, providing all pertinent information requested.

4 Proofread the completed form to ascertain accuracy.

5 Role play the act of faxing the completed form to the patient's insurance carrier.

Purpose: To inform the insurance carrier of the patient's medical condition; to request preauthorization for the requested treatment; to request a verification number; and to confirm the specific number of physical therapy sessions.

6 Place a copy of the completed form in the patient's medical record.

Utilization Management

Patient care review by healthcare professionals who do not provide the care is a necessary component of managed care to control costs. A **utilization review** committee reviews individual cases to make certain that medical care services are medically necessary and to study how providers use medical care resources. This committee reviews all physician referrals, emergency department visits, and urgent care. After review, this department will either approve or deny the referral, so it is important to submit exact documentation and precise statements. You will be able to contact this department directly; never refer a member or patient to this department.

Referrals and Authorizations

Managed care changes on a day-to-day basis. To compete within this market, some insurance companies have added a benefit that will allow a member or patient to self-refer (meaning an authorization is not required to see a specialist). Many plans for senior citizens now have a **self-referral** and a copayment as well as some other insurance coverage. Information on referrals and authorizations will apply if you are working for a primary care physician, an internist, a family practitioner, a general practitioner, a pediatrician, and sometimes an obstetrician or a gynecologist.

Referral is a term used in managed care when a patient is referred from a PCP to a specialist. When completing a referral form (Figure 18-2), it is imperative that all necessary information be included (Procedure 18-2). For example:

Referring physician ⇒ Specialist being referred to ⇒ Diagnosis ⇒ Treatment (medication ⇒ past and present) ⇒ Chart notes (if necessary) ⇒ Minor surgical procedures

If a referral is denied because of insufficient information or no medical necessity, the PCP's office will be notified. Some medical groups will notify both the PCP and the patient. When the PCP's office provides the medical group with the necessary information, the referral will be reviewed again.

A referral can take from a few minutes to a few days to be reviewed and approved or denied. There are three types of referrals:

1. A *regular* referral usually takes 3 to 10 working days for review and approval. This type of referral is used when a patient has not responded to a PCP's treatment and/or medication and the physician believes that the patient must see a specialist to continue treatment.
2. An *urgent* referral will usually take about 24 hours for approval. This type of referral is used when an urgent matter occurs and is not life threatening.
3. A *STAT* referral can be approved by telephone immediately after faxing it to the utilization review department. A STAT referral is used in an emergency situation as indicated by the physician, such as life or death situations, miscarriage, loss of limb, or other conditions of similar magnitude. Usually the physician will refer the patient by telephone and will fax the information with the referral afterward.

A regular referral is the most common and can be inconvenient for the patient. Most managed care plans require contacting the member services department to check the status of a referral. A cardinal rule is to never tell the patient that the referral has been approved unless you have a hard copy of the **authorization**. Authorization is a term used by managed care for an approved referral.

A referral becomes an authorization after it is reviewed by utilization management and/or the medical director and has been approved. When a referral is approved, the PCP's office will receive a copy of the authorization by mail or fax. Always review the authorization thoroughly. The patient will receive a letter with an authorization number and the approved services. The patient must present the authorization to the specialist's office

MANAGED CARE PLAN
TREATMENT AUTHORIZATION REQUEST

TO BE COMPLETED BY PRIMARY CARE PHYSICIAN
OR OUTSIDE PROVIDER

Health Net	☐	Met Life	☐
Pacificare	☐	Travelers	☐
Secure Horizons	☐	Pru Care	☐

Member No. _____

Patient Name: _____ Date: _____

M _____ F _____ Birthdate _____ Home telephone number _____

Address _____

Primary Care Physician _____ Provider ID# _____

Referring Physician _____ Provider ID# _____

Referred to _____ Address _____

_____ Office telephone no. _____

Diagnosis Code _____ Diagnosis _____

Diagnosis Code _____ Diagnosis _____

Treatment Plan: _____

Authorization requested for procedures/tests/visits:

Procedure Code _____ Description _____

Procedure Code _____ Description _____

Facility to be used: _____ Estimated length of stay _____

Office ☐   Outpatient ☐   Inpatient ☐   Other ☐

List of potential consultants (i.e., anesthetists, assistants, or medical/surgical):

_____

Physician s signature _____

TO BE COMPLETED BY PRIMARY CARE PHYSICIAN

PCP Recommendations: _____ PCP Initials _____

Date eligibility checked _____ Effective date _____

TO BE COMPLETED BY UTILIZATION MANAGEMENT

Authorized _____ Not authorized _____

Deferred _____ Modified _____

Authorization Request# _____

Comments: _____

FIGURE 18-2   Example of a referral form. (Modified from Fordney M: *Insurance handbook for the medical office*, ed 7. Philadelphia, 2002, WB Saunders, p 339.)

Obtaining a Managed Care Referral

GOAL: Using the information in the case study, accurately complete a referral form for the managed care patient.

EQUIPMENT AND SUPPLIES

- Patient record
- Referral form
- Patient's insurance information
- Pen/pencil

CASE STUDY

PATIENT NAME: Calina V. Matucek   PATIENT NO. 5432

DATE OF VISIT: 6/02/XX   DOB: 07/28/XX

S. This 27-year-old female, an anthropology instructor at Bremmer College, comes to the clinic today complaining of fatigue, low-grade fever, stomach cramps, intermittent diarrhea, loss of appetite, and an erratic sleep pattern. She reports a 20-lb weight loss in the last two to three months. She is a vegetarian. Ms. Matucek was on an educational sabbatical to Indonesia at the onset of symptoms. She reports that while she was careful to drink bottled water, eating utensils were washed with untreated water. She was treated by a local doctor in Indonesia with an unknown drug (for suspected *Giardia lamblia*) and improved somewhat; however, the symptoms have returned. PFSH: See copy of form in chart.

ALLERGIES: Penicillin and aspirin.

O. Vital signs: T: 99.3; P: 84 and regular; R: 20. B/P: 114/74. Ht: 5 ft 8 in.; wt: 115 lb. HEENT: PERLA. Funduscopic: Benign. Sinuses: Nontender. Neck: Supple, no nodes or masses. Chest: Clear. COR: RRR without murmur. ABD: Somewhat guarded. Cranial nerves II-XII, sensory, motor, cerebellar grossly intact. Pt is pale and appears lethargic. Lab tests: See copies in chart of CBC w/automated diff and C&S taken at the ER on 6/04/xx.

A. (1) Lambliasis, suspected
(2) Anemia, chronic, simple (probably due to the fact that she has been a vegetarian for approx. 10 years).

P. Tylenol as directed for fever. An appointment has been scheduled with Gastroenterology on 6/12/xx.

Elwood P. Waxwood, MD/xx

Dr. Waxwood (phone 555-111-2222) is the primary care physician (PCP) in this case study, and Ms. Matucek is being referred to Terin B. McFlavin, Gastroenterologist (555-876-0987).

PROCEDURAL STEPS

1 Assemble the necessary documents and equipment.

2 Examine the patient record, and determine the service for which the patient is to be referred, including the specialist's name and phone number, and the reason for the referral.

Purpose: To correctly complete the required form for a PCP to refer a managed care patient to a specialist.

3 Role play with a partner the act of telephoning the patient's insurance carrier.

Purpose: To inform the insurance carrier of the patient's medical condition; to request authorization for the referral; to request a verification number; and to confirm the specific number of visits or length of treatment.

4 Complete the referral form, providing all information requested.

5 Proofread the completed form to ascertain accuracy.

6 Place a copy of the completed form in the patient's medical record.

receptionist on the day the services will be provided. An authorization provides the following information to both the PCP and the specialist:

1. An authorization number, which may be alphabetical, numeric, or alphanumeric.
2. The date on which it was received by utilization management, the date on which it was approved, and the expiration date.
   a. An authorization is good for 60 days.
   b. If services are provided after the expiration date, the services will be denied. If this happens, you need to contact utilization management or member services, ask for an extension, and answer a few questions. Sometimes you may have to involve the patient and/or the specialist's office.
   c. If the authorization expires and services have not been provided, you can request an extension. Utilization management will change the expiration date and will fax a copy to the PCP and specialist or will generate a new authorization with a new number.
3. A diagnosis code.
4. The name, address, and telephone number of the contracted specialist where services will be provided. Sometimes the PCP will refer the patient to a specialist but will not receive approval for that specialist and must get approval for another. Always be sure that any specialist to whom your physician refers patients is contracted with the same managed care plan as the PCP.
5. The comments section is the most critical area of a referral, because this area will designate what services are approved.
   a. The specified number of authorized visits to the specialist.
   b. An authorization may be issued for (1) evaluation only, (2) evaluation and treatment plan, (3) evaluation and biopsy, (4) evaluation and one injection, etc.
   c. Authorization for an evaluation only and/or treatment plan. When this authorization appears, the medical assistant must inform the patient that there will not be any treatment—only an evaluation and/or a treatment plan.

CRITICAL THINKING APPLICATION

Many private carriers and managed health plans have precertification or preauthorization requirements. How can Beverly explain the rationale of preapproval to inquiring patients?

Verification of Insurance Benefits

It is important to verify insurance benefits before providing services to patients. To verify benefits, the following steps should be taken:

1. When a patient calls for an appointment, identify what type of insurance the patient has or what managed care organization the patient belongs to.
2. When the patient arrives for the appointment, photocopy both sides of the patient's ID card (because copayments or amounts to be paid may appear on the back for hospital, office, and the emergency department).
3. Give the patient a letter to read and sign outlining the plan requirements and possible restrictions or noncovered items.
4. When referrals are required, explain the procedure to the patient so it is understood that without the referral, it is the patient's responsibility to pay for the physician's services.
5. Collect any copayments or deductibles.

Fee Schedules

A healthcare practitioner has three commodities to sell—time, judgment, and services. In every case, the healthcare practitioner must place an estimate on the value of these services. Fees for medical procedures and services differ from office to office based on the type of practice and the needs of the facility. The physician or physicians establishing the practice normally set the fees for procedures and services. In the past, most physicians worked on a *fee-for-service* basis (e.g., patients were charged for the provider's service based on each individual service performed).

In recent years third-party payors (particularly government and managed healthcare organizations) have greatly influenced what healthcare providers can charge by establishing what is referred to as the *allowable charge*. The allowable charge is the maximum that third-party payors will pay for a particular procedure or service.

When healthcare providers establish a fee schedule, there are other factors influencing what the charge for a particular procedure or service can be.

Relative Value Scale (RVS)

The RVS was pioneered by the California Medical Association in 1956 to help physicians establish rational, relative fees. Other states soon followed suit. Hundreds of the most commonly performed procedures were compiled, given procedure numbers similar to those in the AMA's Current Procedural Terminology (CPT) code list, and assigned a unit value. The assigned unit value represented the value of that procedure in relation to other procedures commonly performed. Although no monetary value was placed on the units, many insurance companies used the RVS to determine benefits by applying a conversion factor to assign a monetary value to the unit value. In 1978 the Federal Trade Commission (FTC) interpreted the California RVS as a fee-setting instrument and prohibited its publication and distribution. The FTC was attempting to make medical practice more competitive by ruling against the setting of fees and by encouraging physicians to advertise.

Resource-Based Relative Value Scale

As discussed earlier in this chapter, HCFA (now CMS) developed the first comprehensive RBRVS-based fee schedule, which was adopted by Medicare in 1992. The RBRVS-based fee schedule adjusts fees for differences in resources used to provide each service. The amount of resources required to perform a service is determined through the use of relative value units (RVUs) assigned to the CPT codes developed by the AMA. This system was implemented to standardize payment with an adjustment for overhead costs in different geographic areas. Since Medicare's introduction of RBRVS, most third-party payors have adopted similar approaches in developing their fees.

Tracking Insurance Claims

Chapter 17 discussed how a medical assistant should keep a log (or register) of insurance claims as they are received and processed. Forms should be date-stamped as they are received, and the information entered into the log. This log will enable the medical assistant to determine at a glance whether a claim form has been completed and mailed. In addition to keeping a log, it is also advisable to establish a routine for claims processing as follows:

- If possible, set aside a definite time for completing insurance claims.
- Have a central location for all insurance forms.
- Have all the necessary manuals, code books, and other needed references readily available.
- Create a master list of codes most often used by the practice, including fourth and fifth digits and/or modifiers, if appropriate.
- Make it a practice to complete the forms as soon as possible after services are rendered, usually at the end of the day.
- Use the CMS-1500 (formerly HCFA-1500) form as often as possible.
- Complete the forms by category (e.g., all Blue Cross, then all Medicare, and so on).
- If using a computer-billing program to print insurance forms, the computer will store insurance information on outstanding claims that can be printed in batches using the CMS-1500 form. Adjust the printer so the information lines up correctly on the form.
- Transmit claims electronically whenever possible.

Electronic Claims

A computerized medical practice uses the computer for processing claims electronically. This may be handled in several ways (e.g., transmitting data via modem, recording data on a computer disk and sending it to the payor or fiscal intermediary).

An obvious advantage of electronic billing is the amount of time saved with its use. The system interrupts the transmission of incomplete or incorrect data, giving the biller the opportunity for on-the-spot correction. The sender knows immediately whether the insurance company is accepting the claim. Another advantage of electronic billing is that it speeds up the date of payment, which results in an increase in cash flow to the practice.

Not all claims are suitable for electronic submission. For example, claims that are complicated and require a cover letter or those that require some kind of attachment must be sent on hard copy (paper) by mail or messenger.

Prospective Payment System

In April 1983, the Social Security Amendments Act of 1983 (Public Law 98-21) was signed into law. Title VI of this law contained the prospective payment system (PPS) for hospitals, which would begin the radical restructuring of the payment system to hospitals for Medicare inpatient services.

As identified by HCFA, now referred to as CMS, a major objective of the PPS was to establish the government as a prudent buyer of healthcare while maintaining beneficiaries' access to quality care. The prudent buyer objective was to be accomplished by paying Medicare providers a predetermined specific rate per discharge for diagnoses rather than on the basis of reasonable costs.

If a hospital does not contract with a regional office (RO), it is not eligible for payment from the Medicare program. The law provides authority to grant waivers from the PPS if a state has an approved hospital reimbursement control system. Additional criteria must be met by a state to receive approval and a waiver from the federal PPS.

Diagnosis-Related Groups (DRGs)

The DRG classification forms the basis for payment under the PPS. It is based on an average cost for treatment of a patient's condition, as opposed to the traditional method of payment based on actual costs incurred in the provision of care. Payment to the hospital of a DRG amount generally constitutes payment in full for services rendered to Medicare patients.

The DRG system, which classifies patients on the basis of diagnosis, was developed by Yale University researchers in the 1970s as a mechanism for utilization review. DRGs are derived from taking all possible diagnoses identified in the ICD-9-CM system, classifying them into 25 major diagnostic categories (MDCs) based on organ system, and further breaking them down into 495 distinct groupings, each of which is said to be medically meaningful. The principal diagnosis is the most critical factor in the assignment of DRGs. All diagnoses must reflect information contained in the patient's medical record.

To assign a case to a DRG, five pieces of information are necessary:

1. The patient's principal diagnosis and up to four complications or comorbidities
2. Treatment procedures performed
3. The patient's age

4. The patient's sex
5. The patient's discharge status

Hospital Coding

Chapters 15 and 16 discussed ICD-9, CPT, and HCPCS codes, which are used for diagnostic and procedural coding in physicians' offices and clinics. Hospitals use a slightly different coding approach. While hospitals do use CPT for coding procedures and volumes 1 and 2 of the ICD-9-CM manual for coding diagnoses on outpatient services, they use volume 3 of ICD-9-CM for coding inpatient services rather than CPT. This volume combines both the alphabetical and tabular lists for surgical and nonsurgical procedures and diagnostic procedures. Some publishers combine all three volumes into one manual, and others publish volume 3 as a separate book.

Another difference in hospital coding is that the patient's **principal diagnosis** is coded rather than the **primary diagnosis**. The principal diagnosis is that which is determined after study to be the major cause of the patient's hospital admission; a primary diagnosis (used in physicians' offices) is the condition considered to be the patient's major health problem. Another basic difference in inpatient diagnostic coding is that the insurance billing specialist codes all "rule out," "suspected," "likely," "questionable," "possible," or "still to be ruled out" situations as if one or more existed.

Finally, hospitals do not use the CMS-1500 claim form. They use the Uniform Bill (UB-92) claim form, also known as the CMS-1450 (Figure 18-3). For more information on hospital coding, refer to the reference listed at the end of this chapter.

HCPCS

Medicare carriers have since converted to CMS's (formerly HCFA's) Common Procedure Coding System (HCPCS, pronounced "Hic-Pics"). HCPCS, part of which is based on the current edition of CPT, is a five-digit alphanumeric coding system that can accommodate the addition of modifiers. There are three levels of codes assigned and maintained by most carriers:

1. Level I codes, which include 95% to 98% of all Medicare Part B procedural codes, and consist only of CPT codes (excluding those for anesthesiology, which is currently designated by surgery codes).
2. Level II codes, which are assigned by CMS (formerly HCFA) and are consistent nationwide. These codes are for physician and nonphysician services not contained in the CPT system. They are alphanumeric ranging from A0000 to V9999. These codes describe items such as drugs and durable medical equipment (DME).
3. Level III codes, which are assigned and maintained by each local fiscal intermediary. These codes represent services that are not included in the CPT system and are not common to all carriers. These codes range from W0000 to Z9999.

The Federal Register

The *Federal Register* is the official daily publication for rules, proposed rules, and notices of federal agencies and organizations, as well as Executive Orders and other Presidential documents. Publications are sponsored by the Office of the Federal Register (OFR) and produced by the Government Printing Office (GPO). The system was established to regulate complex social and economic issues after it was decided that agencies and the general public needed a centralized filing and publication system to keep track of rules and regulations.

Medical assistants can use the *Federal Register* for researching rules and regulations governing health insurance and coding. The *Federal Register* website is very user-friendly; just type in http://fr.cos.com/ to your computer's browser window, and your search engine will take you directly to their home page. From that point a search can be launched by topic, issue, or agency. Medical assistants may want to take a few minutes to browse this interesting website.

Patient Education

Understanding the ramifications of third-party reimbursement is challenging for a patient as well as a medical assistant. However, it is important that patients understand how their insurance works. Many, especially elderly persons, believe that if they have health insurance, all charges for their healthcare will be covered, and they don't always understand the intricacies of deductibles, copayments, medical necessity, and allowable charges.

One of the responsibilities of a medical assistant is to keep the patient informed and answer questions as they arise. Often medical facilities will provide informational brochures to their patients that explain how third-party reimbursement works, giving definitions of some of the more common terms used in the insurance claims process. If patients are well advised and comfortable with insurance facts before treatment begins, the medical experience will go more smoothly, and collection of fees not covered by their carrier will be easier. The medical assistant must use good communication skills, patience, and tact when discussing third-party reimbursement issues with patients.

CRITICAL THINKING APPLICATION

An elderly patient comes to the office complaining that Medicare did not pay her bill in full. "Medicare is supposed to pay 80% of all my medical bills," she insists. What information will Beverly need to get to the bottom of this problem? How will she explain it to this elderly patient in a way that she will understand?

Beverly notices that a new patient is a member of a PPO of which the physician in her office is not a member. How might Beverly explain this situation to the patient? How could she attempt to resolve it?

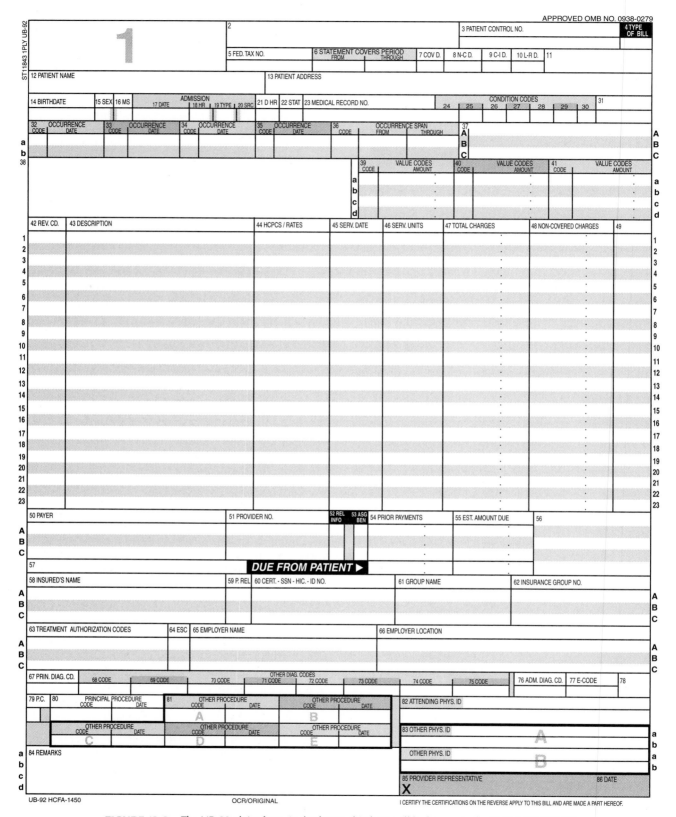

FIGURE 18-3 The UB-92 claim form. In the future, this form will be known as the CMS-1450 (UB-92).

Legal and Ethical Issues

Throughout their careers, medical assistants must remember that an individual's medical record is personal and private. Conversations between patients and their healthcare providers (and staff) are considered privileged communication. Nearly every day a medical assistant is in a position to read and hear information of a private medical nature, and both the caregiver and the patient expect that this information will not leave the medical office.

Unauthorized release of medical information carries over into the insurance claims processing area. Even though the patient expects the insurance form to be filled out and submitted for payment, this cannot be done without proper written release. This medical release form should be kept in the patient's chart, and it should be updated on a regular basis.

Managed care has often been criticized by the news media. Some types of managed care can create a physician-patient barrier that did not exist during the fee-for-service era. An extra effort in human relations by the medical assistant can help to overcome this barrier and put the patient at ease.

SUMMARY OF SCENARIO

Beverly and her peers have their plan in place for being successful with the challenging issues presented in this chapter. Their instructor is impressed with their effort and common sense study methods. In fact, the instructor has asked them to share their three-phase strategy with other members of the class, so they can benefit from it. The "trouble spots" identified by Beverly and her group did not seem so insurmountable when these were separated out and put into perspective.

Managed care and how it differs from traditional indemnity insurance was one of the issues that needed additional study and discussion. The websites they researched shed light on the subject, and the students enjoyed "surfing the Web" for answers to their questions.

There is still a lot of information to digest in this chapter on third-party reimbursement, but Beverly is now much more comfortable with its concepts and no longer feels that understanding the various topics is impossible. A structured study routine coupled with group "brainstorming" and internet research proved to be a successful strategy. The coordination and teamwork involved in the group experience are valuable skills that can be transferred to the workplace once Beverly's career as a medical assistant begins.

SUMMARY OF LEARNING OBJECTIVES

■ Medical assistants should have an understanding of the purpose of health insurance. This will help in the workplace not only by facilitating their knowledge of the subject, but also in educating patients. The trend for insurance policies to encourage preventive medicine can be appreciated.

■ Insurance policies fall into many different categories and are available in many different forms. The ability to differentiate among the various types of insurance policies gives medical assistants a solid background in what is available on the market, what is included in each policy category, and the function of each. It is also important for medical assistants to understand and appreciate that there are still many people in this country that cannot afford and do not receive quality healthcare.

■ Insurance packages are often tailored to the needs of each individual or group, and the ways to combine benefits are limitless. Health insurance policies normally contain a combination of the different benefits discussed in this chapter (e.g., surgical, basic medical, and major medical).

■ Benefits are determined and paid in one of several ways: indemnity schedules, service benefit plans, determination of the UCR fee, and relative value studies. Medical assistants should become familiar with each of these methods and understand the ramifications of all.

■ Healthcare has changed tremendously in recent years, and the cost of quality healthcare has skyrocketed. Efforts have been made in both the public and private sector to introduce various healthcare reform methods in order to contain these costs. Healthcare reform has had little success on a national level; however, state legislatures are beginning to pass laws that have brought improvement. Medical assistants should become well informed on the issues of healthcare reform and keep current by reading pertinent magazines and periodicals and paying close attention to news broadcasts.

■ Managed care is a broad term used to describe a variety of health plans developed to provide healthcare services at lower costs. There is a lot of confusion as to what managed care entails. To fully understand managed care, a medical assistant must know its history and how it evolved. When the medical assistant is employed in a medical facility, he or she will undoubtedly be working with one or more managed care plans. Therefore it is important to know the various types (e.g., HMO, IPS, and PPO) and understand how each one functions. Managed care has had both positive and negative effects on modern medicine. The bottom line is to be well informed.

▪ The maze of managed care options can create confusion in even the best-informed people. PPOs are another popular managed care option where physicians sign a contract with a PPO organization and agree to allow PPO members a discount for healthcare services. It may be difficult for medical assistants to become experts on every type of managed care; however, every medical assistant should research the ones that are the most common in his or her area of practice and concentrate on them.

▪ Other major third-party payors the medical assistant should become familiar with are Blue Cross/Blue Shield, Medicaid, Medicare, CHAMPVA, TRICARE, and workers' compensation. Medicare is the largest third-party insurer in the country,

making quality healthcare affordable for the elderly and select other groups. Medicaid is another government-sponsored healthcare plan for individuals who qualify for these benefits. Workers' compensation covers employees who are injured or who become ill as a result of accidents or adverse conditions in the workplace. Disability programs reimburse individuals for monetary losses incurred as a result of an inability to work for reasons other than those covered under workers' compensation.

▪ Many problems can be prevented for both the patient and the medical office if the medical assistant develops and follows a procedure for verifying insurance benefits before services being rendered. This procedure includes gathering as much information as possible about the demographics of the patient and his or her insurance coverage. A pragmatic and tactful discussion with all new patients explaining the established policy that the medical office adheres to regarding the insurance claims process and the collection of fees not covered by their policy will pay off in the end.

■ It is important for the medical assistant, and patients alike, to realize that fees for medical procedures and services differ from office to office based on the type of practice and the needs of the facility. Until the advent of managed care, most physicians operated on a *fee-for-service* basis where the provider would render his or her services and charge accordingly. In recent years, government and managed care organizations have greatly influenced what healthcare providers can charge. Many third-party payors base reimbursements on what is referred to as the *allowable charge*. Other fee schedule types include the Relative Value Scale (RVS) and the resource-based relative value scale (RBRVS).

INTERNET CONNECTIONS

- Blue Cross/Blue Shield
  http://www.bluecrossblueshieldusa.com/
  http://www/bluecares.com/
- Federal Register
  http://fr.cos.com/
- Kaiser Permanente
  http://www.kaiserpermanente.org/

REFERENCE

Fordney MT: *Insurance handbook for the medical office*, ed 7. Philadelphia, 2002, WB Saunders.

CHAPTER 19

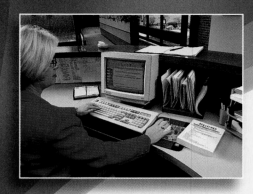

Scenario

Laura Anderson likes working with figures and has always been interested in bookkeeping. In high school she took all the bookkeeping and accounting courses that were offered, and during the summer months she helped out in the accounting department of the family business. In addition to her schooling and on-the-job experience, Laura wants to learn all she can about the financial transactions common to a medical practice. She is especially interested in electronic banking and all of the possibilities that it has to offer. Once her career in medical assisting is launched, Laura hopes to specialize in helping medical offices set up and run electronic banking systems.

Although Laura has had considerable bookkeeping experience, she realizes that there is still a lot to learn about the daily financial duties in a medical office, including accounts payable, working with the business checkbook, making deposits, reconciling bank statements, and many other banking responsibilities.

Taking on the bookkeeping functions of a medical office involves not only responsibilities to the physician and employer, but also to patients and the vendors from whom the medical office purchases supplies. Laura realizes that to perform well in her upcoming career as a medical assistant, she must learn all she can about the topics pertinent to her special interest areas and stay current with the rapidly changing world of finance.

Banking Services and Procedures

Janet Beik

Learning Objectives

- Define and spell the terms listed in the vocabulary.
- Explain how the Internet has changed traditional banking practices.
- State the four requirements of a negotiable instrument.
- Discuss the advantages of using checks.
- Identify the three most common types of bank accounts.
- Explain how you would handle mistakes made in preparing a check.
- List and discuss eight precautions to observe in accepting checks.
- Name and compare the four kinds of endorsements.
- Discuss the actions necessary when a deposited check is returned.
- Demonstrate the procedure for reconciling a bank statement.
- Correctly write checks for bill payment.
- Prepare a bank deposit and appropriate office documents.
- Accurately reconcile a bank statement with the office checking account.

National Curriculum Competencies

ADMINISTRATIVE COMPETENCIES

2a. Prepare a bank deposit
2b. Reconcile a bank statement
2c. Prepare a check

TRANSDISCIPLINARY COMPETENCIES

2b. Perform within legal and ethical boundaries

Vocabulary

bank reconciliation The process of proving that a bank statement and checkbook balance are in agreement.

clearinghouses Networks of banks that exchange checks with each other.

disbursements Money (funds) paid out.

drawee Bank or facility on whom a check is drawn or written.

drawer Person who writes a check.

e-banking Electronic banking via computer modem or over the Internet.

endorser Person who signs his or her name on the back of a check for the purpose of transferring title to another person.

holder Person presenting a check for payment.

m-banking Banking through the use of wireless devices, such as cellular phones and wireless Internet services.

maker (of a check) Any individual, corporation, or legal party who signs a check or any type of negotiable instrument.

negotiable Legally transferable to another party.

payee Person named on a draft or check as the recipient of the amount shown.

payor Person who writes a check in favor of the payee.

power of attorney A legal statement in which a person authorizes another person to act as his or her attorney or agent. The authority may be limited to the handling of specific procedures. The person authorized to act as the agent is known as the *attorney in fact*.

principal A capital sum of money due as a debt or used as a fund for which interest is either charged or paid.

Uniform Commercial Code (UCC) A series of laws (regulations), adopted by most states, that regulate the fields of sales of goods; commercial paper, such as checks; secured transactions in personal property; and particular aspects of banking, letters of credit, warehouse receipts, bills of lading, and investment securities.

F inancial transactions in the professional office nearly always involve banking services and the use of checks. Therefore a medical assistant must understand the responsibilities involved in accepting payments, endorsing and depositing checks, writing checks, and regularly reconciling bank statements. Payments received in the medical office should be deposited as soon as possible—ideally, the same day. The medical assistant may very well be in charge of these financial responsibilities; therefore he or she must understand each transaction and what its function is.

Banking in the New Millennium

With the advent of the Internet, banking as we once knew it has changed. People once had to fight traffic and wait in line at crowded banks; today they can sit in the comfort of their own homes and do their banking on the computer at any time of day. It is now possible to conduct such electronic banking transactions as buying and selling shares, paying bills, and transferring funds between accounts. In addition, customers have access to information about stock market prices and news and historical analyses of shares, which makes buying or selling decisions easier.

In fact, it is no longer necessary to sit in front of a computer terminal to conduct banking transactions. Instead, customers can sit on a bus or a train or be waiting for a flight and still make their investments or carry out other bank services. All of this is possible by just turning on a mobile telephone.

Online Banking

Online banking is a means to perform banking services via the Internet. It is also called *PC banking, home banking, electronic banking,* **e-banking,** or *Internet banking.* There are many facilities to choose from; most of them offer both basic and advanced services. Basic services usually include these:

- Checking account balances
- Transferring funds between accounts
- Paying bills electronically

Some of the advanced services that banks offer include the following:

- Applying for loans
- Downloading account information
- Trading stocks or mutual funds
- Viewing images of transactions (checks and deposits)

There are advantages and disadvantages to online banking. One of the most obvious advantages is the ability to bank at one's own convenience in one's own home or office at any time. This can save considerable time and expense, especially if banking must be done daily. Many people find online banking a convenient and comprehensive method for money management. Other advantages include ease of use, portability, and availability.

Disadvantages of e-banking include learning the software—it is less versatile than physical banking—and service options are often more limited. In addition, some experts believe that there may be a slight increase in risk as compared with conventional banking, although this has been debated by e-banking proponents. Forecasts show, however, that in spite of the disadvantages, banking via the Internet is becoming more popular, with an estimated 20% to 25% of homes and businesses using it.

The cost of online banking varies from bank to bank. Some charge a flat rate (from $5 to $10 per month), with varying fees for additional transactions.

Online Loans

Online lending is becoming more common as well. Loans are available for nearly anything consumers want to purchase—from homes and cars to small business loans and student loans for college tuition. Although online lending still has many loopholes, consumers can save time and money by comparison shopping the dozens of lenders available to find a good rate. Application forms can be downloaded for processing to initiate the process quickly, but the complicated loan process—especially for home mortgages—still requires coordination among many parties, and the sensitive financial and personal information needed for loan approval can raise online security concerns. Despite these issues, many people are "surfing the Web" for loans.

Online Convenience

Convenience is probably the number one reason people and businesses use the Internet for their financial services. There is no frenzied drive to the bank during rush hour, waiting in line, or working around the confines of banking hours. Online banking is available 24 hours a day, 7 days a week. In addition to Internet banking services, consumers can also pay bills online, without the delay of mailing. Credit card holders can check their balance and transaction status. Costly fees can be avoided for financial transactions left until the last minute, because online transactions can be accomplished in a matter of seconds. No need to wait and worry if the mail will get it there in time.

Customer-Oriented Banking

Americans are becoming more and more mobile. They want to conduct business and take care of personal concerns over cell phones on their way to and from work. In addition, the rapid pace of life requires rapid or "instant" solutions: people are buying take-out food at a record rate; some churches even offer drive-up services. It is no wonder that today's mobile consumers want the ability to conduct their financial transactions on the go, every day, at any time.

Banks no longer consider customers to be merely account numbers; to stay competitive, banks are being forced to look at the total customer picture. Some banks even offer a type of interactive voice response system that operates through speech recognition, allowing customers to conduct business through a combination of talking into the telephone and using the telephone keypad. The call centers of some banks employ live customer service personnel to answer questions and fulfill requests for all types of bank transactions.

Another customer-oriented innovation is mobile banking, or **m-banking**, which is emerging through the wireless technology market. Through the use of wireless devices such as cellular phones and wireless Internet services, customers can conduct a variety of financial transactions, set up alerts and notifications when bills are due, and make electronic transfers to pay these bills.

CRITICAL THINKING APPLICATION

Laura is excited about all of the possibilities available with e-banking and M-banking. Where can Laura learn more about electronic banking and its advantages and disadvantages compared with conventional banking?

Checks

A check is a bank draft or order to pay a certain sum of money payable on demand to a specified person or entity. The concept of writing and depositing checks as a method of conducting financial transactions dates back as far as the Roman Empire. Widespread check-writing didn't become popular, however, until the 1500s, when people in Holland began depositing excess cash with Dutch "cashiers," as a safer alternative than keeping money in their homes. These cashiers then paid the debts of the "depositors" on receipt of a written order. The word "check" was coined in England nearly 200 years later, when serial numbers were marked on these written orders of payment as a way to "check" on them. About 90% of all financial transactions in the United States are said to be effected by check.

A check is considered to be a **negotiable** instrument. For a check to be negotiable, it must:
- Be written and signed by a **maker**
- Contain a promise or order to pay a sum of money
- Be payable on demand or at a fixed future date
- Be payable to order or bearer

ADVANTAGES OF USING CHECKS

Using checks for the transfer of funds has many advantages:
- Checks are both safe and convenient, particularly for making payments by mail.
- Expenditures are quickly calculated.
- Specific payments can be easily located from the check record.
- A stop-payment order can protect the payor from loss due to stolen, lost, or incorrectly drawn checks.
- Checks provide a permanent reliable record of disbursements for tax purposes.
- The deposit record provides a summary of receipts.
- Checking accounts protect the money while on deposit.

Types of Checks

A medical assistant is probably familiar with the standard personal check, but there are many additional types of checks used in business transactions. He or she should also be familiar with other types of checks, which will be discussed next.

Bank Draft. A bank draft is a check drawn by a bank against funds deposited to its account in another bank.

Cashier's Check. A cashier's check is a bank's own check drawn on itself and signed by the bank cashier or other authorized official. It is also known as an *officer's* or *treasurer's check*. A cashier's check is obtained by paying the bank cashier the amount of the check, in cash or by personal check. Many banks charge a fee for this service. Cashier's checks are often issued to accommodate the savings account customer who does not maintain a checking account.

Certified Check. A certified check is the depositor's own check, on the face of which the bank has placed the word *certified* or accepted with the date and a bank official's signature. Because the bank deducts the amount of the check from the depositor's account at the time it certifies the check, the bank can guarantee that the amount is available. A certified check, like a cashier's check, can be used when an ordinary personal check might not be acceptable. If not used, a certified check should be redeposited promptly, so that the funds previously set aside are credited back to the depositor's account.

Limited Check. A check may be limited as to the amount written on it and as to the time during which it may be presented for payment—30, 60, or 90 days. The limited check is often used for payroll or insurance checks.

Money Order. Domestic money orders are sold by banks, some stores, and the United States Postal Service. Money orders are often used for paying bills by mail when an individual does not have a checking account. The maximum face value varies according to the source. International money orders may be purchased for limited amounts, indicated in U.S. dollars, for use in sending money abroad.

Traveler's Check. Traveler's checks are designed for persons traveling where personal checks may not be accepted or for use in situations in which it is inadvisable to carry large amounts of cash. Traveler's checks are usually printed in denominations of $10,

$20, $50, and $100, and sometimes $500 and $1000. They require two signatures of the purchaser, one at the time of purchase and the other at the time of use. They are available at banks and some travel agencies. The use of traveler's checks is becoming less common, because major credit cards are widely accepted throughout the world.

Voucher Check. A voucher check has a detachable voucher form. The voucher portion is used to itemize or specify the purpose for which the check is drawn. It is used for the convenience of the **payor** and shows discounts and various other itemizations. This portion of the check is removed before presenting the check for payment and provides a record for the **payee** (Figure 19-1).

The Banking System

The Federal Reserve

Wanting to provide the nation with a safer, more flexible and stable monetary and financial system, Congress created the Federal Reserve in 1913 as the central bank of the United States. It consists of a seven-member Board of Governors with headquarters in Washington, D.C., and twelve Reserve Banks located in major cities throughout the country.

Figure 19-2 shows how the country is divided into the twelve regional Federal Reserve districts. For additional information on the Federal Reserve System and its regional banks, visit its website, listed at the end of this chapter.

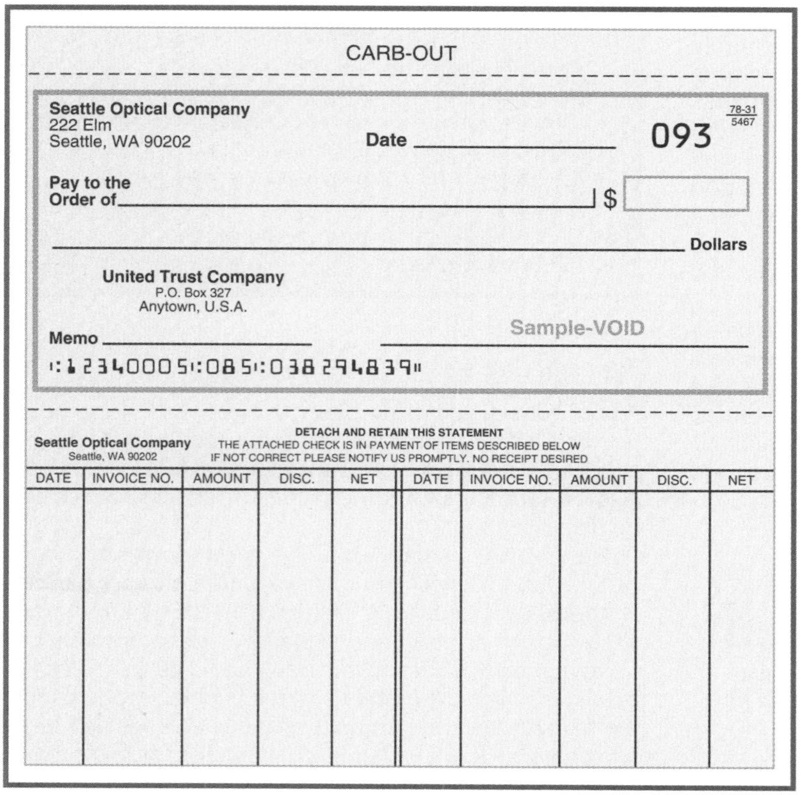

FIGURE 19-1   Page from a bank order book showing a sample voucher check.

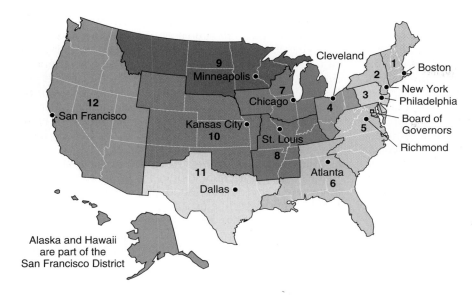

FIGURE 19-2   The twelve federal reserve districts.

Alaska and Hawaii are part of the San Francisco District

ABA Number

The ABA number is part of a coding system originated by the American Bankers Association. It appears in the upper right area of a printed check. The number is used as a simple way to identify the area where the bank on which the check is written is located and the particular bank within the area. The code number is expressed as a fraction (Figure 19-3), for example:

$$\frac{90\text{-}1822}{1222}$$

In the top part of the fraction, before the hyphen, the numbers 1 to 49 designate cities in which Federal Reserve banks are located or other key cities; the numbers from 50 to 99 refer to states or territories. The part of the number following the hyphen is a number issued to each bank for its own identification purposes. The ABA number is used in preparing deposit slips, to identify each check. The bottom part of the fraction includes the number of the Federal Reserve district in which the bank is located and other identifying information.

How Checks are Processed

When a check is presented for payment, the **drawee** (bank or facility on whom the check is drawn or written) pays the specified sum of money written on the face of the check to the **holder** (person presenting the check for payment). Checks received by the bank are turned over daily to a regional clearinghouse, which cancels each one by stamping, mechanically punching, or embossing them. The identifying code numbers, printed on the face of the check with magnetic ink, enables this "clearing" process to be accomplished quickly and efficiently. Checks due from and to all banks outside of a specific region are settled by means of computerized entries. The cancelled check is then either kept by the financial institution or returned to the **drawer** (person who wrote the check). Many banks no longer provide cancelled checks on a regular basis with the onset of internet banking services and most sophisticated computer systems. If the drawer needs proof of payment, a copy of the check can be requested from the bank if they are not returned in the monthly bank statement.

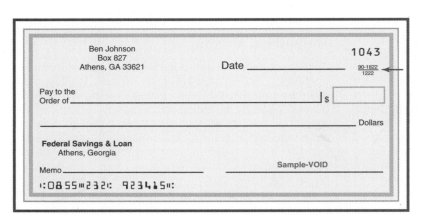

FIGURE 19-3   Sample check. The arrow indicates the American Bankers Association number.

Clearinghouses

As the use of checks grew, the system became confusing because so many different banks were involved. At first, messengers were used for collection; however, this involved a lot of traveling and carrying a lot of cash. Then, in a London coffee shop, a solution came about when two bank messengers discussing the shortcomings of the system realized they both had checks for each other. They decided to exchange them and save some time and effort. This practice evolved into a system of check *clearinghouses*—networks of banks that exchange checks with each other—that is still in use. Today banks in the United States can present checks to the Federal Reserve System or private clearinghouses for regional and national check collection.

Magnetic Ink Character Recognition (MICR)

Characters and numbers printed in magnetic ink are found at the bottom of checks. They represent a common machine language, readable by machines as well as by humans. When a check is deposited, the amount of the check can also be printed in magnetic ink below the signature. MICR identification facilitates processing through a high-speed machine that reads the characters, sorts the checks, and does the bookkeeping.

Bank Accounts

Common Types of Accounts

Checking Accounts. By placing an amount of money on deposit in a bank, a depositor can set up a checking account. Simply stated, a checking account is a bank account against which checks can be written. Many variations in checking accounts have been developed over the years. Instead of a straight, non–interest-bearing account, one might have an insured money market checking account, which bears interest at the daily money market rate if a certain minimum balance is retained. Most banks, however, do not offer interest-bearing checking accounts for businesses.

A physician often requires three different checking accounts:

1. An account for personal and family expenses
2. A separate checking account for office expenses
3. A high-yield interest-bearing account for funds reserved for paying insurance premiums, property taxes, and other seasonal expenses.

A medical assistant's use will probably be limited to the office checking account.

Savings Accounts. Money that is not needed for current expenses can be deposited in a savings account. In most cases, savings accounts earn interest on the amounts deposited; that is, the bank pays the depositor a certain percentage monthly or quarterly for the use of the money in the savings account. An ordinary savings account draws interest at the lowest prevailing rate and has no minimum balance requirement and no check-writing privileges.

Interest. Interest is a charge (or payment) in exchange for the use of money. It is usually figured as a percentage of the **principal**. Simple interest is computed annually; compound interest is figured on the principal as well as any previous interest that has been added to the original sum of money and can be computed using a variety of time increments—daily, monthly, quarterly, and so on. Certain checking accounts draw a small amount of interest—1% or 2% on the average daily balance. Savings accounts usually pay a higher rate of interest than a checking account—2% to 3%. However, these rates fluctuate with the financial market.

Money Market Savings Account. An insured money market savings account requires a minimum balance, anywhere from $500 to $5000; draws interest at money market rates (which is usually a higher percentage rate that a regular savings account); and allows the writing of a specified number of checks (frequently three) per month. There may be a minimum fee charged for each transaction. Such checks are usually written for transfer of funds to a checking account. Some businesses transfer excess funds from their business checking account to a money market account over the weekend or over an extended holiday period to draw interest on the funds (Figure 19-4).

Individual Retirement Accounts (IRAs). IRAs are a type of individual savings plan that are allowed special tax treatment at the federal and sometimes state level. This tax-favored status is what distinguishes an IRA from an ordinary savings account; however, you must follow specific rules to get the tax savings. IRA rules are stricter than those for ordinary savings accounts.

There are several different types of IRAs, such as traditional, Roth, and Education. IRAs are often used as a way to prepare for retirement for several reasons:

- Savings grows tax-deferred
- Tax deductions are realized for contributions (for traditional IRAs)
- Interest earned may not be taxed at withdrawal (for Roth IRAs)

IRAs come in all shapes and sizes. It is important to study and know the rules of each one before deciding which is best for an individual's needs.

CRITICAL THINKING APPLICATION

One of Laura's co-workers wants to open an account at her local bank. She knows Laura has more experience in this field than she, so she asks for her advice. How might Laura advise her on this?

The Business Account

A business bank account is used for business or company operations and managing cash related to day-to-day business functions. There is a wide variety available for businesses today, including checking, savings, and money market accounts, as well as other types of financial elements. When setting up a business account, careful consideration should be given to each of these elements to determine which account best meets the particular needs of a business.

What to Look For in a Business Account. Most businesses want "the most bang for their buck." In other

014143759	R		1	12/20/02
Account Number	Type	Items	Page No.	Statement Date

Statement of Account   14700 CT

001

Current Balance	Previous Statement Date	Previous Balance
2896.34	11/21/02	2886.59

ANSWERS TO YOUR BANKING QUESTIONS 24 HOURS A DAY,
7 DAYS A WEEK.   CALL ANSWERLINE TODAY

****   SUPER INSURED MONEY MARKET ACCOUNT   ****

YOUR OPENING BALANCE OF: 2,886.59

                          NO   DEPOSITS LISTED TOTALING: .00

- OTHER CREDITS -

12-20 SUPER INSURED MONEY MKT. INT. PAID   9.75

                          1   CREDITS LISTED TOTALING: 9.75

                          NO   CHECKS LISTED TOTALING: .00

                          NO   DEBITS LISTED TOTALING: .00

EQUALS YOUR ENDING BALANCE OF: 2,896.34

DAILY ACCOUNT BALANCES

DATE	BALANCE	DATE	BALANCE	DATE	BALANCE
12-20	2896.34				

- - - - - - - - - - - - - - - SUPER INSURED MONEY MARKET STATEMENT - - - - - - - - - - - - - - -

DATE	COLLECTED BALANCE	INTEREST RATES	DATE	COLLECTED BALANCE	INTEREST RATES
11-22	2,886.59	04.40	11-25	2,886.59	04.40
11-26	2,886.59	04.40	11-27	2,886.59	04.40
12-02	2,886.59	04.40	12-03	2,886.59	04.40
12-04	2,886.59	04.15	12-05	2,886.59	04.15
12-06	2,886.59	04.15	12-09	2,886.59	04.15
12-10	2,886.59	04.15	12-11	2,886.59	04.15
12-12	2,886.59	04.15	12-13	2,886.59	04.15
12-16	2,886.59	04.15	12-17	2,886.59	04.15
12-18	2,886.59	04.15	12-19	2,886.59	04.15
12-20	2,886.59	04.15			04.15

FIGURE 19-4   Example of a money market account statement. This type of check-writing has limited privileges.

words, they want to have the most services possible for the least amount of money—just as individuals do with personal accounts. Some of the service components available for business accounts include the following:

- Business checking with interest, accruing interest with either checking or savings accounts
- Free checks and deposits, with a maintained minimum balance (which varies from bank to bank)
- Overdraft protection, accomplished by linking the account to a savings account or to a bank-issued credit or debit card
- Online banking

Perks for Businesses. Many financial institutions are offering perquisites ("perks") for businesses opening accounts at their facility by offering special features. These may include the following:

- Business Express: A computerized cash management system that allows access to account information by telephone.
- "Sweep" account: An account in which excess funds over a minimum balance are "swept" into a higher yielding interest-bearing investment account. Then, when the balance in the account drops below the minimum, funds are "swept" back into it automatically.
- Business checking with "special features": A customized bank account designed for businesses with low to moderate transaction volumes and limited cash balances. This service helps business owners manage their day-to-day business and/or personal finances.
- Cash management account: Combines a checking account with a money market fund and a brokerage account. All cash activities are summarized on one monthly statement. This is ideal for business owners who do not have time for managing their money and/or investments.
- Other special features offered to businesses by banks include automatic bill paying, payroll preparation, and timed business deposits.

Business Checks. The checkbook most widely used in the professional office is a ledger-type book with three checks per page and a perforated stub at the left end of the check (Figure 19-5).

Checks may be in a bound soft cover or punched for a ring binder. The checks and matching stubs are numbered in sequence and preprinted with the depositor's name and account number, along with any additional information, such as address and telephone number. Check quantities of 100 to 300 are usually ordered at one time, and the cost is charged against the account. Numbered deposit slips in separately bound books are also supplied to the depositor.

Computer-Generated Checks. Instead of ordering checks to be printed by the bank, personalized checks can be ordered from printing houses to fit your computer's financial software program (e.g., Quicken). Checks can be prepared on the computer in much the same manner as using a typewriter. The checks may have one or more copies that serve as the record of checks written.

One-Write Check Writing. A one-write system of writing checks can save time and minimize errors in medical office **disbursements**. The office with a pegboard bookkeeping system (see Chapter 14) may wish to include one-write check writing. By using a combination check-writing system, such as the one illustrated in Figure 19-6, one check and one record of checks drawn handle both bill paying and payroll check writing.

When the check is written, a permanent record is created through the carbonized line of the check onto the record of checks drawn and the employee's payroll record, including a record of all deductions. Space is provided for the payee's address, so that the check can be mailed in a window envelope. This not only saves time

but also ensures that the check will go to the right address. Suppliers of basic pegboard systems can also provide a check-writing system such as the one described.

Bill Paying and Check Writing

Establishing a Bill-Paying System

A systematic plan should be established for the writing of checks and the paying of bills. Check writing usually is done on a specific day or days of each month. An exception sometimes arises when it is possible to realize a good discount if payment of a bill is made within a specified time, such as 10 days. Such discounts are usually indicated at the bottom of invoices or billing statements.

When a check is written in payment of a statement or invoice, it is good practice to write on the invoice the number of the check and the date it was paid. Then if any question arises about whether or when the bill was paid, you can readily locate the check stub. The handling and writing of checks must be done with extreme care (Procedure 19-1).

Designated Times. Rather than haphazardly paying bills as they are received in the office, the medical assistant should establish a routine for paying bills at designated times, such as on the fifteenth and thirtieth days of each month. Most vendors allow a 30-day cycle to elapse before adding on interest or late fees.

One method of handling accounts payable is to create a chronological "tickler file" with dividers for each pay cycle (e.g., the 10th of the month, the 20th, and the 30th). Behind each of the dividers, the invoices can be arranged alphabetically, if desired. When the date arrives, the medical assistant can pull all of the bills from that section and prepare the checks.

Paying Bills to Maximize Money. In establishing the procedure for accounts payable, a medical assistant should keep in mind that most vendors allow 30 days to pay. When each invoice is received, check the "terms," which are usually located at the top of the document. A few vendors offer a discount (normally 1% to 2%) if bills are paid within a shorter period of time. If the terms say "Net 30," this means the total amount of the bill is due within 30 days. Remember to allow a certain number of days (2 to 5, depending on where payment is to be sent) for mailing. If the business checking account is an interest-bearing one, do not pay bills before their due date. In this way, the funds in the account will continue to draw interest until it is time to write the check.

Also, if the practice has a weekly service, such as a laundry or cleaning service that bills several times a month, accumulate the invoices and issue only one check per month. Checks are costly, and some banks charge businesses a fee for each transaction.

Automatic Withdrawals and Deductions. Some routine bills that occur monthly or on a regular billing cycle, such as insurance premiums, rent payments, and utility bills, can be set up to be paid automatically through prior arrangements with the bank.

Online Bill-Paying. An online bill-paying account can be established with a bank or other business entity.

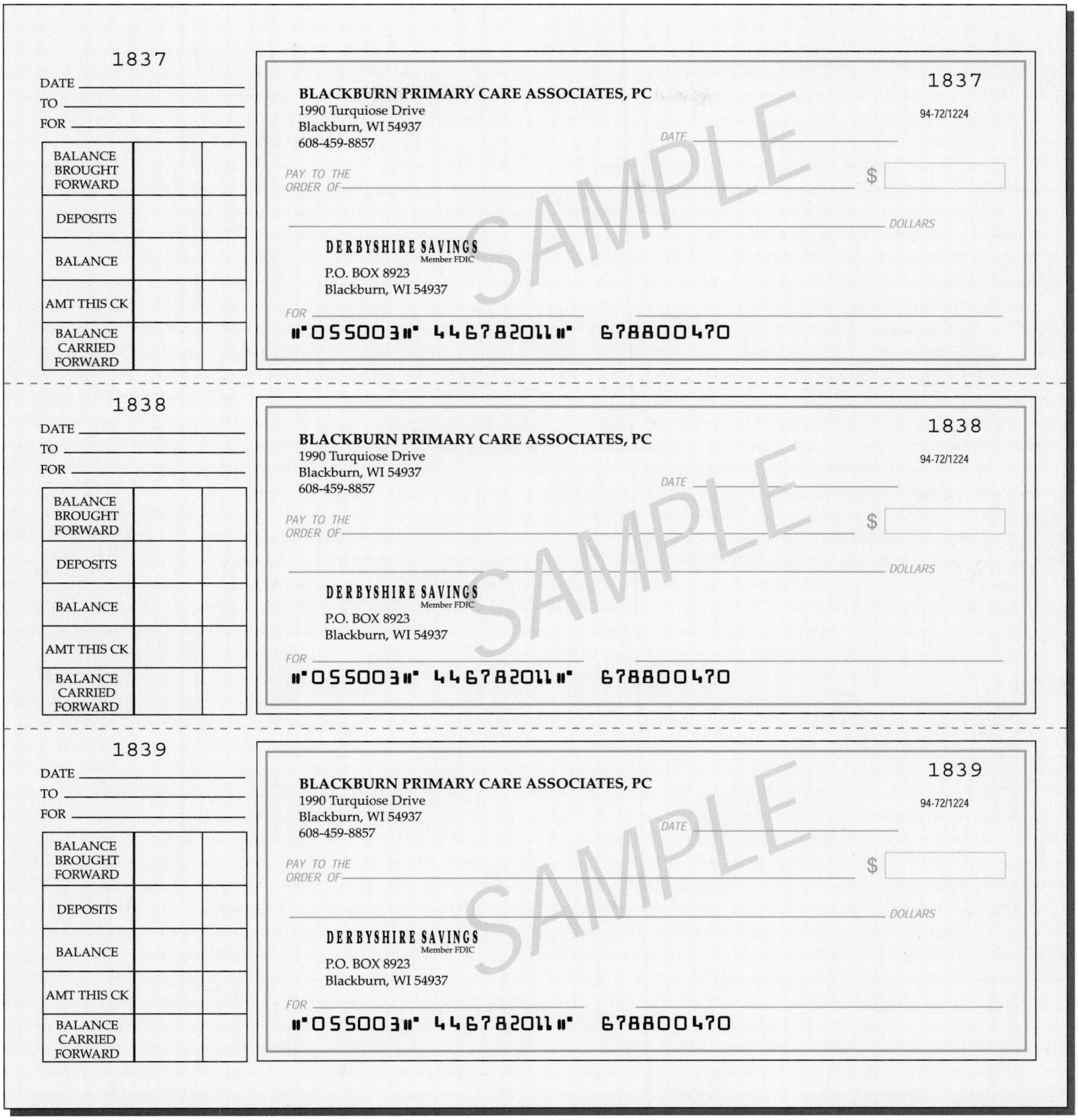

FIGURE 19-5 Example of business checks with stubs. (From Hunt SA: *Fundamentals of Medical Assisting*, Philadelphia, 2002, Saunders, p. 894.)

The bank then pays bills by automatically debiting the customer's account and crediting the merchant's account. More banks are offering this service; however, not all vendors accept electronic transfers in payment of bills. If a business decides to take advantage of online bill-paying, the options should be researched carefully, with consideration of the advantages and disadvantages involved.

Writing Checks

Instructions. Writing checks is a routine and basically simple function; however, there are certain guidelines to follow that prevent potential problems. Figure 19-7 illustrates several correct methods to use when writing checks.

Figure 19-8 shows the correct method for writing a check for an amount less than a dollar (top). The check on the bottom illustrates an incorrect method of check writing. Note the incomplete name and space for altering (e.g., $6.00 could easily be changed to $26.00 or more, and 00 could be made into 88). When writing in the numerical amount of a check, begin as far to the left in the block as possible. When inserting the written amount of the check, again start as far to the left as possible, allowing

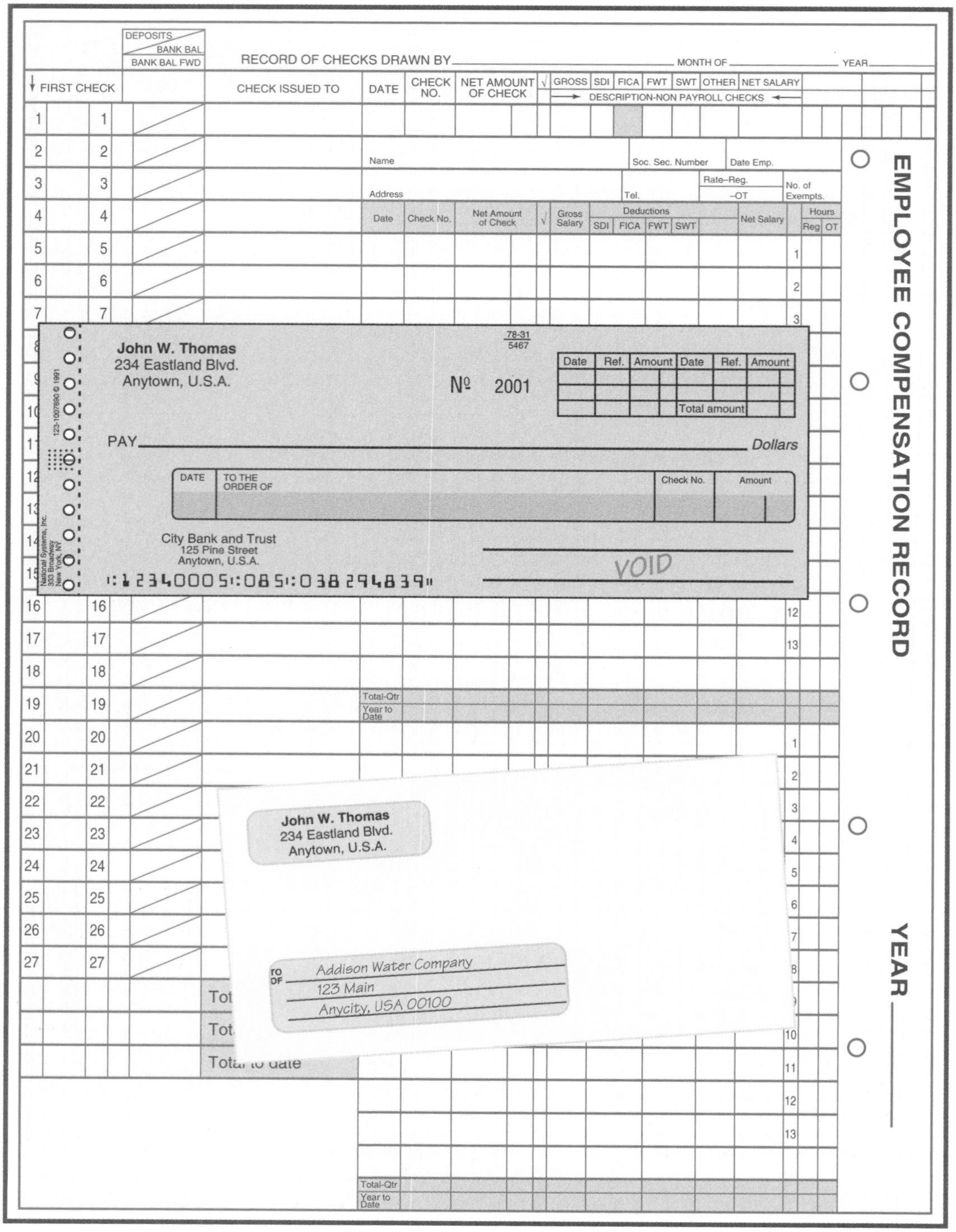

FIGURE 19-6
Pegboard system for check writing. (Courtesy Bibbero Systems, Inc., Petaluma, Calif. 94954, (800) 242-2376, www.bibbero.com.)

no space for added or altered words. Writing checks for less than a dollar is not recommended.

Checkbook Stubs. The check stub (the part that remains in the book after the check has been written and removed) is the depositor's own record of checks written, date, amount, payee, and purpose (Figure 19-9). It is important that the stub be completed before the check is written.

This prevents the possibility of writing a check and neglecting to complete the stub. If the stub is not completed and the check is sent out, you will have no record of the payee and the amount taken from the account until the cancelled check is returned at a later date. Consequently, you will be unable to balance the account or determine the amount on hand until the bank returns those cancelled checks. It is possible to get this information from the bank after the check has been cashed. There may be a charge for this service.

Signing Checks. After all checks have been written, place them along with the invoices or other verifying

PROCEDURE 19-1

Writing Checks in Payment of Bills

GOAL: To correctly write checks for payment of bills.

EQUIPMENT AND SUPPLIES

- Checkbook
- Bills to be paid

PROCEDURAL STEPS

1 Locate the first bill to be paid. Before writing the check, fill out the stub or the place designated for recording expenditures. Include the date, name of payee, amount of check, the new balance to be carried forward, and usually, the purpose of the check.

Purpose: To prevent the possibility of delivering or mailing a check without entering the information in the checkbook.

2 Complete both the check and the stub with pen or typewriter.

Purpose: To avoid danger of alteration for any reason.

3 Date the check the day it is written (do not postdate).

4 Write the name of the payee after the printed words, "Pay to the Order of _____ " with the

necessary information following. Do not use abbreviations unless so instructed.

5 Leave no space before the name and follow it with three dashes if there is space remaining.

6 Omit personal titles from the names of payees.

7 If a payee is receiving a check as an officer of an organization, the name of the office should follow the name. Example: "John F. Jones, Treasurer."

8 Start writing at the extreme left of each space. Leave no blank spaces. Keep the cents notation close to the dollars figure to prevent alteration.

9 Verify that the amount of the check is recorded correctly on the stub, in the box for the dollar ($) amount, and on the line where the amount is written in words.

10 If a check is written for an amount less than 1 dollar, the figures by the $ sign may be circled or enclosed in parentheses ($0.65) to emphasize the amount.

information on the physician's desk for signature. In some practices, the medical assistant who has charge of the financial matters is also allowed to sign the checks. This is accomplished by filing a **power of attorney** at the depositor's bank. The power of attorney may limit the check-signing authorization to a certain amount or to a limited time period.

Handling Corrections. Do not cross out, erase, or change any part of a check. Checks are printed on sensitized paper so that erasures are easily noticeable, and the bank has the right to refuse to pay on any check that has been altered. (See Figures 19-7 and 19-8 for examples of correct and incorrect check writing.) If a mistake is made, write the word "VOID" on the stub and the check, but do not throw out or destroy the check. It should be filed with the canceled checks so that it is available for auditing purposes.

Writing Cash Checks. A cash check is made payable to cash or bearer. Such checks are completely negotiable. Because these checks are easily cashed without positive identification, it is poor policy to write cash checks unless they are to be cashed at the time they are written. Some bank personnel may require that the person receiving the cash endorse the check. Many experts in the banking business advise their customers not to endorse a check written for cash or petty cash; often, if there is a problem, the person who endorses the check is liable. A medical

assistant should never endorse a check written for cash or petty cash, as he or she is not a party in the transaction.

Mailing Checks. When checks are sent through the mail, the check should not be visible through the envelope. Either place the check within a letter or fold it into a plain sheet of paper. Checks may be folded at the right end to conceal the amount of money written. Make certain the envelopes are sealed before mailing, and the medical assistant should personally mail all checks as soon as possible after writing.

Special Problems With Checks

Special problems may arise when a check is written on nonexistent funds or when a payor wishes, for a legitimate reason, to prevent the payee from cashing a check.

Overdraws or Overdrafts. When a depositor draws a check for more than the amount on deposit in the account, the account becomes overdrawn. In most states, it is illegal to issue a check for more than the amount on deposit in the bank. Should this happen through error or oversight, the bank may refuse to honor the check and will return it to the bank that presented it for payment. Such a check is said to "bounce."

If a check is written by an established depositor, the bank may honor the check and notify the depositor that

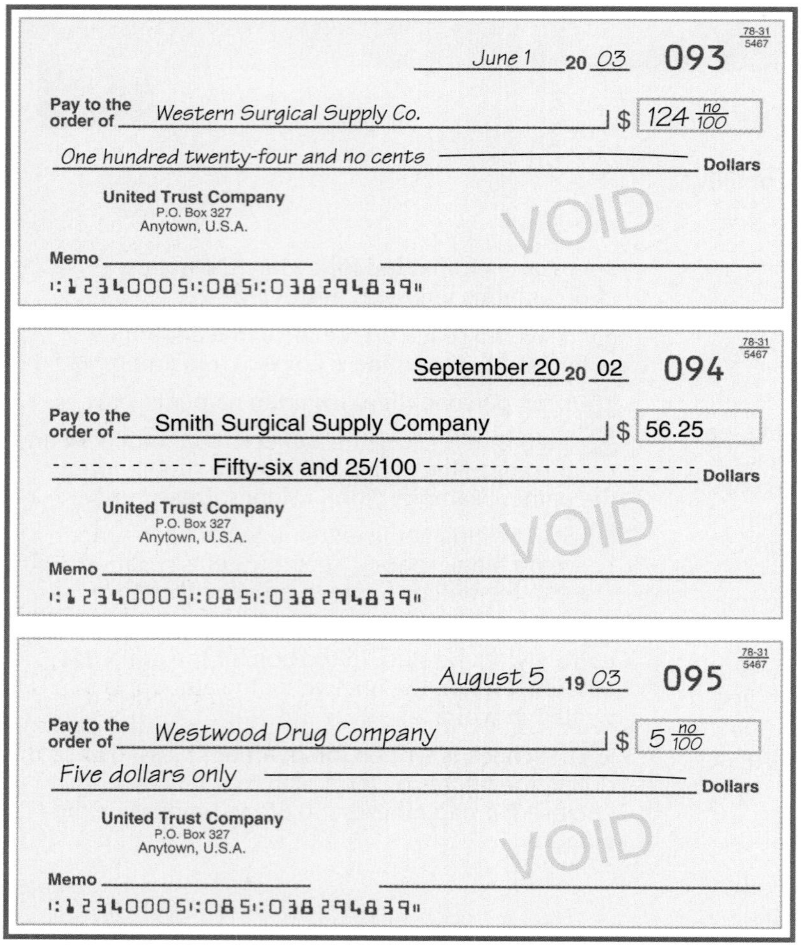

FIGURE 19-7   Correct methods of writing checks.

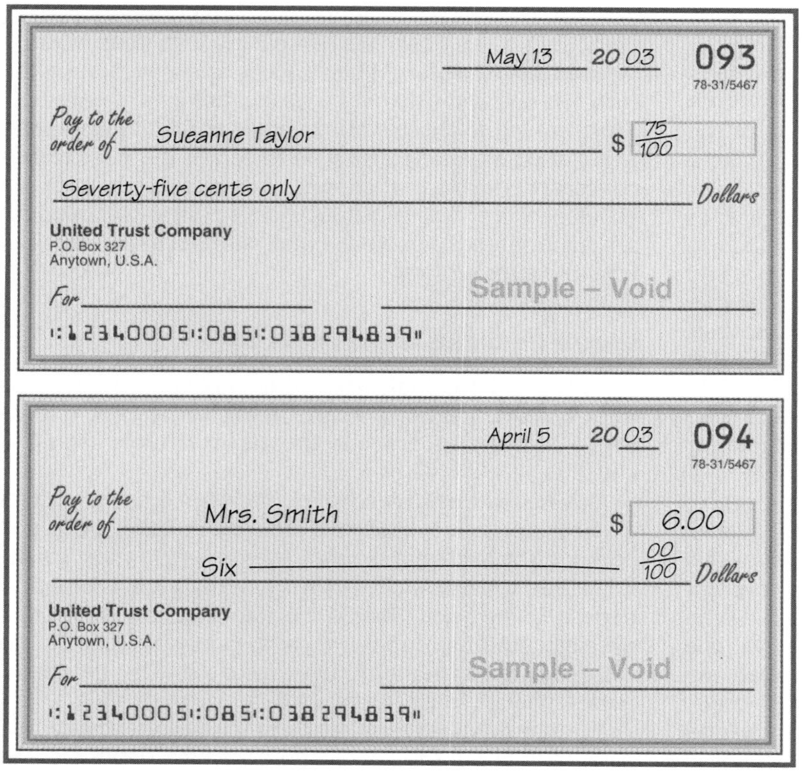

FIGURE 19-8   *Top,* Correct method of writing a check. *Bottom,* Incorrect method of writing a check, with incomplete name and space for altering (e.g., 6.00 could be made into 26.00 or more and 00 could be made into 88).

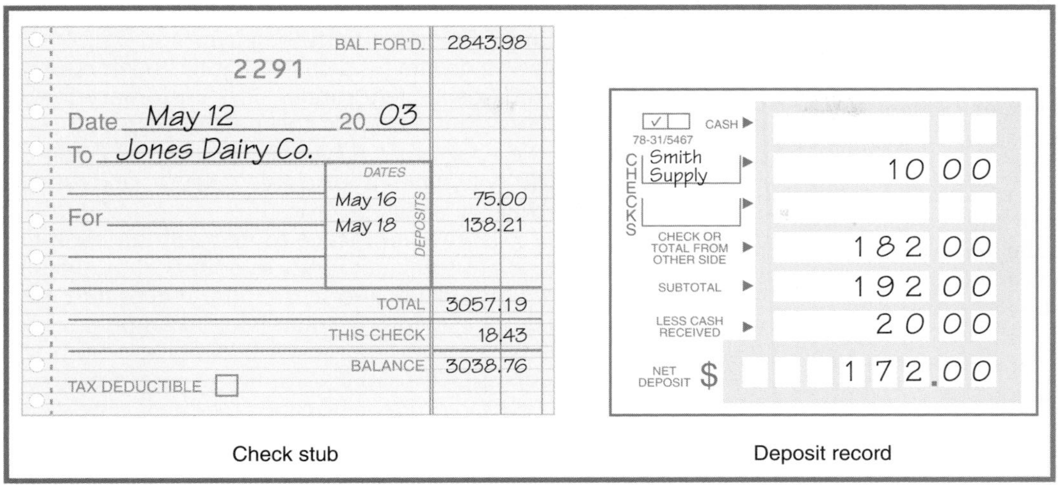

FIGURE 19-9 Methods of filling out a check stub.

the account is overdrawn. If the bank thus pays or covers the check, it issues an overdraft on the depositor's account. Considerable fees (from $10 to $25) are normally charged when an overdraft occurs.

Stop-Payments. A depositor or check writer who wishes to rescind the check has the right to request that the bank stop payment on it. Stop-payment orders should be used only in emergencies. Reasons for stop-payment requests are

- Loss of a check
- Disagreement about a purchase
- Disagreement about a payment

As with overdrafts, most banks charge a fee for stop payment orders.

CRITICAL THINKING APPLICATION

When Laura arrives at the office on Monday morning, she discovers that a check is missing from the business checkbook, and the stub is blank. What actions should Laura take to solve the problem?

Check Washing. Check washing is the fraudulent process of erasing or "washing out" the ink on a check with common household chemicals, such as bleach, benzene, or correction fluid. The person then rewrites the check to himself or herself, increasing the amount payable by hundreds and even thousands of dollars. It is estimated that check-washing fraud amounts to over $800 million a year in this country, and it is increasing at an alarming rate.

The National Check Fraud Center suggests the following to minimize the chance of check fraud:

- Ask your bank to advise your office when new books of checks are ready, then either pick them up or use a parcel delivery service to deliver them.
- Make sure cancelled checks are in a secured area, such as a bank lock box or a wall safe. Don't throw them in the trash.
- Check bank statements immediately after receiving them. If check fraud is not reported within 30 days

of receiving a monthly statement, the bank does not have to reimburse the loss (UCC Code 4-406).
- Print a return address on an envelope. A signature can be traced, duplicated, or forged.
- Don't discard credit card records or bills with trash.

For more information on how to avoid check fraud or what to do when fraud occurs, log onto the National Check Fraud Center's website, listed at the end of this chapter.

Accepting Checks

Precautions in Accepting Checks

A medical assistant is presented with checks for payment of physician's services on a daily basis. In most cases these are personal checks. Study the following Box for guidelines for accepting checks.

GUIDELINES FOR ACCEPTING CHECKS

- Scan the check carefully for the correct date, amount, and signature.
- Do not accept a check with corrections on it.
- If you do not know the person presenting a personal check, ask for identification and compare signatures.
- Accept an out-of-town check, government check, or payroll check only if you are well acquainted with the person presenting it and it does not exceed the amount of the payment.
- Acceptance of a third-party check is generally unwise. A third-party check is one made out to your patient by a party unknown to you. A check from the patient's health insurance carrier is an exception.
- When accepting a postal money order for payment, make certain it has only one

GUIDELINES FOR ACCEPTING CHECKS— cont'd

endorsement. Postal money orders with more than two endorsements will not be honored.

- Do not accept a check marked "Payment in Full" unless it does pay the account in full up to and including the date on which it is received. If a check so marked is less than the amount due, you will be unable to collect the balance on the account once you have accepted and deposited such a check. It is illegal for you to scratch out the words "Payment in Full."
- Accepting checks written for more than the amount due and returning cash for the difference between the amount of the check and the amount owed is poor policy. If the check is not honored by the bank, your office will suffer the loss not only of the amount of the check but also of the amount returned in cash.

Acknowledging Payment in Full

If payment in full is to be recognized in regard to a given check, the statement "Payment in Full to Date" must appear *on the back of the check*, above the endorsement, not on the face of the check. Canceled checks are a receipt for the maker of the check, not for the payee.

CRITICAL THINKING APPLICATION

A new patient wishes to pay for his services at the end of the office visit. The charge is $75. The patient writes the check out for $100 and asks Laura for $25 in currency in return. How should Laura handle the situation?

Returned Checks

Occasionally the bank may return a deposited check because of some irregularity, such as a missing signature or missing endorsement. More often, it is because the payor has insufficient funds on deposit to cover the check.

If a check is stamped "NSF," indicating *nonsufficient funds*, do not delay in contacting the person who gave you the check. If you are unable to contact the maker of a bad check, waste no time in tracking down all leads, such as referrals, numbers you obtained from credit cards, driver's license, and so forth. There are several places to which bad checks may be reported. Credit associations are often a great help when such problems arise. Turn the account over to a qualified collection agency if you do not succeed in collecting on the account yourself within a short time.

If a check is returned to your office marked "No Account" and it is a check that you had deposited promptly, you have obviously been swindled. This check should be given to the police, the local Better Business Bureau, or your collection agency.

Charging Fees. To cover their overhead costs, most banks currently charge both the payor and payee a fee of $15 to $30 dollars for a check that has been returned because of "insufficient funds." It is customary for the medical assistant to notify the person responsible for writing the check that it has been returned. Often the individual will have a plausible excuse and simply request that the check be "run through again." If this is the case, it is a wise practice to first call the bank and ask if there are sufficient funds to do this, thus avoiding additional time delay and fees. Some offices add these charges to the patient's account in an attempt to recoup the expense.

Collecting Returned Checks. There are several options available for collecting returned checks. As mentioned previously, the medical assistant might want to make an initial collection attempt by either telephoning or writing a letter to the patient. Many NSF problems can be cleared up quickly and easily using courtesy and tact, assuming that the situation was simply a mistake or oversight. If this method proves unsuccessful, the office might consider registering with a company that specializes in collecting bad checks. This can be done online or physically, using a local collection agency.

Additional methods of bad-debt collection are discussed in Chapter 14.

Legal Options. After all reasonable options for collecting NSF checks have been exhausted, a medical assistant may employ a collection method using the court system. Small claims court is a special court in which disputes are resolved inexpensively and quickly; it is a commonly used method that avoids costly attorney fees. Filing fees are in the $20 to $30 range, and there is usually a charge for having the papers served. There are restrictions, however. The amount for which the plaintiff (individual or company initiating the suit) can sue in a small claims lawsuit is limited to $5000. Other limitations vary from state to state. Contact the local Clerk of the District Court for the necessary forms and instructions in completing a small claims suit. For more information on filing small claims, refer to the government legal department's website, listed at the end of this chapter.

CRITICAL THINKING APPLICATION

When opening the mail, Laura notices a form from the bank with a check attached. It is a check from Elliott Benson, a new patient seen in the office the previous week, being returned for NSF. How should Laura handle this problem?

It is important that the medical assistant learn how to become "proactive" rather than "reactive" when it comes to problem patients. He or she should discuss fees with the patient on the first visit and gather all the financial and insurance information necessary to make a judgment as to whether the patient is able and willing to pay. An experienced medical assistant can often sense a "red flag" during this initial information-gathering process. If this happens, requesting payment in advance might be wise.

This practice should not be abused, however, and the medical assistant should follow the established office policy or discuss the matter with the office manager or physician when necessary.

Endorsements

An endorsement is a signature plus any other writing on the back of a check by which the **endorser** transfers all rights in the check to another party. Endorsements are made in ink, with either pen or rubber stamp, on the back of the check across the left (or perforated) end.

Why an Endorsement is Necessary

The Uniform Negotiable Instrument Act, applicable in all states, explains the need for an endorsement as follows:

> An instrument is negotiated when it is transferred from one person to another in such a manner as to pass title to another party. If payable to bearer, it is negotiated by delivery. If payable to order, it is negotiated by the endorsement of the holder completed by delivery.

The name of the last endorser of the check shows who last received the money. If a check is cashed for someone who did not endorse it and is returned for some reason, the bank will charge the check to the last endorser, not to the last person receiving the money. For this reason, it is not wise to cash a check made payable to another party without having the endorsement of the person who delivered the check to you for cashing.

Types of Endorsements

There are four principal kinds of endorsements. Blank and restrictive endorsements are the ones most commonly used.

Blank Endorsement. The payee signs only his or her name. This makes the check payable to the bearer. It is the simplest and most common type of endorsement on personal checks but should be used only when the check is to be cashed or deposited immediately.

Restrictive Endorsement. This specifies the purpose of the endorsement. A restrictive endorsement is used in preparing checks for deposit to the physician's checking account. An example is shown in Figure 19-10.

Special Endorsement. This endorsement includes words specifying the person to whom the endorser makes the check payable. For instance, a check naming Helen Barker as the payee may be endorsed to the physician by writing on the back of the check as follows:

> Pay to the order of
> Theodore F. Wilson, M.D.
> Helen Barker

The check is still negotiable but requires Dr. Wilson's signature or endorsement.

Qualified Endorsement. The effect of the endorsement is qualified by disclaiming or destroying any future liability of the endorser. Usually the words "without recourse" are written above by an attorney who accepts a check on behalf of a client but who has no personal claim in the transaction.

Methods of Endorsement

Stamp. As checks from patients and other sources arrive, they should be recorded on the ledger and immediately stamped with the restrictive endorsement "For Deposit Only." This is a safeguard against lost or stolen checks.

Any endorsement should agree exactly with the name on the face of the check. If the name of the payee is misspelled, it is usually necessary for the payee to endorse the check the way the name is spelled on the face, followed by the correctly spelled signature. The Uniform Commercial Code, Section 3-203, states:

> Where an instrument is made payable to a person under a misspelled name or one other than his own, he may endorse in that name or his own or both; but signature in both names may be required by a person paying or giving value for the instrument.

Most banks accept routine stamp endorsement that is restricted to deposit only, if the customer is well known and maintains an established account.

Signature. Some insurance checks or drafts require a personal signature endorsement; a stamped endorsement is not acceptable. This will be stated on the back of the check. In such cases, ask the payee to endorse the check, then stamp immediately below the signature the restrictive endorsement "For Deposit Only."

Making Deposits

The financial duties of a medical assistant include depositing checks and reconciling the bank statements with the checkbook. Checks should be deposited promptly, for these reasons:

- There is the possibility of a stop-payment order.
- The check may be lost, misplaced, or stolen.
- Delay may cause the check to be returned because of insufficient funds.
- The check may have a restricted time for cashing.
- It is a courtesy to the payor.

> Pay to the Order of
> Midwest National Bank
> Main Branch
> For Deposit Only
> CARLOS MACAULEY
> 301-012697

FIGURE 19-10   Example of a restrictive endorsement.

Preparing the Deposit

Deposit slips are itemized memoranda of cash or other funds that a depositor presents to the bank with the money to be credited to the account. All deposits must be accompanied by a deposit slip. A carbon or photocopy of the deposit slip should be kept on file (Procedure 19-2).

There are several types of deposit slips, sometimes called *deposit tickets*. The commercial slip is used for the office checking account. The deposit slips are printed with the number of the account in magnetic ink characters to correspond with the checks. Preprinted deposit slips are ordered along with the checks.

Some write-it-once accounting systems include a deposit slip that the bank will accept as the itemization if it is attached to the customer's numbered deposit slip. The deposit slip should be prepared before you go to the bank, with the money organized and ready to present to the bank teller.

Payment on patient accounts is generally made by check, but some payments are made in currency (paper money). Each type of fund is recorded separately on the deposit slip. The currency is usually listed first. Organize the currency so that all of the bills are facing in the same direction—for example, with the black-ink (portrait) side up. Place the largest-denomination bills on top.

Some banks prefer that checks be recorded individually by the ABA number; others use just the maker's name. If the checks are arranged alphabetically by the names of the patient accounts, with these names included on your office copy of the deposit slip, you will have a ready reference of checks deposited should a question arise regarding a patient's payment. Follow the procedure below for preparing a deposit slip (Figure 19-11):

1. List all checks on the back of the deposit slip.
2. Transfer the total to the front of the slip.
3. Enter the amount of the total deposit on the deposit slip stub.

Money orders, either postal, express, or others, are identified by "PO Money Order" or "Express MO." Remember that money orders cannot have more than two endorsements.

The deposit slip should be carefully totaled and the total entered in the checkbook. Any torn bills should be mended with transparent tape. Clip the currency together, and clip the checks in a separate packet. Then place the entire amount in a heavy envelope for taking to the bank. Deposit the currency and checks daily if possible.

Deposits by Mail

Depositing by mail saves time and is easily accomplished if the deposit consists of checks only. Banks usually supply their customers with special mailing deposit slips and envelopes on request (Figure 19-12).

Some mailing deposit slips have an attached portion that the bank will stamp and return to the customer as a receipt. Others may provide the customer with a receipt card that is sent along with the deposit each time for the bank's notation. The mailer shown in Figure 19-12 has a peel-off receipt for the depositor's records. Mailed deposits are prepared in the same manner as are regular deposits, but certain precautions should be observed.

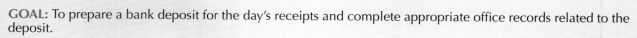

PROCEDURE 19-2

Preparing a Bank Deposit

GOAL: To prepare a bank deposit for the day's receipts and complete appropriate office records related to the deposit.

EQUIPMENT AND SUPPLIES

- Currency
- Six checks for deposit
- Deposit slip
- Endorsement stamp (optional)
- Typewriter
- Envelope

PROCEDURAL STEPS

1 Organize currency.
Purpose: To arrange currency in the best order for speedy and accurate presentation to the teller.

2 Total the currency and record the amount on the deposit slip.

3 Place restrictive endorsements on the checks, using an endorsement stamp or the typewriter.
Purpose: To transfer the title and protect checks from loss or theft.

4 List each check separately on the deposit slip by ABA number and its amount.

5 Total the amount of currency and checks and enter on the deposit slip.

6 Enter the amount of the deposit in the checkbook.
Purpose: To record the current balance in the account.

7 Prepare a copy of the deposit slip for the office record, including the names of the payors.
Purpose: For verification of checks deposited, if necessary.

8 Place the currency, checks, and deposit slip in an envelope for transporting to the bank.

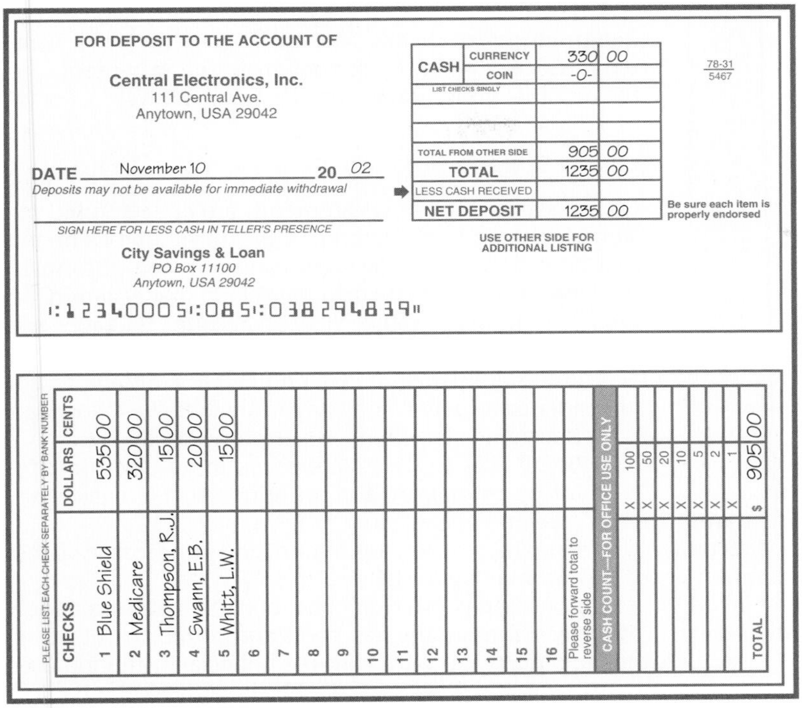

FOR DEPOSIT TO THE ACCOUNT OF

Central Electronics, Inc.
111 Central Ave.
Anytown, USA 29042

DATE _____November 10_____ 20 _02_
Deposits may not be available for immediate withdrawal

SIGN HERE FOR LESS CASH IN TELLER'S PRESENCE

City Savings & Loan
PO Box 11100
Anytown, USA 29042

⑆123400051:085:038294839⑈

CASH	CURRENCY	330	00		78-31
	COIN	-0-			5467
LIST CHECKS SINGLY					
TOTAL FROM OTHER SIDE		905	00		
TOTAL		1235	00		
LESS CASH RECEIVED					
NET DEPOSIT		1235	00		Be sure each item is properly endorsed

USE OTHER SIDE FOR ADDITIONAL LISTING

CHECKS	DOLLARS	CENTS
1 Blue Shield	535	00
2 Medicare	320	00
3 Thompson, R.J.	15	00
4 Swann, E.B.	20	00
5 Whitt, L.W.	15	00
6		
7		
8		
9		
10		
11		
12		
13		
14		
15		
16		
Please forward total to reverse side		
TOTAL	905	00

CASH COUNT—FOR OFFICE USE ONLY
× 100
× 50
× 20
× 10
× 5
× 2
× 1
$

PLEASE LIST EACH CHECK SEPARATELY BY BANK NUMBER

FIGURE 19-11   Front and back of a deposit slip.

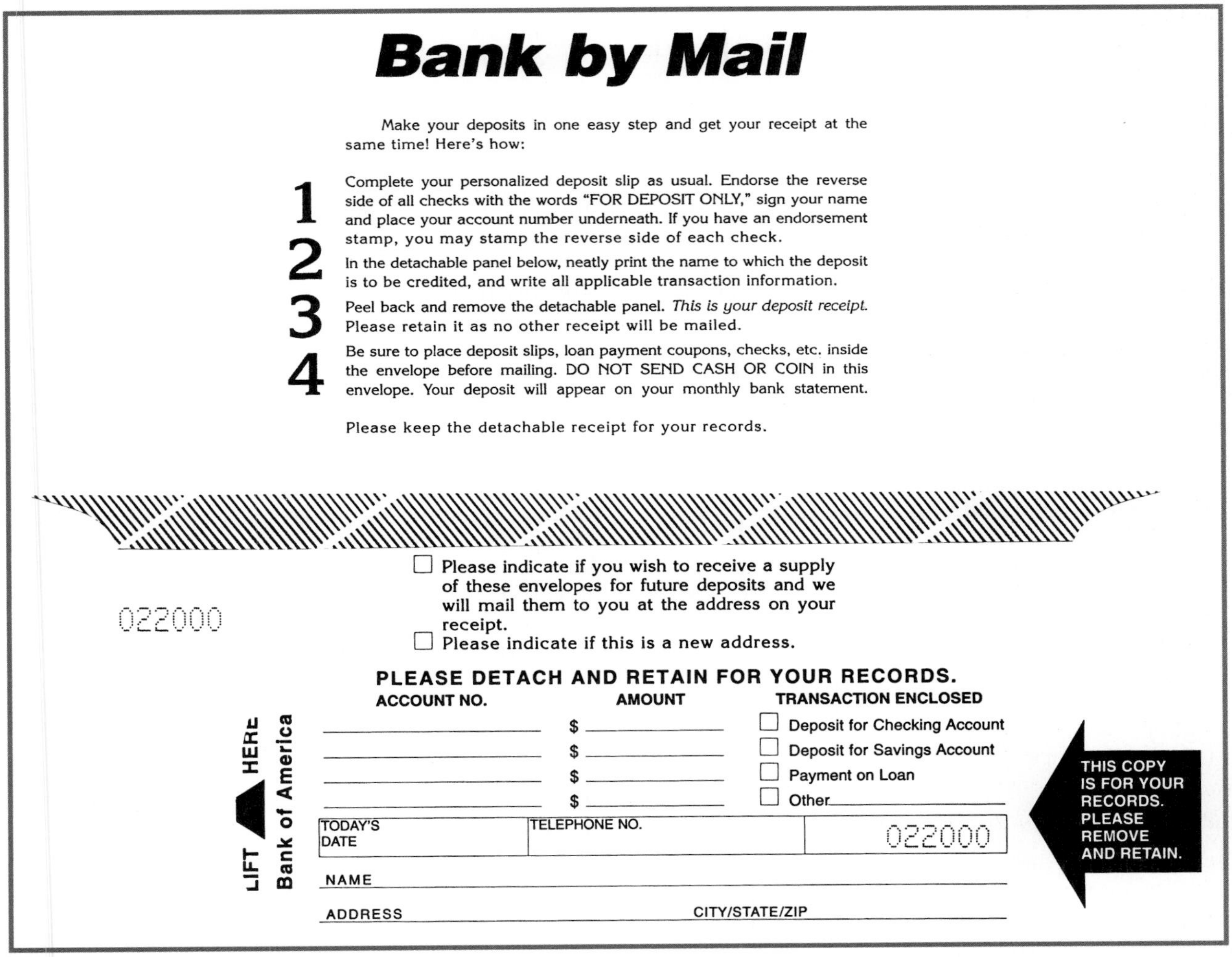

Bank by Mail

Make your deposits in one easy step and get your receipt at the same time! Here's how:

1 Complete your personalized deposit slip as usual. Endorse the reverse side of all checks with the words "FOR DEPOSIT ONLY," sign your name and place your account number underneath. If you have an endorsement stamp, you may stamp the reverse side of each check.

2 In the detachable panel below, neatly print the name to which the deposit is to be credited, and write all applicable transaction information.

3 Peel back and remove the detachable panel. *This is your deposit receipt.* Please retain it as no other receipt will be mailed.

4 Be sure to place deposit slips, loan payment coupons, checks, etc. inside the envelope before mailing. DO NOT SEND CASH OR COIN in this envelope. Your deposit will appear on your monthly bank statement.

Please keep the detachable receipt for your records.

022000

☐ Please indicate if you wish to receive a supply of these envelopes for future deposits and we will mail them to you at the address on your receipt.
☐ Please indicate if this is a new address.

PLEASE DETACH AND RETAIN FOR YOUR RECORDS.

ACCOUNT NO.	AMOUNT	TRANSACTION ENCLOSED
_____	$ _____	☐ Deposit for Checking Account
_____	$ _____	☐ Deposit for Savings Account
_____	$ _____	☐ Payment on Loan
_____	$ _____	☐ Other_____

TODAY'S DATE | TELEPHONE NO. | 022000

NAME

ADDRESS   CITY/STATE/ZIP

LIFT ▲ HERE   Bank of America

THIS COPY IS FOR YOUR RECORDS. PLEASE REMOVE AND RETAIN.

FIGURE 19-12   Example of a bank-by-mail deposit envelope. (Courtesy Valley Bank of Nevada, Las Vegas, Nev.)

DEPOSIT BY MAIL PRECAUTIONS

1. Do not send cash or currency by mail. If this is absolutely necessary, then send it by registered mail.
2. Use only a restrictive endorsement; use a deposit stamp or write the notation "For Deposit Only to the account of _____ ."
3. If you have not obtained mailing deposit slips or your bank does not provide them, make duplicate slips and mail them with your deposit. Ask the bank to stamp one copy and return it to you as a receipt.

Direct Deposits

Direct deposit is a plan in which payments are transferred, usually electronically, by a paying agency directly to the account of a recipient. Direct deposits are commonly used for paying salaries where paychecks are credited to employees' accounts—checking, savings, or any other type of account—at any financial institution.

Other Methods of Deposit

Advances in computer technology have allowed financial institutions to offer other methods of deposit to consumers and business customers. Some ATM machines will accept deposits, and there are checking accounts available that allow the customer to conduct the majority of banking services using the computer and ATM machines. These types of accounts may limit the amount of times the customer can use teller services without a fee.

Online banking allows customers to view their account, make transfers, order checks, pay bills, and perform numerous other transactions by simply logging on to the bank website and accessing the account with a password. Online banking is also an excellent way to research the checks that have cleared the bank and compute accurate bank balances.

Bank Statements and Reconciliation

A statement is periodically sent by the bank to the customer; it shows the status of the customer's account on a given date. This statement indicates the following:
- Beginning balance
- Deposits received
- Checks paid
- Bank charges
- Ending balance

Mailed Statements

Bank statements, similar to the one illustrated in Figure 19-13, are prepared at regular intervals (usually once a month) and are usually mailed to their customers. These statements may or may not include the accompanying cancelled checks, depending on bank policy and account type. The back of each page of the statement usually includes a reconciliation page so that the customer can determine what checks have still not cleared the bank, what deposits are not yet shown on the statement, and the accurate account balance.

Online Statements

Online statements, or e-statements, are an electronic version of a paper bank statement. Financial establishments that offer online banking services in an attempt to make banking easier for their customers claim that e-statements are a user-friendly way of viewing account balances and checking financial images online.

With e-statements, there's no need to continue receiving paper statements. The benefits include the following:
- Receiving statements quickly and easily
- Being able to save statements in an electronic file for examination and printing at the customer's convenience
- Keeping fees low by minimizing unnecessary paper and mailing costs

Various banks offer different options, and fees vary. If the medical assistant has been authorized to set up an online banking account with the financial institution used by the medical facility, he or she should visit the bank to discuss the details of what is involved.

Reconciling the Bank Statement

The bank statement balance and the customer's checkbook balance will usually be different, except in a relatively inactive account. The two balances must be reconciled. The reconciliation discloses any errors that may exist in the checkbook or, on rare occasions, in the bank statement (Figure 19-14).

The bank statement may include an entry for service charges that must be deducted from the checkbook balance. In all types of accounts, the bank may charge a fee for services. Usually in the case of an individual account, it is a flat fee; in a business account, the fee is based on services rendered. If the average or minimum balance is maintained at an established level, the bank may forego a service charge.

Most banks ask to be notified within a reasonable amount of time (e.g., 10 days) of any error found in the statement. The bank statement should be reconciled as soon as it is received. You will usually find a form to follow in carrying out this procedure on the back of the bank statement.

The reconciliation procedure may be put in a formula, as shown in the following box.

BANK STATEMENT RECONCILIATION FORMULA

Bank statement balance	$ _____
Less outstanding checks	$ _____
Plus deposits not shown	$ _____
Corrected Bank Statement Balance	$ _____
Checkbook balance	$ _____
Less any bank charges	$ _____
Corrected Checkbook Balance	$ _____

0821-402054

#821

‖l‖l‖l‖l‖l‖l‖l‖l‖l‖l‖l‖l‖l‖l‖l‖l‖l‖l‖l‖l

N
2

CALL (888) 555-2932
24 HOURS/DAY, 7 DAYS/WEEK
FOR ASSISTANCE WITH
YOUR ACCOUNT.

PAGE 1 OF 2   THIS STATEMENT COVERS: 6/22/02 THROUGH 7/22/02

INTEREST CHECKING 0821-402054	SUMMARY			
	PREVIOUS BALANCE	252.10	MINIMUM BALANCE	142.55
	DEPOSITS	68.74 +	AVERAGE BALANCE	220.00
	INTEREST EARNED	.18 +	ANNUAL PERCENTAGE	
	WITHDRAWALS	109.55 −	YIELD EARNED	.96 %
	CUSTOMER SERVICE CALLS	.00 −		
	INTERLINK/PURCHASE FEE	.00 −	INTEREST EARNED 1994	2.23
	MONTHLY CHECKING FEE AND OTHER CHARGES	.00 −		
	► NEW BALANCE	**211.47**		

USE YOUR EXPRESS CARD TO MAKE UNLIMITED PURCHASES AT RETAILERS DISPLAYING
THE INTERLINK SYMBOL. (A $1 MONTHLY FEE MAY APPLY.)

TRY IT TODAY AT ARCO . . . MOBIL . . . LUCKY . . . RALPHS . . . SAFEWAY & MORE!

CHECKS AND WITHDRAWALS	CHECK 202	DATE PAID 7/05	AMOUNT 15.05	CHECK 203	DATE PAID 7/15	AMOUNT 94.50

DEPOSITS			DATE POSTED	AMOUNT
	CUSTOMER DEPOSIT		7/22	68.74
	INTEREST PAYMENT THIS PERIOD		7/22	.18

BALANCE INFORMATION	DATE 6/22	BALANCE 252.10	DATE 7/05	BALANCE 237.05	DATE 7/15 7/22	BALANCE 142.55 211.47

24 HOUR CUSTOMER SERVICE

EACH ACCOUNT COMES WITH 3 COMPLIMENTARY CALLS PER STATEMENT PERIOD.

CALLS TO 24 HOUR CUSTOMER SERVICE THIS STATEMENT PERIOD: 0

INTEREST INFORMATION	FROM	THROUGH	INTEREST RATE	ANNUAL PERCENTAGE YIELD (APY)
	6/22	7/22	1.00%	1.01%

INTEREST RATE/APY AS OF 7/22/02 IF YOUR BALANCE IS

$ 0 - 4,999 . . . . .1.00%	1.01%
$ 5,000 - 9,999 . . . . .1.00%	1.01%
$ 10,000 AND OVER. 1.00%	1.01%

CALL 1-800-555-2932 IN CALIFORNIA ANYTIME FOR CURRENT RATES.

MEMBER FDIC

STATEMENT

FIGURE 19-13   Example of a regular checking account statement.

THIS WORKSHEET IS PROVIDED TO HELP YOU BALANCE YOUR ACCOUNT

1. Go through your register and mark each check, withdrawal, Express ATM transaction, payment, deposit or other credit listed on this statement. Be sure that your register shows any interest paid into your account, and any service charges, automatic payments, or Express Transfers withdrawn from your account during this statement period.

2. Using the chart below, list any outstanding checks, Express ATM withdrawals, payments or any other withdrawals (including any from previous months) that are listed in your register but are not shown on this statement.

3. Balance your account by filling in the spaces below.

ITEMS OUTSTANDING		
NUMBER	**AMOUNT**	
TOTAL	$	

ENTER

The NEW BALANCE shown on this statement _ $_____

ADD

Any deposits listed in your register $_____
or transfers into your account $_____
which are not shown on this $_____
statement.   +$_____

                TOTAL _ _ _ _ _ _ _ _ +$_____

CALCULATE THE SUBTOTAL _ _ _ _ _ _ _ _ _ $_____

SUBTRACT

The total outstanding checks and withdrawals from the chart at left _ _ _ _ _ _ _ _ _ −$_____

CALCULATE THE ENDING BALANCE

This amount should be the same as the current balance shown in your check register _ _ _ _ _ _ _ _ _ _ _ _ _ _ _ _ _ _ $_____

FIGURE 19-14 Reverse side of a bank statement to be used for reconciling a checking account.

IF YOU SUSPECT ERRORS OR HAVE QUESTIONS ABOUT ELECTRONIC TRANSFERS

If you believe there is an error on your statement or Express ATM receipt, or if you need more information about a transaction listed on this statement or an Express ATM receipt, please contact us immediately. We are available 24 hours a day, seven days a week to assist you. Please call the telephone number printed on the front of this statement. Or, you may write to us at United Trust Company, P.O. Box 327, Anytown, USA.

1) Tell us your name and account number or Express card number.

2) As clearly as you can, describe the error or the transfer you are unsure about, and explain why you believe there is an error or why you need more information.

3) Tell us the dollar amount of the suspected error.

You must report the suspected error to us no later than 60 days after we sent you the first statement on which the problem appeared. We will investigate your question and will correct any error promptly. If our investigation takes longer than 10 business days (or 20 days in the case of electronic purchases), we will temporarily credit your account for the amount you believe is in error, so that you may have use of the money until the investigation is completed.

PROCEDURE 19-3

Reconciling a Bank Statement

GOAL: To reconcile a bank statement with the checking account.

EQUIPMENT AND SUPPLIES

- Ending balance of previous statement
- Current bank statement
- Canceled checks for current month
- Checkbook stubs
- Calculator
- Pen

PROCEDURAL STEPS

1 Compare the opening balance of the new statement with the closing balance of the previous statement.
   Purpose: To determine that the balances are in agreement.

2 Compare the canceled checks with the items on the statement.
   Purpose: To verify that they are your checks and that they are listed in the right amount.

3 Arrange the canceled checks in numerical order and compare with the checkbook stubs.

4 Place a checkmark (✓) on each stub for which a canceled check has been returned.
   Purpose: To locate any outstanding checks.

5 List and total the outstanding checks.

6 Verify that all previous outstanding checks have cleared.

7 Subtract the total of the outstanding checks from the bank statement balance.
   NOTE: Do not include any certified checks as outstanding because their amount has already been deducted from the account.

8 Add to the total in Step 7 any deposits made but not included in the bank statement.
   Purpose: To correct the credits in the bank statement balance.

9 Total any bank charges that appear on the bank statement and subtract them from the checkbook balance. Such charges may include service charges, automatic withdrawals or payments, and NSF checks.
   Purpose: To correct the checkbook balance.

10 If the checkbook balance and the statement balance do not agree, match the bank statement entries with the checkbook entries.

If the two *corrected balances* agree, you may stop there. If they do not agree, subtract the lesser figure from the greater figure; the difference will usually give you a clue to locating the error (Procedure 19-3).

QUESTIONS TO ASK IN SEARCHING FOR A POSSIBLE ERROR

- Is your arithmetic correct?
- Did you forget to include one of the outstanding checks?
- Did you fail to record a deposit or did you record it twice?

Signature Cards

When an account is first opened at a banking facility, the depositor will be required to affix his or her handwritten signature to a card, which is then kept on file at the bank. If a check comes through, and there is some suspicion that the depositor's signature has been forged, the bank personnel compare the signature on the check to the original one on the signature card.

In a business situation, as in a medical office, the physician often delegates the responsibility of paying bills to the medical assistant or other office staff. In this case, any staff member who has been authorized to sign the medical facility's checks must go to the bank and add his or her handwritten signature to the signature card. Only the people whose names appear on the signature card are authorized to sign checks, and it is the bank's responsibility to verify any questionable signatures.

Bonding

To protect their business establishments from embezzlement or other financial loss caused by employees who handle large sums of money, physicians often purchase fidelity bonds. Fidelity bonds reimburse the physician for any monetary loss caused by employees. There are three types of bonding methods:

- *Position-schedule bonding*, which covers a specific position rather than an individual, such as bookkeeper or receptionist
- *Blanket-position bonding*, which covers all employees
- *Personal bonding*, which covers specific individuals

For individuals to be bonded, a personal background investigation is normally necessary.

Patient Education

Medical assistants might want to encourage patients to pay for professional services rendered with a personal check because of the numerous benefits checks offer. If a patient attempts to pay for services with a third-party check (other than an insurance reimbursement), the medical assistant should tactfully explain why this is not a wise practice. Additionally, if a patient makes a mistake when writing a check, it is the responsibility of the medical assistant to point it out and request a new one, as corrections on the face of a check often render the check useless.

When a patient's check is returned from the bank marked "insufficient funds," the medical assistant should immediately call the patient and explain the problem, requesting that he or she correct the matter as soon as possible. It is important to remember, however, that most overdrafts are simply the result of mathematical errors or a delay in deposited funds being available for withdrawal. So the medical assistant should be patient and courteous when discussing NSF issues with patients. Patients need to know, however, that overdrafts are costly not only to them, but also to the medical facility.

Legal and Ethical Issues

If a mistake is made in preparing a check, do not destroy this check. Rather, write "VOID" across the face of the check, make a note on the check stub, and file the check with the cancelled checks for auditing purposes.

A stop-payment order may be placed with the bank in an emergency, such as a check being lost, or a disagreement about a purchase or payment.

Do not accept a check made payable to another party without having the endorsement of the person who gives the check to you. If the check is returned by the bank for any reason, the check will be charged to the last endorser, not the last person to receive the money.

SUMMARY OF SCENARIO

Laura has gained considerable knowledge through her experiences and work with the various aspects of the banking world. The goals she set for completing the assignments and competencies were accomplished in the time frame allowed by the instructor. She is comfortable now that she can readily apply this knowledge to whatever medical facility she works in.

Laura spent extra time outside of class exploring online banking and bill paying on the Internet and found a wealth of information available. Laura now plans to visit several banks in her area to see what kind of e-banking services they offer.

The versatility of the medical assistant's role and the variety of the opportunities available reinforce to Laura that she has made the right decision for her career choice.

SUMMARY OF LEARNING OBJECTIVES

■ The Internet has changed conventional banking as we know it, and it offers expansive opportunities without leaving home. As with everything, however, e-banking has both advantages and disadvantages, and it should be thoroughly researched before an online account is opened.

■ For an instrument (e.g., a check) to be "negotiable," it must meet certain criteria: (1) be written and signed by a maker, (2) contain a promise or order to pay a sum of money, (3) be payable on demand or at a fixed future date, and (4) be payable to order or bearer.

■ There are many advantages to using checks. These advantages include safety and convenience, quick calculation of expenditures, and a permanent record for tax purposes.

■ The three most common types of bank accounts are checking accounts, savings accounts, and money market savings accounts. Each one is slightly different, and each has its special uses.

■ Normally, when a mistake is made on a check, it should be marked "VOID" and a new check should be written. Some banks will accept minor errors if the maker initials the error. Erasures are not allowed, nor is the use of correction fluid.

■ List and discuss eight precautions to observe in accepting checks.

■ The four kinds of endorsements are (1) blank endorsement, in which the payee simply signs his or her name on the back of the check, (2) restrictive endorsement, which specifies which bank and what specific account the funds are to be deposited in, (3) special endorsement, which names a specific person as payee on the back of the check, and (4) qualified endorsement, which disclaims future liability. This type of endorsement is used when the person who accepts the check has no personal claim in the transaction.

■ When a deposited check is returned, the maker should be contacted immediately, informed of the situation, and asked to remedy the situation either by immediately depositing funds in his or her account to cover the check, or to pay the bill by alternative means—cash or money order.

■ The procedure for reconciling a bank statement is simple and straightforward; however, until it is done a few times, it can be confusing. Follow the formula listed in the box on p. 368. If the bank statement and checkbook do not balance, look for possible errors as listed in the box on p. 371.

INTERNET CONNECTIONS

- The Federal Reserve System
  http://www.federalreserve.gov/
- National Check Fraud Center
  http://www.ckfraud.org/washing.html
- State of California Department of Consumer Affairs (for information on small claims court)
  http://www.dca.ca.gov/legal/small_claims/basic_info.htm#what

UNIT four

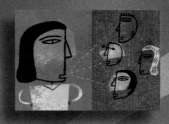

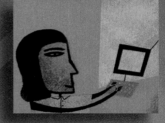

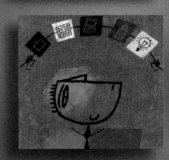

Medical Practice and Health Information Management

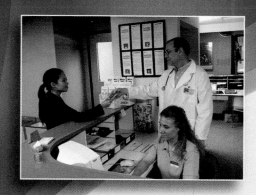

CHAPTER 20

Scenario

Katherine Martinson is the office manager for Dr. Michael Bouchard, a family practitioner in a group practice located in a metropolitan area. The office usually carries a full schedule of patients each day. Katherine has been instrumental in the seamless operation of the practice. Before joining Dr. Bouchard, Katherine worked for a physician in the same group practice, Dr. Grant Bradley, who retired last year. She worked as an administrative medical assistant for 6 years before that. Her strength and ability to motivate employees led Dr. Bouchard to approach her about becoming his office manager once Dr. Bradley retired.

Katherine is the consummate professional but knows the importance of treating each employee as an individual. At weekly staff meetings, the employees offer input on the various procedures followed in the office. Katherine regularly counsels with the staff members, always asking for input as to how the office can function more effectively and implementing many of the suggestions in the day-to-day activities of the office. She knows that employees need to feel a part of the team, and by trying the procedures others suggest she validates them as an asset to the facility.

When there is a position available, Katherine is careful about whom she hires, always checking at least three references per applicant and verifying each place of employment. She trains each employee on every aspect of the job and keeps checklists that reflect the employee has been given instruction on certain skills.

Katherine makes sure that each person has the tools needed to do the job. She also explains overhead costs to employees and helps them to understand what is involved with the daily operation of the practice. With this information, the employees are more conservative about use of supplies and care of equipment. Major changes are presented to the entire staff, and although Dr. Bouchard has the final decision, he and Katherine seek the input of the staff, too. The cooperative attitude between management and the employees of the office provides a good atmosphere for teamwork, and Katherine and the physician are pleased with the results.

Medical Practice Management

National Curriculum Competencies

vocabulary

affable Being pleasant and at ease in talking to others; characterized by ease and friendliness.

agenda A list or outline of things to be considered or done.

ancillary Subordinate; auxiliary.

appraisal To give an expert judgment of the value or merit of; judging as to quality.

blatant Completely obvious, conspicuous, or obtrusive, especially in a crass or offensive manner; brazen.

burnout Exhaustion of physical or emotional strength or motivation, usually as a result of prolonged stress or frustration.

chain of command A series of executive positions in order of authority.

circumvention To manage to get around, especially by ingenuity or stratagem.

cohesive The state of sticking together tightly; exhibiting or producing the cohesion.

disparaging Speak slightly about, with a negative or degrading tone.

embezzlement Stealing from an employer; to appropriate goods, services, or funds for personal use without permission.

extrinsic External to a thing, its essential nature, or its original character.

impenetrable Incapable of being penetrated or pierced; not capable of being damaged or harmed.

incentives Something that incites or spurs to action; a reward or reason for performing a task.

insubordination Disobedient to authority.

intrinsic Originating or due to causes within a body, organ, or part.

mentor A trusted counselor or guide.

meticulous Marked by extreme or excessive care in the consideration or treatment of details.

micromanage To manage with great or excessive control or attention to details.

morale The mental and emotional condition, such as enthusiasm, confidence, or loyalty, of an individual or group with regard to the function or tasks at hand.

motivation The process of inciting a person to some action or behavior.

reprimands Criticisms for a fault; a severe or formal reproof.

retention To keep in possession or use; to keep in one's pay or service.

subordinate Submissive to or controlled by authority; placed in or occupying a lower class, rank, or position.

targeted Directed or used toward a target; directed toward a specific desire or position.

The management of a professional medical office can greatly influence the success of the operation. Good management will allow the physician to see and treat his or her patients in a functional environment with the confidence that the business side of the facility is operating as it should be. A well-managed office is not something that just happens. Great effort and strong teamwork are necessary to ensure that the day-to-day activities are carried out efficiently and that the many details that need attention are handled expeditiously.

Who's In Charge?

If there is only one medical assistant, that person must be able to assume many of the management responsibilities with cooperation from the physician. When there are two medical assistants, one administrative and one clinical, it is often the administrative medical assistant who is expected to assume the management duties. In the office with a larger staff, a line of authority must be established.

A facility with three or more employees should have one person designated as supervisor or office manager. This individual should have management skills and the ability to deal with personnel matters (Table 20-1). Other employees answer to the supervisor, and the supervisor answers to the physician or physicians. This sets up an orderly way for the office staff to consult with the physician regarding administrative or clinical problems, complaints, or grievances. It also allows the physician to check on the operation of the office, disseminate information on policy changes, and correct errors or grievances.

The career of medical assisting becomes more challenging with the passing years, and offers more opportunities for advancement. The recently graduated medical assistant, whose first position possibly was as a receptionist, may systematically be given more responsibilities and may eventually become the office manager of a large staff. There is a shortage in executive-level personnel, one of the most critical areas in healthcare. Specifically there is a need for individuals competent to develop and operate a health maintenance organization or prepaid group practice.

Management problems often can be avoided by carefully defining the areas of authority and responsibility of each employee. Many physicians say that friction between workers is their most common personnel problem. A definite **chain of command** must be established, and the physician must not undermine the supervisor's

TABLE 20-1	Qualities of an Effective Manager

- Uses good judgment
- Has good health
- Has the ability to organize
- Is willing to learn
- Possesses original ideas
- Has leadership ability
- Is fair with all employees
- Is flexible
- Has a sense of fairness
- Cares about employees
- Remains calm during crises
- Is open to constructive criticism
- Has good communication skills
- Uses good listening skills
- Is approachable

authority by **circumvention**. When employees know what is expected of them, they can plan both their daily and long-term work more effectively.

Duties of the Medical Office Manager

The duties carried out by medical office managers vary from place to place and practice to practice. Some physicians take on a much more active role in office management than others. The best management plan for the physician is to hire an office manager who is trustworthy and reliable, and then allow him or her to run the business aspects of the office. This frees the physician to concentrate on taking care of patients (Figure 20-1).

Some of the tasks performed by the medical office manager include:

- Preparing and updating policy and procedure manuals
- Developing job descriptions
- Recruiting new employees
- Orientation and training
- Performance and salary reviews
- Dismissal of employees
- Planning staff meetings
- Maintaining staff harmony
- Establishing work-flow guidelines

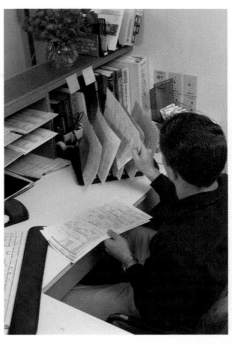

FIGURE 20-1 The office manager ensures that the medical facility runs smoothly so that the physician can concentrate on patient care.

PROCEDURE 20-1

Making Travel Arrangements

GOAL: To make travel arrangements for the physician or another staff member.

EQUIPMENT AND SUPPLIES

- Travel plan
- Telephone
- Telephone directory
- Typewriter or computer
- Typing paper

PROCEDURAL STEPS

1 Verify the dates of the planned trip.
- Desired date and time of departure.
- Desired date and time of return.
- Preferred mode of transportation.
- Number in party.
- Preferred lodging and price range.
- Preferred ticketing method (electronic or paper).

2 Telephone a trusted travel agency to arrange for transportation and lodging reservations.

3 Arrange for traveler's checks, if desired.

4 Pick up tickets/e-receipts or arrange for delivery.

5 Check tickets to confirm conformance with the travel plan.

Purpose: To avoid any error due to misunderstanding and to verify compliance with requests.

6 Check to see that hotel and air reservations are confirmed.

7 Prepare an itinerary, including all the necessary information:
- Date and time of departure.
- Flight numbers or identifying information of other modes of travel.
- Mode of transportation to hotel(s).
- Name, address, and telephone number of hotel(s), with confirmation numbers if available.
- Name, address, and telephone number of travel agency.
- Date and time of return.

8 Place one copy of itinerary in the office file.

Purpose: It may be necessary to contact the traveler or to forward mail.

9 Give several copies of the itinerary to the traveler.

Purpose: The traveler may wish to have extra copies for family or friends.

- Improving office efficiency
- Supervising the purchase and care of equipment
- Educating patients
- Eliminating time-wasting tasks for the physician (Procedure 20-1)
- Marketing the practice
- Customer service

Office management can best be accomplished by developing a thorough office policy and procedure manual. This will be discussed later in the chapter.

The Power of Influence

Managers have a great deal of influence over the people they supervise. A successful manager must be interested in people and enjoy working with them on a daily basis. It is said that if one helps others get what they want in life, the individual usually gets what he or she wants as well. An effective manager discovers the motivation behind employees' drives to be a part of the profession in which they are employed, and then helps them achieve their individual goals. In turn, most employees are enthusiastic about working toward the facility's goals as productive team members.

Successful managers know that their employees should be encouraged to perform at optimal levels, and they are confident enough in their own skills to give credit to those employees who develop ideas and concepts for the team. These managers know how to let their employees help them "look good." A manager with a group of outstanding employees usually is looked upon as an effective leader.

CRITICAL THINKING APPLICATION

- When Katherine first began as Dr. Bouchard's office manager, she found several supportive employees, but a few were concerned about their new boss. How can a new manager help employees be at ease during the first few weeks?
- Katherine scheduled a time with each employee and asked the three things he or she liked best about the office and three things he or she liked the least. How does this help her to manage the office effectively?

The Manager as a Leader

Leaders nurture other people. They take the time to discover what makes people tick and then give them opportunities that will help them rise to new levels of responsibility. Leaders have a strong belief in people, and they express confidence in their abilities, seeing them as successes rather than failures. Often this belief exists before people prove themselves, and that provides motivation to reach their potential.

Perhaps most important, leaders listen to their people. Few things are more frustrating than an employee attempting to talk to a manager who is working on some project or typing on the computer. Listening involves eye contact and questions to ensure that the employee is understood. Being willing to take the time to listen is a step toward success as a manager.

Types of Leaders

There are three basic types of leaders today, including the charismatic leader, the transactional leader, and the transformational leader. Each has positive qualities and all can be successful in business.

Charismatic leaders have a special way of inspiring an unswerving allegiance and devotion from their followers. They encourage people to overcome great obstacles and buy into their vision for the organization or business. They also tend to trust their **subordinates** and earn trust in return.

Transactional leaders are structured and organized. They ensure that their subordinates understand their duties and roles. These leaders are fair and provide rewards when they have been earned. The transactional leader is hardworking, a planner, and strict about budgets and time frames.

Transformational leaders are innovative and able to bring about change in an organization. These leaders are relationship builders. They stress shared values and strive to create a common ground among team members. Transformational leaders are the most effective when an organization is experiencing change and reorganization.

Styles of Management

Some managers are democratic and willing to listen to employees. These managers are fair-minded and ask the opinions of the staff when making decisions. This is a contrast to the autocratic manager, who is more of a dictator, making demands and insisting tasks be done in a certain way—his or her way. The laissez-faire manager is easy-going and does not make a lot of demands on employees. This is a "go with the flow" manager who lets employees work on their own and does not **micromanage**.

Leading During Transitions and Change

Change is a part of the life of every person and every business. Most people are initially hesitant to face change and many people try to avoid it completely. However, a business cannot experience growth without change. The manager who is able to lead subordinates through periods of change will be a valuable asset to the organization. They will need guidance on maintaining focus on the tasks at hand. The manager should remain visible to the employees during times of change and communicate frequently with status reports and updates on policies and procedures.

The book *Who Moved My Cheese?* by Spencer Johnson, MD,* is one of the most innovative stories in recent years. Any manager or employee experiencing a time of change should study this simple, short book. The opening quotes A. J. Cronin, saying:

---

*Johnson S: *Who moved my cheese? An amazing way to deal with change in your work and in your life*. New York, 1988, The Putnam Publishing Group.

"Life is no straight and easy corridor along which we travel free and unhampered, but a maze of passages, through which we must seek our way, lost and confused, now and again checked in a blind alley. But always, if we have faith, a door will open for us, not perhaps one that we ourselves would ever have thought of, but one that will ultimately prove good for us."

Who Moved My Cheese? stresses several points about change that the good manager should remember, including:

*   Change happens.
*   Anticipate change.
*   Monitor change.
*   Adapt to change quickly.
*   Move with the change.
*   Enjoy change.
*   Be ready to change again quickly and enjoy it again.

The simplicity of this advice does not diminish its truth. Change will happen in any person's job and personal life. Those who learn to adapt quickly and move forward will be the ones who survive the casualties of change.

The Role of Power

One definition of power is the ability to influence employees so that they carry out their directives. Leaders use many types of power.

Coercive power is manipulative, and the leader often makes threats or uses fear to accomplish goals. The fear of losing a job is one manipulation of power.

Granting rewards is a more positive use of power. When the leader is able to give employees some type of reward for a job well done, most strive to reach goals.

Expert power is a factor when the leader is knowledgeable about a subject. Employees respect leaders who know their job and how things should be done. Most people look up to a person who has a high degree of knowledge about a given subject. When working for someone who knows nothing about procedures or the services offered, employees frequently are frustrated.

Legitimate power is that of position or status. It does not really matter who the President of the United States is—the office itself carries the weight of power. Therefore the individual who serves as President holds legitimate power.

Referent power is granted from subordinates to those who lead by example. It is a power based on the admiration of the leader. Mentors, parents, and teachers are often the objects of referent power.

CRITICAL THINKING APPLICATION

*   Katherine is a respected office manager in the facility where she works, but there are several other managers who are not as well liked. What makes a good office manager?
*   Everyone has worked for at least one supervisor that they were not fond of. What traits make a poor office manager?

Abuse of Power and Authority

Unfortunately, many managers have the capacity to abuse the power they have. There are several ways to do this. A manager who puts up barriers and erects emotional walls with the employees will have difficulty forming a **cohesive** team. Some managers use other people as tools to get what they want, while others stick to their own level or stature, relating only to the inner circle of decision makers in the facility.

When there are no checks and balances in an organization, it is easy to abuse power. It is difficult to work with a manager who cannot look inside himself or herself and see mistakes. Some managers stress rules and conformity, leaving no gray areas where subordinates are concerned. Some show a false humility and pretend to care, but most employees can see right through this half-effort at a relationship. Others only hire "yes" people, who agree with everything that the manager says. All of these are abuses of power and indications of a poor manager.

The Power of Motivation

What motivates a person to reach a goal? In the list below, distinguish which motivators are effective in helping an individual reach goals:

*   A challenge
*   Money
*   Praise
*   Satisfaction
*   Freedom
*   Fear
*   Family
*   Insecurity
*   Competition
*   Fulfillment
*   Integrity
*   Honor
*   Reputation
*   Responsibility
*   Prestige
*   Needs
*   Love

All of the motivators listed above could prompt an employee to action. There are two general types of motivation. **Intrinsic** motivation is internal or originates within someone. Intrinsic motivation is long term and can be a lifelong goal. **Extrinsic** motivation is external and more material in nature. Generally, extrinsic motivation is more short lived and less satisfying than intrinsic motivation.

CRITICAL THINKING APPLICATION

*   Katherine knows that employees have different reasons and motivations for working. Some must work to help support their families, and others work simply because of a love for their field. How can Katherine discover her employees' motivations for working?
*   How does this knowledge benefit the office manager?
*   Can this knowledge help Katherine achieve her own goals?

Creating a Team Atmosphere

Teamwork is critical in the medical profession. In the physician's office the manager must promote an atmosphere in which the employees are willing to work together toward common goals. Low **morale** may exist in the office because of recent changes in policies or procedures, changes in staff or management, terminations of recent employees, lack of business, or any number of other reasons. The wise manager will take steps to constantly improve employee morale, including scheduling frequent meetings and keeping the employees abreast of changes and developments that affect them (Figure 20-2). Employees like to be kept "in the loop." Some managers attempt to shield employees from negative information, but this practice can cause rumors to circulate and make morale even worse.

Managers can improve morale by scheduling activities that involve the families of employees and making an obvious effort to include employees in various events. One of the most effective ways to improve employee morale is to communicate. Regular staff meetings are critical for good communication and smooth operation of the medical facility.

FIVE ESSENTIAL ELEMENTS OF A TEAM

- *Mutual accountability:* Each person on the team holds the others accountable for the success of the organization.
- *Common purpose and performance goals:* Short-term and intermediate goals must relate to the long-term goals of the group.
- *Small size:* Most successful teams have a small number of members, and fewer than 10 is optimum.
- *Common approach:* All of the team members must learn to work together toward the goal.
- *Complementary skills:* A variety of talent, skill, and ability are needed for a successful team.

From Katzenbach JR, Smith DK: Wisdom of teams: creating the high-performance organization. Boston, 1992, Harvard Business School Publishing.

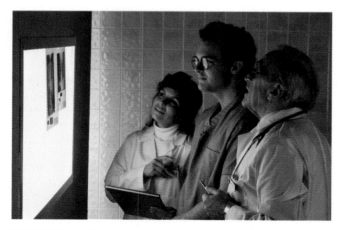

FIGURE 20-2 Communication is vital when building a team. Employees appreciate good communication with management. Sharing good and bad news openly with employees leads to fewer rumors and nervous workers.

Use of Incentives and Employee Recognition

The staff of the physician's office should feel satisfaction with the working conditions and atmosphere in the facility. The office manager plays a part in ensuring that this happens.

Incentives give the employees reason to perform over and above the level expected of them. For instance, if the staff meets or exceeds a goal that has been set, the physician may elect to provide tickets to a sports or entertainment event for the entire staff. A paid day off is always a great incentive for accomplishing a goal. Some physicians have an incentive program that is related to the collections for the office in a given period. These ideas provide a goal for the employees to work toward and an opportunity to expand their efforts as a team.

Recognition is a strong method of improving employee morale and encouraging outstanding performance. Certificates for peak performance in a given area are a great way to motivate employees. For instance, the office manager may decide to award a certificate each month to the employee who provides the best customer service. Patients could even be involved by allowing them to nominate employees for this honor. When an award is at stake, most employees will enjoy participating and striving toward the goals that have been set.

CRITICAL THINKING APPLICATION

- One of Katherine's employees, Jewel, is very sensitive about performing perfectly on the job. She is an excellent employee, but she does have a few weaknesses. However, she has received a lot of recognition for the good things she has done at work. Katherine still feels that she needs to discuss the areas where Jewel is performing weakly with her but knows that it will upset her. How might Katherine deal with this sticky situation?
- How can Katherine reassure Jewel that she is pleased with her overall performance?

Problem Employees

Occasionally, problem employees disrupt the flow of efficiency in the physician's office. Counseling these employees to find the source of their difficulties is the first step toward resolution. Many employees can be redirected to become productive staff members with a little patience and understanding on the part of the manager. However, some employees have negative attitudes that seem **impenetrable**.

The manager must never hesitate to counsel the employee who is not performing at the expected level, and this includes employees with attitude problems. A set regimen of counseling should be established. Many offices allow one verbal warning before written **reprimands** go into the employee files. If the manager does not make a habit of writing formal reprimands, there may be insufficient documentation of problems with the employee once the manager is ready to terminate him or her. Even small offenses, such as being tardy, should at least be noted in the employee's file. The manager should never be in a position that the termination of an employee cannot be justified by written documents.

Preventing Burnout

Burnout is defined as exhaustion of physical or emotional strength or motivation, usually as a result of prolonged stress or frustration. Medical professionals are particularly susceptible to burnout because of the intensity of their jobs. Even small decisions could affect the life of a patient. Therefore the office manager should take measures to help employees avoid burnout (Table 20-2).

Some of the causes of burnout include a stressful, disorganized home or work environment; poor human relations skills; a feeling of being out of control of one's life; excessive expectations from supervisors or family members; long work hours or time away from family and friends; and not being able to relax either at home or in the work environment.

Keeping the Management Relationship Professional

When people work together for an extended period, they often become **affable** and sometimes relationships develop into close friendships. This is a normal occurrence, but the office manager must be careful about becoming too close to his or her employees. When there is a friendly relationship, it is sometimes difficult to reprimand an employee when this is needed. Some employees will take advantage of a good relationship with the office manager and may begin to arrive late or call in sick more than usual. A healthy respect for each other must be maintained. The manager can have a good rapport with employees without becoming overly friendly, and this is the best policy. Some facilities have strict rules about fraternization with subordinates outside of the work facility. It is advisable to keep the relationship on a professional level at all times.

TABLE 20-2	Tips for Preventing Burnout

- Ask for help.
- Devote specific times for self-introspection or meditation.
- Understand what can be changed and what cannot be changed.
- Get some exercise.
- Organize and prioritize tasks.
- List tasks that are displeasing and delegate to others, if possible.
- Understand personal limitations.
- Take short vacations at least twice a year.
- Identify goals and try to perform only tasks that lead to reaching goals.
- Consider options, including changing jobs.
- Personalize work space with pictures and comforting items.
- Get a good understanding of a position and the stress involved before accepting it.

CRITICAL THINKING APPLICATION

- The clinical medical assistants usually celebrate payday by going to eat after work every other Friday. After about 6 months on the job, they invited Katherine to join them. Should she go with the employees? Why or why not?
- Most offices plan parties for Christmas or at other times during the year. Are these good for employee morale or should they be avoided?

Selecting the Right Staff Members

The most important asset to any medical office is the staff that cares for the patients. From the doctor to the receptionist, all play a vital role in the well-being of those who visit the office. Selecting staff members that can be molded into a cohesive team is not an easy task. Care should be taken to choose employees who have the necessary skills and the right personality for the office. Never try to select employees who are all alike. A variety of personality types work better than several similar personalities.

Understanding the Needs of the Office

The office manager should discuss with the physician the type of employee needed when an opening arises. Ask what qualities he or she desires in the person who occupies that particular position and what tasks the person will be responsible for. Once the need has been established and the duties confirmed, the office manager can begin the recruiting process.

One of the most effective methods of finding new employees is through word of mouth. Ask other office managers, physicians, or medical professionals if they are aware of a person looking for employment who has the skills needed in the office. It is a good idea to keep a file of resumes that can be accessed when an opening exists in the office. Often the physician or office manager may know of a person working in another area of the clinic or perhaps in a nearby hospital who may be interested in a job change. Be careful in approaching a person who is already employed. There is no harm in asking if a person is interested, but if the reply is negative, do not pursue the issue further.

Employment agencies can be used to find staff members, but they may charge a fee for their services. The office manager may wish to contact a local medical assistant school to secure an extern. If the extern proves to be an asset to the office, then he or she may be offered the permanent position. Newspaper ads are another option for finding employees, but many resumes may be submitted from people who are not qualified, especially when the economy is not at its best. When creating an ad for the newspaper, list the basic requirements for the position. Briefly describe the office and location, and the personality type being sought. Some offices list a few of the benefits offered to attract applicants and may disclose a salary range as well.

Reviewing Resumes and Applications

Once several resumes or applications have been submitted, the office manager should set aside quiet time to review the documents. Place them into one of three stacks—stack one should contain resumes of individuals who will be called for an interview, stack two those of possible candidates but not the strongest, and stack three those of applicants who will not be called.

During this preliminary review process, look for several items. First, be sure the documents are neatly prepared and completely legible (Figure 20-3). The person hired will probably write in the patient charts, so this is a good opportunity to ensure that his or her handwriting can be read clearly. Second, look for gaps between positions. Be sure that any lengthy time of unemployment is explained. The application should be filled out completely, and no notations of "see resume" should be included. The application provides important information and an applicant who does not fill it out in its entirety might be classified as lazy and prone to taking shortcuts. Watch for inconsistencies or oversights, including information that seems incomplete. Also look for resumes that are **targeted** toward the job opening available in the clinic. Targeted resumes are written specifically for a certain position. With today's computer capabilities, job seekers can target their resumes for each job applied for, and this strategy tells the manager that the applicant has enough interest in the job to demonstrate that he or she meets the requirements.

Once the entire stack of documents has been reviewed and separated, return to the stack of potential interviews. Careful judgment and objectivity must be used in the search for an employee who is suitable for the practice. Before interviewing any applicant, the manager needs to know several details:
- What personal qualities and abilities must the applicant have?
- What responsibilities are involved with the position?
- What is the salary range that the physician is willing to offer?
- How soon the position will be open?

Once these facts are clear, the manager should review the final resumes and applications with the following questions in mind:
- Do the applicant's appearance and personal grooming meet the standards set forth in the policy manual?
- Has the applicant been employed previously? What duties were performed?
- If previously employed, how long was the applicant in the last position? Why did the applicant leave?
- What are the applicant's skills? Do these meet the requirements for the position as set forth in the office procedure manual?
- Does the applicant seem to accept and enjoy responsibility?
- What is the applicant's formal education? Is he or she registered or certified? If not, is the applicant interested in taking the examination?
- Is the applicant a member of a professional organization? Does he or she attend meetings?

Arranging the Personal Interview

If the applicant sent a letter asking for an interview, note whether the letter was correctly typed, included essential contact information, and whether he or she also provided an attractive resume. It is amazing how many resumes do not include a contact telephone number. By telephoning the applicant, there will be an opportunity to judge his or her telephone voice. The manager may wish to prescreen applicants with the telephone call, asking several questions about the person's education and experience. Because the employee probably will speak with patients on the telephone, clarity of speech will be important. Those who perform well during the prescreening should be scheduled for an interview.

CRITICAL THINKING APPLICATION

- Katherine was impressed with Carol Limpken's resume and application, but when scheduling an interview on the telephone she noticed that Carol's grammatical abilities were not as professional as Katherine would like. Should this influence Katherine's decision to hire Carol?
- Why is speech such an important issue in the medical office?

Set a time for the personal interview when the applicant can be given undivided attention. An applicant who is being considered for employment should have an opportunity to see the office when there is a fairly normal amount of activity. The prospective employee who is interviewed in a peaceful, quiet office on the physician's day out may not be prepared for the activity on a normal working day.

Before interviewing any applicant, be thoroughly familiar with the federal, state, and local fair employment practice laws affecting hiring practices. Both men and women receive protection from on-the-job discrimination, sexual harassment, mandatory lie detector tests, and unfair discharge. Title VII of the Civil Rights Act of 1964, as amended by the Equal Employment Opportunity Act of 1972, prohibits inquiries into an applicant's race, color, sex, religion, and national origin. Inquiries regarding medical history, arrest records, or previous drug use are also illegal. Most states have laws designed to protect the rights of job applicants, and these laws may impose additional restrictions.

If an application has not been submitted, have the applicant complete it at the time of the interview. The application form can serve as a check of the applicant's penmanship and thoroughness as well as become a permanent record if the individual is hired. Tell the candidate if the form should be completed in the applicant's own handwriting, and be sure to state this on the instructions. Check to see if the applicant was **meticulous** about following instructions and filling in all the blanks. This provides the manager with an indication of the individual's capacity for following directions.

APPLICATION FOR POSITION / Medical or Dental Office
AN EQUAL OPPORTUNITY EMPLOYER

(In answering questions, use extra blank sheet if necessary)

No employee, applicant, or candidate for promotion, training or other advantage shall be discriminated against (or given preference) because of race, color, religion, sex, age, physical handicap, veteran status, or national origin.

PLEASE READ CAREFULLY AND WRITE OR PRINT ANSWERS TO ALL QUESTIONS. DO NOT TYPE.

Date of Application

A. PERSONAL INFORMATION

Name - Last	First	Middle	Social Security No.	Area Code/Phone No. ( )

Present Address: - Street   (Apt #)   City   State   Zip   How Long At This Address?:

Previous Address: - Street   City   State   Zip   Person to notify in case of Emergency or Accident - Name:

From: To: Address: Telephone:

B. EMPLOYMENT INFORMATION

For What Position Are You Applying?:   ☐ Full-Time ☐ Part-Time ☐ Either   Date Available For Employment?:   Wage/Salary Expectations:

List Hrs./Days You Prefer To Work   List Any Hrs./Days You Are Not Available: (Except for times required for religious practices or observances)   Can You Work Overtime, If Necessary? ☐ Yes ☐ No

Are You Employed Now?: ☐ Yes ☐ No   If So, May We Inquire Of Your Present Employer?: ☐ No ☐ Yes, If Yes: Name Of Employer: Phone Number: ( )

Have You Ever Been Bonded? ☐ Yes ☐ No   If Required For Position, Are You Bondable? ☐ Yes ☐ No ☐ Uncertain   Have You Applied For A Position With This Office Before? ☐ No ☐ Yes   If Yes, When?:

Referred By / Or Where Did You Learn Of This Job?:

Can You, Upon Employment, Submit Verification Of Your Legal Right To Work In The United States?: ☐ Yes ☐ No
Submit Proof That You Meet Legal Age Requirement For Employment? ☐ Yes ☐ No   Language(s) Applicant Speaks or Writes (If Use Of A Language Other Than English is Relevant To The Job For Which The Applicant Is Applying:

C. EDUCATIONAL HISTORY

Name & Address Of Schools Attended (Include Current)	Dates From	Thru	Highest Grade/Level Completed	Diploma/Degree(s) Obtained/Areas of Study
High School				
College				Degree/Major
Post Graduate				Degree/Major
Other				Course/Diploma/License/ Certificate

Specific Training, Education, Or Experiences Which Will Assist You In The Job For Which You Have Applied.

Future Educational Plans

D. SPECIAL SKILLS

CHECK BELOW THE KINDS OF WORK YOU HAVE DONE:

☐ BLOOD COUNTS	☐ DENTAL ASSISTANT	☐ MEDICAL INSURANCE FORMS	☐ RECEPTIONIST
☐ BOOKKEEPING	☐ DENTAL HYGIENIST	☐ MEDICAL TERMINOLOGY	☐ TELEPHONES
☐ COLLECTIONS	☐ FILING	☐ MEDICAL TRANSCRIPTION	☐ TYPING
☐ COMPOSING LETTERS	☐ INJECTIONS	☐ NURSING	☐ STENOGRAPHY
☐ COMPUTER INPUT	☐ INSTRUMENT STERILIZATION	☐ PHLEBOTOMY (Draw Blood)	☐ URINALYSIS
OFFICE EQUIPMENT USED: ☐ COMPUTER	☐ DICTATING EQUIPMENT	☐ POSTING	☐ X-RAY
		☐ WORD PROCESSOR	☐ OTHER:

Other Kinds Of Tasks Performed Or Skills That May Be Applicable To Position: Typing Speed   Shorthand Speed

(PLEASE COMPLETE OTHER SIDE)

FIGURE 20-3   Application for employment. Candidates for jobs in the medical office should complete applications accurately, leaving no blanks or unanswered questions. (Courtesy Bibbero Systems, Inc., Petaluma, Calif., 94954, (800) 242-2376, www.bibbero.com.)   *continued*

E. EMPLOYMENT RECORD

LIST MOST RECENT EMPLOYMENT FIRST
May We Contact Your Previous Employer(s) For A Reference? ☐ Yes ☐ No

1) Employer

Work Performed. Be Specific:

Address   Street   City   State   Zip Code

Phone Number ( )

Type of Business | Dates Mo. Yr.   Mo. Yr.
From   To

Your Position | Hourly Rate/Salary
Starting   Final

Supervisor's Name

Reason For Leaving

2) Employer

Worked Performed. Be Specific:

Address   Street   City   State   Zip Code

Phone Number ( )

Type of Business | Dates Mo. Yr.   Mo. Yr.
From   To

Your Position | Hourly Rate/Salary
Starting   Final

Supervisor's Name

Reason For Leaving

3) Employer

Worked Performed. Be Specific:

Address   Street   City   State   Zip Code

Phone Number ( )

Type of Business | Dates Mo. Yr.   Mo. Yr.
From   To

Your Position | Hourly Rate/Salary
Starting   Final

Supervisor's Name

Reason For Leaving

F. REFERENCES — FRIENDS / ACQUAINTANCES NON-RELATED

(1) Name   Address   Telephone Number (☐ Work ☐ Home) Occupation Years Acquainted

(1) Name   Address   Telephone Number (☐ Work ☐ Home) Occupation Years Acquainted

Please Feel Free To Add Any Information Which You Feel Will Help Us Consider You For Employment

READ THE FOLLOWING CAREFULLY, THEN SIGN AND DATE THE APPLICATION

"I certify that all answers given by me on this application are true, correct and complete to the best of my knowledge. I acknowledge notice that the information contained in this application is subject to check. I agree that, if hired, my continued employment may be contingent upon the accuracy of that information. If employed, I further agree to comply with Company/Office rules and regulations."

Signature: _____   Date: _____

FIGURE 20-3—Cont'd   For legend see previous page.

The Interview

First make certain that the applicant feels at ease (Figure 20-4). Shake his or her hand and ask a few social questions before starting the interview. In general, follow good manners and see that the person to be interviewed is comfortable. Most people feel some butterflies in their stomach when interviewing, but the manager will get a better idea of the person's capabilities if he or she is relaxed and able to discuss strengths and background openly with the manager.

Begin with a few open-ended questions that cannot be answered with a simple "yes" or "no," such as "What were your duties during your last position?" When interviewing a recent graduate who does not have experience, ask questions such as, "What subject did you perform well in at school?" When speaking with the candidate, make a mental note of whether he or she displays essential personal qualities, such as the ability to converse easily, the capacity to listen, and a bright smile. The applicant should be interested enough in the position to ask intelligent questions and appear interested in the office and the physician's specialty.

Avoid inquiries that involve the applicant's privacy. The questions should be related to the available position and the applicant's ability to do the job. An interview is a two-way exchange of information between the applicant and the interviewer. If the applicant appears to be one who will receive serious consideration, explain what will be expected as an employee. Office policies regarding appearance, working hours, overtime, time off, and vacations may be discussed at this stage. Salary and other fringe benefits should be discussed once the manager is ready to offer the job. If the manager fails to mention these items, the applicant may be hesitant to inquire.

Some employers request a credit check before offering employment, especially if the individual will be handling practice finances. It can safely be assumed that one who is unable to handle personal financial affairs will be a poor risk in handling office finances.

Review the job description for the position being filled. The person being interviewed must understand the required duties and responsibilities of the job. Ask if the applicant has any questions, and close the interview on a positive note. Let the candidate know when a decision will be made and what further contact the office will initiate.

During the hiring proceedings, the manager may wish to invite the prospective employee to lunch with the staff or for coffee in the more relaxed atmosphere of the employee lounge. This presents an opportunity to discover whether the applicant's personality will mesh with the atmosphere of the office. Employees appreciate being asked their opinion on those who are potential team members.

An extensive list of interview questions can be found in Chapter 25.

Follow-Up Activities

When the interview is over, take a few moments immediately to rate the applicant. Jot down some notes so that the applicant will be remembered easily when the final decisions are being made as to who will be hired. Do not trust the impressions to memory, especially if several applicants have been interviewed. Never write harmful personal statements; instead, be objective and fair. Should the potential employee ever have cause to bring the physician to court for discrimination in hiring practices, there should be no **disparaging** information written down that would reflect in a negative way on the physician or office manager.

It is always advisable to carefully check all references and to follow through on any leads for information. It is best to use the telephone in checking references, because people are sometimes less than candid in a letter; furthermore, letter writing is time consuming and a reply may never be sent. If the email address for a reference is provided, this is an excellent way to check a reference, and the printed version may be added to the applicant's file.

Prepare a checklist before placing the call. When speaking with the person called, be sure to "listen between the lines." Note the tone of the replies to the questions. Do not ask questions that might incriminate the person answering them. The following questions are effective as an introduction:

1. When did (the applicant) work for you?
2. For how long?
3. What were the duties and responsibilities?
4. Did the employee assume responsibility well?

Some employers will provide information only on the date of hire, job title, and date of termination of the employment. Respect the company's policy and do not press for further information.

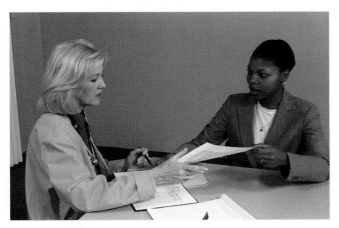

FIGURE 20-4   Put the applicant at ease. Job applicants perform at their peak when relaxed and calm.

CRITICAL THINKING APPLICATION

- While checking Carol's references, Katherine speaks to her last employer who makes the statement, "she is *not* eligible for rehire." The former employer placed strong emphasis on the word "not." All of Carol's other references were glowing. Should Katherine decide not to hire Carol on the basis of this employer's comment?
- How might Katherine find out more about the situation with the last employer?

Any person who is granted an interview should send a thank-you letter to the person who interviewed him or her. Watch the mail to see if any of the applicants perform this important follow-up task.

A second interview may be granted when the field is narrowed to two or three candidates. The physician may wish to participate in these interviews. Some offices conduct a group interview with several staff members present. Remember that these interviews become more and more stressful for the candidate, and the manager should expect some nervousness.

Making the Selection

When a decision has been reached to hire someone, it is best to bring the successful candidate back into the office to offer the position and negotiate the final details. Remember to notify all others who have interviewed for the position, so that they can look for other positions. They may have hesitated to accept other interviews, and it is unfair to keep individuals who are seeking employment hoping for a telephone call from the physician's office. Good etiquette requires dropping them a note or calling to say that the position is filled. Thank the individual for applying, and offer to keep his or her application on file. The office manager may wish to wait until the first-choice candidate has actually accepted the offer before notifying anyone else that the job has been filled. Don't expect the potential employee to answer the offer on the spot. Twenty-four hours is a reasonable time to consider the offer.

Orientation and Training–Critical Factors for Successful Employees

Recruitment does not end with the hiring. The orientation and training will help new employees to understand what is expected and to develop to their full potential (Figure 20-5). One of the most critical errors in bringing new staff members aboard is not providing them with a fair orientation and training period. The office manager should develop a checklist of the paperwork needed for newly hired staff and all of the information that should be covered with the new employee at the onset of the job.

Some managers assign a **mentor** to assist the new employee during the initial probationary period. This is a guide whom the new staff member can approach with questions and concerns (Figure 20-6). It is a good practice to use this type of "buddy" system, because the new person does not feel isolated and alone during the first few weeks on the job.

Acquaint the new employee with such aspects of the office as:
- Staff members and their names
- Physical environment and layout of the office
- Nature of the practice and specialty
- Types of patients seen in the office
- Office policies
- Long-range expectations

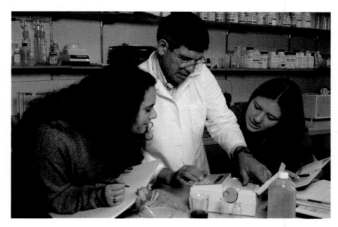

FIGURE 20-5 Training the employee well contributes greatly toward his or her success.

All new employees should be required to read the office policy and procedure manual. It is advisable for the manager to require the employee to sign a statement verifying that the manuals were read.

Be sure that all federal and state regulations are met where new employees are concerned. The Occupational Safety and Health Administration (OSHA) training must be provided to employees at risk of exposures before beginning any duties. Certain documents that verify the employee's right to work in the United States must be examined also. It is wise to insist on a fully completed personnel file before allowing the employee to work even 1 hour.

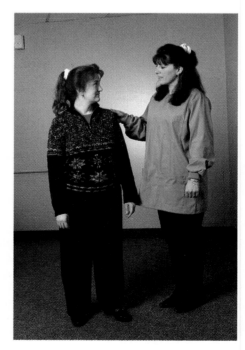

FIGURE 20-6 Mentors are valuable to the new employee. A mentor provides assistance to new employees who are learning their duties and growing accustomed to the medical office.

Job Descriptions

The job description is a tool designed to inform employees about the duties they are expected to perform. Well-written job descriptions list the essential functions of the job and reveal the chain of command that the employee should follow when questions or concerns arise. These documents provide a good guideline for employees so that they will understand exactly what is expected of them and what they are responsible for at work.

The job description should include a statement that says the employee must perform any additional duties as assigned by the supervisor. With this statement in place, the employee cannot say "that is not my job." All employees should be willing to pull together and assist with any tasks, but this statement gives added weight to assignments that are not specified in the written job description.

An effective manager understands the phrase "inspect what you expect." When duties are assigned, the manager should ensure that the tasks were completed correctly and in a timely manner. New employees should be monitored to make certain that their delegated tasks are getting done and getting done right. Without inspection, the manager cannot know that the new employee is meeting expectations. Once employees have earned a degree of trust, inspecting their work is not as necessary as in the beginning.

Staff Development Training

Continuous training and staff development are vital aspects of any medical office. Constant advancements and technological changes take place, and employees must be kept up to date on the changes. Meetings should be held at least quarterly to ensure that the staff is using the latest techniques and current regulations when dealing with issues that confront the medical facility.

Delegation of Duties

Delegating duties to subordinates allows managers to concentrate on the most critical aspects of their own jobs. Delegation also provides an opportunity for the employees to grow and learn new skills. Some managers are hesitant to assign duties to employees because they feel the tasks are too important not to complete themselves. However, this type of manager will soon be overrun with tasks and unable to complete them. Managers should place trust in employees who have earned it and allow them to prove their abilities.

Discover the strengths of individual employees and then assign them tasks that will use those strengths. If a medical assistant was hired to do administrative duties but is good with phlebotomy, encourage and allow the employee to assist with venipunctures whenever needed.

Using Performance Evaluations Effectively

A new employee should be granted a probationary period. Sixty to ninety days has been traditional, but many employers believe that 2 weeks is sufficient to determine whether the employee will be able to learn and adapt to the position.

A definite date for a performance review at the end of the probationary period should be set at the time of employment. This review should not be squeezed in between patient visits or be given a token few minutes at the end of a day. There should be ample time to relax and talk. At this time, tell the new employee how well expectations have been met and whether there are any deficiencies. Then give the employee an opportunity to ask questions. Sometimes an employee fails to perform because of never having been told what was expected. Although the probationary period does not always allow time to fully train an individual for a specific position, it is fair to assume that the potential for being a satisfactory employee can be judged at this time. Now is the time to talk out any problems and make suggestions for improvement.

The performance **appraisal** includes a judgment of both the quality and quantity of work, personal appearance, attitudes and team spirit, dependability, self-discipline, **motivation**, attendance, punctuality, and any other qualities essential to satisfactory performance of the job in question (Figure 20-7). The supervisor is responsible for ongoing performance appraisals of all employees, complimenting whenever possible and appropriate and offering helpful criticism when necessary. A formal performance appraisal at the end of the probationary period and at regular 6-month intervals thereafter, with a report to the physician employer, is helpful in the employee's salary review.

When negative information is to be relayed to the employee during a performance appraisal, sandwich the negative comment between two positive ones whenever possible. For instance, tell the employee:

"Jewel, you are a pro at greeting patients and making them feel at home. I would like to see you improve your time management skills, however, because I feel you are spending too much time with each individual patient. I must confess that they feel a part of the clinic family. Just watch the time and keep making them feel so welcome!"

Managers also may use the "feel, felt, found" approach when talking with employees about their performance. Consider the example below:

"Jewel, I feel the same way you do about the patients taking up a lot of our time. I know there are some that want to talk with us for hours, and I have felt the pressure of wanting to make them feel comfortable but having so much to do,

PERFORMANCE EVALUATION AND DEVELOPMENT PLAN
(OFFICE AND CLERICAL)

NAME: _____   DATE OF EVALUATION: _____

DATE OF HIRE: _____   DEPARTMENT: _____

JOB TITLE: _____   SUPERVISOR: _____

DATE APPOINTED THIS JOB: _____   MANAGER: _____

LAST REVIEW DATE: _____   LAST REVIEW RATING: _____

NEXT REVIEW DATE: _____   CURRENT REVIEW RATING: _____

PURPOSE

The purpose of this evaluation is to:

1. SET GOALS WITHIN SCOPE OF PRESENT JOB.
2. COMMUNICATE OPENLY ABOUT PERFORMANCE.
3. EVALUATE PAST PERFORMANCE.
4. DISCUSS FUTURE DEVELOPMENT PLANS FOR GROWTH.

INSTRUCTIONS

1. Supervisor to review form prior to completion. If specific items are not applicable they should be left blank.

2. Supervisor and employee to review job description prior to review.

3. In "COMMENTS" section supervisor may indicate which factors should be more heavily weighted in this particular evaluation.

4. Comments should be specific and job-related. All appropriate evaluation factors should be commented on to some degree.

I. POSITION OBJECTIVES AND MAJOR RESPONSIBILITIES. Summarize specific responsibilities of the job.

_____

_____

_____

II. ACCOMPLISHMENTS AND/OR IMPROVEMENTS. What specific accomplishments and/or improvements has employee made since last review with respect to set goals?

_____

_____

_____

PLEASE CONSIDER THE EMPLOYEE'S DEMONSTRATED PERFORMANCE AND MARK THE CIRCLE WHICH MOST CLOSELY DESCRIBES THAT PERFORMANCE.

4 - Performance consistently far exceeds expectations and requirements.
3 - Performance consistently exceeds normal expectations and job requirements.
2 - Performance consistently meets expectations and job requirements
1 - Performance usually meets expectations and minimum job requirements.
0 - Performance does not meet job requirements.

– CONTINUED, NEXT PAGE –

FORM # 72-119 © 1987 BIBBERO SYSTEMS, INC. PETALUMA, CA

TO REORDER CALL TOLL FREE:
800-BIBBERO /(800 242-2376) OR
FAX: (800) 242-9330 MFG IN U.S.A.

FIGURE 20-7   Performance evaluation and development plan. Performance evaluations should be considered tools that will help employees reach their personal goals and the goals of the organization. (Courtesy Bibbero Systems, Inc., Petaluma, Calif., 94954, (800) 242-2376, www.bibbero.com.)

7. DEPENDABILITY: CONSIDER ATTENDANCE, PUNCTUALITY, IDLE TIME AND RELIANCE WHICH CAN BE PLACED ON EMPLOYEE TO PERSEVERE AND CARRY THROUGH TO COMPLETION ALL ASSIGNED TASKS

○ 0   ○ 1   ○ 2   ○ 3   ○ 4

_____
_____
_____

8. COMPLIANCE WITH COMPANY POLICIES: DOES THE EMPLOYEE COMPLY WITH RULES AND REGULATIONS WHICH APPLY TO SAFETY, FAIR EMPLOYMENT PRACTICES AND GENERAL ADMINISTRATIVE PROCEDURE.

○ 0   ○ 1   ○ 2   ○ 3   ○ 4

_____
_____
_____

9. SPECIFIC PERFORMANCE

	1	2	3	4	COMMENTS
A. Ability to handle scheduling:					
B. Willingness to work OT when necessary:					
C. Handling of calls and follow-up:					
D. Maintenance of equipment:					
E. Ability to handle patient complaints:					
F. Tact in dealing with patients:					
G. Speed (in specific technical procedures):					
H. Secretarial accuracy:					
I. Professional terminology:					
J. Assisting procedures:					
K. Laboratory techniques:					
L. X-ray techniques:					
M. Physical therapy:					
N. Collections:					
O. Medical Insurance:					
P. Bookkeeping:					

10. PERSONAL

	1	2	3	4	COMMENTS
A. Grooming:					
B. Professional conduct:					
C. Energy, enthusiasm:					
D. Ability to handle stress:					

ADDITIONAL COMMENTS: _____
_____
_____
_____
_____

FORM # 72-119 © 1987 BIBBERO SYSTEMS, INC. PETALUMA, CA

FIGURE 20-7—Cont'd   For legend see previous page.

too. I have found that if I explain that I have a meeting or another patient to assist, they are very understanding and not offended. Perhaps you can try that approach, too."

Peer Evaluations

Some innovative companies use peer evaluations of employees to get a different view of the work performed by a worker. Asking co-workers to assist in the evaluation process can promote teamwork and cooperation. The rare employee will offer a poor evaluation because of a personal problem with another staff member but, for the most part, employees will provide fair, unbiased evaluations, knowing that they will also be evaluated when it is their turn.

360° evaluations are excellent tools for evaluating any employees, including managers. This evaluation usually consists of a questionnaire that is given to those who work closely with the employee, and they provide input regarding the performance of the person being evaluated.

Poor Evaluations Made Easier

No supervisor enjoys giving an evaluation that is not a positive one. It is difficult to know where to begin when the employee has not performed as expected or hoped. Perhaps the best way to open the conversation is to say, "This is not going to be a positive evaluation, and we have several items to discuss." The manager should have good documentation of the problems that led to the poor evaluation. If so, these can be reviewed with the employee with specific times, dates, and descriptions of incidents. If the manager does not document these issues, the conversation can become an argument and grow quite heated. Firm dates and times leave little room for defense and place the manager on the offensive.

CRITICAL THINKING APPLICATION

- While giving an evaluation on a particularly poor employee who Katherine plans to terminate, the employee begins screaming and accusing Katherine of discrimination and harassment. How should Katherine handle this situation?
- What are Katherine's options if the employee does not stop the inappropriate behavior?

Terminating Employees

The necessity for dismissing an employee is unpleasant at best, but if the ground rules are decided on in advance, written into the policy manual, and explained to all employees, the problem is partially solved. The policies must be applied equally and impartially to all. The final decision for dismissal probably will be made by the physician but may be based on the recommendation of the office manager or supervisor. The person who does the hiring should do the firing.

The probationary employee who does not prove satisfactory should be dismissed at the end of the probationary period, with tact and a full explanation of the reasons for dismissal. In all fairness, an individual should be told why the employment is ended and not be given weak excuses or untruths that do not help to correct deficiencies. If the manager is not straightforward in giving the reason for dismissal, the employee will not have the opportunity to grow and improve his or her performance.

An employee who has been in service for some time and is offering unsatisfactory performance should be warned and given an explanation of the specific improvements expected (Figure 20-8). If a second chance does not produce improvement in performance or attitude, then dismissal must follow. It should be done privately, with tact and consideration.

Most practice consultants believe that firing should come close to the end of the day, after all other employees have left, and that the break should be clean and immediate. If the office policy provides for 2 weeks' notice, the physician may wish to offer 2 weeks' pay, unless the circumstances that led to the dismissal were extremely **blatant**. A dismissed employee should never be allowed to train or influence a replacement.

The exit meeting should be planned just as carefully as the employment interview. Be honest with the employee. Discuss the employee's assets as well as liabilities and give the reasons for the termination. There is no need to dwell on the employee's deficiencies. These should have been thoroughly discussed at the warning interview, and the employee need only be told that the necessary improvements have not been made. Do listen to the employee's feedback, unless it becomes abusive. This may reveal some important administrative problems that need correction.

After dismissing an employee, do not leave that person in the office unattended. Request and get the office keys and any other equipment in the employee's possession before the dismissed employee leaves the building. Most states have strict payday laws that will not allow holding the final paycheck for any reason. Do not offer to give the employee a good reference unless it can be done sincerely.

Certain breaches of conduct, such as **embezzlement** and **insubordination** or violation of patient confidentiality, are grounds for immediate dismissal without warning.

Occasionally, an employee voluntarily terminates a job without giving a valid reason. The physician or office manager may wish to follow up with a letter to the former employee to seek out any problem that may have prompted the resignation.

CRITICAL THINKING APPLICATION

- Katherine has two employees who have never seemed to get along. One of the employees has a history of being vindictive and manipulative, but never in an obvious enough way for Katherine to have sufficient proof to reprimand her in writing. One day, this employee comes to Katherine's office to report that she saw the other employee, who has an exemplary record, taking drugs from the supply cabinet. How does Katherine react to this situation?
- What steps should Katherine take from here?

TERMINATION / REHIRE EVALUATION FORM

Employee Name_____ Social Security No. _____

Department _____ Title _____

Termination Date _____

Reason for Termination: _____Resigned _____Laid Off_____Retired

Evaluation of Job Performance	Excellent	Very Good	Average	Poor	Unacceptable
Quality (accuracy, etc.)	☐	☐	☐	☐	☐
Quantity (productivity, consistency, etc.)	☐	☐	☐	☐	☐
Knowledge of Duties	☐	☐	☐	☐	☐
Reliability (absenteeism)	☐	☐	☐	☐	☐
Punctuality	☐	☐	☐	☐	☐
Ability to Cooperate with Co-workers	☐	☐	☐	☐	☐
Relationship with Patients	☐	☐	☐	☐	☐
Overall Attitude (willingness and commitment)	☐	☐	☐	☐	☐
Initiative	☐	☐	☐	☐	☐
Judgment	☐	☐	☐	☐	☐

Recommendation for Rehiring: _____

_____

_____

Comments:_____

_____

_____

_____

_____

_____

_____

_____

_____ Date _____

Supervisor's Signature

FORM # 72-123   PERSONNEL RECORDS ORGANIZING SYSTEMS • © 1987 BIBBERO SYSTEMS, INC. • PETALUMA, CA.
TO REORDER CALL TOLL FREE: (800) BIBBERO (800-242-2376) OR FAX (800) 242-9330   MFG IN U.S.A.

FIGURE 20-8   Termination form. Document the reasons for terminating employees and be sure that there is supporting documentation showing warnings and previous counseling efforts. (Courtesy Bibbero Systems, Inc., Petaluma, Calif., 94954, (800) 242-2376, www.bibbero.com.)

Fair Salaries and Raises

Medical office managers should recruit employees who will remain with the office for a long period of time. There are always situations when a part-time worker returns to college, or someone working during the summer months goes back to school. However, good employee **retention** is a goal to work toward.

In order to keep good employees, they must be paid a fair salary and will expect regular raises if they are performing as expected. The office manager can find information about salary comparisons on the Internet. Check the job duties and descriptions found on the web, and see if the salary that the medical facility is offering is comparable to other salaries for similar jobs in the area.

Merit raises are increases based on an employee's commendable performance. Cost of living increases are given when earned, usually after specific periods or annually, and are based on national statistics and trends. An employee who is being promoted may be awarded a salary increase, also. When the office pays a fair salary for the work being done, the physician will retain happy employees.

Staff Meetings

There must be some formal mechanism for keeping the office manager and other key employees current on the daily business affairs of the practice. One of the most common complaints from office personnel is that of being unable to discuss problems with the physician. The solution to this problem may be to hold regular staff meetings, which may be scheduled as frequently as weekly but should be no less often than quarterly (Figure 20-9). Some of the best ideas on improvement come from the office staff, and expressing ideas should be encouraged.

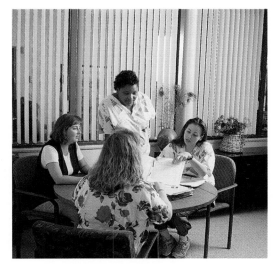

FIGURE 20-9 Periodic staff meetings are important tools for improving communication and resolving problems.

The simplest technique is to set aside a specific time for regular meetings at an hour when the most people can attend with the least disruption (Procedure 20-2). The meetings need not be long or overly formal, but to be effective they must be planned and organized. There must be a leader, and a secretary should be appointed to take notes. The effectiveness of the leader, a person who can balance firmness with fairness, is an important aspect of the meeting. This is usually either the physician or the office manager/supervisor. All members of the staff should be encouraged to submit ideas for discussion.

Draw up a simple **agenda** listing the issues to be discussed and prepare any supporting data needed for the meeting. There are many kinds of staff meetings. They may be purely informational, problem solving, or brainstorming. They may be work sessions for updating manuals, training seminars, or whatever is necessary to that individual practice. Or, meetings may be scheduled to discuss new ideas and any changes in office procedures. Some meetings are held simply to resolve specific problems. The staff meeting must not be allowed to deteriorate into a gripe session. Individual complaints should be handled privately.

The meeting must have a set agenda, with time for topics that need discussion on a regular basis, as well as time to handle any current problems. The agenda might be similar to that of any business meeting:

1. Reading of the last meeting's minutes
2. Discussion of any unfinished business
3. Discussion of any problems in the clinical area
4. Discussion of any problems in the administrative area
5. Discussion of any problems in common areas
6. Adjournment

Some physicians like to combine the staff meeting with a breakfast or lunch. The time or place is not important as long as it is neutral and meets the needs of the practice. Meetings should be conducted regularly, democratically, and without interruption. There must be follow-up to the items discussed; otherwise, the only result will be frustration and a reluctance to discuss problems at future meetings.

Seeing the Whole Picture

The office manager must keep a bird's-eye view on the office operations. He or she must look at the whole picture when difficulties arise. Remember, there are always two sides to every story, and there is usually truth intermingled with falsity. Do not form the habit of taking every word that an employee says as being 100% accurate. This is not meant to suggest that all employees are not truthful, but to encourage the office manager to look at all sides before making critical decisions.

See issues from the employees' point of view. Try to understand their perspective when dealing with everyday situations in the medical facility. Do not become closed-minded as a manager, unable to grasp what the employees see as important.

Arranging a Group Meeting

GOAL: To plan and execute a productive meeting that will result in achieved goals.

EQUIPMENT AND SUPPLIES

- Meeting room
- Agenda
- Visual aids and equipment
- Handouts
- Stopwatch or clock
- Computer or word processor
- Paper
- List of items for the agenda

PROCEDURAL STEPS

1 Determine the purpose of the meeting and draft a list of the items to be discussed. Include the desired results of the meeting.

Purpose: To keep the focus on the issues at hand and make the meeting a productive one.

2 Determine where the meeting will be held, the time and date of the meeting, and the individuals who should attend.

Purpose: To have the demographic information about the meeting on hand prior to posting a notice. Only necessary staff members should attend, so that those not directly involved in the issues to be discussed will be allowed to continue their regular duties.

3 Send a memo, email, or letter to the individuals who should attend the meeting at least 10 days in advance, if possible. Send a copy to any supervisors who should be kept informed about the issues to be raised in the meeting.

Purpose: To allow for rescheduling if the key personnel cannot attend on the originally planned time and date. To keep managers informed of important details in areas for which they are ultimately responsible.

4 Be sure that the notice includes the following information:
- Date
- Time
- Place
- Directions, if not in a common meeting room or if away from the office
- Speakers and/or meeting topics
- Cost and registration information, if applicable

- List of items individuals should bring to the meeting

Purpose: To fully inform those who should attend the meeting of the demographic information and their responsibilities.

5 Finalize the list of items to discuss and place them in priority order.

Purpose: To keep the focus of the meeting on the issues at hand and to avoid discussion of nonrelated items. To make certain that the time spent in the meeting is productive for all involved.

6 Delegate any tasks that others can accomplish and follow-up to be sure that they fulfill their duties prior to the meeting.

Purpose: To ensure that all needed information and items are available for the meeting.

7 Assign a staff member the task of keeping notes and keeping time during the meeting.

Purpose: To have notes as to what happened so that a permanent record of what was discussed and the decisions that were made can be written after the meeting.

8 Make a list of all items that need to be taken to the meeting, including equipment such as microphones, projectors, screens, computers, disks containing presentations, etc.

Purpose: To be fully prepared and have all needed items in place during the meeting.

9 Compile the final agenda for the meeting.

10 On the meeting day, transport all items needed to the meeting room. Begin and end the meeting on time. Stay on track and follow the agenda.

Purpose: Following the plan and being considerate of the time that staff members devote to meetings will promote a positive attitude for meetings and will encourage group participation.

11 Follow-up whenever necessary on items discussed in the meetings. Distribute a synopsis of the meeting to all of the individuals who attended and keep a copy in a binder or folder.

Purpose: To have a permanent record of the meeting and items discussed and decided.

Other Office Manager Responsibilities

Patient Information Folder

Only a very small percentage of practices have a booklet that explains the information basic to the operational and service aspects of the practice. Yet, the physician and staff can easily compile a patient information folder cooperatively during a staff meeting. Experience has shown that if such a folder is given to every new patient, the number of incoming telephone calls can be reduced by an average of 20% to 30%. It also can reduce misunderstandings and forgotten instructions. The folder must of necessity be tailored to the specific practice.

The patient information folder should be an introduction to the practice and, if possible, mailed to a new patient before the first visit. A supply also may be left with referring physicians' offices to be given to patients coming to your office. It should be designed to fit easily into a No. 10 business envelope.

The cover should show the name of the practice, its location, and the practice logo, if there is one. Consider using a photo of the medical building for easy identification by the new patient, and a map to the office.

A statement of philosophy frequently is included in the introduction, followed by a description of the practice, such as in the example below:

"The doctors and staff would like to welcome you to our office. We work as a team with the goal of providing prompt and thorough care of your problems. We are always working to improve our care and service in any way possible. Our practice is limited exclusively to the musculoskeletal system and its disorders. Therefore it is important for each patient to have a primary care physician such as a pediatrician, family physician, or internist to oversee the primary medical care for the entire patient. Our role is most effective as a consultant to your primary care physician."

Describe the office policy regarding appointments and cancellations, telephone calls, and the function of the answering service. If a separate business telephone line is available, be sure to include this information, as in the following example:

"This office has two receptionists available to answer telephone calls during regular office hours. The office is very busy, and occasionally you will be asked to hold for a brief period. Please be patient with this. If you wish to speak to a doctor, your call usually will be returned during the next available break period or at the end of the office day. We receive many calls during the day, and it is unfair to the patients who have scheduled appointments to continually interrupt the doctor for telephone calls. Therefore the receptionist usually will take a message, and your call will be returned as soon as possible. Please inform the receptionist if your problem is urgent and she will let the doctor know this."

Describe any **ancillary** or laboratory services provided, how test results are reported, and your policy on prescription renewals. Patients need to know the provisions for emergency procedures: What hospitals does the practice use regularly? What is the night and weekend coverage? Hospitalization procedures and postoperative care and follow-up may also be included:

"One of the doctors in the group is always on call for emergency situations. You may reach him by calling our office telephone number (714) 555-2323, and the answering service will put you in touch with the doctor on call at that time. Our doctors are on staff at St. Joseph Hospital (714) 555-3333 and, for children, Children's Hospital of Orange County (714) 555-4444. In case of emergency, call 911."

List all physicians in the practice; state their educational backgrounds, training, and board certifications; and define their specialties. List the names of key clinical and administrative staff members, such as registered nurses and nurse practitioners, medical assistants, the office manager, and the business manager. Provide the practice address, a map of how to get there, and information about the parking facilities.

Do not just stack these folders in the reception room for patients to pick up. Have the receptionist write the patient's name on the folder and hand it to the patient when he or she registers for the first appointment and suggest that the patient keep it for future reference.

Financial Policy Folder

A separate small folder covering the financial policies of the office can eliminate many questions and possible misunderstandings. Tailor the financial policy folder to the specific practice. Keep it small enough to fit into the billing envelope and send it out with the first monthly statement. If the practice sends out a welcome package before the patient's first visit, include the financial policy folder. Otherwise, present one at the first visit.

Spell out policies regarding billing and collection procedures, and make it clear that patients are responsible for the uninsured portion of the fees. If payment is expected at the time of service, put this in the folder. Keep the language simple and straightforward so that the message is clear:

"We ask that our services be paid for at the time they are rendered. You will be provided with an encounter form so that you may bill your insurance company and be reimbursed for services paid at the time of your visit. Simply attach the encounter form to your insurance form and mail it to the insurance company. The appropriate diagnoses and charges will be on the encounter form. There is usually a greater charge for the initial visit, because this involves more time than follow-up visits. If you are sent to an outside office for laboratory testing or special x-rays, you will be billed separately from that office. We will be available to help if special circumstances arise involving difficulty with forms or receiving reimbursement. We will bill your insurance if you have a special situation such as surgery, prepaid health plans, Medicaid, CCS, or Senior Savers. We will complete disability papers as promptly as possible. However, you must obtain the necessary forms from your employer or the disability office."

The financial policy folder should also clearly state that the ultimate responsibility for payment lies with the patient.

Patient Instruction Sheets

In most medical offices there are patient procedures that occur over and over again. Instead of attempting to instruct a patient orally each time, why not develop clearly stated instruction sheets that can be reviewed with the patient and then give the patient the written instructions to take home? The following are suggestions for patient instruction sheets:

- Preparation for x-ray or laboratory tests
- Preoperative and postoperative instructions
- Diet sheets
- Performing an enema
- Dressing a wound
- Taking medications
- Using a cane, crutches, walker, or wheelchair
- Care of casts
- Exercise therapy

Moving a Practice

The thought of moving into a shiny new spacious office can be exciting. However, unless the move is planned in advance, moving day and the weeks that follow can be a nightmare.

Planning the New Quarters. Do some careful measuring to see how the furniture and equipment that will be moved will fit into the new quarters. If possible, draw the rooms to scale and show where each item is to be placed by the mover. Include the location of available electrical outlets in the floor plan. If new furniture, carpets, or equipment is needed, try to have them in place before moving day. Do not expect to have the new carpet installed the day of the move.

Establishing a Moving Date. Decide what day the move will take place and whether the office will close for 1 day or several. Select a mover and confirm the date. Patients must be notified of the move. As soon as the moving date is established, post a notice in the office and draw the patients' attention to it. Send announcement cards to the active patients. Many physicians place a notice in the local newspapers.

Notifying Utilities and Mailers. At least 60 days in advance of the move, start a change-of-address notification campaign. Notify publishers of journals and suppliers of catalogs. Cards for changes of address are available from the post office. Six weeks' notice generally is required on subscriptions, and postage due on forwarded journals can be very expensive. Notify the telephone company and utility companies well in advance so that there will be no break in service. File a change of address card with the local post office. Order stationery and business cards with the new address.

Packing. The moving company will supply packing cartons. Have each employee be responsible for packing and labeling the items from his or her own work area. Tag each carton with a number and keep a master list of what is in each numbered carton. This will help to find items that are needed. Also, if a carton should be lost or mislaid, a record of what was in it will be available. If time allows, just before moving is a good time to cull material from the files and discard old journals, supply catalogs, and any obsolete supplies or equipment.

Moving Day Strategy. Prepare a written outline of the moving day strategy, indicating each person's responsibility, and give each member of the office staff a copy. It

may be wise to work in shifts to avoid confusion, but have one person stationed at the new address to direct the movers when they arrive.

Follow-Up. After the move, be sure to mention the new address when patients call for appointments. This often is neglected, especially after a few months have passed, and is very upsetting to the patient who tries to check in at the former address.

Closing a Practice

A medical practice may be closed because of retirement, death, a change in geographic location, or a change in profession. If the closing is unexpected, as in the case of sudden death of the physician, much of the burden falls on the staff. If the closing is voluntary and planned for, the physician may wish to consult an attorney or the local medical society for guidelines. The following information is useful in either event.

Advance Notice to Patients. The physician who anticipates retirement can begin cutting back the practice months in advance. Patients can be notified as they come in that the practice will be closing on a specified date and asked to begin arrangements for care from another physician. The physician also can ask that patients pay at the time of service, to minimize accounts receivable at the time of retirement.

Avoiding Abandonment Charge. To avoid a charge of abandonment, the physician should notify active patients by letter that the practice is being discontinued. The letter should be sent out at least 3 months in advance, if possible. If a patient has been discharged or has not been given care by the physician for at least 6 years, there is no obligation to send the notice.

Public Announcement. About 1 month after the physician begins telling patients of the closing, an announcement should be placed in a local newspaper, giving the closing date of the office, explaining any arrangements made for continuing care, and thanking patients for their support over the years.

Other Notices. Hospital affiliations should be informed early, particularly if the physician will be leaving the community. If the office space is being rented, be sure to notify the landlord in observance of the rental contract if there is one. Insurance carriers must be advised of the change. The state medical licensure board should be contacted. If the practice is incorporated, an attorney should be consulted about dissolving the corporation.

Patient Transfer and Patient Records. If another physician is taking over the practice, tell the patients about the new physician. However, be sure to explain that a patient's records will be transferred to the physician of his or her choice and that the request for transfer of records must be in writing. For convenience, the physician can have a form available that needs only the patient's signature.

Although the records belong to the physician, they can be transferred legally to another physician only with the consent of the patient. Any records not transferred should be stored, either in bulk or on microfilm or disk, until the statutes of limitations for malpractice and abandonment have run out.

Financial Concerns When a Practice Closes. Income tax returns and supporting documents should be kept for at least 3 years after the tax return was filed. Appoint someone to take care of any remaining outstanding accounts receivable.

Disposition of Controlled Substances. Check with the Drug Enforcement Administration (DEA) for current regulations on disposal of controlled substances and the physician's certificate of registration. Do not simply toss them out. The certificate will have to be sent to the DEA for cancellation, and then it will be returned. It may be necessary to produce an inventory of all controlled substances on hand when the practice is terminated, along with duplicate copies of the official order forms that were used to obtain them. Return any unused forms to the DEA. Do not use leftover prescription blanks for note pads. Burn or shred them to avoid misuse.

Professional Liability Insurance. The physician who is discontinuing active medical practice can safely drop the professional liability insurance. However, do not destroy any of the previous policies. Most professional liability claims are covered by the policy that was in effect at the time the alleged act of negligence took place. The suit may be filed many years later, and it is important that the old policy be available.

Furnishings and Equipment. Unfortunately, used office furniture and equipment do not bring much in the marketplace. If another physician is taking over the practice, the value of the furnishings and equipment can be negotiated. Many physicians donate their libraries to the local hospital and declare the gift as an income tax deduction. This is an item to check with the accountant.

A physician may reward loyal employees with severance pay. On average, this equals at least 1 month's salary plus prorated compensation for any unused vacation time. A letter of reference usually is offered.

There are many details to take care of in closing a medical practice. Contact the local medical society for further guidance.

Closing Comments

Successful office managers care about their employees and the vision for the office. They must be strong promoters of the office mission statement. The areas of authority and responsibility must be clearly defined to avoid management problems. A solid office policy and procedure manual will assist the office manager in running an efficient office.

Leadership is an important quality for any manager, and the medical office manager is no exception. The manager should develop good leadership skills, be fair and open-minded, and treat employees and patients as he or she would want to be treated. These actions will help to ensure a pleasant, productive working environment.

Patient Education

Educate patients about the policies and procedures in the office by providing patient information folders or brochures. When these documents are prepared and given to the patients formally, the patient is better informed and fewer calls will come to the office.

Legal and Ethical Issues

Office managers must stay abreast of current employment laws and regulations for all of the different agencies that govern the medical office. Joining an office manager's association will help the manager keep the office up to date and in compliance. Periodic checks on the websites of various organizations, such as OSHA, will help the manager to stay aware of the most recent changes in policies and rules.

Documentation is a critical aspect of the office manager's duties. The manager should keep detailed notes on the performance of employees and always discuss poor performance with employees. Never allow bad habits to go unmentioned. To the extent that it is possible, treat employees in a similar fashion and extend fairness to all.

SUMMARY OF SCENARIO

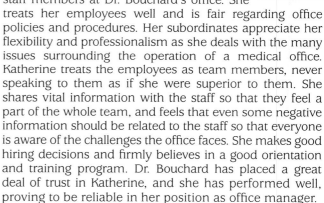

Katherine has made an impact on all of the staff members at Dr. Bouchard's office. She treats her employees well and is fair regarding office policies and procedures. Her subordinates appreciate her flexibility and professionalism as she deals with the many issues surrounding the operation of a medical office. Katherine treats the employees as team members, never speaking to them as if she were superior to them. She shares vital information with the staff so that they feel a part of the whole team, and feels that even some negative information should be related to the staff so that everyone is aware of the challenges the office faces. She makes good hiring decisions and firmly believes in a good orientation and training program. Dr. Bouchard has placed a great deal of trust in Katherine, and she has performed well, proving to be reliable in her position as office manager.

SUMMARY OF LEARNING OBJECTIVES

■ Management is an important aspect of running a professional medical office. The physician counts on the office manager to run the business aspects of the office so that he or she can focus efforts on good patient care. A high degree of trust is placed with the office manager.

■ A good office manager is fair and flexible. Good communications skills are necessary, as well as attention to details. The manager should care about the employees and have a sense of fairness. The ability to remain calm in a crisis is important, as is the use of good judgment and ability to organize tasks.

- Charismatic leaders inspire allegiance and dedication while encouraging individuals to overcome great obstacles. The transactional leader is structured and organized, hardworking, and a planner. The transformational leader is excellent during times of transition and is effective at building relationships.

- Power can be both a positive and negative entity. Power should not be used in a manipulative or coercive manner. Expert power is based upon a high degree of knowledge about a certain subject. Using rewards is one form of invoking power, and legitimate power is that of position or status. Referent power is granted from subordinates to those who lead by example.

- Employees are motivated by various factors, including money, praise, insecurity, honor, prestige, needs, love, fear, satisfaction, and many others. The effective manager attempts to discover what motivates employees to do a good job.

- Intrinsic motivation comes from within the employee. Extrinsic motivation has an outside source.

- Asking for help, first and foremost, can prevent burnout. Managers often take on too many duties and do not delegate as much as they should. Exercise and rest help prevent burnout, as well as understanding one's own personal limitations. Focused goals are important and help keep the manager working toward the most critical tasks.

- Resumes and applications should be reviewed for accuracy and completeness. Gaps in employment dates should be explained fully and the office manager should verify any references given. Documents should be legible and the information contained should be consistent without oversights.

- The telephone voice of an applicant is important because most employees have occasion to answer the telephone while at work. The employee's voice should be clear and easily understandable. Good grammar skills must be used to reflect a professional image.

- After interviewing a prospective candidate, the office manager should verify the facts on the resume and application and check several references. A comparison should be made between the candidates and the top two or three chosen for a possible second interview. It is wise to involve other staff members when choosing new employees for the office.

- Mentors assist new employees by offering information regarding policies and procedures. The mentor can be a helpful advocate that the new employee can approach when there are questions about any aspect of the medical office.

- Staff meetings may be held to relay information, solve a problem, or brainstorm ideas. Some meetings are designed as work sessions, while others may be scheduled to discuss new policies or changes in procedures.

INTERNET CONNECTIONS

- 360° Evaluation
  www.shine-360-degree-feedback.co.uk
- Baudville Recognition—Putting Applause on Paper
  www.baudville.com
- Panoramic Feedback
  www.panoramicfeedback.com
- Professional Association of Healthcare Office Management
  www.pahcom.com
- Salary Comparison and Calculator
  www.salary-comparison-and-calculator.com
- Successories
  www.successories.com
- Who Moved My Cheese?
  www.whomovedmycheese.com

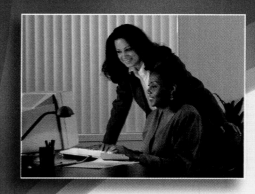

CHAPTER 21

Scenario

Monica Ray is a medical assistant who is also pursuing a bachelor's degree in marketing. She has worked for Drs. Julie and Robert Todd for 2 years and, based upon her interest in marketing, the physicians have agreed to allow her to develop some new strategies for their obstetrics and gynecology office.

Monica is highly computer literate and can design web pages. She plans to incorporate several ideas she has seen on other physicians' websites, including a method of online scheduling. Monica is quite creative and she is excited about the challenge of providing such a service to the patients of the clinic.

Monica knows that planning is involved in any project, such as the facility's Internet presence. She plans to speak to every employee of the office to get input as to the design and content of the site. Patients will be able to provide her with additional suggestions as to what they would like to see, as well.

This new development for the office is just one way that Monica hopes to incorporate more formal customer service techniques. She plans to share the information she is learning in the classroom with the physicians and staff at the clinic. Monica and the doctors are fortunate that the staff is enthusiastic about these plans and eager to try new methods of customer service. The physicians plan to set specific goals with the help of the employees and to devise a reward system for reaching them. An exciting few months are ahead for this innovative group of medical professionals!

Medical Practice Marketing and Customer Service

Vocabulary

marketing The process or technique of promoting, selling, and distributing a product or service.
objectives Something toward which effort is directed; an aim, goal, or end of action.
outreach The process of using marketing and education strategies to reach and involve diverse audiences through the use of key messages and effective programs.
prosthetic The surgical or dental specialty concerned with the design, construction, and fitting of prostheses, which are artificial devices that replace missing parts of the body.
tangible Capable of being appraised at an actual or approximate value; capable of being precisely identified or realized by the mind.
target market A specific group of individuals to whom the marketing plan is focused.

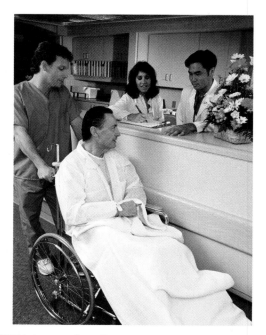

FIGURE 21-1 Friendly staff members are the best marketing tools. A smile is an excellent way to make patients feel welcome in the medical facility.

Each medical office should have a mission statement that defines the reason for the existence of the office. The physician's philosophy of medicine and reasons for pursing medicine as a career will greatly influence the mission statement. With this statement in place, the staff must develop goals that will assist them in meeting the mission. The goals can be met through a **marketing** and **outreach** plan for the practice and by providing excellent customer service to patients and visitors of the facility.

Developing Marketing Strategies

If a business is to grow, marketing strategies must be developed. A marketing strategy is designed to promote the services offered by the organization and encourage new business. Three steps are generally followed when preparing to implement or change medical marketing strategies:

- Evaluate what is being done now to increase patient flow.
- Decide what objectives are important and how meeting these objectives will be measured.
- Develop a plan with various means of marketing the practice and a specific methodology for implementing each phase.

CRITICAL THINKING APPLICATION

- Monica knows that the office has never attempted any formal marketing in the past. Because no one at her office is familiar with this task, who might she contact for advice and assistance?
- Even though her fellow staff members are not familiar with marketing, could they provide workable ideas?
- What are some ideas for marketing a medical practice?

Knowing the Target Market

During the strategic phase of developing a marketing plan, the physician and office manager must identify the **target market** for the services provided by the clinic. The target market is the group or groups of individuals that the office wishes to reach. Reaching the target market means that the specific groups are made aware of the clinic and what it has to offer. With managed care restrictions and regulations, competition for patients has become keen between physicians, and a facility that does not pursue growth runs a great risk of not surviving.

Several questions must be answered when discussing the target market. Consider the following:

- What specific outcomes do we hope to accomplish?
- What are the needs and desires of our target market?
- What are the characteristics of a typical member of the target market?
- How can the target market be reached in the most cost-effective ways?

Staff meetings are excellent times to brainstorm about reaching target markets. The staff can relate the needs of the patients who are currently coming to the medical office. If patients have made suggestions, they should be discussed and weighed as to which would most benefit the patient population of the facility (Figure 21-1).

CRITICAL THINKING APPLICATION

- What community resources could Monica seek as she is determining the target market of the practice?
- What information does she need to begin her search?

Suggestion boxes are a great way to solicit patient input. Ask patients for ideas as to how the clinic could operate in a smoother fashion and what additional services they would like to have. Check the suggestion box frequently. If the patient leaves his or her name on the suggestion form, it is a good customer service move to reward the patient for the suggestion. Mail the patient a coupon for a free lunch at a local restaurant or a free car wash at a local detailing shop. Involving other businesses in marketing efforts helps both attract new customers.

The "Four P's." The "four p's" of marketing include *p*roduct, *p*lacement, *p*rice, and *p*romotion. A physician's office offers medical services as a product. Some offices have **tangible** retail products that they also offer, such as vitamins or **prosthetic** devices. Placement involves the actual location of the medical office. It may be located in an urban area close to large neighborhoods of young professionals, or in a rural area with a few people living several miles apart. Placement can refer also to the setup of the office, the specific suite in a shopping strip where the office is located, or even the placement of retail objects on a shelf. Placement can greatly influence the traffic to the facility.

Price is simply the amount of money charged for goods and services provided. Promotion refers to the methods used to get the product or services to the consumers, or patients, in the case of the medical office.

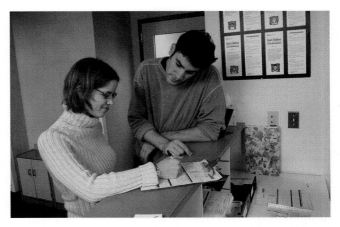

FIGURE 21-2   Offer services that are important in the geographical area of the office. College students may need to see a physician for minor illnesses, and they will appreciate offices that provide short office visits at a reasonable fee.

CRITICAL THINKING APPLICATION

- How can Monica investigate the charges for similar procedures at other clinics in her area?
- Why is this information important to Monica?

Deciding What Services to Offer. Once the physician and office manager have identified the target market, decisions can be made regarding what services should be offered to the patients. For instance, suppose the office is situated in a neighborhood of young families. There is a strong possibility that both parents work outside the home, so evening hours would be beneficial to these patients. The physician may decide to extend office hours to 8:00 PM twice a week and to open from 9:00 to 12:00 noon on Saturdays. If there are several schools in the area, particularly junior high and high schools, the physician may wish to offer a special price on sports physicals during the fall. Schools often require physicals, and if the physician offers them at a reasonable price, the entire family may decide to seek medical care from the physician.

If the office is located in a college town, the physician may wish to offer a special student rate for short office visits (Figure 21-2). If there are a number of senior citizens in the area, a senior citizen discount might be appropriate. Input from patients and staff members will be valuable in deciding what services to offer in the medical facility.

Developing a Plan

There are several specific planning steps that the facility may use for events, marketing strategies, and any number

of other ideas that the physician would like to implement. They are:

1. Assessment
2. Research
3. Plan
4. Execution
5. Evaluation

Assessment is the phase of planning in which the problem or goals are reviewed. This is another excellent time for brainstorming. Research allows the physician or office manager to investigate the needs of the target market and then decide what the medical office can do to meet those needs. Planning the concept follows and, once a firm plan is in place, it is executed or carried out. Afterward, evaluate what went well and what problems occurred so that future efforts will be even more successful.

Promoting the Practice

The physician and office manager should constantly watch for ways to promote the medical practice and keep its name in the public eye. Some of these methods are free of charge, and others will need detailed budgeting and planning.

Tapping into Free Resources

Many good promotional activities are relatively free to the physician. One of the most popular and beneficial to the physician is a professional website. If the physician or office staff has sufficient knowledge for website construction, then there is little or no cost to the doctor if one of the free website services is used.

Some newspapers offer an advice column wherein different types of professionals give general medical advice to those who write in with questions. Physicians volunteer to answer these questions in print and, in return, the office address, the office telephone number, and often the physicians' pictures are featured. This is an excellent way to generate patient calls and inform the public about the specialties and types of cases the physician handles.

CRITICAL THINKING APPLICATION

- Monica knows there are many opportunities and free resources in her area. Where should she begin to look?
- How might Monica's clinic partner with other businesses and services to provide excellent care and help each other at the same time?

Community Involvement

Getting involved in the local community is another way to promote a medical practice. Some physicians sponsor Little League Football, baseball teams, or bowling leagues. Some entire staffs participate in charity events and marathons, wearing t-shirts with the clinic name imprinted on the back.

The physician or staff may have specific charities that they support on an annual basis, or they may participate in United Way activities, which distribute funds to many different types of worthy organizations through payroll deductions and other gifts. Some medical facilities have volunteer programs in which employees receive recognition for participation in various activities. A good example includes blood donations. Many blood centers offer pins and recognition certificates for the number of pints of blood that volunteers donate. The office staff may set a goal to reach a certain number of donated pints in a year, and as recognition certificates are collected, the staff may wish to display them in a prominent place in the office. This is an indication to patients that the staff is concerned about the community and is volunteer minded. From a public relations standpoint, this is valuable to the medical office, because patients tend to expect medical professionals to be volunteer oriented.

Health fairs are a great avenue for promoting the services offered by the clinic, obtaining name recognition, and increasing public visibility. Some health fairs are huge, highly publicized events, while others are small, often held at a local shopping mall or grocery store. All of these events could be worthy projects for the physician and the medical office.

CRITICAL THINKING APPLICATION

- What community organizations might help Monica in her efforts to make the office an integral part of the community?
- What resources and community organizations are available in your area that would be good avenues for practice marketing and community service?

Advertising Plans and Agencies

Most physician offices do not use advertising agencies to promote their practices, but there are occasions when an agency might be useful (Figure 21-3). If a very special event is scheduled that needs extensive planning, then a public relations firm or advertising agency might be consulted. Unfortunately, the cost of these groups is usually high and beyond the reach of sole practitioners or small group practices. However, the investment may be well spent when an event is critical and attendance is important to its success.

There is a difference between advertising and public relations. Advertising could be defined as "creating or changing attitudes, beliefs, and perceptions by influencing people with purchased broadcast time, print space, or other forms of written and visual media." Broadcast time could be in the form of television commercials, radio broadcasts, or audiovisual aids. Print could be in a newspaper, magazine, or trade journal, while written and visual media may be a flier, brochure, or billboard. Public relations offerings are influential as well, using news broadcasts, radio reports, and magazine or newspaper articles to reach people. Most public relations efforts are free, but it is often difficult to get others interested enough in the activities the medical office is planning to warrant coverage.

Communication as a Marketing Tool

Many medical offices use communications tools to market the practice and improve customer service. Sending a monthly newsletter through mail or electronically provides health information and news about upcoming events. The newsletter can be very personalized for the office and might even include news about patients and the medical staff, as long as permission is obtained.

Sending birthday cards is an excellent public relations tool. Some offices sign the greetings at staff meetings and they are placed in a tickler file for the proper mailing date. Sending holiday greetings is another method of wishing patients well.

Automated call distribution is becoming a popular means of communicating with large numbers of people. A computer dials multiple numbers at the same time and plays a recorded message, which can be the actual physician reading a message. Although many people block such calls to their homes and an equal number hang up, the success rate of automatic call distribution is actually quite good.

Many individuals listen and respond to the calls, especially if they come from someone they know giving important information. For instance, if a medical clinic were planning to move to another part of the city, a program could be initiated to notify all patients with telephone numbers that the office will be moving after a certain date. The message could include the address of the new location, and even prompt patients to "press 1" if they need to schedule an appointment. The same principle could be applied to news about an upcoming health fair, a special seminar about a certain illness, or even an article that will be in the Sunday paper about the clinic.

FINDING A GOOD ADVERTISING AGENCY

1. *Define your objective in hiring an ad agency.* What do you want to achieve? What should be different after the agency goes to work for you? What kind of working relationship do you prefer?
2. *Check out sources.* Consider work you have seen or heard that has impressed you. Call friends and colleagues you trust and get their recommendations. Attend professional or trade association meetings, and talk to members who have used agencies before. Seek out their opinions, and note whose names come up often (both pro and con). Watch for articles about ad agencies in area papers, trade magazines, and related publications, such as chamber of commerce newsletters.
3. *Once you have a list of candidates, screen them by telephone.* Ask about their backgrounds, projects they have worked on, the results they have had, their fees, and anything else important to you. Then set up interviews with the three or four firms that impressed you the most.
4. *Interview the finalists.* Find out the following:
   - *Do they have experience working with your industry?* What is their track record when working with companies like yours? Do they understand your business and the nuances of what you do? If not, are they willing to research the information they need?
   - *Is there chemistry?* You can tell if there is a good "fit" with an ad agency. A good agency will express interest in getting to know you as an individual and learning more about your company. They will be good listeners and quick learners. They will make good suggestions and react quickly to your questions and opinions. They should demonstrate the ability to anticipate what is best for your business and be prepared to disagree with you if they feel you are on the wrong track.
   - *Do they show originality and creativity?* Based on the agency's previous work, do you feel these people understand how best to "sell" your product or service? If you operate a home healthcare agency, for example, you probably do not want an ad campaign that features technology over tenderness. Sensing your clientele, the agency should know enough about you to put together the appropriate message.
   - *Are they reliable and budget conscious?* No amount of chemistry and creativity can make up for a missed deadline or an estimate that is way off. Be sure the agency has not only the creative skills needed but also the time and commitment to devote to your needs. Whether you are the biggest or smallest client in their stable, you should be able to count on consistent attention to detail. Their staff should be available to answer your questions and be accountable for delays and expenses.

FIGURE 21-3 Selecting an advertising or public relations agency. (From Anderson L: Star makers. *Entrepreneurial magazine,* April 1997.)

Promoting a New Practice

Most physicians who open a new practice place an ad in local newspapers to announce the event. Usually a picture of the physician is included, and a map to the exact location may be available on the ad. Some physicians purchase clinics from others who are moving or retiring, but many will open a freestanding clinic in a new building, and the word about the new facility must be spread for the business to be a success.

Providing business cards for all employees is a good way to increase public knowledge about the facility. Some offices offer incentives for patient referrals from the staff or other patients, but the physician must ensure that there are no state statutes or ethical standards that prohibit this. The incentive could be a simple coffee cup with the clinic's logo on it or a book about a healthcare issue. Recognition is the important factor where referrals are concerned. A thank you card is the minimal acceptable "thanks" for patient referrals.

Some physicians hold an open house when the new facility opens. Often, those individuals who assisted with the business from its inception will attend the open house to lend support to the owners. Bankers, attorneys, accountants, and other physicians will often show their support by attending the open house. Pictures from this event should be placed on the facility's website or in the monthly newsletter.

Building a Practice Website

There are four basic steps involved in building a website for the medical practice. These steps include the following:
- Define the objectives of the website.
- Design the pages.

- Locate a web server where the pages can be uploaded.
- Upload the page to the web server.

Defining Objectives. When defining **objectives**, important decisions about specific goals must be considered. The physician and staff should discuss who the audience for the website will be and what will be included on the site. Most websites designed for physician offices and clinics are informational, developed mostly for patient and public use. Once the objectives are clearly defined, specific content can be written to place on the website.

Designing the Pages. Once the objectives are clear, begin developing ideas as to what the site will look like on the computer screen. Color choices, animation, and fonts will enhance the look that is being created and make a strong statement about the medical facility. The menus should be designed so that viewers can navigate easily through the site. Most users appreciate a means to go back to the page previously viewed and grow frustrated with sites that have an excessive number of pop-up boxes. Consistency is important, so it is a good idea to keep the same design theme on each page of the website.

The most important part of the website is the text. It has been said that every word in a book must add to the story, and this is a good way to look at the text in a website. Avoid repetition and remain clear about what is being communicated on the site. Headings and titles help to clarify the theme of each page. Use a spell checker before uploading the message and making it available for public viewing.

Photographs, graphics, music, and video can add fun to the website, but be careful not to overdo them. Graphics are often large files that take time to download. Most people will not wait more than about 10 seconds for a web page to load before clicking elsewhere. When designing web page graphics, remember that smaller is better. Graphics can be found by searching for "index of GIF files" or "GIF library." Once an appropriate file is found, it should be copied onto the hard drive by "right clicking" the graphic and selecting "save picture as." Music can be found by searching for "mid" or "midi." The search can even specify a certain singer, song, or composer. Always respect any copyrights that are designated on any file used. Many websites offer these files for free.

For a more professional-looking website, consider purchasing web development software, such as Macromedia's Dreamweaver or Microsoft's Front Page. These feature-rich products are fairly inexpensive and can help the medical assistant create very attractive, easy-to-maintain websites. Most products integrate tutorial and "help" features that explain how to use them.

Hyperlinks are words or graphics on a web page that, when clicked, take the viewer to another page or another website. To add a hyperlink, simply highlight the text field or graphic, select the hyperlink icon, and specify the destination address (uniform resource locator [URL]). Always specify the full URL.

The main page should always be assigned the file name "index.htm" or "default.htm." Other pages on the website can be assigned any name; however, keep the names short and avoid using special characters.

Locating a Web Server. At this point, the design of the website is complete, but the files reside on the computer hard drive, not on the Internet. Now the pages are ready to be uploaded, or published, to a web server that will allow them to be viewed on the Internet. The Internet service provider (ISP) that the office uses for email and online services may offer free web space to its customers. If not, there are a number of companies that will provide web space at no charge, but the user usually will be required to use banners on the site that advertise the ISP or other services. If no banner ads are desired, the medical facility may wish to use a paid provider. Some web hosting companies provide other services free of charge, like simple web page editors and email addresses.

Uploading the Website to the Web Server. When using a free web server, instructions and passwords will be sent to the user that describe how to upload files to the server. The password is necessary so that other people cannot alter the files. Copying the files from the local hard disk to the web server is a simple process. The hosting site will prompt the user for the name of the directory on the hard drive where the files are stored and for the names of the specific files to be uploaded. To avoid confusion, make certain that the files saved on the server have the same file names that were used on the hard drive.

Once all of the files have been uploaded, test the page on the web server and make certain that it functions properly and that all files have been uploaded correctly. It is also a good idea to test the page using a different computer to ensure that graphic files are being read from the server and not from the local hard drive.

Evaluating the Website. Include an email address where viewers of the website can interact with the creator with comments. This way problems with the site can be readily identified and corrected. It is also advisable to check the site every few days to make certain that it is functioning properly.

Counters often can be added to the website that will indicate how many people viewed it. This helpful tool will allow the medical facility to track how many people are viewing which pages.

Quality Customer Service in the Medical Practice

Treating the Patient as a Customer

The best way to increase the number of patients in a medical office is through word of mouth. When patients are satisfied with the treatment they receive, they will refer other patients to the physician. However, if they are dissatisfied, they will tell everyone they know!

Because patients often have a choice as to who provides their healthcare services, it is important that the physician's office become the patient's *first choice*. Some patients have such loyalty to a certain physician that even if their healthcare coverage would no longer pay for visits, they would continue to see that doctor. This happens because of the attitude of the physician and his or her office staff.

CRITICAL THINKING APPLICATION

- Monica is considering a "Frequently Asked Questions" section of the website. How might this help patients?
- What kinds of questions might be asked in this section?
- How might including this section benefit employees?

Helpful Attitudes. The physician and staff probably emote a helpful attitude in every contact with the patient. They sincerely ask, "How may I help you?" and then take steps to assist the patient in whatever way possible. Instead of pointing in the general direction of the radiology department, they take the patient there and introduce him or her to the receptionist. Instead of telling a patient on the telephone, "Ann handles the insurance billing—I'll transfer you to her," say, "One moment, Mrs. Brown, let me see if Ann is at her desk." Then place Mrs. Brown on hold, call Ann, and let her know that she has a call. Then return to Mrs. Brown and tell her that Ann is at her desk and transfer the call at that time. Be courteous and kind to every patient and visitor to the office. Good customer relations must be one of the primary goals of the medical facility. Patients count on the staff members to be reliable and available to help them to the best of their abilities.

CUSTOMER SERVICE AT NORDSTROMS

Use your good judgment in all situations. There will be no additional rules.

From the Nordstrom, Inc., Employee handbook. Courtesy Nordstrom, Inc.

Phrases that Undermine Successful Customer Service. There are several phrases that could be considered the "deadly sins" of customer service. These phrases should never be used when relating to patients and visitors:

- "I don't know."
- "I don't care."
- "I can't be bothered."
- "Ask someone else."
- "It's not my job."
- "It's not my fault."
- "I know that."
- "I'm right, you're wrong."

All of these phrases will give the patient or visitor a negative view of both the office and those who work in the facility.

Identifying with the Patient. Patients appreciate staff members who can identify with the problems they are facing. This is especially effective when a patient is upset or angry. For example, if a patient comes to the office complaining that charges were placed on his account for procedures that were not performed, the medical assistant may respond with a phrase similar to the following:

"Mr. Roberts, I understand that you are upset about these additional charges. I know I would be upset if I were billed for something I didn't receive. Let me help you though, by doing this . . . "

Identifying with the patient shows an understanding on the part of the staff member, no matter how upset the patient may be. Always acknowledge and restate the patient's concern. It proves that the medical assistant was listening and is interested in resolving the problem.

Remember, it costs much more to find new customers than to keep existing customers happy. Providing helpful, personal service impresses even the most difficult patient. To patients and visitors to the clinic, whomever they speak to represents the whole company. Perceptions and opinions will likely be formed based on experiences with only one person. Each individual employee must be aware that to the patient, each employee is the healthcare facility.

What Do the Patients Expect?

First, patients expect to be treated using the golden rule. They expect their concerns to be met with responsiveness, which means that the medical assistant should have a caring attitude. They also expect that the professionals in the medical office are knowledgeable about their field or specialty. An insurance biller should know more than just the basics of insurance filing. The office manager should have a certain degree of authority to handle problems and complaints. Patients also expect confidentiality and trust from the staff of the medical office. They expect an organized office that runs on schedule, and that if a staff member promises to do something, it is as good as done (Figure 21-4).

Remembering the Internal Customer

Most of us do not have problems figuring out who the external customers are in a medical practice. Patients, their families and friends, and visitors to the office are external customers. But who is the internal customer?

Internal customers are employees and staff members of the facility. Although they work for the business, they also are served by the business. If they are not pleased with the atmosphere of the medical facility, they are sure to look elsewhere for employment. Keeping the internal customer is just as important as keeping the external customer.

Closing Comments

Providing good customer service is a commitment that must be made by every employee of the medical facility, every single day. There will be times that the customer is not right, but he or she should be treated with dignity and respect at all times. Additionally, the expert customer service provider will have the knack for making the customer think he or she was right all along! The medical office is no exception to the requirements for providing good service to its patients, and doing so will result in an excellent reputation for the clinic, built by those who matter most—the patients.

Todd Family Medical Clinic

Julie Todd, M.D.   Robert Todd, M.D.
3343 Smithson Place
Dallas, Texas 75229

We are interested in the customer service you received today as a patient of our clinic. Please return this form by mail and help us evaluate our service to you!

Date of contact or visit: _____   Day of week: _____

Name of employees with which you made contact (if known):

How was this contact made?   ☐ by phone   ☐ by mail   ☐ in person

This is a (please check appropriate box)   ☐ complaint   ☐ comment

Description of situation:

Has the problem been resolved to your satisfaction, if any?   ☐ yes   ☐ no

If not, how can we resolve the problem?

Please rate the following based on your experience with our staff:

	Excellent	Good	Fair	Poor
Greeting to you by name	☐	☐	☐	☐
Familiarity with your account	☐	☐	☐	☐
Courtesy and willingness to help	☐	☐	☐	☐
Quickness in answering the phone	☐	☐	☐	☐
Time placed on hold	☐	☐	☐	☐
Quickness in locating your chart	☐	☐	☐	☐
All of your questions answered	☐	☐	☐	☐
Phone transfers kept to a minimum	☐	☐	☐	☐

Other suggestions and comments:

Name (optional): _____   Phone Number (optional): _____

FIGURE 21-4 Customer service evaluation form for the medical office. By using this form for patient feedback, the medical office manager can better assess patient expectations.

Patient Education

Endless opportunities for patient education exist through the practice's marketing and public relations efforts. Most physicians agree that a part of their obligation to the medical profession is to educate patients about healthcare issues. The public relations and practice's marketing staffs can work together to provide information to patients of the facility and to the general public.

Many physicians attend health fairs, where brochures and pamphlets can be distributed about conditions such as diabetes, heart disease, hypertension, and other disorders. Screenings for cholesterol and blood pressure checks are good ways to market a practice and gain new patients.

The medical assistant who knows how to build and maintain a simple website can be of great value to the physician. The practice website could provide opportunities for educating the patient, as well as special sections for upcoming events, an online newsletter, appointment setting, and even a separate patient education section. The website address should be included on stationery, business cards, and other documents used to promote the facility.

Legal and Ethical Issues

The physician must take care that patients do not use the information in brochures or on the practice website as medical advice or a substitute for the physician's counsel. When attaching links to other websites, be sure they are reputable. The patient may consider information on the practice's website to be an extension of the advice of the physician, so make sure that everything on the website is accurate.

The physician should review carefully all printed information that is used to promote the medical facility. Be sure that no misleading statements are included. A disclaimer should be used to remind patients that the information given in brochures and on websites is only general information. Patients should discuss specific medical issues with the physician.

SUMMARY OF SCENARIO

Monica knows that without growth, many businesses eventually fail. She is confident that with a simple marketing plan, the clinic will experience steady, continuous expansion. She has spoken to all of the office staff members and gained input from both employees and the patients of the clinic. Many offered excellent suggestions that Monica can incorporate into her marketing plan.

One of her first activities was to develop an annual calendar of special events and outreach efforts. A monthly newsletter and the practice website will be the main thrusts of her marketing plan. The newsletter will be avail-able both in print and online. The patients in the office database who have email addresses will receive automatically a computer-generated email message containing a link that will take them directly to the online newsletter. Inside, patients will find health information and details about upcoming events.

Monica also planned one special activity for each month of the year. She scheduled a blood drive, a Christmas toy drive, and mini–health fair. Because both Dr. Julie and Dr. Robert Todd are dedicated to students who wish to pursue medicine, Monica even planned a career day for high school students interested in becoming physicians, inviting representatives from the medical school that the Todds attended. Because this is considered a public service, Monica was able to get press coverage on the local radio station and in the newspaper at no cost.

Monica visited a new restaurant located close to the office that serves heart-healthy dishes, met with the manager, and discussed ways that the two businesses could help each other. They decided to provide a "buy one entrée, get one free" coupon to patients who referred other patients to the clinic. In turn, Dr. Robert Todd agreed to hold his free nutrition seminars at the restaurant. This arrangement has proven to work well for both businesses.

Monica plans to track responses to each event to determine what efforts were the most effective. The website will allow her to count the number of times it is accessed, as well as which pages were the most popular within the website. She will keep the physicians informed and be open to their suggestions throughout the year. Monica is anxious to see results of her marketing efforts and feels confident of success.

SUMMARY OF LEARNING OBJECTIVES

■ When preparing to implement marketing strategies, first evaluate what currently is being done toward the marketing effort. Then, decide what the objectives of the marketing plan are and how they will be measured. Last, develop a specific plan and timeline for implementing each phase.

■ A target market is a very specific group of people or individuals that the medical facility wishes to serve. The geography where the individuals live, the lifestyle they are accustomed to, and the personality of the individuals all are ways to classify them into a specific target market. When identifying a target market ask, "Who is our patient?", "What does our patient want?", and "Why is it wanted?" These questions will help the medical facility to design a marketing plan to meet the needs of these individuals.

■ Suggestions from patients and employees should always be welcomed in the medical office. Often these people see the facility from a different point of view, and their suggestions can enhance the atmosphere and services that are offered.

■ A marketing plan must always address the "four p's," which are product, placement, price, and promotion. The product in a medical office would include the services, and any actual retail items that might be sold. Placement relates to the location of the office and its convenience to the patients, and the placement of retail items in the facility. Price represents the charges for goods and services, and promotion entails the ways in which the services are promoted to the general public and the target market.

■ When developing a marketing plan, the facility should first assess the efforts that have been made in the past and then research the results of those efforts. Next the plan is developed, which should include very specific steps for each aspect of the endeavor. After the plan is executed, the staff must evaluate its effectiveness and then determine whether the goals were met. The evaluation is important in planning future marketing strategies.

■ Involvement in the community is an excellent way to give to the medical profession and to remain in the public eye. These efforts can result in new patients for the facility. The public sees medical professionals as caring and compassionate, so volunteer activities reinforce this attitude and help to meet patient expectations.

■ Advertising is defined as a medium that creates or changes attitudes, beliefs, and perceptions through purchased broadcast time, printed material, or other forms of communication. Public relations are similar but rely more on news broadcasts or reports, magazine or newspaper articles, and radio reports to reach the audience.

■ The new medical practice can be promoted by placing an announcement in the newspaper about its opening. Some physicians hold an open house, inviting the public to visit the office. A website is an excellent promotional tool and should be listed on business cards and stationery. Community service and volunteer activities that mention the practice will also help to spread the word about the services that are available.

■ Identifying with the patient is an effective customer service tool. The medical assistant should express his or her understanding about the patient's concerns. Then, tell the patient that the situation can be resolved and how it will be resolved. Four magic words in customer service are, "Let me help you."

■ External customers are those who visit the facility, such as patients. However, staff members and employees are internal customers, who wish to derive a sense of satisfaction in working for the medical office. The internal customers are just as important as the external customers.

INTERNET CONNECTIONS

- American Marketing Association
  www.ama.org
- Medical MultiMEDIA Group
  www.medicalmultimediagroup.com
- The Patient Education Institute
  www.patient-education.com
- United Way
  www.unitedway.org

FREE WEB PAGES ARE AVAILABLE WITH:

- www.angelfire.lycos.com
- www.dreamwater.com
- www.freewebspace.com
- www.geocities.com
- www.webspawner.com

CHAPTER 22

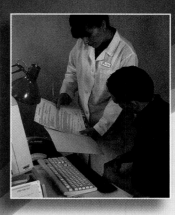

Scenario

Laura Kelly graduated from her medical assistant training 1 year ago and is now employed at a regional hospital in the quality assurance department as an administrative assistant. She enjoys working with statistics, is very detail oriented, has excellent computer skills, and is able to comprehend the lengthy regulatory text, such as that set forth in the Health Insurance Portability and Accountability Act (HIPAA) rules and guidelines. She has proven to be a valuable employee as the hospital has begun to comply with privacy laws.

Laura thought that quality assurance involved only patient satisfaction when she began working for the hospital. She has learned that this is just a small part of the total quality picture of the facility. The hospital has developed a patient questionnaire to solicit input from patients, and she enjoys talking with them about their experiences. Laura rarely encounters complaints, and she is proud to work for a medical facility that has practitioners who are concerned about giving exceptional care to patients. She now understands that there are many aspects to providing quality in a healthcare facility.

Laura also realizes that health information encompasses much more than the patient's chart. She knows that health statistics are vital to research and that physicians rely on statistical information when prescribing drugs, giving treatments, and performing other services. Providers frequently contact Laura to determine how many cases of a certain disease or disorder occurred at the hospital during a given period. The hospital database is very sophisticated and allows her to access many types of statistics quickly. Her office also monitors who enters the database and what information is accessed. This is one method of ensuring that privacy is maintained.

Laura has attended continuing education workshops that allow her to gain information that will help the staff to stay in compliance with the numerous regulations that govern the facility. She is eager to learn and assist her employers in keeping the hospital safe for all patients and visitors.

Health Information Management

Learning Objectives

- Define and spell the terms listed in the vocabulary.
- Describe several ways that health information is used.
- Contrast the nine characteristics of quality health data.
- Explain the four concerns of quality assurance.
- Discuss the importance of the HIPAA.
- Explain the functions of the National Center for Health Statistics (NCHS).
- Discuss the types of statistics kept by the NCHS.
- Define total quality management.
- Explain the function of Joint Commission on Accreditation of Healthcare Organizations (JCAHO).
- Discuss the importance of healthcare standards in medical facilities.

National Curriculum Competencies

2d. Document appropriately

2e. Perform risk management procedures

4a. Apply managed care policies and procedures

4b. Apply third party guidelines

Vocabulary

authenticated Proof of; with regard to medical records, it applies to a signature, initials, or computer keystroke by the maker of the record who verifies that the record is correct.

circumvent To manage to get around, especially by ingenuity or stratagem.

contraindication Something, as a symptom or condition, that makes a particular treatment or procedure inadvisable.

disparities Containing or made up of fundamentally different and often incongruous elements; markedly distinct in quality or character.

encrypt To convert from one system of communication to another; encode.

erroneous Containing or characterized by error or assumption.

gradient A change in response with distance from the stimulus.

nosocomial Originating or taking place in a hospital.

quality assurance Activities designed to increase the quality of a product or service through process or system changes that increase efficiency or effectiveness.

sentinel event An unexpected occurrence involving death or serious physical or psychologic injury, or the risk thereof.

standards Established by authority, custom, or general consent as a model or example; something set up and established by authority as a rule for the measure of quantity, weight, extent, value, or quality.

transpose To change the relative place or normal order of; to alter the sequence.

Prior to the 1990s, practitioners in the healthcare field were barely familiar with the term *health information management*. Today, it is a well-respected profession that employs thousands of individuals across the United States. As more medical facilities move toward computer-based medical records, more trained health information management professionals are needed. The medical assistant may wish to pursue employment in this growing field.

The health information management profession is supported by a national organization called the American Health Information Management Association. This association's House of Delegates developed a statement in 1994 that defines the profession. The statement reads:

"Health information management is the profession that focuses on healthcare data and the management of healthcare information resources. The profession addresses the nature, structure, and translation of data into usable forms of information for the advancement of health and healthcare of individuals and populations. Health information professionals collect, integrate, and analyze primary and secondary healthcare data; disseminate information; and manage information resources related to research, planning, provision, and evaluation of healthcare services."

Evolution of the Profession

In 1928, the American College of Surgeons realized that accurate medical records promoted good medical care. This desire for quality led to the establishment of the Association of Record Librarians of North America. Years later in 1970, the organization changed its name to the American Medical Record Association. Medical records professionals found employment in hospitals, health clinics, insurance companies, and other organizations that utilized medical records.

In 1991, the organization became known as the American Health Information Management Association. Advances in technology have brought the health information management profession from a paper environment into a highly sophisticated computer age, where physicians can access patient and statistical data in seconds.

CRITICAL THINKING APPLICATION

- Laura is eligible to join the American Health Information Management Association, and her employer will pay for her dues. How might joining this professional organization benefit Laura?
- How would the hospital benefit from Laura's membership in the organization?

The Use of Healthcare Data

Many people and various organizations use healthcare data in a multitude of ways (Figure 22-1). Primarily, healthcare data are used to plan care for patients and ensure that they receive continuity of care from one healthcare provider to another. However, the information provided through healthcare records is useful in other capacities.

For example, when a drug is being evaluated, statistics must be kept to help the manufacturers of the product determine its effectiveness. Information on side effects and other **contraindications** is reviewed and used to make the product safer and more marketable. Sometimes, the drug must be changed and then returned to clinical trials.

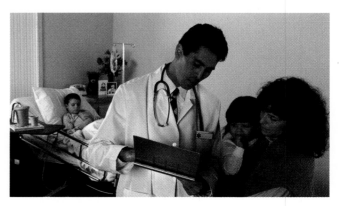

FIGURE 22-1 Physicians rely on health information to provide quality care to their patients.

Healthcare organizations gather information on the number of patients who enter the facility with the same diagnosis. This and other information helps them to plan what types of equipment will be needed to meet the needs of the patient population. For instance, if the geographic area where the facility is located contains a large number of patients with cardiac disease, a hospital may need to add a cardiac intensive care unit. If the facility is located in a neighborhood where there are many young families, the obstetrics and pediatrics departments may be expanded. Healthcare data and statistics guide planning for the needs of next week and for the next decade.

CRITICAL THINKING APPLICATION

- Laura has noticed that the hospital keeps extensive records on the admitting diagnosis and the discharge diagnosis. Why is this information important?
- If a certain physician is admitting numerous patients with the same diagnosis and is a family practitioner, what concerns might this raise for the facility?

Third-party payors use healthcare information to determine whether claims should be paid. The data provide proof that a certain procedure or treatment was medically necessary and therefore should be reimbursed (Figure 22-2). Government and regulatory agencies use data to make certain that healthcare facilities are in compliance with the various statutes and standards that govern them.

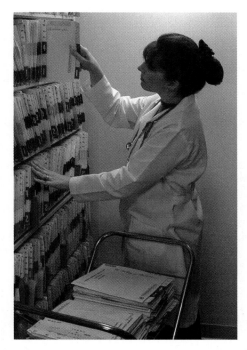

FIGURE 22-2 Healthcare providers often rely on statistics when treating their patients. Most statistical information is gleaned from patient charts.

Data also are used by facilities in determining whether quality healthcare is being provided to patients.

What Are Quality Data?

The information that is contained in a database is only as reliable as the person who entered it into the computer. Most database systems require information to be saved after it is entered by clicking an additional button. Without saving, the time and effort spent in entering the data have been wasted.

*Health Information: Management of a Strategic Resource** identifies nine characteristics of quality health data. These characteristics are validity, reliability, completeness, recognizability, timeliness, relevance, accessibility, security, and legality.

Validity

The validity of health data is synonymous with accuracy. Accuracy is one of the most important characteristics of data, whether in paper-based or computer-based records. Great care must be taken when characters are typed on the keyboard, so that letters or numbers are not **transposed.**

Reliability

The healthcare professional must be able to rely on the data presented. If a patient's medical chart is marked such that he or she has no allergies, the medical assistant must be able to trust that information and give an injection with the confidence that the patient is not allergic to the medication. Reliability also pertains to the degree to which the information in the database can be trusted.

Completeness

The information must not only be accurate, it must also be complete. If the medical assistant gives an injection yet fails to document it in the patient's chart, then the record is incomplete. If a computer system is designed to upload new information into the database every night and the system malfunctions, there is a strong possibility that the records contained within the system are incomplete, possibly missing vital information needed to care for the patient.

Recognizability

All users of health information must be able to interpret the data that are presented in the health record. The facility should have a consistent use of abbreviations so that no misunderstandings occur when reviewing a patient's chart.

*Abdelhak M, Grostick S, Hanken MA, Jacobs E: *Health information: management of a strategic resource*, ed 2. Philadelphia, 2001, WB Saunders.

Timeliness

Health data must be entered into the chart or database as soon as it happens. The medical assistant should never commit information to memory intending to enter it later. Reports from laboratories or medical tests also should be placed in the chart as soon as the information is reviewed by the physician, so that decisions made are supported by the latest information on the patient's condition.

Relevance

The information contained in the database must be relevant to be useful. Needless and meaningless statistics about patient treatments or drug interactions do not benefit providers and users of health information.

Accessibility

One of the advantages of a computer-based patient record is that it is accessible to multiple users at the same time. The facility must take care to provide access only to individuals who are authorized to view the records. The computer system should have a login capability, which prompts for a password. In addition, the system should keep records of who accesses information by time and date. Paper-based patient records should be returned to their proper place when they are not in use so that they will be accessible to all staff members.

Security

Although only certain employees are allowed to access health information, precautions must be taken to prohibit access to intruders. Firewalls are similar to filters that allow only certain types of data to enter or exit. Information can be **encrypted**, which means that it is changed into a code that can only be read once unencrypted. These precautions are necessary because of the sensitivity of patient information. Also, care must be taken to ensure that no one can change the information already contained in the record.

Legality

Many statutes govern medical records. The laws concerning record retention vary from state to state. Medical records cannot be altered but should be corrected according to accepted guidelines. The record must be completely legible and **authenticated** properly (Figure 22-3).

CRITICAL THINKING APPLICATION

- One of Laura's duties involves making sure that medical records have been authenticated. Why is the authentication of records important?
- One physician, Dr. Norman, is consistently careless about record authentication. How can the hospital encourage him to complete this critical duty?

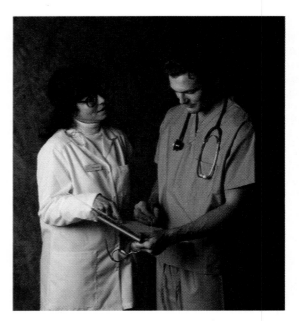

FIGURE 22-3   Physicians must authenticate medical records by initialing or signing their entries. Some computer systems automatically authenticate records.

The Challenges of Quality Assurance Problems

Many of the larger medical facilities today have entire departments that are devoted to **quality assurance**. Quality assurance is defined as the activities designed to increase the quality of a product or service through process or system changes that increase efficiency or effectiveness. Although many people assume that quality is determined solely by the patient, there is much more involved in quality assurance than just the patient's satisfaction with services rendered. Quality assurance also is concerned with the *overuse, underuse, misuse,* and *variations in use* of different healthcare services.

Healthcare services that are excessive and unnecessary cause costs to rise. Treatments and services that are overused include hysterectomies, tympanostomy tubes, and antibiotics. Medical studies have shown that up to 16% of all hysterectomies performed in 1993 were unnecessary and up to 23% of tympanostomy tube operations performed between 1991 and 1992 were unnecessary. Antibiotics are prescribed widely for common colds and acute bronchitis, but the drugs do not benefit these illnesses.

The underuse of services and treatments can be equally costly. Mammograms and cervical cancer screening tests can detect medical problems yet are not taken advantage of by enough at-risk patients (Figure 22-4). The use of beta blockers has been proven to reduce mortality in patients who have had heart attacks by as much as 43%, but often they are not prescribed for these patients. Diabetic patients should have their eyes checked regularly, but many do not. All of these are examples of the underuse of services that can affect the quality of healthcare.

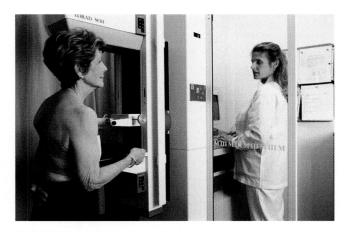

FIGURE 22-4 Healthcare professionals must encourage at-risk patients to have screening tests done, such as those for breast and cervical cancer.

CRITICAL THINKING APPLICATION

- How might a hospital employee encourage patients to have screening tests done, such as mammograms and for cervical cancer?
- What marketing strategies could Laura assist in developing that will result in more patients taking advantage of health screening opportunities?
- How do these services benefit the health facility?

Some healthcare services are misused. These errors can cause death, delay of correct diagnosis, unnecessary injuries, and increased healthcare costs. Examples of misuse can include laboratory tests that provide **erroneous** results. Medication errors can be fatal to patients or cause complications to the illnesses from which they are already suffering. Hospital injuries and **nosocomial** infections promote further complications. A study at the Harvard School of Public Health published in 1994 estimated that up to 180,000 needless deaths occurred each year as a result of preventable errors.

There are wide variations in services in different parts of the country. Discharge rates (which indicate that the patient left the hospital without expiring) are higher in some areas of the United States than others. Individuals who seek medical care are more conscientious and likely to seek health services in different geographic areas. All of these issues contribute to the concept of quality healthcare.

Health Insurance Portability and Accountability Act

As technology advanced and more health records became computerized, legislation dealing with privacy became imperative. HIPAA of 1996 was developed, in part, to help ensure the confidentiality of medical records. The statute, which became law in August of 1996, applies to those records that are created or maintained by healthcare providers, health plans, and healthcare clearinghouses that engage in certain electronic transactions.

The Office for Civil Rights, a division of the Health and Human Services Department, regulates HIPAA.

In August of 2002, the Department of Health and Human Services Secretary Tommy Thompson announced the final ruling relating to HIPAA's privacy act, which became effective April 14, 2003. Under the privacy rule:

- Patients must give specific authorization before entities covered by the regulation could use or disclose protected information in most nonroutine circumstances—such as releasing information to an employer or for use in marketing activities. Doctors, health plans, and other covered entities would be required to follow the rule's standards for the use and disclosure of personal health information.
- Covered entities generally will need to provide patients with written notice of their privacy practices and patients' privacy rights. The notice will contain information that could be useful to patients choosing a health plan, doctor, or other provider. Patients would generally be asked to sign or otherwise acknowledge receipt of the privacy notice from direct treatment providers.
- Pharmacies, health plans, and other covered entities must first obtain an individual's specific authorization before sending marketing materials. At the same time, the rule permits doctors and other covered entities to communicate freely with patients about treatment options and other health-related information, including disease management programs.
- Specifically, improvements to the final rule strengthen the marketing language to make clear that covered entities cannot use business associate agreements to **circumvent** the rule's marketing prohibition. The improvement explicitly prohibits pharmacies or other covered entities from selling personal medical information to a business that would market its products or services under a business associate agreement.
- Patients generally will be able to access their personal medical records and request changes to correct any errors. In addition, patients generally could request an accounting of nonroutine uses and disclosures of their health information.

Many healthcare organizations have concern about the costs of implementing and maintaining measures that will comply with the privacy regulations. However, the benefits of the act far outweigh the inconveniences of remaining in compliance. Patients have the right to expect complete confidentiality with regard to their health records (Figure 22-5).

CRITICAL THINKING APPLICATION

- Laura is concerned about the number of employees in her facility who are allowed to access patient information. For instance, all nurses have access to health information on all patients. Is this a good policy? Why or why not?
- Should all physicians have access to all patient records? Why or why not?

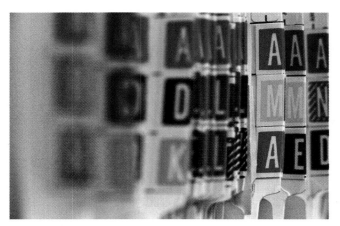

FIGURE 22-5 Patients must have the assurance that their medical records are only accessed by authorized individuals.

National Center for Health Statistics

The NCHS is a division of the Centers for Disease Control. The agency is the primary provider of health information statistics used to guide the actions and policies that relate to the health of the American public. The functions of the NCHS include:

- Documentation of the health status of the population and of important subgroups
- Identification of **disparities** in health status and use of healthcare by race, ethnicity, socioeconomic status (SES), region, and other population **gradients**
- Description of experiences with the healthcare system
- Monitoring of trends in health status and healthcare delivery
- Identification of health problems
- Support of biomedical and health services research
- Provision of information for making changes in public policies and programs
- Evaluation of the impact of health policies and programs

Statistics are of vital importance to many entities that are interested in the healthcare industry. Some of the available statistics through the NCHS are related to:

- Teenage pregnancy
- Incidence of HIV infection
- Alcohol and drug use
- Births
- Deaths
- Communicable diseases
- Infant health and mortality
- Leading causes of death
- Life expectancy
- Sexually transmitted diseases
- Suicide

Total Quality Management

Total quality management is management and control activities based on the leadership of top-level management, supported by the involvement of all employees and departments from planning and development to sales and service. These management and control activities focus on quality assurance. Qualities that satisfy the customer are built into products and services during the above processes.

For total quality management practices to be effective, all employees must make a commitment to provide patients with the best care possible. This includes top-level management as well as the staff members who work directly with the patients.

The Total Quality Management Concept. Much of the thrust of today's interest in total quality management originated from the teachings of W. Edwards Deming. Deming obtained a doctorate in mathematical physics from Yale University in 1928. He is perhaps best known for the work he did with Japanese managers and engineers regarding quality management. Deming compiled 14 points for managers to institute that were designed to place the emphasis on quality rather than quantity.

The following is an excerpt from Deming's book *Out of the Crisis** and briefly describes the Fourteen Points for Management.

- Create constancy of purpose toward improvement of product and service, with the aim to become competitive, to stay in business, and to provide jobs.
- Adopt the new philosophy. Western management must awaken to the challenge, must learn their responsibilities, and take on leadership for change.
- Cease dependence on inspection to achieve quality. Eliminate the need for inspection on a mass basis by building quality into the product or service in the first place.
- End the practice of awarding business on the basis of price tag. Instead, minimize total cost. Move toward a single supplier for any one item, on a long-term relationship of loyalty and trust.
- Constantly improve the system of production and service, to improve quality and productivity, and thus constantly decrease costs.
- Institute training on the job.
- Institute leadership. The aim of supervision should be to help people and machines and gadgets to do a better job. Supervision of management is in need of overhaul as well as supervision of production workers.

*Deming WE: *Out of the crisis.* Cambridge, Mass, 1986, Massachusetts Institute of Technology.

- Drive out fear, so that everyone may work effectively for the company.
- Break down barriers between departments. People must work as a team, to foresee problems of production and in use that may be encountered with the product or service.
- Eliminate slogans, exhortations, and targets for the work force asking for zero defects and new levels of productivity. Such exhortations only create adversarial relationships. Eliminate quotas and substitute leadership. Eliminate management by objective. Eliminate management by numbers and numerical goals. Substitute leadership.
- Remove barriers that rob the hourly worker of his right to pride of workmanship. The responsibility of supervisors must be changed from sheer numbers to quality.
- Remove barriers that rob people in management and in engineering of their right to pride of workmanship. This means the abolishment of the annual merit rating and of management by objective.
- Institute a vigorous program of education and self-improvement.
- Put everybody in the company to work to accomplish the transformation. The transformation is everybody's job.

Deming believed that these points would assist managers in bringing quality to the facility or business in which they were used (Figure 22-6). They are widely used in countless business and service organizations today.

Joint Commission on Accreditation of Healthcare Organizations

JCAHO is a nonprofit organization that assists healthcare facilities by providing accreditation services. The facilities participate in obtaining accreditation voluntarily, but over 17,000 healthcare facilities in the United States are accredited by and comply with JCAHO standards.

For many years, healthcare facilities were interested in meeting the minimum **standards** that would reflect quality healthcare. Recently, there has been a shift from simply meeting minimum standards to exceeding standards and providing optimal healthcare to patients (Figure 22-7). Standards are a set of criteria that the facility must adhere to and be able to prove their compliance.

Risk Management

A risk is any occurrence that could result in patient injury or any type of financial loss to the healthcare facility. The policies and procedures that facilities develop are designed to manage risk and prevent situations that can cause harm to persons or property for which the healthcare facility could be held liable.

Risk management programs in healthcare facilities should focus on financial loss prevention and reduce the possibility of negative publicity resulting from **sentinel events**. JCAHO defines a sentinel event as an "unexpected occurrence involving death or serious physical or psychological injury, or the risk thereof." Sentinel events must be investigated thoroughly and their contributing

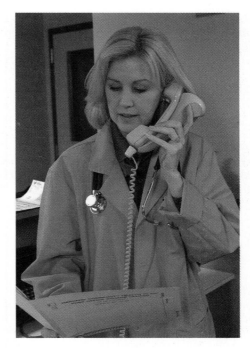

FIGURE 22-6   Quality management is a vital part of accreditation of healthcare organizations, and all physicians should be dedicated to providing optimal quality care to patients.

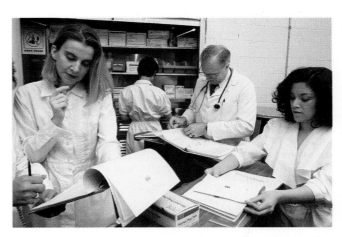

FIGURE 22-7   Accreditation of a healthcare facility takes teamwork and a commitment to quality assurance.

factors rectified so that they are avoided in the future. Records are kept of the sentinel events that happen in a facility, especially those that involve injury to patients.

Closing Comments

Health information management is a critical aspect of today's healthcare facility. Although regulations may seem stringent, the value of protecting the patient's privacy is immeasurable. Patients have the right to expect that their health information is kept confidential. The medical assistant should focus on meeting privacy guidelines and take great care when working with medical records and information.

Patient Education

HIPAA received a great deal of publicity. Patients had long been concerned about their rights to privacy regarding access to health information.

Many patients may have questions about HIPAA and the extent of their rights to limit access to their records. Be prepared to answer their questions or guide them to the right source for information.

Legal and Ethical Issues

The medical assistant must be familiar with the laws surrounding privacy issues and be able to guide patients as they have concerns. Seminars that will target the compliance issues that affect the physician's office often are available to the medical assistant. Most employers are willing to pay for such seminars so that the office can remain in strict compliance with legal issues. Remember that the medical profession is one of constant change. The medical assistant must have a positive attitude about the learning process, especially when new rules and regulations take effect.

SUMMARY OF SCENARIO

Laura is learning more about health information management each day that she goes to work. She has earned the respect of her supervisors, who often give her a lengthy, complicated document concerning regulations and ask her to read and summarize it for the staff. She has a knack for weeding out the actual requirements amid the excess of legalese.

Laura has developed good relationships with many of the staff physicians at the hospital. She has approached several of them about record authentication, and her bright personality helps to foster a sense of cooperation between the medical staff and the hospital staff. She has even begun to give coupons good for one lunch in the cafeteria when physicians form the habit of authenticating their records in a timely manner. The physicians appreciate the recognition for completing their duties on schedule.

Laura has given thought to continuing her education in the health management field and possibly gaining certification in this area. She knows that this will lend credibility to the knowledge that she has gained on the job. Her supervisors are pleased with her performance and know they can count on Laura to complete any task she is assigned on time with accurate results. Laura looks forward to a long career at the hospital and being of service to the patients and staff alike in the years to come.

SUMMARY OF LEARNING OBJECTIVES

- Both physicians and employees of medical facilities use health information in many ways. The information helps to ensure continuity of care from provider to provider. It assists manufacturers in determining side effects of drugs. It provides statistical information regarding primary and secondary diagnoses. Health information also helps the medical facility plan for future needs and capital equipment.

- There are nine characteristics of quality health data. Validity refers to the accuracy of the information, while reliability means that the information can be counted on to be accurate and medical decisions can be made based on the information. Completeness simply means that the information is available in its entirety, and recognizability refers to the data being understood by the users. Timely information allows the provider to make decisions based on the latest data about a patient or a treatment. Relevance refers to the usefulness of the health information, and accessibility means that the information is easily available to the provider when it is needed. Security encompasses the effort to keep unauthorized people from accessing health information. Legality refers to the correctness of the information and its authentication by the healthcare provider.

- Four concerns that surround quality assurance include the overuse, underuse, misuse, and variations in use of healthcare services. Overused services are excessive and cause cost increases. An example includes using the emergency room for nonemergencies. Underuse means that patients do not take advantage of many services they should be using, especially if they are at-risk patients. Misuse of services often reflects errors, such as lab errors or misdiagnoses. Variations in services simply means that in various parts of the country, individuals use services in different ways, which can influence the quality of care overall in the United States.

- HIPAA is a milestone in support of patient privacy issues. There are several facets of the act, but the most widely publicized sections deal with the right to patient privacy. The act will give a degree of control to patients and allow them information about who accesses their records. Patients must also give specific authorization for the use and dissemination of the information contained in the medical record.

- The NCHS is a part of the Centers for Disease Control. Health statistics are important, because they enable providers to better treat their patients. For instance, if a certain area has a high number of outbreaks of a particular disease, the physician may be better prepared to cope with patients with the symptoms of that disease, treating them faster and promoting a full recovery. Health statistics provide information about these types of issues. The NCHS helps to compile information such as the number of HIV infections, teen pregnancies, and other vital health data that is useful to medical professionals.

■ Some of the statistics kept by the NCHS include alcohol and drug use information, births, deaths, communicable diseases, infant health and mortality, and life expectancy.

■ Total quality management is management and control activities based on the leadership of top-level management, supported by the involvement of all employees and departments in an effort to provide quality assurance.

■ JCAHO is a nonprofit organization that offers accreditation services to healthcare facilities that wish to excel in healthcare services. Accreditation is voluntary; however, over 17,000 healthcare facilities in the United States are accredited by this agency.

■ Without strong healthcare standards, quality cannot exist. The focus of quality assurance has shifted in recent years from just meeting the minimum standards to providing optimal quality. People expect quality healthcare when they get treatment. Today's organizations that seek accreditation or focus their efforts on quality will exceed standards, not just meet them.

INTERNET CONNECTIONS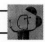

- Agency for Healthcare Research and Quality
  www.ahrq.gov
- Joint Commission on Accreditation of Healthcare Organizations
  www.jcaho.org
- National Center for Health Statistics
  www.cdc.gov/nchs

CHAPTER 23

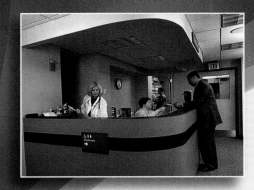

Scenario

Brenda Newman is the office manager for Dr. Susan Wilkins, a neurologist who is beginning her second year of practice. Dr. Wilkins is financially savvy and takes care with the money she has invested in her business. She encourages her employees to plan for the future, and offers them a retirement plan as well as opportunities for investing in mutual funds through payroll deduction. Her accountant, Grant Schmidt, assists Dr. Wilkins with the financial aspects of her practice, and is always willing to counsel the employees of the clinic about finances.

Mr. Schmidt has taught Brenda several methods of keeping track of the practice finances. Brenda is interested in learning more about general accounting rules and bookkeeping. She is able to perform computerized accounting duties and is also able to use a pegboard system. She is able to work with patients when they need to make payment arrangements, and has an excellent collection ratio.

Dr. Wilkins is cost conscious and does not order random supplies and equipment. Instead, she and Brenda plan the inventory for a 6-month period, and have needed to only order supplies every 6 months. By ordering in precise amounts, Dr. Wilkins saves money and uses the extra funds for staff development events and seminars. Each month, the budget is reviewed to ensure that the office is on track with expenses.

The team effort between Dr. Wilkins, Brenda, and Mr. Schmidt results in a balanced budget for the clinic, and subsequently the staff is able to enjoy more benefits and perks.

Management of Practice Finances

Vocabulary

accounts payable Debts incurred and not yet paid.

accounts receivable Amounts owed to the physician.

accounts receivable trial balance A method of determining that the journal and the ledger are in balance.

accrual basis of accounting Method of accounting in which income is recorded when earned, and expenses are recorded when incurred.

assets The entire property of a person, association, corporation, or estate applicable or subject to the payment of debts.

balance sheet A financial statement for a specific date that shows the total assets, liabilities, and capital of the business.

bookkeeping The recording of business and accounting transactions.

cash basis of accounting Method of accounting in which income is recorded when received, and expenses are recorded when paid.

cash flow statement A financial summary for a specific period that shows the beginning balance on hand, the receipts and disbursements during the period, and the balance on hand at the end of the period.

disbursements journal A summary of accounts paid out.

equities The money value of a property or of an interest in a property in excess of claims or liens against it.

fiscal year An accounting period of 12 months.

in balance The total ending balances of patient ledgers equal total of accounts receivable control.

invoice A paper describing a purchase and the amount due.

liabilities Something that is owed; a debt.

packing slip An itemized list of objects in a package.

petty cash fund A fund maintained to pay small unpredictable cash expenditures.

statement A request for payment.

statement of income and expense A summary of all income and expenses for a given period.

trial balance A method of checking the accuracy of accounts.

A physician's business records are the key to good management practice. The medical assistant who can keep accurate financial records and who will conduct the administrative side of the practice in a businesslike fashion is genuinely needed and appreciated.

Financial records that are complete, correct, and current are essential for:

- Prompt billing and collection procedures
- Professional financial planning
- Accurate reporting of income to federal and state agencies

What Is Accounting?

Accounting is a system of recording, classifying, and summarizing financial transactions. **Bookkeeping** is mainly the recording part of the accounting process. The book-keeping must be done daily and is the responsibility of the administrative medical assistant in a small practice, and the office manager or financial manager in a larger practice.

Accounting Bases

There are two general bases, or methods, for accounting: the cash basis and the accrual basis. Most physicians use the **cash basis of accounting**, which means that charges for services are entered as income when payment is received, and expenses are recorded when they are paid. Merchants, on the other hand, generally use an **accrual basis of accounting**. Income is considered earned when services have been performed or goods have been sold, even though payment may not have been received. Expenses are recognized and recorded when incurred, even though they have not been paid.

Financial Summaries

The financial records of any business should at all times show:

- How much was earned in a given period
- How much was collected
- How much is owed
- The distribution of expenses incurred

From the daily entries, the accountant can prepare monthly and annual summaries that provide a basis for comparing any given period with another similar period. Periodic analyses of the financial records can result in improved business practices, better management of time, curtailment or elimination of unprofitable services, and better budgeting of expenses. With the appropriate software these analyses can be accomplished using the computer. The medical assistant may notice notations of AP/AR, which stand for **accounts payable** and **accounts receivable**.

CRITICAL THINKING APPLICATION

- Brenda has noticed several errors on encounter forms lately. These errors seem to be a result of not using a calculator when adding the charges once the patient checks out. Brenda has approached the person who assists the patients in this area, but has not seen any improvement in the errors. How might she convince the employee to follow precautions in adding charges?
- How might Mr. Schmidt educate the staff about the importance of accurate financial records?

The Cardinal Rules of Bookkeeping

There are many rules that apply to bookkeeping that the medical assistant must learn. First, use good penmanship so that the records are clearly legible, even years later. Use the same pen style and ink consistently. Keep columns of figures straight and write well-formed figures (a careless 9 may look like a 7; an open 0 may resemble a 6). Carry decimal points correctly.

Enter all charges and receipts immediately in the daily record or journal. Write a receipt in duplicate for any currency received (Figure 23-1). Writing receipts for checks is optional, but a consistent pattern should be followed. Post all charges and receipts to the patient ledger daily. Checks should be endorsed for deposit as soon as received. Verify that the total of the deposit plus the amount on hand equal the total to be accounted for in the daily journal. Petty cash funds should be used to pay for small unpredictable expenses. Pay all other expenses by check. A cancelled check is the best proof of payment. Bills should be paid before their due dates, after checking them for accuracy. Place date of payment and number of check on paid bills.

Do not erase, write over, or blot out figures. If an error is made, a straight line should be drawn through the incorrect figure and the correct figure written above it. Bookkeeping procedures are not complicated, but they do require concentration to avoid errors. There is no such thing as *almost* correct financial records. The books either balance or they do not balance. The bookkeeping is either right or wrong. This is not the place to be creative or take shortcuts.

The medical assistant should set aside a certain time each day for bookkeeping tasks, if possible. Do not attempt to work on financial records when busy attending patients or when there are other distractions.

Kinds of Financial Records

Daily Journal. The daily journal day sheet is the chronological record of the practice—the financial diary. All information regarding services rendered, charges, and receipts is first recorded in the daily journal. It is important that every transaction be recorded.

In addition to professional services rendered in and out of the office, there may be income from other sources, such as rentals, royalties, interest, and so forth.

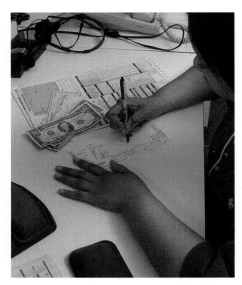

FIGURE 23-1   Accurate records reflect competency in the medical office. The medical assistant should use a calculator when adding figures and be careful not to transpose numbers.

Usually a special place is provided in the journal for such income. Any income that is not practice related should be recorded separately from patient receipts.

Checkbook. Receipts are usually deposited in the checking account, and a record of the deposit is entered in the journal and on the check stub. A copy of each deposit slip should be kept with the financial records. Bills are usually paid by check or online bill-paying services, and a record of the payment is entered on the check stub and in the disbursements section of the general journal.

CRITICAL THINKING APPLICATION

- Brenda has noticed two checks missing from the business checkbook. Dr. Wilkins is out of town for a week and unable to be contacted. How might Brenda determine where the checks are or to whom they were written?
- What steps can be taken to resolve the problem of not knowing the amount of a missing check?

Disbursements Journal

Manual Posting. In simplified accounting systems, the **disbursements journal** usually consists of a section at the bottom of each day sheet and a check register page at the end of each month, plus monthly and annual summaries. It must show:
- Every amount paid out
- Date and check number
- Purpose of payment

Computer Posting. Use the cash or check payments screen. Enter payment information and the computer can print the check, or enter information after the check has been manually prepared.

Petty Cash Records. A **petty cash fund** and voucher system should be established to take care of minor unpredictable expenditures such as postage due, parking fees, small contributions, emergency supplies, and miscellaneous small items. In the average facility, $25 to $50 is sufficient for the petty cash fund. If a larger sum is available, there is a tendency to pay too many bills out of petty cash instead of writing a check.

When the check for this fund is exchanged at the bank for small bills and coins, the money is placed in a cashbox or drawer that can be locked or kept in the safe at night. One person only should be in charge of the petty cash fund. This person must be able to account for the full amount of the fund at any time.

CRITICAL THINKING APPLICATION

- Brenda has noticed that on several occasions, employees have borrowed money from the petty cash fund. Is this an acceptable practice? Why or why not?
- How might Brenda keep an accounting of money taken from the petty cash drawer if she is not the person actually in control of it?

Payroll Records. The payroll record is an auxiliary disbursement record. A separate page or card for each employee, as well as a summary record, should be kept. This procedure is discussed in more detail later in this chapter.

Comparison of Common Bookkeeping Systems

Success in bookkeeping requires a thorough understanding of the system and what it is expected to accomplish. There are many variations in bookkeeping systems, from simple to complex, no one of which can meet the needs of every physician. The basic principles are the same for all; only the system of recording varies. The three most common systems found in the professional office are:

- Single-entry
- Double-entry
- Pegboard or write-it-once

An overview of the three systems is presented here. More detailed instruction for the pegboard system, the most widely used manual system in medical practices, is found in Chapter 14.

Single-Entry System

Single-entry bookkeeping is inexpensive, is simple to use, and requires very little training. It is the oldest and simplest of bookkeeping systems and includes at least three basic records:

- A general journal, also called a daily log, daybook, day sheet, daily journal, or charge journal.
- A cash payment journal, which in its simplest form is a checkbook.
- An accounts receivable ledger, which is a record of the amounts owed by all the patients. The accounts receivable ledger may be a bound book, a loose-leaf binder, a card file, or loose pages in a ledger tray.
- There may also be auxiliary records for petty cash and payroll records.

The records of charges and receipts are usually entered into a bound journal with a page for each day of the year, monthly summary pages, and an annual summary. Daily pages have columns for entering each transaction that show the patient's name, the service performed and the charge, any payments received, and the totals for charges and receipts. The daily totals are entered on the monthly summary, and the monthly totals are carried forward to the annual summary.

The same bound book may also have space for recording cash payments, or the checkbook may be the only cash payment journal. Monthly and annual summaries would be done from the checkbook.

The accounts receivable ledger usually consists of an account card for each patient on which are entered the charges and payments from the general journal. The patients' statements are prepared from these cards. In a single-entry system, each entry is made separately.

Although the single-entry system may satisfy the requirements for reporting to government agencies, it does have some drawbacks:

- Errors are not easily detected.
- There are no built-in controls.
- Periodic analyses are inadequate for financial planning.

The single-entry system was at one time widely used in healthcare facilities but has been largely replaced by more complete accounting systems.

Double-Entry System

Double-entry bookkeeping is also inexpensive but requires a trained and experienced bookkeeper or the regular services of an accountant. The transactions may be recorded manually or by computer. In addition to the basic journals used in a single-entry system, there may be numerous subsidiary journals. The system is based on the accounting equation:

Assets = Liabilities + Proprietorship (Capital)

Every transaction requires an entry on each side of the accounting equation, and the two sides must always be in balance. For this reason the system is called double-entry bookkeeping. It is the most complete of the three systems. An understanding of the basics of double-entry bookkeeping will help to clarify the principles of all systems.

Assets are the properties owned by a business, such as bank accounts, accounts receivable, buildings, equipment, and furniture. The rights to these assets are called **equities**. The equity of the owner is called *capital*, *proprietorship*, or *owner's equity*. The equities of the creditors to whom money is owed are called **liabilities**. The owner's equity or capital is what remains of the value of the assets after the creditor's equities or liabilities have been subtracted.

For example, if the physician purchased equipment for $1000, paid $250 down, and gave a promissory note for $750, the accounting equation would be:

$$\text{Assets} \quad \$1000 = \begin{array}{l} \text{Liabilities} \quad \$750 \\ + \\ \underline{\text{Capital} \quad \underline{\quad 250}} \\ \$1000 \end{array}$$

$$\underline{\$1000}$$

The total value of the asset is $1000. The owner's equity is $250, and the creditor's equity is $750. The accounting terms *capital*, *proprietorship*, *owner's equity*, and *net worth* are used interchangeably.

Few medical assistants are trained in accounting. If a double-entry system is used, a practice management consultant or the accountant who does most of the actual bookwork and reports usually sets it up. The medical assistant in this instance generally maintains only the daily journal, from which the accountant takes the figures once a month.

The double-entry system provides a more comprehensive picture of the practice and its effect on the physician's net worth. Errors show up readily, and there are many built-in accuracy controls; however, because of the time and skill required, it is not frequently used in the small practice.

Pegboard or Write-It-Once System

The pegboard is the most commonly used manual method of accounting in the physician's office. It is discussed at length in Chapter 14.

CRITICAL THINKING APPLICATION

- Mr. Schmidt has taught Brenda all three types of accounting systems. Which seems to be the easiest system to use in the medical office? What is the basis for this choice?

End-of-the-Day Summarizing

Most computer accounting systems will perform end-of-the-day summarizing automatically. If the office uses the pegboard system, the bottom of the day sheet has three sections to be completed that will show that the accounts have balanced for the day.

The first section is the proof of posting section, which deals with the transactions that occurred today on the day sheet. In the second section, the month-to-date accounts receivable proof, today's totals are being added to the month-to-date totals, and should balance to the penny. The last section is the year-to-date accounts receivable proof, which adds the accounts, including today's totals, to the year-to-date total.

Most systems also have a deposit ticket, which can be double-checked when adding the cash receipts and the checks. This is handy when preparing the day's deposit.

The totals at the bottom of the second and third sections must be an exact equal. When the end-of-the-day summarizing does not balance, the medical assistant should first check the addition of each column, both horizontally and vertically. This will result in finding most errors (Figure 23-2). Be sure that the instructions are followed to the letter. To avoid frustrating mistakes, it is best to use a calculator, even when adding small numbers.

Trial Balance of Accounts Receivable

A trial balance should be done once per month *after* all posting has been completed and *before* preparing the monthly statements. The purpose of a trial balance is to disclose any discrepancies between the journal and the ledger. It does not prove the accuracy of the accounts. For example, if a charge or payment was posted to the wrong account, or if the wrong amount was entered in the journal and then posted to the ledger, the totals would still "balance," but the accounts would not be accurate.

To begin, pull all the account cards that have a balance, enter each balance on the adding machine, and total the figures. This should equal the accounts receivable balance figure on the control. If there is no daily control, total all of the charges, all of the payments, and all of the adjustments for the month, and then do the computation illustrated below. The end-of-the-month accounts receivable figure must agree with the figure arrived at by adding all

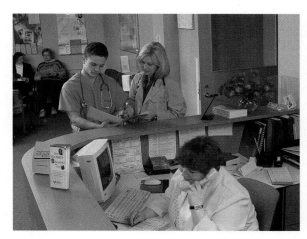

FIGURE 23-2   Ask the physician when unsure about financial information. When an unfamiliar statement arrives, check with the physician to be sure it should be paid.

the account card balances. The accounts are then said to be **in balance**. If the two totals do not agree, the error must be located.

Example of Balancing End-of-Month Accounts Receivable

Accounts receivable at first of month	$ _____
Plus total charges for month	$ _____
Subtotal	$ _____
Less total payments for month	$ _____
Subtotal	$ _____
Less total adjustments for month	$ _____
Accounts receivable at end of month	$ _____

Locating and Preventing Errors

After checking the tape and verifying that there is no error in calculation, the first step in locating an error in the trial balance is to find the difference between the two totals. Then search the daily journal pages and the account cards for an entry of the identical amount. Check each one found, and verify that it was posted correctly. Of course, there may be more than one error that adds up to this amount.

If there is only one error, and the amount of the error is divisible by 9, a figure may have been transposed. For example, if the difference is $81 (a number divisible by 9), the person who posted to the account may have written $209 instead of $290. If the amount of the error is divisible by 2, the amount may have been posted to the wrong column, reversing a debit and a credit.

A common error is made by entering the wrong amount in the previous balance column or in figuring the new balance. This kind of error will show up on the pegboard daily proof but could easily go undetected in the single-entry system. Carrying forward the wrong amount results in another common error total from one day to the next (e.g., carrying forward the beginning accounts receivable total rather than the ending accounts receivable total). There is always a chance of sliding a number, which means writing the first digit in the wrong column, such as writing 400 for 40 or 60 instead of 600.

Many bookkeepers avoid errors in the cents column by using a line (—) instead of writing two zeros when only even dollars are involved. For example, instead of writing $12.00, the bookkeeper will write $12.—. This eliminates the possibility of misreading zeros as other numbers. It also speeds the adding process when columns must be totaled.

If the medical assistant is unable to locate any numerical error, there is the possibility that an account card was lost or overlooked or was transferred as paid in full.

CRITICAL THINKING APPLICATION

- What should Brenda do if she has repeatedly reviewed records in search of an error and is still unable to find it?
- Who should this be reported to?

Accounts Payable Procedures

Invoices and Statements

When an item is not paid for at the time of purchase, the vendor usually includes a **packing slip** with delivery of the merchandise. A packing slip describes the items enclosed. The vendor may also enclose an **invoice**. An invoice describes the items and shows the amount due. Always check to verify that the items listed on the packing slip and invoice are included in the delivery.

Invoices should be placed in a special folder until paid. The facility may be making more than one purchase from the same vendor during the month. Some vendors request that payment be made from the invoice; others expect to send a **statement** later. A statement is a request for payment.

Paying for Purchases

At the time of payment, compare the statement with the invoice to verify accuracy, fasten the statement and invoice together, write the date and check number on the statement, and place it in the paid file.

CRITICAL THINKING APPLICATION

- Brenda does not recall ordering a certain item from the office supply company. However, it was included in her last shipment and listed on the packing list. How can she recount whether the item was ordered?
- How would Brenda correct this problem if the item was in fact not ordered?

Recording Disbursements

Both the pegboard and the single-entry bookkeeping systems provide pages for recording disbursements. This is sometimes called a check register. On these pages, disbursements are distributed to specific expense accounts such as:

- Auto expense
- Dues and meetings
- Equipment
- Insurance
- Medical supplies
- Office expenses
- Printing, postage, and stationery
- Rent and maintenance
- Salaries
- Taxes and licenses
- Travel and entertainment
- Utilities
- Miscellaneous
- Personal withdrawals

Each check should be entered on the disbursement page, showing the date, the name of the company to which the check was written, the number and amount of the check, and the payment allocated to one or more of the expense accounts. It is important to separate personal expenditures from business expenses. Business expenses are tax deductible and are considered in determining net income from the practice, but personal expenditures are not. Although personal expenses are not deductible in determining net income from the practice, some qualify as personal deductions in computing personal income tax, so a careful accounting should be kept. Deductible expenses would include property taxes, interest paid out, contributions, and so forth.

Accounting for Petty Cash

The petty cash fund is a revolving fund (Procedure 23-1). It does not change in amount except to increase or decrease the established fund. To establish the petty cash fund, a check is written payable to Cash or Petty Cash and entered in the disbursements journal under Miscellaneous. This is the only time that the petty cash check is charged to Miscellaneous.

Each time the fund is replenished, the amount of the check is spread among the various accounts for which the money was used. This is determined from a record of expenditures. The headings of the columns should correspond to headings in the disbursements journal to which they will be posted.

A pad of petty cash vouchers is kept in or near the cash box. For every disbursement from the fund, the petty cashier should either have a receipt or prepare a voucher. The total of the petty cash vouchers and receipts plus the amount of cash in the box must always equal the original amount of the fund.

At the end of the month, or sooner if the fund is depleted, a check is written to Cash for replenishing the fund, but instead of being charged to Miscellaneous as previously, the amount of the check is divided among the various accounts affected.

PROCEDURE 23-1

Accounting for Petty Cash

GOAL: To establish a petty cash fund, maintain an accurate record of expenditures for 1 month, and replenish the fund as necessary.

EQUIPMENT AND SUPPLIES

- Form for petty cash fund
- Pad of vouchers
- Disbursement journal
- Two checks
- List of petty cash expenditures

PROCEDURAL STEPS

1 Determine the amount needed in the petty cash fund.

2 Write a check in the determined amount.
Purpose: To establish a fund.

3 Record the beginning balance in the petty cash fund.

4 Post the amount to Miscellaneous on the disbursement record.
Purpose: To account for the original amount in the fund.

5 Prepare a petty cash voucher for each amount withdrawn from the fund.
Purpose: The vouchers will be used for internal audit.

6 Record each voucher in the petty cash record and enter the new balance.
Purpose: To record current balance and determine the need for replenishing the fund.

7 Write a check to replenish the fund as necessary.
Note: The total of the vouchers plus the fund balance must equal the beginning amount.

8 Total the expense columns and post to the appropriate accounts in the disbursement record.
Purpose: To record expenditures in the correct expense category.

9 Record the amount added to the fund.

10 Record the new balance in the petty cash fund.

Avoid the habit of borrowing from the petty cash fund. This admonition applies to the physician as well as to the medical assistant. If the physician requests cash from the fund, request a personal check or an office check in exchange for cash from the fund. It is also poor policy to use the petty cash fund for making change. In facilities where patients frequently pay with currency, a separate change fund should be kept.

Periodic Summaries

Financial summaries are compiled on monthly and annual bases. They may be prepared either by the medical assistant manually or on the computer or by the accountant. Common summary reports include:

- Statement of income and expense
- Cash flow statement
- Trial balance
- Accounts receivable trial balance and aging analysis
- Balance sheet

The **statement of income and expense** is also known as the profit and loss statement and covers a specific period. It lists all the income received and all expenses paid during the period. The total income is called gross income or earnings. The income after deduction of all expenses is the net income.

A **cash flow statement** starts with the amount of cash on hand at the beginning of the month (or for any specified period). It then lists the cash income and the cash disbursement made throughout the period, and concludes with a statement of the amount of cash remaining on hand at the end of the period.

A **trial balance** is necessary to determine that the books are in balance. All of the columns on the disbursements journal must be totaled at the end of the month. The combined totals of all the expense columns must be equal to the total of the checks written. If the figures do not balance, it is necessary to recheck every entry until an error is found.

The **accounts receivable trial balance** is done before sending out the monthly statements. First, record the total of the accounts receivable ledger at the end of the previous month; then add the charges for the current month and subtract the adjustments and the payments received. The remainder should equal the total of the accounts receivable ledger at the end of the current month.

The **balance sheet**, also known as a statement of financial condition, shows the financial picture of the practice on a specific date. Often, it is done only on an annual basis. The balance sheet is set up using the accounting equation:

Assets = Liabilities + Proprietorship

The title of the statement had its origin in the equality of the elements—the balance between the sum of the assets and the sum of the liabilities and proprietorship.

At the end of the accounting year, it is very simple to combine the monthly reports to compile the annual summaries. The annual summaries simplify the reporting of income for tax returns.

Payroll Records

Handling payroll records, whether for one employee or dozens of employees, involves frequent reporting activities (Procedure 23-2). Government regulations require the withholding of taxes from employees and payment of certain taxes due from both employees and employers. To comply with government regulations, complete records must be kept for every employee. All records of employment taxes must be kept for at least 4 years. These should be available for review by the Internal Revenue Service (IRS). Such records include the following:

- Social Security number of the employee
- Number of withholding allowances claimed
- Amount of gross salary
- All deductions for Social Security and Medicare taxes; federal, state, and city or other subdivision withholding taxes; state disability insurance; and state unemployment tax, where applicable

CRITICAL THINKING APPLICATION

- Brenda hired a new employee on Friday, who reported to work on Monday. The new employee states that she cannot produce her Social Security card. Can Brenda allow the individual to work?
- Investigate the procedures for verifying a Social Security number.

Payroll Reporting Forms

Each employee and each employer must have a tax identification number. The Social Security number is the employee's tax identification number. Any person who does not have a Social Security number should apply for one, using Form SS-5 available from any Social Security Administration office.

The employer applies for a number for federal tax accounting purposes using Form SS-4, available at Social Security Administration offices. In states that require employer reports, a state employer number must also be obtained.

PROCEDURE 23-2

Processing an Employee Payroll

GOAL: To process payroll and compensate employees, making deductions accurately.

EQUIPMENT AND SUPPLIES

- Checkbook
- Computer and payroll software, if applicable
- Pen
- Tax withholding tables
- Federal Employers Tax Guide

PROCEDURAL STEPS

1 Be sure that all information has been collected on the employees, including a copy of the Social Security card, a W-4 form, and an I-9 form.
Purpose: To make certain that the employee is eligible to work in the United States, and to determine what withholding amounts should be deducted from paychecks.

2 Review the time cards for all employees. Determine if any employees need counseling due to late arrivals or habitual absences.
Purpose: To address problem issues immediately and help to correct habits that can lead to employee termination.

3 Figure the salary or hourly wages that are due the employee for the period worked.
Purpose: To ascertain the amount owed to the employee.

4 Figure the deductions that must be taken from the paycheck. This usually includes, but is not limited to:
- Federal, state, and local taxes
- Social Security withholdings
- Medicare withholdings
- Other deductions, such as insurance, savings, and so forth
- Donations to organizations, such as the United Way

Purpose: To comply with federal, state, and local laws and deduct amounts for insurance, savings plans, and so forth.

5 Write the check for the balance due the employee. Most software programs can print the checks and explanations of deductions.

6 Have employees sign for their paychecks, if that is the policy of the office.

Before the end of the first pay period, the employee should complete an Employee's Withholding Allowance Certificate (Form W-4) showing the number of withholding allowances claimed (Figure 23-3). Otherwise, the employer must indicate withholding on the basis of a single person with no exemptions.

The employee should complete a new form when changes occur in marital status or in the number of allowances claimed. Each employee is entitled to one personal allowance and one for each qualified dependent. The employee may elect to take fewer or no allowances, in which case the tax withheld will be greater and a refund may be due when the employee's annual tax report is filed (Figure 23-4). If an employee claims more than 10 withholding allowances or an exemption from withholding and his or her wages would normally be more than $200 per week, the employer is required to send copies of these W-4 forms to the IRS.

A supply of all the necessary forms for filing federal returns, preprinted with the employer's name, will be furnished to an employer who has applied for an employer identification number. Extra forms may be obtained from the IRS office.

CRITICAL THINKING APPLICATION

- Mr. Schmidt has explained to Brenda that the more withholding deductions an employee claims, the less tax is taken from the paycheck. If Brenda's new employee wishes to claim seven deductions, and she only has three children and is single, could she do so legally?
- Why or why not?
- Why might it be risky to claim all of the deductions a person is legally entitled to?

Income Tax Withholding. Employers are required by law to withhold certain amounts from employees' earnings. These amounts must be reported and forwarded to the IRS to be applied toward payment of income tax. The amount to be withheld is based on the following:

- Total earnings of the employee
- Number of withholding allowances claimed
- Marital status of the employee
- Length of the pay period involved

The *Federal Employer's Tax Guide* includes tables to be used in determining the amount to be withheld. There is one table for single persons and unmarried heads of households and one for married persons. The tables cover monthly, semimonthly, biweekly, weekly, and daily or miscellaneous periods.

Employers Income Tax. The physician who is practicing as an individual is not subject to withholding tax but is expected to make an estimated tax payment four times a year. The accountant prepares four copies of Form 1040-S, Declaration of Estimated Tax for Individuals, for the ensuing year when the annual income tax return is prepared. The first form and the quarterly estimated tax for the next year are filed at the same time as the tax return. The remaining three forms, with the estimated tax due, must be filed on June 15, September 15, and January 15. It may be the business manager's responsibility to see that these returns are filed when due. The employer also contributes to Social Security and Medicare in the form of a self-employment tax.

Social Security, Medicare, and Income Tax Withholding. The Federal Insurance Contributions Act (FICA) provides for a federal system of old age, survivors, disability, and hospital insurance. The tax rate is reviewed frequently and is subject to change by Congress. As of 2001, the wage base for Social Security tax is $84,900 and the tax rate is 6.2% each for employers and employees. All wages are subject to the Medicare tax at a rate of 1.45% each for both employees and employers.

Quarterly Returns

Each quarter of the year, all employers who are subject to income tax withholding (including withholding on sick pay and supplemental unemployment benefits) of Social Security and Medicare taxes must file an Employer's Quarterly Federal Tax Return on or before the last day of the first month after the end of the quarter (Figure 23-5). Due dates for this return and full payment of the tax are April 30, July 31, October 31, and January 31. If deposits equaling full payment of taxes due have been made, the due date for the return is extended 10 days.

Annual Returns

The employer is required to furnish two copies of Form W-2, the Wage and Tax Statement, to each employee from whom income tax or Social Security tax has been withheld or from whom income tax would have been withheld if the employee had claimed no more than one withholding allowance. The forms should be given to employees by January 31. If employment ends before December 31, the employer may give the W-2 form to the terminated employee any time after employment ends. If the employee asks for Form W-2, the employer should give the employee the completed copies within 30 days of the request or the final wage payment, whichever is later.

Employers must file Form W-3, the Transmittal of Income and Tax Statement, annually to transmit wage and income tax withheld statements (Form W-2) to the Social Security Administration. These forms are processed by the Social Security Administration, which then furnishes the IRS with the income tax data that it needs from those forms. Form W-3 and its attachments must be filed separately from Form 941 on or before the last day of February after the calendar year for which the W-2 forms are prepared.

Federal Unemployment Tax

Employers also contribute under the Federal Unemployment Tax Act (FUTA). Generally, credit can be taken against the FUTA tax for amounts paid into a state unemployment fund up to a certain percentage. Employers are re-

Form W-4 (2002)

Purpose. Complete Form W-4 so your employer can withhold the correct Federal income tax from your pay. Because your tax situation may change, you may want to refigure your withholding each year.

Exemption from withholding. If you are exempt, complete only lines 1, 2, 3, 4, and 7 and sign the form to validate it. Your exemption for 2002 expires February 16, 2003. See **Pub. 505,** Tax Withholding and Estimated Tax.

Note: *You cannot claim exemption from withholding if (a) your income exceeds $750 and includes more than $250 of unearned income (e.g., interest and dividends) and (b) another person can claim you as a dependent on their tax return.*

Basic instructions. If you are not exempt, complete the **Personal Allowances Worksheet** below. The worksheets on page 2 adjust your withholding allowances based on itemized deductions, certain credits, adjustments to income, or two-earner/two-job situations. Complete all worksheets that apply. **However, you may claim fewer (or zero) allowances.**

Head of household. Generally, you may claim head of household filing status on your tax return only if you are unmarried and pay more than 50% of the costs of keeping up a home for yourself and your dependent(s) or other qualifying individuals. See line **E** below.

Tax credits. You can take projected tax credits into account in figuring your allowable number of withholding allowances. Credits for child or dependent care expenses and the child tax credit may be claimed using the **Personal Allowances Worksheet** below. See **Pub. 919,** How Do I Adjust My Tax Withholding? for information on converting your other credits into withholding allowances.

Nonwage income. If you have a large amount of nonwage income, such as interest or dividends, consider making estimated tax payments using **Form 1040-ES,** Estimated Tax for Individuals. Otherwise, you may owe additional tax.

Two earners/two jobs. If you have a working spouse or more than one job, figure the total number of allowances you are entitled to claim on all jobs using worksheets from only one Form W-4. Your withholding usually will be most accurate when all allowances are claimed on the Form W-4 for the highest paying job and zero allowances are claimed on the others.

Nonresident alien. If you are a nonresident alien, see the **Instructions for Form 8233** before completing this Form W-4.

Check your withholding. After your Form W-4 takes effect, use Pub. 919 to see how the dollar amount you are having withheld compares to your projected total tax for 2002. See Pub. 919, especially if you used the **Two-Earner/Two-Job Worksheet** on page 2 and your earnings exceed $125,000 (Single) or $175,000 (Married).

Recent name change? If your name on line 1 differs from that shown on your social security card, call 1-800-772-1213 for a new social security card.

Personal Allowances Worksheet (Keep for your records.)

A Enter "1" for **yourself** if no one else can claim you as a dependent . . . . **A** _____

B Enter "1" if:
- You are single and have only one job; or
- You are married, have only one job, and your spouse does not work; or
- Your wages from a second job or your spouse's wages (or the total of both) are $1,000 or less.

. . **B** _____

C Enter "1" for your **spouse.** But, you may choose to enter "-0-" if you are married and have either a working spouse or more than one job. (Entering "-0-" may help you avoid having too little tax withheld.). . . . . **C** _____

D Enter number of **dependents** (other than your spouse or yourself) you will claim on your tax return . . . . **D** _____

E Enter "1" if you will file as **head of household** on your tax return (see conditions under **Head of household** above) . **E** _____

F Enter "1" if you have at least $1,500 of **child or dependent care expenses** for which you plan to claim a credit . . **F** _____

(**Note:** *Do not include child support payments. See Pub. 503, Child and Dependent Care Expenses, for details.*)

G **Child Tax Credit** (including additional child tax credit):
- If your total income will be between $15,000 and $42,000 ($20,000 and $65,000 if married), enter "1" for each eligible child plus **1 additional** if you have three to five eligible children or **2 additional** if you have six or more eligible children.
- If your total income will be between $42,000 and $80,000 ($65,000 and $115,000 if married), enter "1" if you have one or two eligible children, "2" if you have three eligible children, "3" if you have four eligible children, or "4" if you have five or more eligible children. **G** _____

H Add lines A through G and enter total here. Note: *This may be different from the number of exemptions you claim on your tax return.* ▶ **H** _____

For accuracy, complete all worksheets that apply.
- If you plan to **itemize or claim adjustments to income** and want to reduce your withholding, see the **Deductions and Adjustments Worksheet** on page 2.
- If you have **more than one job** or are **married and you and your spouse both work** and the combined earnings from all jobs exceed $35,000, see the **Two-Earner/Two-Job Worksheet** on page 2 to avoid having too little tax withheld.
- If **neither** of the above situations applies, **stop here** and enter the number from line H on line 5 of Form W-4 below.

------------------------------ **Cut here and give Form W-4 to your employer. Keep the top part for your records.** ------------------------------

Form W-4

Department of the Treasury
Internal Revenue Service

Employee's Withholding Allowance Certificate

▶ **For Privacy Act and Paperwork Reduction Act Notice, see page 2.**

OMB No. 1545-0010

2002

1 Type or print your first name and middle initial Last name	2 Your social security number

Home address (number and street or rural route)

3 ☐ Single ☐ Married ☐ Married, but withhold at higher Single rate.
Note: *If married, but legally separated, or spouse is a nonresident alien, check the "Single" box.*

City or town, state, and ZIP code

4 If your last name differs from that on your social security card, check here. You must call 1-800-772-1213 for a new card. ▶ ☐

5 Total number of allowances you are claiming (from line **H** above **or** from the applicable worksheet on page 2) **5** _____

6 Additional amount, if any, you want withheld from each paycheck . . . . **6** $ _____

7 I claim exemption from withholding for 2002, and I certify that I meet **both** of the following conditions for exemption:
- Last year I had a right to a refund of **all** Federal income tax withheld because I had **no** tax liability **and**
- This year I expect a refund of **all** Federal income tax withheld because I expect to have **no** tax liability.

If you meet both conditions, write "Exempt" here . . . . ▶ **7** _____

Under penalties of perjury, I certify that I am entitled to the number of withholding allowances claimed on this certificate, or I am entitled to claim exempt status.

Employee's signature
(Form is not valid unless you sign it.) ▶

Date ▶

8 Employer's name and address (Employer: Complete lines 8 and 10 only if sending to the IRS.)

9 Office code (optional)

10 Employer identification number

Cat. No. 10220Q

FIGURE 23-3   IRS Form W-4: Employee's Withholding Allowance Certificate.

Form W-4 (2002)   Page **2**

Deductions and Adjustments Worksheet

Note: *Use this worksheet only if you plan to itemize deductions, claim certain credits, or claim adjustments to income on your 2002 tax return.*

1 Enter an estimate of your 2002 itemized deductions. These include qualifying home mortgage interest, charitable contributions, state and local taxes, medical expenses in excess of 7.5% of your income, and miscellaneous deductions. (For 2002, you may have to reduce your itemized deductions if your income is over $137,300 ($68,650 if married filing separately). See **Worksheet 3** in Pub. 919 for details.) . . . **1** $ _____

2 Enter:
{ $7,850 if married filing jointly or qualifying widow(er)
$6,900 if head of household
$4,700 if single
$3,925 if married filing separately } . . . . **2** $ _____

3 **Subtract** line 2 from line 1. If line 2 is greater than line 1, enter "-0-" . . . . **3** $ _____

4 Enter an estimate of your 2002 adjustments to income, including alimony, deductible IRA contributions, and student loan interest **4** $ _____

5 **Add** lines 3 and 4 and enter the total. Include any amount for credits from **Worksheet 7** in Pub. 919. **5** $ _____

6 Enter an estimate of your 2002 nonwage income (such as dividends or interest) . . . . **6** $ _____

7 **Subtract** line 6 from line 5. Enter the result, but not less than "-0-" . . . . **7** $ _____

8 **Divide** the amount on line 7 by $3,000 and enter the result here. Drop any fraction . . . . . . **8** _____

9 Enter the number from the **Personal Allowances Worksheet,** line H, page 1 . . . . . . **9** _____

10 **Add** lines 8 and 9 and enter the total here. If you plan to use the **Two-Earner/Two-Job Worksheet,** also enter this total on line 1 below. Otherwise, **stop here** and enter this total on Form W-4, line 5, page 1 . **10** _____

Two-Earner/Two-Job Worksheet

Note: *Use this worksheet only if the instructions under line H on page 1 direct you here.*

1 Enter the number from line H, page 1 (or from line 10 above if you used the **Deductions and Adjustments Worksheet**) **1** _____

2 Find the number in **Table 1** below that applies to the **lowest** paying job and enter it here . . . . . **2** _____

3 If line 1 is **more than or equal to** line 2, subtract line 2 from line 1. Enter the result here (if zero, enter "-0-") and on Form W-4, line 5, page 1. **Do not** use the rest of this worksheet . . . . **3** _____

Note: *If line 1 is **less than** line 2, enter "-0-" on Form W-4, line 5, page 1. Complete lines 4–9 below to calculate the additional withholding amount necessary to avoid a year end tax bill.*

4 Enter the number from line 2 of this worksheet . . . . **4** _____

5 Enter the number from line 1 of this worksheet . . . . **5** _____

6 **Subtract** line 5 from line 4 . . . . **6** _____

7 Find the amount in **Table 2** below that applies to the **highest** paying job and enter it here . . . . . **7** $ _____

8 **Multiply** line 7 by line 6 and enter the result here. This is the additional annual withholding needed . . **8** $ _____

9 Divide line 8 by the number of pay periods remaining in 2002. For example, divide by 26 if you are paid every two weeks and you complete this form in December 2001. Enter the result here and on Form W-4, line 6, page 1. This is the additional amount to be withheld from each paycheck . . . . **9** $ _____

Table 1: Two-Earner/Two-Job Worksheet

Married Filing Jointly				All Others			
If wages from **LOWEST** paying job are—	Enter on line 2 above	If wages from **LOWEST** paying job are—	Enter on line 2 above	If wages from **LOWEST** paying job are—	Enter on line 2 above	If wages from **LOWEST** paying job are—	Enter on line 2 above
$0 - $4,000	0	44,001 - 50,000	8	$0 - $6,000	0	75,001 - 95,000	8
4,001 - 9,000	1	50,001 - 55,000	9	6,001 - 11,000	1	95,001 - 110,000	9
9,001 - 15,000	2	55,001 - 65,000	10	11,001 - 17,000	2	110,001 and over	10
15,001 - 20,000	3	65,001 - 80,000	11	17,001 - 23,000	3		
20,001 - 25,000	4	80,001 - 95,000	12	23,001 - 28,000	4		
25,001 - 32,000	5	95,001 - 110,000	13	28,001 - 38,000	5		
32,001 - 38,000	6	110,001 - 125,000	14	38,001 - 55,000	6		
38,001 - 44,000	7	125,001 and over	15	55,001 - 75,000	7		

Table 2: Two-Earner/Two-Job Worksheet

Married Filing Jointly		All Others	
If wages from **HIGHEST** paying job are—	Enter on line 7 above	If wages from **HIGHEST** paying job are—	Enter on line 7 above
$0 - $50,000	$450	$0 - $30,000	$450
50,001 - 100,000	800	30,001 - 70,000	800
100,001 - 150,000	900	70,001 - 140,000	900
150,001 - 270,000	1,050	140,001 - 300,000	1,050
270,001 and over	1,150	300,001 and over	1,150

FIGURE 23-3—Cont'd   For legend see previous page.

SINGLE Persons—WEEKLY Payroll Period
(For Wages Paid in 2002)

If the wages are—		And the number of withholding allowances claimed is—										
At least	But less than	0	1	2	3	4	5	6	7	8	9	10
		The amount of income tax to be withheld is—										
$0	$55	$0	$0	$0	$0	$0	$0	$0	$0	$0	$0	$0
55	60	1	0	0	0	0	0	0	0	0	0	0
60	65	1	0	0	0	0	0	0	0	0	0	0
65	70	2	0	0	0	0	0	0	0	0	0	0
70	75	2	0	0	0	0	0	0	0	0	0	0
75	80	3	0	0	0	0	0	0	0	0	0	0
80	85	3	0	0	0	0	0	0	0	0	0	0
85	90	4	0	0	0	0	0	0	0	0	0	0
90	95	4	0	0	0	0	0	0	0	0	0	0
95	100	5	0	0	0	0	0	0	0	0	0	0
100	105	5	0	0	0	0	0	0	0	0	0	0
105	110	6	0	0	0	0	0	0	0	0	0	0
110	115	6	0	0	0	0	0	0	0	0	0	0
115	120	7	1	0	0	0	0	0	0	0	0	0
120	125	7	1	0	0	0	0	0	0	0	0	0
125	130	8	2	0	0	0	0	0	0	0	0	0
130	135	8	2	0	0	0	0	0	0	0	0	0
135	140	9	3	0	0	0	0	0	0	0	0	0
140	145	9	3	0	0	0	0	0	0	0	0	0
145	150	10	4	0	0	0	0	0	0	0	0	0
150	155	10	4	0	0	0	0	0	0	0	0	0
155	160	11	5	0	0	0	0	0	0	0	0	0
160	165	11	5	0	0	0	0	0	0	0	0	0
165	170	12	6	0	0	0	0	0	0	0	0	0
170	175	13	6	1	0	0	0	0	0	0	0	0
175	180	13	7	1	0	0	0	0	0	0	0	0
180	185	14	7	2	0	0	0	0	0	0	0	0
185	190	15	8	2	0	0	0	0	0	0	0	0
190	195	16	8	3	0	0	0	0	0	0	0	0
195	200	16	9	3	0	0	0	0	0	0	0	0
200	210	17	10	4	0	0	0	0	0	0	0	0
210	220	19	11	5	0	0	0	0	0	0	0	0
220	230	20	12	6	0	0	0	0	0	0	0	0
230	240	22	13	7	1	0	0	0	0	0	0	0
240	250	23	15	8	2	0	0	0	0	0	0	0
250	260	25	16	9	3	0	0	0	0	0	0	0
260	270	26	18	10	4	0	0	0	0	0	0	0
270	280	28	19	11	5	0	0	0	0	0	0	0
280	290	29	21	12	6	0	0	0	0	0	0	0
290	300	31	22	14	7	1	0	0	0	0	0	0
300	310	32	24	15	8	2	0	0	0	0	0	0
310	320	34	25	17	9	3	0	0	0	0	0	0
320	330	35	27	18	10	4	0	0	0	0	0	0
330	340	37	28	20	11	5	0	0	0	0	0	0
340	350	38	30	21	12	6	1	0	0	0	0	0
350	360	40	31	23	14	7	2	0	0	0	0	0
360	370	41	33	24	15	8	3	0	0	0	0	0
370	380	43	34	26	17	9	4	0	0	0	0	0
380	390	44	36	27	18	10	5	0	0	0	0	0
390	400	46	37	29	20	11	6	0	0	0	0	0
400	410	47	39	30	21	13	7	1	0	0	0	0
410	420	49	40	32	23	14	8	2	0	0	0	0
420	430	50	42	33	24	16	9	3	0	0	0	0
430	440	52	43	35	26	17	10	4	0	0	0	0
440	450	53	45	36	27	19	11	5	0	0	0	0
450	460	55	46	38	29	20	12	6	0	0	0	0
460	470	56	48	39	30	22	13	7	1	0	0	0
470	480	58	49	41	32	23	15	8	2	0	0	0
480	490	59	51	42	33	25	16	9	3	0	0	0
490	500	61	52	44	35	26	18	10	4	0	0	0
500	510	62	54	45	36	28	19	11	5	0	0	0
510	520	64	55	47	38	29	21	12	6	0	0	0
520	530	65	57	48	39	31	22	14	7	1	0	0
530	540	67	58	50	41	32	24	15	8	2	0	0
540	550	68	60	51	42	34	25	17	9	3	0	0
550	560	70	61	53	44	35	27	18	10	4	0	0
560	570	71	63	54	45	37	28	20	11	5	0	0
570	580	74	64	56	47	38	30	21	12	6	0	0
580	590	76	66	57	48	40	31	23	14	7	1	0
590	600	79	67	59	50	41	33	24	15	8	2	0

FIGURE 23-4   Pages from the 2002 Withholding Tax Table.

sponsible for paying the FUTA tax; it must not be deducted from employees' wages. For 1998 the FUTA tax was 6.2% of the first $7,000 in wages paid to each employee during the calendar year.

For deposit purposes, the FUTA tax is figured quarterly, and any amount due must be paid by the last day of the first month after the quarter ends. The formula for determining the amount due is set forth in the Federal Employer's Tax Guide.

An annual FUTA return must be filed on Form 940 on or before January 31 following the close of the calendar year for which the tax is due (Figure 23-6). Any tax still

MARRIED Persons—MONTHLY Payroll Period
(For Wages Paid in 2002)

| If the wages are— | | And the number of withholding allowances claimed is— | | | | | | | | | | |
At least	But less than	0	1	2	3	4	5	6	7	8	9	10
		The amount of income tax to be withheld is—										
$0	$540	$0	$0	$0	$0	$0	$0	$0	$0	$0	$0	$0
540	560	1	0	0	0	0	0	0	0	0	0	0
560	580	3	0	0	0	0	0	0	0	0	0	0
580	600	5	0	0	0	0	0	0	0	0	0	0
600	640	8	0	0	0	0	0	0	0	0	0	0
640	680	12	0	0	0	0	0	0	0	0	0	0
680	720	16	0	0	0	0	0	0	0	0	0	0
720	760	20	0	0	0	0	0	0	0	0	0	0
760	800	24	0	0	0	0	0	0	0	0	0	0
800	840	28	3	0	0	0	0	0	0	0	0	0
840	880	32	7	0	0	0	0	0	0	0	0	0
880	920	36	11	0	0	0	0	0	0	0	0	0
920	960	40	15	0	0	0	0	0	0	0	0	0
960	1,000	44	19	0	0	0	0	0	0	0	0	0
1,000	1,040	48	23	0	0	0	0	0	0	0	0	0
1,040	1,080	52	27	2	0	0	0	0	0	0	0	0
1,080	1,120	56	31	6	0	0	0	0	0	0	0	0
1,120	1,160	60	35	10	0	0	0	0	0	0	0	0
1,160	1,200	64	39	14	0	0	0	0	0	0	0	0
1,200	1,240	68	43	18	0	0	0	0	0	0	0	0
1,240	1,280	72	47	22	0	0	0	0	0	0	0	0
1,280	1,320	76	51	26	1	0	0	0	0	0	0	0
1,320	1,360	80	55	30	5	0	0	0	0	0	0	0
1,360	1,400	84	59	34	9	0	0	0	0	0	0	0
1,400	1,440	88	63	38	13	0	0	0	0	0	0	0
1,440	1,480	92	67	42	17	0	0	0	0	0	0	0
1,480	1,520	96	71	46	21	0	0	0	0	0	0	0
1,520	1,560	100	75	50	25	0	0	0	0	0	0	0
1,560	1,600	106	79	54	29	4	0	0	0	0	0	0
1,600	1,640	112	83	58	33	8	0	0	0	0	0	0
1,640	1,680	118	87	62	37	12	0	0	0	0	0	0
1,680	1,720	124	91	66	41	16	0	0	0	0	0	0
1,720	1,760	130	95	70	45	20	0	0	0	0	0	0
1,760	1,800	136	99	74	49	24	0	0	0	0	0	0
1,800	1,840	142	105	78	53	28	3	0	0	0	0	0
1,840	1,880	148	111	82	57	32	7	0	0	0	0	0
1,880	1,920	154	117	86	61	36	11	0	0	0	0	0
1,920	1,960	160	123	90	65	40	15	0	0	0	0	0
1,960	2,000	166	129	94	69	44	19	0	0	0	0	0
2,000	2,040	172	135	98	73	48	23	0	0	0	0	0
2,040	2,080	178	141	103	77	52	27	2	0	0	0	0
2,080	2,120	184	147	109	81	56	31	6	0	0	0	0
2,120	2,160	190	153	115	85	60	35	10	0	0	0	0
2,160	2,200	196	159	121	89	64	39	14	0	0	0	0
2,200	2,240	202	165	127	93	68	43	18	0	0	0	0
2,240	2,280	208	171	133	97	72	47	22	0	0	0	0
2,280	2,320	214	177	139	102	76	51	26	1	0	0	0
2,320	2,360	220	183	145	108	80	55	30	5	0	0	0
2,360	2,400	226	189	151	114	84	59	34	9	0	0	0
2,400	2,440	232	195	157	120	88	63	38	13	0	0	0
2,440	2,480	238	201	163	126	92	67	42	17	0	0	0
2,480	2,520	244	207	169	132	96	71	46	21	0	0	0
2,520	2,560	250	213	175	138	100	75	50	25	0	0	0
2,560	2,600	256	219	181	144	106	79	54	29	4	0	0
2,600	2,640	262	225	187	150	112	83	58	33	8	0	0
2,640	2,680	268	231	193	156	118	87	62	37	12	0	0
2,680	2,720	274	237	199	162	124	91	66	41	16	0	0
2,720	2,760	280	243	205	168	130	95	70	45	20	0	0
2,760	2,800	286	249	211	174	136	99	74	49	24	0	0
2,800	2,840	292	255	217	180	142	105	78	53	28	3	0
2,840	2,880	298	261	223	186	148	111	82	57	32	7	0
2,880	2,920	304	267	229	192	154	117	86	61	36	11	0
2,920	2,960	310	273	235	198	160	123	90	65	40	15	0
2,960	3,000	316	279	241	204	166	129	94	69	44	19	0
3,000	3,040	322	285	247	210	172	135	98	73	48	23	0
3,040	3,080	328	291	253	216	178	141	103	77	52	27	2
3,080	3,120	334	297	259	222	184	147	109	81	56	31	6
3,120	3,160	340	303	265	228	190	153	115	85	60	35	10
3,160	3,200	346	309	271	234	196	159	121	89	64	39	14
3,200	3,240	352	315	277	240	202	165	127	93	68	43	18

FIGURE 23-4—Cont'd   For legend see previous page.

due is payable with the return. Form 940 may be filed on or before February 10 following the close of the year, if all required deposits were made on time and if full payment of the tax due is deposited on or before January 31.

State Unemployment Taxes

All of the states and the District of Columbia have unemployment compensation laws. In most states, the tax is imposed only on the employer, but a few states require employers to withhold a percentage of wages for unem-

Form **941**
(Rev. January 2002)
Department of the Treasury
Internal Revenue Service (99)

Employer's Quarterly Federal Tax Return

▶ **See separate instructions revised January 2002 for information on completing this return.**

Please type or print.

Enter state code for state in which deposits were made **only** if different from state in address to the right ▶ (see page 2 of instructions).

Name (as distinguished from trade name)

Trade name, if any

Address (number and street)

Date quarter ended

Employer identification number

City, state, and ZIP code

OMB No. 1545-0029

T	
FF	
FD	
FP	
I	
T	

If address is different from prior return, check here ▶

IRS Use

1 1 1 1 1 1 1 1 1 1 1   2   3 3 3 3 3 3 3   4 4 4   5 5 5

6   7   8 8 8 8 8 8 8   9 9 9 9 9   10 10 10 10 10 10 10 10 10 10

If you do not have to file returns in the future, check here ▶ ☐   and enter date final wages paid ▶

If you are a seasonal employer, see **Seasonal employers** on page 1 of the instructions and check here ▶

1	Number of employees in the pay period that includes March 12th . ▶	**1**
2	Total wages and tips, plus other compensation	**2**
3	Total income tax withheld from wages, tips, and sick pay	**3**
4	Adjustment of withheld income tax for preceding quarters of calendar year	**4**
5	Adjusted total of income tax withheld (line 3 as adjusted by line 4—see instructions)	**5**
6	Taxable social security wages . . . . . **6a** × 12.4% (.124) = **6b**	
	Taxable social security tips . . . . . . **6c** × 12.4% (.124) = **6d**	
7	Taxable Medicare wages and tips . . . **7a** × 2.9% (.029) = **7b**	
8	Total social security and Medicare taxes (add lines 6b, 6d, and 7b). Check here if wages are not subject to social security and/or Medicare tax . . . . ▶ ☐	**8**
9	Adjustment of social security and Medicare taxes (see instructions for required explanation) Sick Pay $ _____ ± Fractions of Cents $ _____ ± Other $ _____ =	**9**
10	Adjusted total of social security and Medicare taxes (line 8 as adjusted by line 9—see instructions)	**10**
11	**Total taxes** (add lines 5 and 10)	**11**
12	Advance earned income credit (EIC) payments made to employees	**12**
13	Net taxes (subtract line 12 from line 11). **If $2,500 or more, this must equal line 17, column (d) below (or line D of Schedule B (Form 941))**	**13**
14	Total deposits for quarter, including overpayment applied from a prior quarter	**14**
15	**Balance due** (subtract line 14 from line 13). See instructions	**15**
16	**Overpayment.** If line 14 is more than line 13, enter excess here ▶ $ _____	

and check if to be: ☐ Applied to next return   **or**   ☐ Refunded.

- **All filers:** If line 13 is less than $2,500, you need not complete line 17 or Schedule B (Form 941).
- **Semiweekly schedule depositors:** Complete Schedule B (Form 941) and check here . . . . ▶ ☐
- **Monthly schedule depositors:** Complete line 17, columns (a) through (d), and check here. . . . . ▶ ☐

17	**Monthly Summary of Federal Tax Liability.** Do not complete if you were a semiweekly schedule depositor.		
(a) First month liability	**(b)** Second month liability	**(c)** Third month liability	**(d)** Total liability for quarter

Third Party Designee

Do you want to allow another person to discuss this return with the IRS (see separate instructions)?   ☐ **Yes.** Complete the following.   ☐ **No**

Designee's name ▶   Phone no. ▶ ( )   Personal identification number (PIN) ▶

Sign Here

Under penalties of perjury, I declare that I have examined this return, including accompanying schedules and statements, and to the best of my knowledge and belief, it is true, correct, and complete.

Signature ▶   Print Your Name and Title ▶   Date ▶

For Privacy Act and Paperwork Reduction Act Notice, see back of Payment Voucher.   Cat. No. 17001Z   Form **941** (Rev. 1-2002)

FIGURE 23-5   IRS Form 941: Employer's Quarterly Federal Tax Return.

Form 941
Payment Voucher

Purpose of Form

Complete Form 941-V if you are making a payment with **Form 941,** Employer's Quarterly Federal Tax Return. We will use the completed voucher to credit your payment more promptly and accurately, and to improve our service to you.

If you have your return prepared by a third party and make a payment with that return, please provide this payment voucher to the return preparer.

Making Payments With Form 941

Make payments with Form 941 only if:

1. Your net taxes for the quarter (line 13 on Form 941) are less than $2,500 and you are paying in full with a timely filed return or

2. You are a monthly schedule depositor making a payment in accordance with the **accuracy of deposits** rule. (See section 11 of **Circular E,** Employer's Tax Guide, for details.) This amount may be $2,500 or more.

Otherwise, you must deposit the amount at an authorized financial institution or by electronic funds transfer. (See section 11 of Circular E for deposit instructions.) Do not use the Form 941-V payment voucher to make Federal tax deposits.

Caution: *If you pay amounts with Form 941 that should have been deposited, you may be subject to a penalty. See Circular E.*

Specific Instructions

Box 1—Employer identification number (EIN). If you do not have an EIN, apply for one on **Form SS-4,** Application for Employer Identification Number, and write "Applied for" and the date you applied in this entry space.

Box 2—Amount paid. Enter the amount paid with Form 941.

Box 3—Tax period. Darken the capsule identifying the quarter for which the payment is made. Darken only one capsule.

Box 4—Name and address. Enter your name and address as shown on Form 941.

● Make your check or money order payable to the United States Treasury. Be sure to enter your EIN, "Form 941," and the tax period on your check or money order. Do not send cash. Please do not staple this voucher or your payment to the return or to each other.

● Detach the completed voucher and send it with your payment and Form 941 to the address provided on the back of Form 941.

▼ **Detach Here and Mail With Your Payment** ▼   Form **941-V** (2002)

Form 941-V   Department of the Treasury Internal Revenue Service (99)

Payment Voucher

▶ **Do not staple or attach this voucher to your payment.**

OMB No. 1545-0029

2002

1 Enter your employer identification number

2 Enter the amount of the payment | Dollars | Cents

3 Tax period

⟋ 1st Quarter   ⟋ 3rd Quarter

⟋ 2nd Quarter   ⟋ 4th Quarter

4 Enter your business name (individual name if sole proprietor)

Enter your address

Enter your city, state, and ZIP code

FIGURE 23-5—Cont'd   For legend see previous page.

---

ployment compensation benefits. An employer may be subject to federal unemployment tax and not subject to state unemployment tax. In some states, for instance, the employer with fewer than four employees is not subject to the state unemployment tax. The regulations for a specific state should be checked.

State Disability Insurance

Some states require that employees be covered by disability or sick-pay insurance. The employer may be required to withhold a certain amount from the employee's salary to pay for this insurance.

Form **940**

Department of the Treasury
Internal Revenue Service (99)

**You must
complete
this section.** ▶

Employer's Annual Federal
Unemployment (FUTA) Tax Return

▶ **See separate Instructions for Form 940 for information on completing this form.**

OMB No. 1545-0028

20**01**

T	
FF	
FD	
FP	
I	
T	

Name (as distinguished from trade name)   Calendar year

Trade name, if any

Address and ZIP code   Employer identification number

A Are you required to pay unemployment contributions to only one state? (If "No," skip questions B and C) .   ☐ **Yes** ☐ **No**

B Did you pay all state unemployment contributions by January 31, 2002? ((1) If you deposited your total FUTA tax when due, check "Yes" if you paid all state unemployment contributions by February 11, 2002. (2) If a 0% experience rate is granted, check "Yes." (3) If "No," skip question C.) . . . .   ☐ **Yes** ☐ **No**

C Were all wages that were taxable for FUTA tax also taxable for your state's unemployment tax? . . . . .   ☐ **Yes** ☐ **No**

If you answered "No" to any of these questions, you must file Form 940. If you answered "Yes" to all the questions, you may file Form 940-EZ, which is a simplified version of Form 940. (Successor employers see **Special credit for successor employers** on page 3 of the instructions.) You can get Form 940-EZ by calling 1-800-TAX-FORM (1-800-829-3676) or from the IRS Web Site at **www.irs.gov**.

If you will not have to file returns in the future, check here (see **Who Must File** in separate instructions), **and complete and sign the return** . . . . ▶ ☐

If this is an Amended Return, check here. . . . . ▶ ☐

Part I	**Computation of Taxable Wages**

1 Total payments (including payments shown on lines 2 and 3) during the calendar year for services of employees **1**

2 Exempt payments. (Explain all exempt payments, attaching additional sheets if necessary.) ▶ --
---   **2**

3 Payments of more than $7,000 for services. Enter only amounts over the first $7,000 paid to each employee. (See separate instructions.) Do not include any exempt payments from line 2. The $7,000 amount is the Federal wage base. Your state wage base may be different. **Do not use your state wage limitation**.   **3**

4 Add lines 2 and 3 . . . .   **4**

5 **Total taxable wages** (subtract line 4 from line 1) . . . . ▶ **5**

Be sure to complete both sides of this form, and sign in the space provided on the back.

For Privacy Act and Paperwork Reduction Act Notice, see separate instructions.   ▼ **DETACH HERE** ▼   Cat. No. 11234O   Form **940** (2001)

Form **940-V**

Department of the Treasury
Internal Revenue Service

Form 940 Payment Voucher

Use this voucher only when making a payment with your return.

OMB No. 1545-0028

20**01**

Complete boxes 1, 2, and 3. Do not send cash, and do not staple your payment to this voucher. Make your check or money order payable to the **"United States Treasury."** Be sure to enter your employer identification number, "Form 940," and "2001" on your payment.

1 Enter your employer identification number.

2

Enter the amount of your payment. ▶

Dollars	Cents

3 Enter your business name (individual name for sole proprietors).

Enter your address.

Enter your city, state, and ZIP code.

FIGURE 23-6 Employer's Annual Federal Unemployment Tax (FUTA) Return.

Form 940 (2001) Page **2**

Part II   **Tax Due or Refund**

1	Gross FUTA tax. Multiply the wages from Part I, line 5, by .062 . . . . **1**
2	Maximum credit. Multiply the wages from Part I, line 5, by .054 . . | **2**
3	Computation of tentative credit (**Note:** *All taxpayers must complete the applicable columns.*)

(a) Name of state	(b) State reporting number(s) as shown on employer's state contribution returns	(c) Taxable payroll (as defined in state act)	(d) State experience rate period		(e) State experience rate	(f) Contributions if rate had been 5.4% (col. (c) x .054)	(g) Contributions payable at experience rate (col. (c) x col. (e))	(h) Additional credit (col. (f) minus col.(g)) If 0 or less, enter -0-.	(i) Contributions paid to state by 940 due date
			From	To					

3a	Totals . . . ▶	
3b	**Total tentative credit** (add line 3a, columns (h) and (i) only—for late payments, also see the instructions for Part II, line 6) . . . . ▶	**3b**
4		
5		
6	**Credit:** Enter the smaller of the amount from Part II, line 2 or line 3b; or the amount from the worksheet in the Part II, line 6 instructions	**6**
7	**Total FUTA tax** (subtract line 6 from line 1). If the result is over $100, also complete Part III . .	**7**
8	Total FUTA tax deposited for the year, including any overpayment applied from a prior year . .	**8**
9	**Balance due** (subtract line 8 from line 7). Pay to the **"United States Treasury."** If you owe more than $100, see **Depositing FUTA Tax** on page 3 of the separate instructions . . . . . . ▶	**9**
10	**Overpayment** (subtract line 7 from line 8). Check if it is to be: ☐ **Applied to next return** or ☐ **Refunded** . . . . ▶	**10**

Part III   **Record of Quarterly Federal Unemployment Tax Liability** (Do not include state liability.) **Complete only if line 7 is over $100.** See page 6 of the separate instructions.

Quarter	First (Jan. 1–Mar. 31)	Second (Apr. 1–June 30)	Third (July 1–Sept. 30)	Fourth (Oct. 1–Dec. 31)	Total for year
Liability for quarter					

Third Party Designee	Do you want to allow another person to discuss this return with the IRS (see instructions page 4)? ☐ **Yes.** Complete the following. ☐ **No**
	Designee's name ▶ Phone no. ▶ ( ) Personal identification number (PIN) ▶

Under penalties of perjury, I declare that I have examined this return, including accompanying schedules and statements, and, to the best of my knowledge and belief, it is true, correct, and complete, and that no part of any payment made to a state unemployment fund claimed as a credit was, or is to be, deducted from the payments to employees.

Signature ▶   Title (Owner, etc.) ▶   Date ▶

Form **940** (2001)

FIGURE 23-6—Cont'd   For legend see previous page.

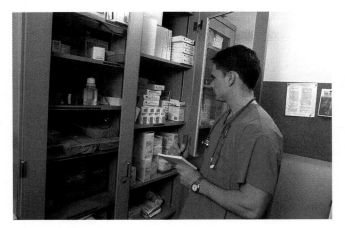

FIGURE 23-7   Inventory supplies and equipment before developing the annual budget. Once a good inventory has been completed, more accurate projections can be made for the expenses of the coming year.

Budgets

Growing businesses must develop budgets that help to plan finances over a certain period. Medical offices should compile a new budget before the beginning of each **fiscal year**. The best way to begin a budget is to look at the expenses from the previous year (Figure 23-7 and Procedures 23-3 and 23-4). These expenses should be divided into categories and then a total derived for each category. Each month should represent approximately $\frac{1}{12}$ of the total budget, not including large capital expenses.

Within the individual categories, examine expenses for those that could be eliminated or those that were underbudgeted. For example, if $3,345 was spent on office supplies and the budget was $3,000, either more money needs to be allotted for this category or cuts in spending are necessary. If $3,345 was spent and the budget was $4,000, the excess may be placed in another category for the next year.

PROCEDURE 23-3

Establishing and Maintaining a Supply Inventory and Ordering System

GOAL: To establish an inventory of all expendable supplies in the physician's office and follow an efficient plan of order control using a card system.

EQUIPMENT AND SUPPLIES

- File box
- Inventory and order control cards
- List of supplies on hand
- Metal tabs
- Reorder tabs
- Pen or pencil

PROCEDURAL STEPS

1 Write the name of each item on a separate card (Figure 1*).

ORDER	(ITEM NAME)	3-ply Disposable Drape Sheets (white) 7459										ON ORDER
ORDER QUANTITY	300							REORDER POINT	100			
ORDER	QTY	REC'D	COST	PREPAID	ON ACCT	ORDER	QTY	REC'D	COST	PREPAID	ON ACCT	
1/25	300	2/10	64.95	X								

INVENTORY COUNT	JAN	FEB	MAR	APR	MAY	JUNE	JULY	AUG	SEPT	OCT	NOV	DEC
20 _00_	200											
20 _00_												

ORDER SOURCE
The Colwell Company
201 Kenyon Road
Champaign, IL 61820

UNIT PRICE
100 - $23.95
300 - $64.95

FORM 2450 COLWELL CO., CHAMPAIGN, ILLINOIS

Figure 1

Purpose: To establish a record of all items in inventory.

2 Write the amount of each item on hand in the space provided.
Purpose: To establish beginning inventory.

3 Place a reorder tag at the point where the supply should be replenished (Figure 2*).
Purpose: The tag will serve as an alert that supply is low.

4 Place a metal tab over the *order* section of the card.
Purpose: The metal tab will be a reminder to include this item in the next order.

5 When the order has been placed, note the date and quantity ordered and move the table to the *on order* section of the card.

6 When the order is received, note the date and quantity in the appropriate column, remove the tab, and refile the card.
Note: If the order is only partially filled, let the tab remain until the order is complete.

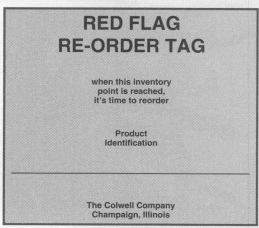

RED FLAG RE-ORDER TAG

when this inventory point is reached, it's time to reorder

Product Identification

The Colwell Company
Champaign, Illinois

Figure 2

*Courtesy of Colwell Systems, Champaign, Illinois.

PROCEDURE 23-4

Preparing a Purchase Order

GOAL: To prepare an accurate purchase order for supplies or equipment.

EQUIPMENT AND SUPPLIES

- List of current inventory
- Purchase order
- Pen
- Phone
- FAX machine

PROCEDURAL STEPS

1 Review the current inventory and determine what items need to be ordered.
Purpose: To determine what is needed so that the office will not be overstocked or understocked.

2 Complete the purchase order accurately, filling in all applicable spaces and blanks with the information requested.
Purpose: An accurately completed purchase order helps to eliminate mistakes in the order and in shipments.

3 List the items to be ordered, including quantity, item numbers, size, color, price, and extended price. Be sure that all applicable information is included.
Purpose: To help ensure accurate orders.

4 Provide the physician's signature, DEA certificate, and medical license when needed.
Purpose: Some items require these documents to verify that the physician is eligible to order them.

5 Call in, FAX, mail, or submit the order electronically to the vendor. Keep a copy for your records. Keep any verification provided that the order was received.
Purpose: To document exactly what was ordered on what date and provide proof that the order was received.

6 Note on the inventory which items are on order.
Purpose: To keep other staff members from preparing duplicate orders.

7 Keep a copy of the order in the appropriate place in the office filing system.
Purpose: To reference the order if needed and have a copy of the items ordered to compare with the packing list once the items arrive at the office.

CRITICAL THINKING APPLICATION

- Brenda has developed a preliminary budget. She realizes that several pieces of equipment need to be replaced in the coming year. However, Dr. Wilkins has expressed that she does not wish to make any capital purchases. How might Brenda approach Dr. Wilkins about the needed equipment?
- How might leasing equipment benefit the office? How can Brenda determine if this would be more or less expensive?

By monitoring expenses on a monthly basis, the physician can see if the facility is over budget, under budget, or right on target. Categories that have been overspent can be reconciled by taking funds from another category (for instance, category B) and adding them to the overspent category (category A). However, the amount taken must be subtracted from category B and added to category A. Those subtracted funds are no longer available in category B. Specific notes should be kept when categories are overspent, so that an adjustment may be made for the next fiscal year.

The following categories should be considered for the physician's operating budget:

- Insurance
- Rent
- Depreciation
- Loan payments
- Advertising/promotions
- Legal/accounting
- Miscellaneous expenses
- Supplies
- Salaries/wages
- Utilities
- Dues/subscriptions/fees
- Taxes
- Repairs/maintenance
- Medical equipment
- Administrative equipment
- Medication/pharmacy expenses

The physician should investigate whether leasing equipment might be a better option for the facility. Some leasing programs are very progressive and provide service contracts at no additional cost. Since depreciation costs are high, leasing might be the best answer to a new equipment need.

Insurance

Insurance coverage is one of the physician's major expenses. Almost every physician carries some type of malpractice insurance for protection against the cost of legal liabilities. Property and fire insurance are mandatory, and most physicians carry Workers' Compensation Insurance to cover employee injuries and accidents. The medical assistant may be asked to shop for the best insurance rates at the time of renewals.

Closing Comments

The physician will come to rely heavily on the person who manages the finances of the office. It is important that this individual keep information confidential. The entire staff must be conscious of the costs involved in operating a medical office and should adhere to their respective budgets as closely as possible. By being conservative, the physician may be willing to spend more money on pay increases and benefits to reward his or her employees.

Patient Education

There may be times when patients do not fully understand the costs involved in providing quality medical care. The medical assistant may need to educate the patient about the basic costs involved with the procedures that are performed in the office. Patients do not need a lengthy explanation, but may be set more at ease in knowing that the physician does not set his or her fees arbitrarily. The physician's office is a small business, like thousands of other small businesses, and should be able to pay its overhead and expenses.

Legal and Ethical Issues

The keeping of the financial records is a position of great trust and responsibility. Some physicians require the person placed in charge of the office finances to be bonded. This means that the facility has done a security check on an individual and the person was found worthy to be placed in a position of responsibility. A bond is issued by an entity on behalf of a second party, guaranteeing that the second party will fulfill an obligation or series of obligations to a third party. In the event that the obligations are not met, the third party will recover its losses via the bond.

Records must be accurate and completed on a daily basis. Daily journals should be kept indefinitely in support of tax returns.

SUMMARY OF SCENARIO

Brenda has learned much about the financial management of a physician's office. She is never hesitant to call the practice accountant, Mr. Schmidt, whenever a question arises. As she gains more experience, she understands the budgeting process, cost management, and the various methods of accounting practice.

There are many things that can affect the finances of a medical practice. However, the physician who is fairly conservative about spending and careful with investments should remain a stable part of the community's healthcare professionals. Dr. Wilkins lives by this philosophy and encourages her employees to manage money wisely, too. This attitude among all the staff members promotes a sense of teamwork and cooperation for the benefit of all.

SUMMARY OF LEARNING OBJECTIVES

■ The financial records of any business should at all times show how much was earned in a given period, how much was collected, how much is owed, and the distribution of expenses incurred.

■ Accounts payable refers to the amounts of money owed by a business and not yet paid, whereas accounts receivable refers to amounts owed to the business that are not yet paid.

■ The three most common bookkeeping systems in use today are the single-entry system, double-entry system, and pegboard system. The single-entry method is the oldest accounting method, and utilizes a general journal, a cash payment journal, and an accounts receivable ledger. Payroll records and petty cash records may also be included. The double-entry system, which is more difficult to use than the single-entry system, requires an entry on each side of the accounting equation, and each side must always balance. The pegboard system requires a moderate initial investment to implement, but allows the user to perform several accounting functions at one time. It is often called the write-it-once system.

■ A trial balance will reflect discrepancies between the journal and the ledger. It does not reveal errors in the individual accounts, but will show errors in the overall balances of accounts.

■ The Internal Revenue Service requires that several employment records be kept for at least 4 years. These records include the Social Security number of the employee; the number of withholding allowances claimed; the amount of gross salary; all deductions for Social Security and Medicare taxes; federal, state, and city or other subdivision withholding taxes; state disability insurance; and state unemployment tax.

■ Several deductions are taken from the employee's wages as required by law. These deductions are based on the total earnings of the employee, the number of withholding allowances claimed, the marital status of the employee, and the length of the pay period involved.

■ There are five common reports used for accounting in the small business office: the statement of income and expense, the cash flow statement, the trial balance, the accounts receivable trial balance, and the balance sheet.

■ The Employee's Withholding Allowance Certificate, or Form W-4, specifies the number of withholding allowances that the employee is claiming. The more allowances that are claimed, the less money that is taken from the employee's paycheck.

■ The Federal Insurance Contributions Act requires that a certain amount of money be deducted from an employee's wages and designated for Medicare and Social Security programs. The current percentages are 1.45% for the Medicare contribution and 6.2% for Social Security. Both the employer and employee contribute these amounts.

■ The physician's office must set a budget each fiscal year to prepare for all of the expenses that will be involved in running the office. Without a well-planned budget, the physician cannot control expenses. The expenditures from the past year should be evaluated when planning the new budget, paying particular attention to the expense categories that exceeded expected amounts.

INTERNET CONNECTION

• Healthcare Financial Management Organization
  www.hfma.org

UNIT five

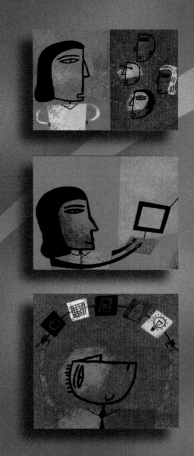

Assisting With Medical Specialties

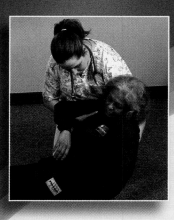

CHAPTER 24

Scenario

Cheryl Skurka, CMA, has been working for Dr. Peter Bendt for about 6 months. During that time a number of patient emergencies have occurred in the office, and even more potentially serious problems have been managed by the phone screening staff. Cheryl is concerned that she is not prepared to assist with emergencies in the ambulatory care setting. Cheryl decides to ask Dr. Bendt for assistance, and he suggests she work with the experienced screening staff to learn how to manage phone calls from patients calling for assistance.

Assisting With Medical Emergencies

Deborah B. Kennedy

Learning Objectives

- Define and spell the terms listed in the vocabulary.
- Describe the medical assistant's responsibilities in an emergency.
- Identify supplies and equipment for emergency situations.
- Summarize the general rules for managing emergencies.
- Demonstrate screening techniques and documentation guidelines for ambulatory care emergencies.
- Determine appropriate action and documentation procedures for common ambulatory care emergencies.
- Recognize and respond to life-threatening emergencies in the ambulatory care setting.
- Identify and assist a patient with an obstructed airway.
- Apply patient education concepts to medical emergencies.
- Discuss the legal and ethical concerns regarding medical emergencies.
- Provide rescue breathing and perform adult CPR.
- Assist a patient with an obstructed airway.
- Demonstrate the use of an automated external defibrillator.
- Administer oxygen through a nasal cannula to a patient in respiratory distress.
- Assist and monitor a patient who has fainted.
- Control a hemorrhagic wound.

National Curriculum Competencies

CLINICAL COMPETENCIES
4i. Obtain CPR certification and first aid training

TRANSDISCIPLINARY COMPETENCIES
1d. Demonstrate telephone techniques

Vocabulary

asystole The absence of a heartbeat.
cyanosis Blue color of the mucous membranes and body extremities caused by lack of oxygen.
dyspnea Difficult or painful breathing.
ecchymosis A hemorrhagic skin discoloration commonly called bruising.
emetic A substance that causes vomiting.
fibrillation Rapid, random, ineffective contractions of the heart.
hematuria Blood in the urine.
mediastinum Space in the center of the chest under the sternum.
myocardium The muscular lining of the heart.
necrosis Pertaining to the death of cells or tissue.
photophobia Visual sensitivity to light.
polydipsia Excessive thirst.
polyuria Excreting large amounts of urine.
transient ischemic attack Temporary neurological symptoms because of a gradual or partial occlusion of a cerebral blood vessel.

First aid is defined as the immediate care given to a person who has been injured or has suddenly taken ill. It includes well-chosen words of encouragement, a willingness to help, a promotion of confidence by the demonstration of competence, and the performance of temporary physical care to alleviate pain or a life-threatening situation. Knowledge of first aid and related skills can often mean the difference between life and death, temporary and permanent disability, and rapid recovery and long-term hospitalization.

Frequently a medical assistant may be responsible for initiating first aid in the office and continuing to administer first aid until the physician or trained medical team arrives. Every medical assistant should successfully complete a course in cardiopulmonary resuscitation (CPR) and continue to hold a current CPR card as long as employed (see Procedure 24-2). Basic knowledge of CPR and life-support skills needs to be updated on a regular basis because of changes in procedures as new techniques are developed. For example, just recently both the Red Cross and the American Heart Association recommended the inclusion of automated external defibrillator (AED) training for all healthcare workers (see Procedure 24-1). Medical assistants need to be consistently trained on current emergency approaches and should encourage their local professional chapters to offer workshops on the management of emergencies in the ambulatory care setting.

THE MEDICAL ASSISTANT'S ROLE IN PERFORMING EMERGENCY PROCEDURES

1. Perform only the emergency procedures in which you are trained.
2. If an emergency occurs in the office, notify the physician.
3. If a physician cannot be located, contact the local EMS team.

Medical assistants are not responsible for diagnosing emergencies but are expected to make decisions on the management of emergencies based on their medical knowledge and training. If there is any doubt about how to manage a particular situation or emergency phone call, refer to the physician, office manager, or a more experienced member of the healthcare team.

Making the Facility Accident-Proof

Usually it is the medical assistant's responsibility to make the office as accident-proof as possible by keeping cupboard doors and drawers closed, wiping up spills immediately, and picking up dropped objects. All medications should be kept out of sight; dangerous drugs should be kept in locked cupboards. If there are children in the office, all sharp objects and potentially toxic substances must be kept out of reach. A medical assistant should never leave a seriously ill patient or a restless, depressed, or unconscious patient unattended.

Planning Ahead

Every healthcare facility should have a policy with specific procedures for the management of emergencies on site. When starting a new job, part of the orientation process is to review the site's policy and procedures manual. Be sure to clarify any questions you may have about how emergencies are managed in that particular facility.

Staff members should discuss possible emergencies that may occur and have an emergency action plan for rapid, systematic intervention. For instance, local industries may present unique problems that call for very specialized care. Plan for these, and ask the physician's advice on what procedures to follow and what supplies to have on hand. If there are several employees, each should be assigned specific duties. Organization and planning make the difference between systematic care for the patient and complete chaos.

Using Community Emergency Services

Most communities have an emergency medical services (EMS) system. This system includes an efficient communications network, such as the emergency telephone number 911, well-trained rescue personnel, properly equipped ambulances, an emergency facility that is open 24 hours a day to provide advanced life support, and hospital intensive care for the victims.

There are more than 300 poison control centers in the United States ready to provide emergency information for treating victims of poisonings. Many of the centers have toll-free lines. Every office is required to post a list of local emergency numbers. This list should be in plain sight and should be known to all office personnel. Include on the list

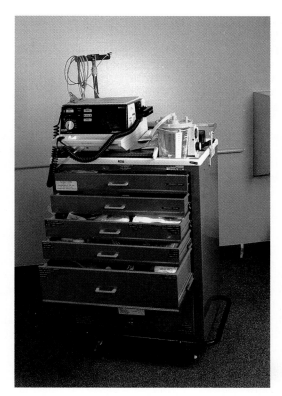

FIGURE 24-1 Office emergency cart with defibrillator. Drawers are marked for easy retrieval of emergency supplies.

the local EMS system, poison control center, ambulance and rescue squad, fire department, and police department numbers.

Supplies and Equipment for Emergencies

Emergency Supplies

Emergency supplies consist of a properly equipped "crash cart" or bag of first aid items needed for a variety of emergencies (Figure 24-1). The contents will vary to some degree, according to the type of emergencies each office encounters. Emergency supplies should be kept in an easily accessible place that is known to all personnel in the office, with inventories of supplies completed on a regular basis. Medication and sterile supplies expiration dates must be checked either weekly or monthly, including the status of available oxygen tanks and related supplies, and the cart should be replenished with fresh supplies after every use.

BASIC EMERGENCY SUPPLIES

Equipment

Adhesive tape in 1- and 2-inch widths
Airways—variety types and sizes
Alcohol wipes
Ambu-bag with assorted sizes of facial masks
Antimicrobial skin ointment
Cotton balls and cotton swabs
CPR masks—both adult and pediatric
Defibrillator
Elastic bandages in 2- and 3-inch widths
Flashlight with batteries
Gauze pads, 2 × 2- and 4 × 4-inch widths and roller bandage—both sterile and nonsterile
Gloves, sterile and nonsterile, in multiple sizes
Hot and cold packs (instant type)
Intravenous catheters, tubing, solutions (variety of types), and tourniquet
Personal protective equipment (PPE), including impervious gowns, splash-guards or goggles, and booties
Portable oxygen tank with regulator and mask
Scissors
Sharps container
Sphygmomanometer—both pediatric and adult regular and large sizes
Splints—various sizes
Sterile dressings—miscellaneous sizes, including two abdominal pads
Steristrips or suturing material
Suction machine and catheters
Syringes and needles in assorted sizes and gauges
Venipuncture supplies and butterfly units

Medications

Activated charcoal, bottle of 30 to 50 g
Amobarbital (Amytal)
Apomorphine
Antihistamine, injectable and oral
Atropine
Dextrose
Diazepam (Valium)
Digoxin (Lanoxin), injectable
Epinephrine (Adrenalin), injectable
Furosemide (Lasix)
Glucagon and/or glucose tablets
Ipecac syrup
Isoproterenol (Isuprel), aerosol inhaler and injectable
Lidocaine (Xylocaine), injectable
Metaraminol (Aramine)
Nitroglycerine tablets
Phenobarbital, injectable
Sodium bicarbonate, injectable
Sterile water for injection

Emergency pharmaceutical supplies should include certain basic drugs. These include epinephrine, which has multiple uses in emergency situations. As a vasoconstrictor, it controls hemorrhage, relaxes the bronchioles to relieve acute asthma attacks, and is an emergency heart stimulant used to treat shock. Epinephrine should be in a ready-to-use cartridge syringe and needle unit. These are supplied in 1.0-ml cartridges.

Other drugs used are atropine, digoxin (Lanoxin), and lidocaine (Xylocaine). Atropine decreases secretions, increases respiration and heart rate, and is a smooth muscle relaxant. It dilates the pupils and is a general cerebral stimulant. Atropine relieves gastrointestinal cramps and hypermotility and may also be used to relieve pain locally. Digoxin is used to treat congestive heart failure (CHF) and is good for emergency use because it has a relatively rapid action. Lidocaine is used intravenously to decrease heart arrhythmia and as both a local and topical anesthetic.

Apomorphine is a fast-acting and effective **emetic** and is used in cases of poisoning when a stomach pump cannot be employed. Syrup of ipecac is also an emetic and one that many physicians recommend be kept on hand in the home for use in emergencies.

Antihistamines are used in the treatment of allergic reactions and anaphylaxis. Isoproterenol, an antispasmodic, is used for bronchial spasms, and is also a cardiac stimulant. Some trade names for this product are Isuprel, Medihaler-Iso, and Norisodrine.

Other medications that may be found in a crash cart are metaraminol (Aramine) (50%, in a prefilled syringe), for severe shock; amobarbital sodium (Amytal) and diazepam (Valium), for convulsions and as sedatives; and furosemide (Lasix), for CHF. Glucagon is primarily used to counteract severe hypoglycemic reactions in diabetic patients taking insulin.

Defibrillators

A medical assistant may be required to assist the team with defibrillation of emergency patients. Defibrillation is indicated when a patient has no pulse and is in ventricular **fibrillation**. Defibrillators are devices that send an electrical current through the **myocardium** by means of hand-held paddles or self-adhesive pads applied to the chest. This electrical shock causes momentary **asystole**, giving the heart's natural pacemaker an opportunity to resume the heart rate at a normal rhythm. The automated external defibrillator (AED) has a computerized system that analyzes a cardiac rhythm and delivers voice-prompt instructions on how to operate the device (Figure 24-2 and Procedure 24-1). The AED uses self-adhesive pads that record and monitor the cardiac rhythm, and the device instructs the rescuer when to deliver the electrical charge. The apex-anterior position is the most commonly used paddle position, with the anterior (sternum) paddle or pads placed to the right of the upper sternum and the apex one to the left of the patient's left nipple at the left midaxillary line (Figure 24-3). For defibrillating a female patient, the apex paddle or pad is placed either next to or underneath the left breast.

General Rules for Emergencies

There are two types of emergencies that a medical assistant will face in the ambulatory care setting: office emergencies and home emergencies. Common office emergencies and their management will be discussed later in this chapter. Besides dealing with actual emergency situations on-site, a medical assistant is frequently the first person to interact with patients facing potential emergencies at home. It is estimated that one third of the telephone calls received in a physician's office are for some type of problem that requires attention. An immediate decision must be made on how to manage that problem—either with home care advice, scheduling an appointment, or in extreme emergencies, notifying EMS. When faced with an emergency, either on the phone or in the facility, the medical assistant should follow some general rules:

1. It is most important to stay calm. Reassure the patient and make him or her as comfortable as possible.
2. Assess the situation to determine the nature of the emergency. Decide whether the need is immediate. This decision requires calm judgment and medical knowledge.
3. Obtain as much information as possible to determine the appropriate action.
4. Immediately refer any concerns to the office supervisor or physician.

Telephone Triage Screening

Every time the phone rings in a healthcare setting, there could be a potential life or death situation on the other end of the line. One of the most important tasks performed by medical assistants every day is answering the phones and managing patient needs efficiently and appropriately. *Triage* is the process of sorting patients, in this case patient phone calls, according to the patients' need for care. There are emergency action principles that serve as a guide for managing emergency phone calls in the ambulatory care setting.

- If the patient's situation is life threatening, activate EMS/911.
  - *Never put the caller with a life-threatening emergency on hold, and always be the last to hang up.*
  - Remain on the line until help arrives and you have talked to EMS personnel.
- Immediately record the name of the caller and that of the patient, location, and phone number in case the connection is lost.
- If you are unsure how to manage the emergency situation, contact the physician.
- If the patient is referred to an emergency department or emergency room (ED or ER), call the emergency department to notify them of the patient's arrival and make a follow-up call to determine the patient's condition.
- Gather as much information as possible about what is wrong with the patient and when the problem started. Obtain details regarding the patient's condition including:
  - Level of consciousness: Alert, responsive, lethargic, or confused? Did the patient lose consciousness at any time? If so, how long?
  - Character of respirations (and pulse if the caller is able to determine this): Normal, rapid, shallow, or difficult?

PROCEDURE 24-1

Using an Automated External Defibrillator (AED)

GOAL: To defibrillate adult victims with cardiac arrest. The majority of adult victims in sudden cardiac arrest are in ventricular fibrillation. Survival rates for victims with ventricular fibrillation are as high as 90% when defibrillation occurs within the first minute of collapse. Survival rates for cardiac arrest caused by ventricular fibrillation decrease by 7% to 10% with every minute that defibrillation does not occur.

EQUIPMENT AND SUPPLIES

- Practice AED
- Approved mannequin

PROCEDURAL STEPS (To be performed on an approved mannequin only.)

AED arrives after CPR has been started and two cycles of compressions and breaths have been completed.

1 Place the AED near the victim's left ear. Turn the AED on.

2 Attach electrode pads as pictured on the AED. Place electrodes at the sternum and apex of the heart. Make sure pads have complete contact with the victim's chest and they do not overlap (see Figure 24-3).

3 All rescuers must clear away from the victim. Press the ANALYZE button. The AED will analyze the victim's coronary status, will announce if the victim is going to be shocked, and automatically charges the electrodes (Figure 1*).

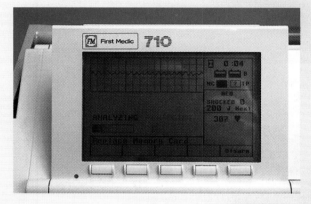

Figure 1

4 All rescuers must clear away from the victim. Press the SHOCK button if the machine is not automated. May repeat one to two more analyze-shock cycles.

5 If the machine gives the "no shock indicated" signal, assess the victim. Check the carotid pulse and breathing status and keep the AED attached until emergency medical services arrives.

---

*From Aehlert B: *ACLS quick review study guide*, ed 2. St Louis, 2001, Mosby.

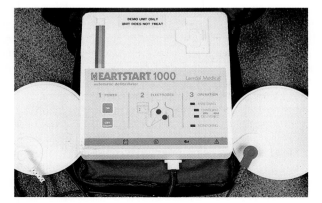

FIGURE 24-2 Fully automated external defibrillator. (From Aehlert B: *ACLS quick review study guide*, ed 2. St Louis, 2001, Mosby.)

- Is there bleeding? If so, how much, from where?
- Is there a suspected head or neck injury? If so, has the patient been moved? Is there a suspected fracture? Where?
- Does the patient have a history of this problem?
- Any other symptoms, such as fever, vomiting, diarrhea, or pain?
- Details regarding what has been done for the patient:
  - Medication: What, when? Dose, effectiveness?
- Thoroughly document the information gathered and any actions taken, including notification of EMS, whether the patient was sent to the emergency department or an appointment was scheduled, all home care recommendations, and whether the physician was notified and when.

Based on the outcome of the telephone interaction, a decision is made about when the practitioner will see the

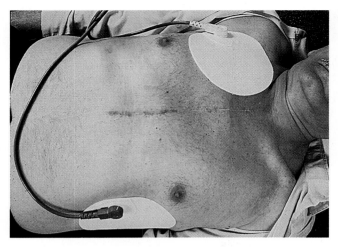

FIGURE 24-3 Connect the adhesive pads to the AED cables, and then apply the pads to the patient's chest at the upper-right sternal border and the lower-left ribs over the cardiac apex. (From Aehlert B: *ACLS quick review study guide*, ed 2. St Louis, 2001, Mosby.)

2. Allergies, current medications, and pertinent health history
3. Name of any person with the patient
4. Vital signs and chief complaint
5. Sequence of events, beginning with how the problem occurred, any changes in the patient's overall condition, and any observations made regarding the patient's condition
6. Details regarding procedures or techniques performed on the patient

patient. Emergency calls require either activation of EMS or immediate attention as soon as the patient arrives. Urgent calls require a same-day appointment if the patient has an acute condition or is in severe discomfort. This would include a young child with a high fever or a patient complaining of moderate to severe abdominal pain. The new patient will have to be worked into the day's schedule, which may cause a delay in currently scheduled appointments. Patients with other less urgent problems can be scheduled for appointments within the next 3 to 4 days.

> ### CRITICAL THINKING APPLICATION
>
> Cheryl is working with the phone triage staff when they receive a call from the mother of a 5-year-old patient; the mother reports that her son fell and cut his arm. What type of information should Cheryl gather about the injury? How should the incident be documented?

Management of On-Site Emergencies

An emergency can occur at any time to anyone. *Always follow standard precautions.* When an emergency occurs, it is impossible to determine the level of infection. All body fluids must be considered infectious, and the appropriate precautions must be employed. If the situation is life threatening, activate EMS and stay with the patient until you are relieved by the EMS provider or the physician.

> ### DOCUMENTATION OF AN ON-SITE EMERGENCY
>
> 1. Patient's name, address, age, and health insurance information

> ### CRITICAL THINKING APPLICATION
>
> Cheryl is working the front desk when a patient comes into the office limping and says she fell in the parking lot and hurt her ankle. Role-play the situation with a classmate and make a list of at least 10 questions Cheryl should ask the patient.

Life-Threatening Emergencies

If a patient in the facility exhibits any signs of nonresponsiveness, the clinician must be brought to the patient immediately. If there is no clinician in the facility, EMS should be activated. Even in situations in which a physician is present, the physician may order you to call 911 for immediate emergency care. Before beginning assessment of the patient, *put on gloves*, because any emergency situation may necessitate exposure to blood or body fluids.

Nonresponsive Patient

If the patient is nonresponsive, the physician must be notified immediately. The physician may instruct the medical assistant to activate EMS.

Caring for a patient who is nonresponsive first requires assessing the patient's respirations to determine the presence of breathing. Position the patient on the back and apply the head tilt–chin lift movement to open the airway. If there is a suspected head or neck injury, the neck should be manipulated as little as possible, so open the airway with the jaw thrust maneuver. Both of these actions relieve possible obstruction of the trachea by the tongue. Check for breathing by looking for a rise in the chest and either listening or feeling for air exchange (Figure 24-4). Breathing may suddenly cease for a variety of reasons, including shock, disease, and trauma. If no breaths are detected, artificial ventilation must be started immediately since death may occur within 4 to 6 minutes. There should be barrier devices on hand for artificial respirations (Figure 24-5) and should be used if rescue breaths are required (Procedure 24-2).

After giving the patient two slow breaths, check for cardiac circulation at the carotid pulse in the adult and

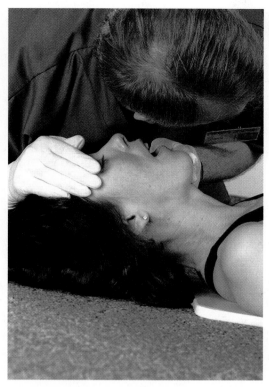

FIGURE 24-4   Checking for breathing in an unconscious patient.

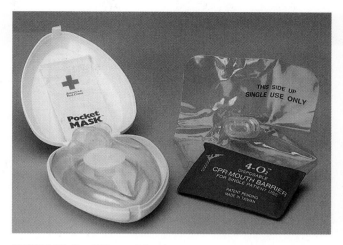

FIGURE 24-5   CPR mouth barriers.

child or the brachial pulse in the infant (Figure 24-6). If the pulse is present, continue ventilating the lungs every 5 seconds in the adult or one breath every 3 seconds in a child or infant. If the pulse is absent, begin cycles of chest compressions followed by two slow breaths.

When both breathing and pulse stop, the victim has suffered sudden death. There are many causes of sudden death, including heart disease, choking, drowning, poisoning, suffocation, electrocution, and smoke inhalation. CPR

PROCEDURE 24-2

Performing Adult Rescue Breathing and One-Rescuer CPR

GOAL: To restore a victim's breathing and blood circulation when respiration and/or pulse stop.

EQUIPMENT AND SUPPLIES

- Disposable gloves
- CPR ventilator mask
- Approved mannequin

PROCEDURAL STEPS (To be performed on an approved mannequin only.)

1 Establish unresponsiveness. Tap the victim and ask, "Are you OK?" Wait for victim to respond.
Purpose: To determine whether the victim is conscious.

2 Activate the emergency response system. Put on gloves and get ventilator mask.
Purpose: As soon as it is determined that an adult victim requires emergency care, immediately activate EMS. Most adults with sudden, nontraumatic cardiac arrest are in ventricular fibrillation. The time from collapse to defibrillation is the single most important predictor of survival.

3 Tilt the victim's head and lift the chin. Look, listen, and feel for signs of breathing. Place your ear

over the mouth and listen for breathing. Watch the rising and falling of the chest for evidence of breathing (Figure 1*).

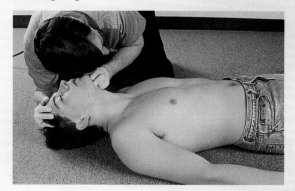

Figure 1

Purpose: To open the airway and determine if the victim is breathing.

4 If breathing is absent or inadequate, place the ventilator mask over the victim's mouth and give two slow breaths (2 seconds per breath), holding the ventilator mask tightly against the face while tilting the victim's chin back to open the airway (Figure 2*). Allow time for exhalation between breaths.

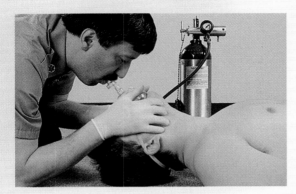

Figure 2

Purpose: The chin must be tilted back to open the airway and an airtight seal must be present so that air cannot escape around the mask.

5 Check the carotid pulse. If a pulse is present, continue rescue breathing (one breath every 5 seconds, about 10 to 12 breaths per minute). If no signs of circulation are present, begin cycles of 15 chest compressions (at a rate of about 100 compressions per minute) followed by two slow breaths (Figure 3*).

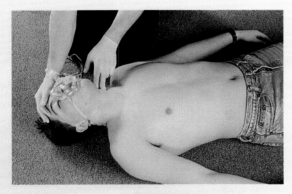

Figure 3

6 Kneel at the victim's side opposite the chest. Move your fingers up the ribs to the point where the sternum and the ribs join. Your middle fingers should fit into the area and your index finger should be next to it across the sternum.

7 Place the heel of your hand on the chest midline over the sternum, just above your index finger (Figure 4*).

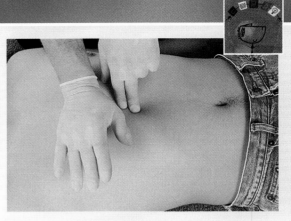

Figure 4

8 Place your other hand on top of your first hand and lift your fingers upward off of the chest (Figure 5*).

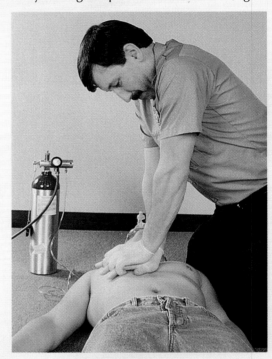

Figure 5

Purpose: This position gives you the most control, allowing you to avoid injuring the victim's ribs as you compress the chest.

9 Bring your shoulders directly over the victim's sternum as you compress downward, and keep your arms straight.

10 Depress the sternum 1½ to 2 inches for an adult victim. Relax the pressure on the sternum after each compression but *do not remove your hands* from the victim's sternum.

Purpose: The depth of compression is needed to circulate blood through the heart. Movement of the hands may cause injury to the victim.

PROCEDURE 24-2—Cont'd

11 After performing 15 compressions (at a rate of about 100 compressions per minute), open the airway and give two slow breaths.

12 After four cycles of compressions and breaths (15:2 ratio, about 1 minute) recheck breathing and carotid pulse. If there is a pulse but no breathing, continue rescue breathing (one breath every 5 seconds, about 10 to 12 breaths per minute) and reevaluate the victim's breathing and pulse every few minutes. If there are no signs of circulation, continue 15:2 cycles of compressions and ventilations, starting with chest compressions. Continue giving CPR until EMS relieves you.

13 Remove gloves and the ventilator mask valve and dispose in the biohazard container. Disinfect the ventilator mask per manufacturer recommendations. Wash hands.

14 Document the procedure and patient condition.

*From Henry M, Stapleton E: *EMT prehospital care*, ed 2. Philadelphia, 1997, WB Saunders.

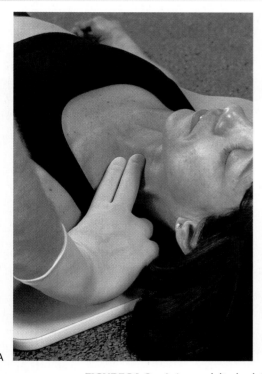

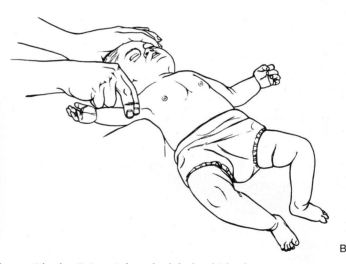

FIGURE 24-6   **A**, In an adult, check for carotid pulse. **B**, In an infant, check for brachial pulse.

must be started immediately in an attempt to prevent death or permanent damage to body organs, especially the brain. After four cycles of compressions and ventilations in the adult patient, recheck the pulse. If there are no signs of circulation, continue CPR until help arrives. If there is a pulse but no breathing, continue rescue breathing and occasionally monitor the pulse until help arrives.

Refer to the American Red Cross *Standard First Aid Manual* or *American Heart Association CPR Manual*, or the organizations' websites listed at the end of this chapter, for specific procedures and precautions in the management of respiratory and cardiac emergencies. As stated earlier, all healthcare professionals must have a current certification in CPR.

Heart Emergencies

Chest pain or *angina* can be associated with heart and lung disease, as well as a few other conditions. It can be quite serious; a patient with chest pain is treated as a cardiac emergency until a physician has ruled this out. The patient is often sweating and may have a gray, ashen appearance. The lips and fingernails may be blue, which is a sign of **cyanosis** (Figure 24-7). Frequently the patient will clutch the chest in pain. This pain may radiate from the **mediastinum** down the left arm and up the left side of the neck. The pulse may be rapid and weak and the patient often complains of nausea.

If a patient presents with any of these symptoms, report this to the clinician immediately. If the physician is not available, activate EMS. Use a wheelchair to move the

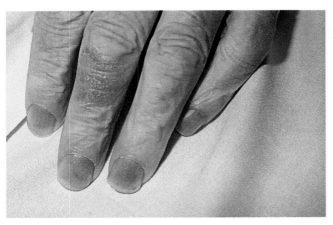

FIGURE 24-7 Cyanosis of nail beds. (From Henry MC, Stapleton ER: *EMT prehospital care*, ed 2. Philadelphia, 1997, WB Saunders.)

patient to an examination room. Breathing will be easier if the patient's head is slightly elevated or in Fowler's position. Keep the patient quiet and warm. Loosen all tight clothing. Take vital signs, including both apical and radial pulses. The physician may order oxygen started on the patient to relieve **dyspnea** (Procedure 24-3). Bring the emergency cart into the room and open the medication drawer so the physician is able to quickly prepare the medications needed. This may be epinephrine (Adrenalin), atropine, digitalis, calcium chloride, or morphine.

If the patient is conscious, ask about any medication that he or she has recently taken or is carrying. If the patient has an established heart disorder, the patient may be carrying nitroglycerin tablets. Nitroglycerin tablets are administered sublingually and may be given with the patient's consent (Figure 24-8). If the physician is in the office or is on the way, connect the patient to the electrocardiograph and record a few tracings. It may be necessary to start mouth-to-mouth resuscitation if there is no evidence of breathing. If chest pain progresses to cardiac arrest and loss of circulation, CPR must be performed.

PROCEDURE **24-3**

Administering Oxygen

GOAL: To provide oxygen for a patient in respiratory distress.

EQUIPMENT AND SUPPLIES
- Portable oxygen tank
- Pressure regulator
- Flow meter
- Nasal cannula with connecting tubing

PROCEDURAL STEPS

1 Gather equipment and wash hands.

2 Identify the patient and explain the procedure.
   Purpose: Patients must be taught to apply the nasal cannula with a nasal prong in each nostril and the tab resting above the upper lip. Patients who will be using oxygen at home need to be taught how to open the oxygen tank and to avoid open flames and not to smoke when oxygen is in use, since it is combustible.

3 Check the pressure gauge on the tank to determine the amount of oxygen in the tank.

4 If necessary, open the cylinder on the tank one full counterclockwise turn and attach the cannula tubing to the flow meter.

5 Adjust the administration of the oxygen according to the physician's order. Check to make sure the oxygen is flowing through the cannula.

6 Insert the cannula tips into the nostrils and adjust the tubing around the back of the patient's ears (Figure 1).

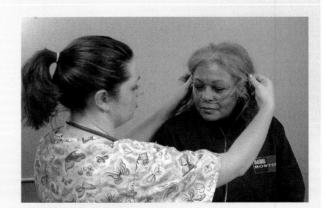

Figure 1

7 Make sure the patient is comfortable and answer any questions.

8 Wash hands.

9 Document the procedure, including the number of liters of oxygen being administered and the patient's condition. Continue to monitor the patient throughout the procedure and document any changes in condition.

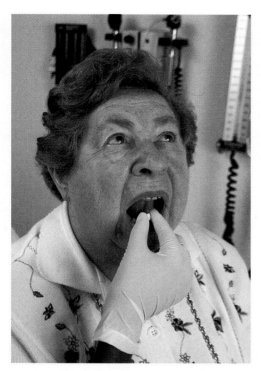

FIGURE 24-8   Nitroglycerin is administered beneath patient's tongue.

Signs of a Heart Attack. A heart attack, or *myocardial infarction*, is usually caused by a blockage of the coronary arteries that decreases the amount of blood being delivered to the myocardium. The most common signal of a heart attack is an uncomfortable pressure, squeezing, fullness, or pain in the center of the chest. This may spread to the shoulder, neck, jaw, or arms. The pain may not be severe. Other symptoms include sweating (*diaphoresis*), nausea or indigestion, shortness of breath (SOB), cold and clammy skin, and a feeling of weakness (*general malaise*).

SYMPTOMS OF HEART ATTACK IN WOMEN

Recent studies have revealed that women may experience different symptoms than the indicators traditionally cited for heart attack. These include the following:
- Back pain or aching and throbbing in the biceps or forearms
- Shortness of breath (SOB)
- Clammy perspiration
- Dizziness (*vertigo*)—unexplained lightheadedness or *syncopal* episodes
- Edema—especially of the ankles and/or lower legs
- Fluttering heartbeat or tachycardia
- Gastric upset
- Feeling of heaviness or fullness in the mediastinum

CRITICAL THINKING APPLICATION

Samantha Amos tells Cheryl when she enters the office that she has not been feeling well lately. She complains of aching in her arms, difficulty breathing, occasional dizziness, and swollen feet. Mrs. Amos does not have a history of heart disease. What should Cheryl do?

Choking

Choking is usually caused by a foreign object, often a bolus of food, lodged in the upper airway. The victim may clutch the neck between the thumb and index finger (Figure 24-9). This universal distress signal should be viewed as a sign that the victim needs help. If the victim has good air exchange or only partial airway obstruction and can speak, cough, or breathe, do not interfere but encourage the patient to continue coughing until the object is expelled. Monitor the patient for signs of respiratory distress, such as pallor and cyanosis. If the patient has a pronounced wheeze or a very weak cough, he or she has a partial airway obstruction with poor air exchange and may need help. If the patient is unable to speak, breathe, or cough, a complete airway obstruction exists and quick action must be taken to clear the airway. With a complete obstruction the patient will eventually lose consciousness from lack of oxygen to the brain. This condition may lead to respiratory and cardiac arrest. If the object is not removed, the victim may die within 4 to 6 minutes (Procedure 24-4).

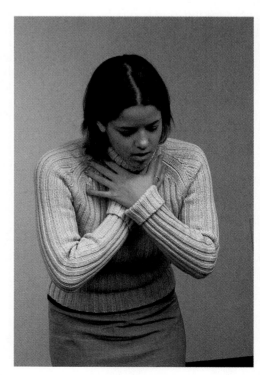

FIGURE 24-9   Universal sign of choking.

PROCEDURE **24-4**

Responding to an Adult With an Obstructed Airway

GOAL: To remove an airway obstruction and restore ventilation.

EQUIPMENT AND SUPPLIES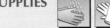
- Disposable gloves
- Ventilation mask (for unconscious victim)
- Approved mannequin to practice unconscious foreign body airway obstruction (FBAO)

PROCEDURAL STEPS (Unconscious maneuver to be performed on an approved mannequin only.)

1 Ask "Are you choking?" If victim indicates yes, ask "Can you speak?" If unable to speak, tell the victim you are going to help.
Purpose: If the victim is unable to speak, is coughing weakly, and/or is wheezing, there is an obstructed airway with poor air exchange and the obstruction must be removed before respiratory arrest occurs.

2 Stand behind the victim with feet slightly apart.
Purpose: With an obstructed airway, the victim may lose consciousness at any time. The rescuer must be prepared to safely lower the unconscious victim to the floor.

3 Reach around the victim's abdomen and place an index finger into the victim's navel or at the level of the belt buckle. Make a fist of the opposite hand (do not tuck the thumb into the fist) and place the thumb side of the fist against the victim's abdomen above the navel. If the victim is pregnant, place the fist above the enlarged uterus. If the victim is obese, it may be necessary to place the fist higher in the abdomen. It may be necessary to perform chest thrusts on a victim who is pregnant or obese.
Purpose: The fist should be placed in the soft tissue of the abdomen to avoid injury to the sternum or rib cage.

4 Place the opposite hand over the fist and give abdominal thrusts in a quick upward movement (Figure 1).
Purpose: Abdominal contents pushing against the diaphragm force trapped air out of the lungs and with it the obstruction.

5 Repeat the abdominal thrusts until the object is expelled or the victim becomes unresponsive.

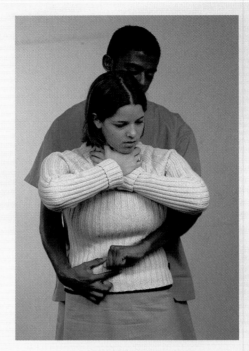

Figure 1

UNRESPONSIVE VICTIM

6 Activate the emergency response system.
Purpose: If the obstruction is not relieved, the victim may go into respiratory arrest, which can lead to cardiac arrest.

7 Put on gloves if available and get ventilation mask. Open the victim's mouth and perform a finger sweep to determine if the foreign object is in the mouth and to remove it (Figure 2).

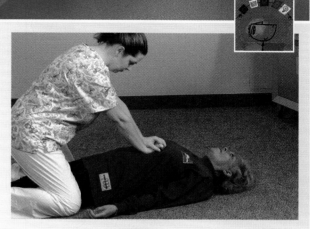

Figure 3

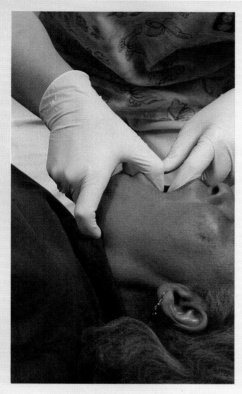

Figure 2

8 Open the airway with a head-tilt, jaw-thrust maneuver and attempt to ventilate using the barrier device with two slow breaths. If breaths do not go in (chest does not rise), retilt the head and try to ventilate again.

   Purpose: If breaths do not go in, retilt the head to make sure that the airway is open.

9 If ventilation is unsuccessful, move to the victim's feet and kneel across the victim's thighs. Place the heel of one hand above the navel but below the xiphoid process of the sternum. Place the other hand on top of the first, with the fingers elevated off of the abdomen. Administer five abdominal thrusts (Figure 3).

10 Move back beside the head of the victim and repeat the finger sweep. If the obstruction is not found, continue cycles of two rescue breaths, five abdominal thrusts, and finger sweep until either the obstruction is removed or EMS arrives.

11 If the obstruction is removed, assess the victim for breathing and circulation. If a pulse is present, but there is no breathing, begin rescue breathing. If there is no pulse, begin CPR.

   Purpose: The obstruction must be removed before air can be administered into the lungs for distribution to the body.

12 Once either patient is stabilized or EMS has taken over care, remove gloves and the ventilator mask valve and dispose in the biohazard container. Disinfect the ventilator mask per manufacturer recommendations. Wash hands.

13 Document the procedure and patient condition.

The procedure for removal of a foreign airway obstruction is exactly the same for a child, *except* never perform a blind finger sweep on an unconscious child, because this may push a foreign body deeper into the airway. After administering the five abdominal thrusts, open the mouth and look for the obstruction. If the object is visible, remove it from the child's mouth and assess vital signs. If the object is not visible, administer two rescue breaths and repeat the series until the object is dislodged or help arrives.

To dislodge a foreign object from the airway of an infant, place the baby face down over your forearm and across your thigh. The head should be lower than the trunk, and you should support the head and neck of the baby with one hand. Using the heel of your other hand, deliver four blows to the back, between the infant's shoulder blades (Figure 24-10, *A*). Turn the infant to his or her back, with the head lower than the trunk. Using two fingers, deliver four thrusts to the midsternal area at the infant's nipple line (Figure 24-10, *B*). Examine the infant's mouth, and if the object is visible, pluck it out with your fingertips, but never perform a finger sweep on an infant. A baby's oral cavity is too small for a finger sweep; such an action may only lodge the obstruction farther into the

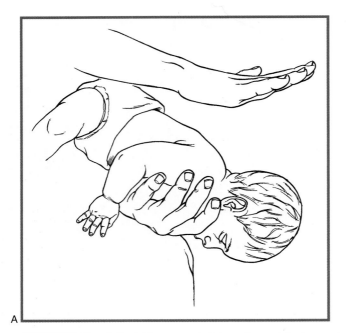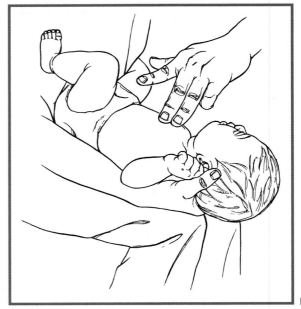

FIGURE 24-10 **A,** Back blows are administered to an infant supported on the arm and thigh. **B,** Chest thrusts are administered in the same position as for cardiac compressions. (From Henry MC, Stapleton ER: *EMT prehospital care,* ed 2. Philadelphia, 1997, WB Saunders.)

airway. If the obstruction is not visible, administer two rescue breaths by covering both the baby's nose and mouth with your mouth. Repeat the sequence until the foreign body is expelled or help arrives.

It is possible to perform the abdominal thrust maneuver on yourself if you are choking and there is no one nearby to help you. Press your fist into your upper abdomen with quick upward thrusts or lean forward and press the abdomen quickly against a firm object, such as the back of a chair.

Cerebrovascular Accident (Stroke)

A cerebrovascular accident (CVA), or stroke, is a disorder of the cerebral blood vessels that results in an impairment of the blood supply to part of the brain. This interruption in normal circulation of blood through the brain leads to some degree of neurological damage, either temporary or permanent, depending on the severity of the oxygen deprivation to the brain cells.

A minor stroke or **transient ischemic attack** (TIA) usually does not cause unconsciousness, and symptoms depend on the location of the circulatory problem in the brain as well as the amount of brain damage. TIA symptoms are temporary and may include headache, confusion, vertigo, ringing in the ears (*tinnitus*), temporary paralysis or weakness of one side of the body, transient limb weakness, slurred speech, and vision problems. TIA episodes indicate the patient is at risk for a major stroke.

Symptoms of a major stroke include unconsciousness, paralysis on one side of the body, difficulty in breathing and swallowing, loss of bladder and bowel control, unequal pupil size, and slurring of speech.

The patient who has suffered a major stroke should be protected against any further injury. Notify the physician

and/or activate EMS. Keep the patient lying down and lightly covered. Maintain an open airway. Position the head so that any secretions will drain from the side of the mouth to prevent choking. Do not give the patient anything to eat or drink. Vital signs should be measured at regular intervals and recorded for the physician.

CRITICAL THINKING APPLICATION

Thomas Antonio, a 67-year-old patient, calls to report that when he woke up this morning the left side of his face was drooping and he had difficulty seeing out of his left eye. The symptoms went away in about 2 hours and he is feeling fine now. There are not any openings in the schedule for 2 days. When should Cheryl make Mr. Antonio an appointment? What questions should Cheryl ask Mr. Antonio?

Shock

Shock is a state of collapse resulting from failure of the circulatory system to deliver enough oxygenated blood to the body's vital organs. An injury, hemorrhage, infection, anesthesia, drug overdose, burns, pain, fear, or emotional stress causes this physiological reaction. Shock may be immediate or delayed, may be mild or severe, and is potentially fatal. There are many different types of shock, but the signs and symptoms are universal. The most common indicators of shock are a pale, gray, or cyanotic appearance; moist but cool skin; dilated pupils; weak and rapid pulse; marked hypotension; shallow and rapid respirations; lethargy or restlessness; and extreme thirst.

TYPES AND CAUSES OF SHOCK

Anaphylactic—a severe allergic reaction
Insulin—overdose of insulin causing severe
  hypoglycemia
Psychogenic or mental—excessive fear, joy,
  anger, or emotional stress
Hypovolemic—excessive loss of blood
Cardiogenic—myocardial infarction,
  pulmonary embolism, or severe CHF
Neurogenic—dilation of blood vessels
  resulting from brain or spinal cord injuries
Septic—systemic infection

If a patient exhibits signs of shock, ensure an open airway and check for breathing and circulation. Place the patient supine with the legs elevated to return the blood from the legs to the vital organs. Loosen all tight clothing and cover the patient with a blanket for warmth. Do not move the patient unnecessarily. Fluids may be given by mouth if the patient is alert. Because shock can develop into a life-threatening situation, it is advisable to administer only basic first aid care and to have the patient transported to the hospital.

Common Office Emergencies

The remainder of the chapter highlights typical emergencies seen either in the ambulatory care setting or in telephone triage situations. Table 24-1 summarizes common emergencies, the questions that should be asked, and possible home care advice.

Fainting (Syncope)

Fainting or *syncope* is a common emergency problem. Syncope is usually caused by a transient loss of blood flow to the brain, such as a sudden drop in blood pressure, which results in a temporary loss of consciousness. It can occur without warning, or the patient may appear pale; may feel cold, weak, dizzy, or nauseated; and may have numbness of the extremities before the incident. The greatest danger to the patient is an injury from falling during the attack. Therefore, if the patient presents with syncopal symptoms, immediately place the patient in a supine position. Loosen all tight clothing and maintain an open airway. Apply a cold washcloth to the forehead. Measure the patient's pulse, respiration rate, and blood pressure and report the findings to the physician. Keep the patient in a supine position for at least 10 minutes after consciousness has been regained. A complete patient history helps diagnose the possible causes of the attack, such as history of heart disease or diabetes. Document the entire episode and the patient's recovery time (Procedure 24-5).

If the patient does not recover quickly, the physician may activate EMS for transportation to the hospital. Syncope might be a brief episode in the development of a serious underlying illness, such as an abnormal heart rhythm, that may increase in severity or lead to sudden cardiac death.

Poisoning

Accidental poisonings result in the largest number of deaths in children in the United States. All poisonings are considered medical emergencies. Poisoning can occur by mouth, absorption, inhalation, or injection. Over-the-counter medications such as acetaminophen, detergents and bleach, plants, cough and cold medicines, and vitamins cause the majority of poison cases seen in young children. Other typical household poisons include drain cleaners, turpentine, kerosene, furniture polish, and paints (Figure 24-11). Signs and symptoms of poisoning vary greatly and include burns on the hands and mouth, stains on the victim's clothing, open bottles of medicines or chemicals, changes in skin color, nausea or stomach cramps, shallow breathing, convulsions, heavy perspiration, dizziness or drowsiness, and unconsciousness.

WHAT TO ASK WHEN A POISONING IS REPORTED

- The name of the poison taken and any information on the label
- How much was taken
- How long ago the poison was taken
- Whether vomiting has occurred
- Any pertinent symptoms, such as difficulty breathing or an altered state of consciousness
- The name, weight, and age of the victim
- Any first aid given

Instruct the caller *not* to hang up and *not* to leave the victim unattended. Call the local poison control center and forward all directions to the caller. Syrup of ipecac, which will cause vomiting within 15 to 20 minutes, should only be used if ordered by the physician or poison control center, because some substances can cause damage when vomited. Do not induce vomiting if the victim is stuporous, unconscious, or having a convulsion because of the risk of aspiration. If syrup of ipecac is recommended, give 2 teaspoons to infants 9 to 12 months old after the child drinks about 4 ounces of warm water. For a child 1 to 4 years old, administer 1 tablespoon after the child drinks 4 to 8 ounces of warm water. If the patient is to be seen by the physician or sent to the hospital, tell the caller to bring the container of poison or sample of vomitus with them so the chemical contents of the substance can be verified.

CRITICAL THINKING APPLICATION

A young mother calls in a panic to report her 18-month-old daughter swallowed at least half a bottle of cough syrup. The child is fussy and very sleepy, and the mother wants to give her ipecac immediately. What should Cheryl do?

TABLE 24-1	Telephone Triage Approach	
Emergency Situation	**Triage/Screening Questions**	**Home Care Advice**
Syncope	Was the patient injured?	Does not necessarily indicate a serious disease. If injured from a fall, the patient may need to be treated.
	Does the patient have a history of heart disease, seizures, or diabetes?	The patient should get up very slowly to prevent a recurrence, take it easy, and drink plenty of fluids.
		If the patient is to be seen, someone should accompany him or her to the clinician's practice.
Animal bites	What kind of animal (pet or wild)?	The health department or police should be notified.
	How severe is the injury?	
	Where are the bites?	Every effort must be made to locate the animal and monitor its health.
	When did the bite occur?	If the skin is not broken, wash well and observe for signs of infection.
Insect bites and stings	Does the patient have a history of anaphylactic reaction to insect stings?	If there is a history of anaphylaxis and the patient has an EpiPen, it should be administered immediately and EMS notified.
	Does the patient have difficulty breathing, have a widespread rash, or have trouble swallowing?	Activate EMS if the patient is having systemic symptoms.
		An antihistamine (Benadryl) relieves local pruritus.
Asthma	Does the patient show signs of cyanosis?	If a patient with asthma is unable to speak in sentences, has poor color, and is struggling to breathe even after inhaler use, he or she should be seen immediately or EMS should be activated.
	Has the patient used the prescribed inhalers?	
Burns	Where are the burns located, and what caused them?	Activate EMS for burns on the face, hands, feet, and perineum or those caused by electricity or a chemical, or burns associated with inhalation.
	Are there signs of shock (moist clammy skin, altered consciousness, rapid breathing and pulse)?	Activate EMS if there are signs of shock.
		The patient must receive a tetanus shot if it has been more than 10 years since the last one.
	Are there signs of infection (foul odor, cloudy drainage) in a burn more than 2 days old?	Schedule an urgent appointment if signs of infection are reported.
Wounds	Is the bleeding steady or pulsating?	Pulsating bleeding usually indicates arterial damage; activate EMS.
	How and when did the injury occur?	If the injury was caused by a powerful force, other injuries may exist.
	Does the patient have any bleeding disorders or is the patient on anticoagulant drugs?	Patient taking anticoagulants, with diabetes or anemia; schedule an urgent appointment.
	Is the wound open and deep?	A gaping, deep wound requires sutures.
Head injury	Did the patient pass out or have a seizure? Is the patient confused, vomiting, or is there clear drainage from nose or ears?	If the answer is "yes" to any of these symptoms, EMS should be activated.

PROCEDURE 24-5

Caring for a Patient Who Has Fainted

GOAL: To provide emergency care for and assessment of a patient who has fainted.

EQUIPMENT AND SUPPLIES

- Sphygmomanometer
- Stethoscope
- Watch with second hand
- Blanket
- Foot stool or box
- Physician may order oxygen:
  - Portable oxygen tank
  - Pressure regulator
  - Flow meter
  - Nasal cannula with connecting tubing

PROCEDURAL STEPS

1 If warning is given that the patient feels faint, have the patient lower the head to the knees to increase blood supply to the brain (Figure 1*). If this does not stop the episode, either have the patient lie down on the examination table or lower the patient to the floor. If the patient collapses to the floor when fainting, treat with caution due to possible head or neck injuries.

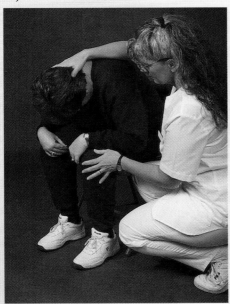

Figure 1

2 Immediately notify the physician of the patient's condition and assess the patient for life-threatening emergencies such as respiratory or cardiac arrest. If the patient is breathing and has a pulse, monitor the patient's vital signs.

3 Loosen any tight clothing and keep the patient warm, applying a blanket if needed.

4 If there is no concern about a head or neck injury, elevate the patient's legs above the level of the heart (Figure 2*).

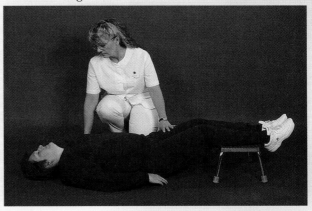

Figure 2

Purpose: Elevating the legs will assist with venous blood return to the heart. This may relieve symptoms of fainting by elevating the blood pressure and increasing blood flow to vital organs.

5 Continue to monitor vital signs and apply oxygen via nasal cannula if ordered by the physician.

6 If vital signs are unstable or the patient does not respond quickly, activate emergency medical services.

Purpose: Fainting may be a sign of a life-threatening problem.

7 If the patient vomits, roll the patient on his or her side to avoid aspiration of vomitus into the lungs.

8 Once the patient has completely recovered, assist the patient into a sitting position. *Do not* leave the patient unattended on the examination table.

9 Document the incident including a description of the episode, patient symptoms, vital signs, length of time, and any complaints. If oxygen was administered, document the number of liters and length of administration.

---

*Figures from Bonewit-West K: *Clinical procedures for medical assistants*, ed 5. Philadelphia, 2000, WB Saunders.

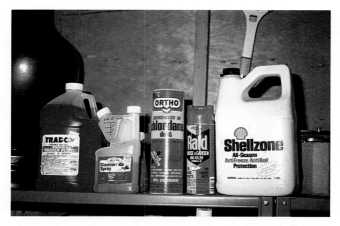

FIGURE 24-11 Hazardous household materials. (From Henry MC, Stapleton ER: *EMT prehospital care*, ed 2. Philadelphia, 1997, WB Saunders.)

Animal Bites

Potential complications from animal bites include rabies, tetanus, and local skin infections. Any animal bite that is extensive or deep should be seen by a physician. Human infection with rabies is rare, but if the bite occurs from a domestic animal, it is recommended that the animal be kept quarantined and under observation for 10 days to monitor for signs of the disease. The animal should not be killed, because a positive rabies identification is almost impossible to make if the animal has been dead for a period of time. If the bite is from a bat, raccoon, or any other wild animal, the animal is assumed to be rabid and the patient must undergo a series of rabies vaccine injections. Local skin infections can be prevented by immediately cleansing the area with antimicrobial soap and water. If the bite (including human) breaks the skin, the patient's tetanus immunization status must be checked and, if needed, a booster or the entire four-dose tetanus series must be administered.

Insect Bites and Stings

The bite or sting of an insect can be irritating and painful because of the chemical material injected from the insect, but it usually is not serious. Typical symptoms—inflammation, itching (*pruritus*), and edema—are local and confined to the area of the bite. Rarely, a severe allergic reaction occurs, which is a potentially dangerous situation that can lead to anaphylaxis. Signs and symptoms of a generalized reaction include a dry cough, feeling of tightening in the throat or chest, swelling or itching around the eyes, widespread hives, wheezing, dyspnea, and hypotension. Difficulty in talking is a sign of edema in the throat. In this situation, there is the possibility of imminent complete airway obstruction. This is a sign of a true emergency. Epinephrine and oxygen should be ready for immediate administration on the physician's orders. Antihistamines may be used, as well as corticosteroids, but the action of these agents is considerably slower than that of epinephrine. If the patient develops acute anaphylactic shock, death may occur within 1 hour unless medical intervention is initiated.

If the stinger is still lodged in the skin, scrape it off with a dull knife or fingernail. Be careful not to squeeze the stinger, because that will inject more venom into the skin. Apply ice in a towel or a plastic bag around the area to relieve the pain and slow the absorption of the venom. Calamine lotion or hydrocortisone cream may be applied to relieve itching. If the patient has a history of allergies, especially to insect venom, he or she should have access to an EpiPen injection system and use it immediately after the sting occurs and be transported to the nearest hospital for immediate care.

TICK REMOVAL

Ticks can cause a number of diseases, including Rocky Mountain spotted fever and Lyme disease. They embed their heads in the skin to obtain blood and should be removed intact by the following method:
- Grasp the body of the tick with tweezers and pull steadily and gently.
- Do not apply a match or cigarette to the area.
- If the entire tick is not removed, an office appointment must be made.

Asthma Attacks

Asthma is a condition characterized by expiratory wheezing, coughing, a feeling of tightness in the chest, and shortness of breath. During an asthma attack two different physiological responses occur. The lining of the respiratory tract becomes inflamed, edematous, and produces mucus, which results in a narrowing of the air passages. At the same time, bronchospasms occur that also constrict the airways. Attacks vary greatly between patients, and treatment must be individualized to minimize or eliminate chronic symptoms. If the patient has been prescribed an inhaler, it should be used at the first indication of symptoms.

Seizures

Seizures may be idiopathic or may result from trauma, injury, or metabolic alterations, such as hypoglycemia or hypocalcemia. A *febrile* seizure is transient and occurs with a rapid rise in fever over 101.8° F (38.8° C). Febrile seizures occur in children between 6 months and 5 years of age. There are many different types of seizures, but they all are caused by a disruption in the electrical activity of the brain.

If a patient suffers a grand mal seizure, which involves uncontrolled muscular contractions, the most important factor is protecting the patient from possible injury. Clear anything from the area around the patient that could cause accidental injury and observe the patient until the seizure ends. Do *not* place anything in the patient's mouth, because it may damage the teeth or tongue. Do *not* hold the patient down, because that may result in muscle and bone injuries. If the patient remains unconscious after the seizure has subsided, position the patient in a side-lying position to maintain an open airway and to allow drainage of excess saliva. After the seizure is over, let the patient rest or sleep, but never leave the patient alone. Follow the physician's directives and assist in every way that you can. If the physician is not in the office, check the protocol section in the office procedure manual.

Call 911 for emergency assistance if the following occurs:

- The patient has not regained consciousness within 10 to 15 minutes.
- The seizure does not stop within a few minutes.
- The patient begins a second seizure immediately after the primary one.
- The patient is pregnant.
- There are signs of head trauma.
- The patient is a known diabetic.
- The seizure was triggered by a high fever in a child.

Abdominal Pain

Abdominal pain is a symptom caused by many different problems and may range from acute discomfort to life-threatening complications. The clinician should see every patient who reports abdominal pain; the question is how soon the patient should be seen. A patient with acute onset of severe and persistent abdominal pain, especially when this is accompanied by fever, should receive medical attention as soon as possible. There are a variety of causes for abdominal pain including intestinal infections, appendicitis, ectopic pregnancy, inflammation, hemorrhage, obstruction, and tumors.

Treatment in the ambulatory care setting varies with the cause of the pain:

- Keep the patient warm and quiet.
- Have an emesis basin available.
- Administer nothing by mouth (NPO).
- Do not apply heat to the abdomen unless so instructed by the physician.
- Check and record the patient's vital signs and follow the physician's directives.

TRIAGE/SCREENING GUIDELINES FOR URGENT PATIENT APPOINTMENT FOR ABDOMINAL PAIN

- Symptoms related to shock
- Severe, constant pain or waves of pain
- Bloody or tarry stools
- Fever greater than 101° F
- Pregnancy or a missed menstrual period
- Continuous vomiting or severe constipation
- Urinary symptoms such as frequency or **hematuria**
- Chest pain, SOB, or continuous cough
- Serious illness such as diabetes, heart disease, or cancer

Sprains and Strains

Sprains are tears of the ligaments that support a joint, and strains are injuries to a muscle and its tendons. Both injuries may also cause damage to blood vessels and surrounding nerve tissue. With a sprain the victim develops edema and **ecchymosis** around the injury, and any movement of the joint, especially a twisting one, results in pain. There usually is no swelling or discoloration with a strain and only mild tenderness unless the injured muscle or tendon is used. Tendon strains and ligament sprains take several weeks to heal, whereas muscle tears usually heal in 1 to 2 weeks, because muscle has such a rich blood supply. These injuries are treated by elevating the affected area, applying mild compression, and rapidly applying ice. Swelling will be reduced if the ice is applied within 20 to 30 minutes of the injury. After 24 to 36 hours, alternately applying mild heat and ice is usually indicated. The patient may be advised to immobilize the part.

Fractures

A fracture is a break or crack in a bone and can result from trauma or disease. Fractures are very painful, and the patient will have difficulty moving the injured part of the body. When a patient with a fracture is brought into the office, the medical assistant should make the patient as comfortable as possible. Place the patient in a position that does not place strain on the area. Notify the physician immediately and proceed according to the orders given. Emergency treatment for fractures includes preventing movement of the injured part through splinting, elevation of the affected extremity, application of ice, and control of any bleeding. If a patient with an open fracture is seen in the ambulatory care setting, he or she should be transported to the emergency department.

Burns

Burns are among the most frequent causes of injuries in the United States. Burn injuries can result from flame, heat, scalds, electricity, chemicals, or radiation. The skin surface may be reddened, blistered, or charred. The depth and extent of burns are the major determinants in classifying the severity of a burn. The extent of the pain is directly proportional to the extent of the surface area burned, as well as the depth and nature of the burn.

To triage a burn injury, it is necessary to understand what caused the burn, its location and approximate size, the depth of the burn, and whether any additional injuries also occurred. The percentage of the body surface area burned can be estimated using the Rule of Nines (Figure 24-12). Partial-thickness burns over 15% of the total body surface and full-thickness burns of less than 2% can be treated in the ambulatory care setting if the patient can be seen immediately. Patients with larger body surface area involvement or other complications should be immediately transported to a hospital, preferably one with a burn unit.

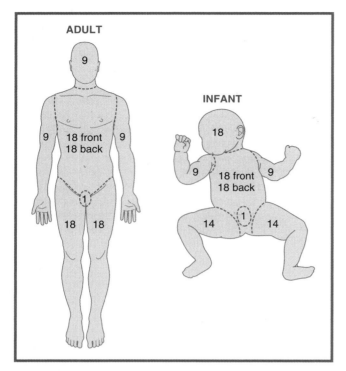

FIGURE 24-12   Rule of Nines classification of burns.

Lacerations

Lacerations are a common presentation in a primary care physician's office. A lacerated wound displays a jagged or irregular tearing of the tissues. The severity depends on the mechanism, site, and extent of the injury and the presence of foreign bodies or contamination in the wound. The injury that caused the laceration may also have caused damage to blood vessels, nerves, bones, joints, and organs within the body cavities.

When the patient arrives at the facility, apply gloves and notify the physician immediately. Have the patient lie down. Cover the injured area with a sterile dressing; use a dressing that is thick enough to absorb the bleeding (Procedure 24-6). Reassure the patient and explain your actions as much as possible. Ask the patient when he or she received the last tetanus inoculation and record the date in the patient's record. If it has been more than 10 years, the physician will probably want a booster injection given.

Wounds that are not bleeding severely and that do not involve deep tissue damage should be cleansed with antimicrobial soap and water to remove bacteria and other foreign matter. If the laceration is extremely dirty, the physician may want the area irrigated with a sterile normal saline solution.

A butterfly closure strip may be used over small lacerations to hold the edges together. If the wound is superficial and has straight edges, it may be closed with a microporous tape, which eliminates the discomfort of suturing and suture removal. After the clinician has completed patient care, apply sterile absorbent gauze

directly to the wound. The dressing selected may vary in size and thickness according to the wound.

Figure 24-13 shows a patient handout from an emergency department on potential danger signs as well as instructions for follow-up care. Patient education forms should be printed in different languages for non–English-speaking patients.

Nosebleeds (Epistaxis)

Nosebleed, or *epistaxis*, is a hemorrhage that usually results from the rupture of small vessels within the nose. Nosebleeds can be caused by injury, disease, hypertension, strenuous activity, high altitudes, exposure to cold, overuse of anticoagulant medications such as aspirin, or nasal recreational drug use. Bleeding from the anterior nostril area is usually venous while that in the posterior region is usually arterial and more difficult to stop. Treatment of epistaxis varies according to the amount of bleeding and the presence of other conditions or the use of anticoagulant medications.

If the bleeding is mild to moderate and from one side of the nose, the patient should sit up, lean forward, and apply direct pressure to the affected nostril by pinching the nose. Continue constant pressure for 10 to 15 minutes to allow clotting to take place. Repeat if bleeding cannot be controlled, insert a clean pad of gauze into the nostril, and notify the physician. If the physician is not available, proceed with standard EMS protocols. Bleeding that is bilateral and continuous or in a patient with a bleeding disorder or on anticoagulant therapy should be considered a medical emergency.

Head Injuries

The severity of a head injury can vary greatly. The history of the injury—details on what and how it happened—is vital to determining management. With a head injury, the patient may appear normal; may experience dizziness, severe headache, mental confusion, or memory loss; or may even be unconscious. The loss of consciousness may be brief or prolonged; it may appear immediately or may be delayed. The victim may experience vomiting; loss of bladder and bowel control; and bleeding from the nose, mouth, or ears. The pupils of the eyes may be unequal and non-reactive to light.

All head injuries must be considered serious. Notify the physician or contact EMS immediately. If there is evidence of neck injury, stabilize the neck and do not attempt to move the victim. Do not administer anything by mouth. Keep the patient warm and quiet. Watch the pupils of the eyes, and record any changes. Obtain vital signs and record the extent and duration of any unconsciousness. If the patient is at home or is sent home after physician assessment, he or she should be watched closely for 24 hours after the injury for any change in mental status.

Foreign Bodies in the Eye

The eye is a delicate organ whose unique structure demands special handling. This kind of emergency is most uncomfortable, and it is often extremely difficult

PROCEDURE **24-6**

Controlling Bleeding

GOAL: To stop hemorrhaging from an open wound.

EQUIPMENT AND SUPPLIES

- Gloves, sterile if available
- Appropriate personal protective equipment according to OSHA guidelines including:
  - Impermeable gown
  - Goggles
  - Impermeable mask
- Sterile dressings
- Bandaging material
- Biohazard waste container

PROCEDURAL STEPS

1 Wash hands and apply appropriate personal protective equipment.
Purpose: To meet OSHA standard precautions.

2 Assemble equipment and supplies.

3 Apply several layers of sterile dressing material directly to the wound and exert pressure.
Purpose: Direct pressure to the wound will slow down or stop bleeding. Sterile supplies are needed to prevent wound infection.

4 Wrap the wound with bandage material. Add more dressing and bandaging material if bleeding continues.

5 If bleeding persists and the wound is located on an extremity, elevate the extremity above the level of the heart. Notify the physician immediately if bleeding cannot be controlled.

6 If bleeding still continues, apply pressure to the appropriate artery. If bleeding is in the arm, apply pressure to the brachial artery by squeezing the inner aspect of the upper mid-arm. If bleeding is in the leg, apply pressure to the femoral artery on the affected side by pushing with the heel of the hand into the femoral crease at the groin. *If bleeding cannot be controlled, it may be necessary to activate the emergency medical system.*

7 Once the bleeding is controlled and the patient is stabilized, dispose of contaminated materials into the biohazard waste container.

8 Disinfect the area, remove gloves, and dispose into biohazard waste.

9 Wash hands.

10 Document the incident including the details of the wound, when and how it occurred, patient symptoms, vital signs, physician treatment, and the patient's current condition.

---

to keep the patient from rubbing the eye. Tell the patient not to touch the eye in any way. If the physician has given prior permission, apply a few drops of ophthalmic topical anesthetic in the eye to relieve the patient's pain. The patient should be placed in a darkened room to wait for the physician, because **photophobia** is common with eye irritations. If there is a contusion and swelling, cold, wet compresses will help. Ask the patient to close both eyes and cover them with eye pads until the physician arrives. The physician may order an eye irrigation to remove the object. Unless the foreign object is clearly visible, do not attempt to search for it or to remove it.

Heat and Cold Injuries

Exposure to extremes in temperature can cause minor to severe injuries. Heat injuries occur most often on humid, hot days and result in cramps, heat exhaustion, or heat stroke. Heat-related muscle cramps are the initial sign of a heat-related emergency while *heat exhaustion* is a more serious condition. Patients with heat exhaustion appear flushed and report headaches, nausea, vertigo, and weak-

ness. *Heat stroke*, the most dangerous form of heat-related injury, results in a shutdown of body systems. Patients with heat stroke have red, hot, dry skin; altered levels of consciousness; tachycardia; and rapid, shallow breathing. This is a true medical emergency. If heat-related problems are recognized in the early stages and adequately treated, the patient does not usually develop heat stroke. Management of heat-related illnesses includes getting the person out of the heat; loosening clothing or removing perspiration-soaked clothing; and giving the person cool drinks if he or she is alert. An effective way to lower the victim's temperature is to apply cool, wet cloths and to fan the moist skin so evaporation occurs and heat is released from the body.

There are two types of cold-related injuries: frostbite and hypothermia. *Frostbite*, which is the actual freezing of tissue, occurs when the skin temperature falls to a range of 14° to 25° F. Prolonged exposure of the skin to cold causes damage similar to a burn. The tissue may appear gray or white, swollen, have clear blisters, or in full-thickness frostbite, show signs of tissue **necrosis**, including blackened areas and severe deformity. The more advanced

LACERATIONS

What you need to know . . .

It is important to prevent infection and to allow your cut to heal. Call your doctor or return to him or her immediately if any of the "danger signs" occur.

Return for recheck in _____ days
Return for suture removal in _____ days

Danger signs to watch for . . .

1. Increasing pain, swelling, redness, and warmth in the injured area.
2. Pus in or around the cut.
3. Fever greater than 100°F (38°C).
4. Blood soaking through the dressing.

If any of these signs occur, contact your doctor or return to the Emergency Department.

What to do at home . . .

1. Take all medicines exactly as directed.
2. Raise the injured area above your heart level for 1 to 2 days.
3. Keep the wound and bandage clean and dry. For cuts on the face, a bandage is often not necessary. All finger dressings must be changed within 24 hours.
4. Remove the bandage/dressing in 24 hours.
5. After 24 hours, you may shower or bathe. Begin cleaning the wound with clear water twice each day to remove crusting and scabbing. Then apply ointment (Polysporin).
6. Prevent sunburn. Use a sunscreen for 6 months (e.g., Pre-Sun or Eclipse).
7. If you have a private doctor or are a member of an HMO (e.g., Kaiser), you should call for an appointment for your recheck and suture removal. If you can't get an appointment, you are welcome to return here to complete your care.

Please remember . . .

1. The exam and treatment you have just received are not intended to provide complete medical care. You need to call your doctor to schedule a follow-up visit.

2. The X-rays or E.C.G. taken today will be reviewed by a specialist. If there is any change in your diagnosis, we will contact you.

FIGURE 24-13 Educational materials about lacerations for home care of a wound.

the frostbite, the more serious the tissue damage, and the more likely the body part will be lost. There is no feeling in tissue that is frozen, but as thawing occurs, the patient reports itching, tingling, and burning pain. Mild frostbite can be managed by applying constant warmth to the affected areas either by immersing the area in warm water (no warmer than 105° F) or wrapping it in warm, dry clothing. Friction should never be used, because this would increase tissue damage. If blisters have formed or if there is evidence of full-thickness frostbite, the patient should be transported to the nearest emergency room.

Hypothermia is a medical emergency that may result in death unless the patient receives immediate assistance. Systemic hypothermia is a core body temperature of less than 95° F, preferably taken with an Ototemp (tympanic thermometer). Symptoms of hypothermia include shivering, numbness, apathy, and loss of consciousness. If hypothermia is suspected, activate EMS and care for any life-threatening conditions until help arrives. Remove the victim's wet clothing and wrap the victim in blankets while moving him or her to a warm place. If the victim is alert, give warm liquids and apply heating pads (using a barrier to avoid burns) to help slowly warm the core body temperature.

Dehydration

A person dehydrates when he or she excretes more water than is taken in. Dehydration can be a very serious health emergency, leading to convulsions, coma, and even death. Infants, young children, and older adult patients are at greatest risk for developing serious complications from dehydration. Severe dehydration may be caused by excessive heat loss, vomiting, diarrhea, or lack of fluid intake. Symptoms include vertigo; dark yellow urine or no urine output for 8 to 10 hours; extreme thirst; lethargy or confusion; and abdominal or muscle cramps. If the patient exhibits any of these symptoms and is not able to retain fluids, schedule an urgent appointment or referral to the emergency department. Replacing lost fluids is vital, so the patient should be encouraged to drink water, tea, sports drinks, fruit juice, or Pedialyte.

Diabetic Emergencies

Diabetes mellitus is caused by either a malfunction in the production of insulin in the pancreas or an inability of the cells to use insulin. Insulin is required on the cellular level so that glucose can be used for energy. Two different diabetic emergencies are caused by either *hyperglycemia* (high blood glucose levels) or *hypoglycemia* (low blood glucose levels).

Insulin shock is caused by severe hypoglycemia, because the diabetic patient either has taken too much insulin, has not eaten enough food, or has exercised an unusual amount. Symptoms have a rapid onset and include tachycardia, profuse sweating (*diaphoresis*), headache, irritability, vertigo, fatigue, hunger, seizures, and coma. It is important to provide glucose immediately, preferably in the form of glucose tablets, because they have a known concentrated quantity of glucose.

Diabetic coma results from severe hyperglycemia, because the body is not producing enough insulin, or may be caused by ingestion of too much food, stress or trauma, or an infection. Symptoms of impending diabetic coma develop slower than those from insulin shock; these include general malaise, dry mouth, **polyuria**, **polydipsia**, nausea, vomiting, SOB, and acetone- or "fruity"-smelling breath. If the patient or a caregiver when calling for an appointment reports these symptoms, notify the physician immediately, because the patient would typically be admitted to the hospital.

In an emergency situation, if a patient who has been diagnosed with diabetes mellitus exhibits signs and symptoms of a diabetic emergency, the patient should be given glucose. If the problem is caused by insulin shock (hypoglycemia), the patient will improve quickly after receiving glucose; if it is caused by diabetic coma (hyperglycemia), a small amount of added glucose will not affect the patient's condition, and he or she will need to be transported to the hospital regardless.

Patient Education

Emergencies can occur in the home, while on vacation, or in the physician's office. Patients need to learn how to handle emergency situations both by example and through instruction. The medical assistant must remain calm, triage the situation, call for help, and be prepared to administer appropriate first aid intervention. Brochures regarding home safety are also invaluable.

All patients, even children, should understand how to contact emergency medical services. This is especially important for families with members who have chronic diseases that are potentially life-threatening, such as heart conditions, severe allergic reactions, and asthma. Patients should be encouraged to post emergency numbers, such as the local EMS number, poison control center, and number of their primary care physician, next to the telephone. Families with young children need to "child-proof" their homes, being especially careful to keep potentially poisonous substances stored where children cannot get into them. "Mr. Yuk" stickers placed on poisonous containers can be an excellent educational tool for young children.

Remember to keep your American Red Cross and American Heart Association certifications current. Take advantage of community workshops to maintain and extend your skills. Post a list of community safety workshops in an area where it can be seen by patients, and encourage them to attend. Your participation in emergency care workshops and your encouragement to have others participate may help to save lives.

Legal and Ethical Issues

Most states have enacted Good Samaritan laws to encourage healthcare professionals to provide medical assistance at the scene of an accident without fear of being sued for negligence. These statutes vary greatly, but all have the intent of protecting the caregiver. It is helpful for the medical assistant to understand the legal responsibilities and the rights of the caregiver. A physician or other healthcare professional is not legally obligated to give emergency care at the site of an accident, regardless of the ethical and moral considerations. Legal liability is limited to gross neglect of the victim or willfully causing further injury to the victim. As a caregiver, you are required to act as a reasonable person and cannot be held liable for personal injury resulting from an act of omission. The Good Samaritan statutes provide for the evaluation of the caregiver's judgment but are *only in effect at the site of an emergency*, not at your place of employment.

If you have never been trained in CPR, you cannot be expected to perform the procedure at the emergency site. However, in many states, a healthcare provider with CPR training and skills who is present at the scene can be declared negligent if cardiac arrest occurs and he or she does not administer CPR to the victim.

If the victim is conscious or if a member of his or her immediate family is present, obtain a verbal consent for the emergency care procedure before you begin. Consent is implied if the patient is unconscious and no family member is present.

Many types of emergencies can be handled in the physician's office. In an emergency situation, decisions that must be made quickly can determine whether the patient lives. A medical assistant must be prepared to act calmly and efficiently in emergency situations.

SUMMARY OF SCENARIO

Cheryl has learned through her work with the triage team and involvement in emergency care situations in the office how important it is to gather complete information about emergency situations as well as to act calmly and knowledgeably when managing all patient problems. She knows she must maintain her certification in CPR and continue to participate in workshops on emergency care to be prepared for the wide variety of patient problems seen in the ambulatory care setting. Working with the triage team has also reinforced the need to document all interactions on the telephone as well as during patient visits. Cheryl will continue to refer to the triage team or Dr. Bendt when she has questions, but she feels more confident in managing emergency situations at work.

SUMMARY OF LEARNING OBJECTIVES

■ A medical assistant should be familiar with the healthcare facility's policy and procedures on the management of emergencies and maintain certification in CPR. Perform only the procedures in which you are trained, always notify the physician or activate EMS if the physician is unavailable. The medical assistant must make sure the facility is accident proof to prevent patient injuries on site, participate in planning for emergency situations, and post emergency telephone numbers for reference during an emergency.

■ A physician's office must have a centrally located crash cart or emergency bag for all emergency supplies, equipment, and medication. This material must be consistently inventoried and maintained. The chapter provided a detailed list of materials that should be readily available for an on-site emergency, including a defibrillator if indicated by the physician's practice.

■ Managing emergencies requires a calm, efficient approach to the situation. Assess the nature of the emergency and determine whether EMS should be activated or whether the patient requires an immediate or urgent appointment. Gather as many details as possible about the situation and refer to the physician when in doubt.

■ Telephone screening is one of a medical assistant's most important tasks. Emergency action principles should be used to determine the level of a patient's emergency. These include determining whether the situation is life threatening and obtaining contact information about the patient as well as all pertinent information regarding the injury and patient signs and symptoms. This information must be shared with the physician, and all details must be documented on the patient's chart.

■ Always follow standard precautions when caring for a patient with a medical emergency. Documentation of emergency treatment should include information about the patient; vital signs; allergies, current medications, and pertinent health history; the patient's chief complaint; the sequence of events, including any changes in the patient's condition since the incident; and any physician's orders and procedures performed.

■ Life-threatening emergencies require immediate assessment, referral to the physician, and, if the physician is not present, activation of EMS. While waiting for assistance, determine the presence of breathing and circulation. Administer rescue breaths or CPR if this is indicated. Depending on the patient's signs and symptoms, monitor the patient for signs of a heart attack; administer the Heimlich maneuver if there is an obstructed airway; evaluate for signs of a CVA; and assess for shock. Ask for assistance when indicated and perform appropriate skills based on the patient's presenting condition.

■ Common ambulatory care emergencies require an assessment, either by phone or on-site, of the patient's current condition and need for a physician's evaluation. Typical emergencies seen in a healthcare facility include syncope, accidental poisoning, animal bites, insect stings, asthma attacks, seizure activity, abdominal pain, orthopedic injuries, burns, lacerations, epistaxis, head and eye injuries, heat and cold injuries, dehydration, and diabetic emergencies. Each of these situations requires the medical assistant to calmly gather pertinent information from the patient and follow through with the facility's policy and physician orders on management of the emergency.

■ Patients should know how to contact emergency personnel, and families with young children should have poison control telephone numbers posted. Educating patients about how to care for minor emergencies at home is an important part of telephone triage in the ambulatory care setting. Encouraging patients to participate in community safety workshops and becoming CPR certified may help them to avoid emergencies as well as save lives.

■ Good Samaritan laws vary from state to state but are designed to protect any individual, whether a healthcare professional or lay person, from liability if he or she provides assistance at the site of an emergency. The law does not require a medically trained person to act, but if emergency care is given in a reasonable and responsible manner, the healthcare worker is protected from being sued for negligence. This protection, however, does not extend into the workplace.

INTERNET CONNECTIONS

- American Heart Association
  http://www.americanheart.org
- American Red Cross
  http://www.redcross.org

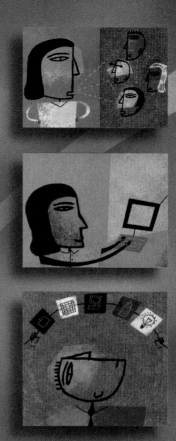

Career
Development

CHAPTER 25

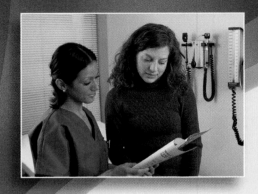

Scenario

Lisa Walker is 1 month away from graduating from her medical assisting program. She has been an excellent student and is looking forward to beginning her career in the medical field. Lisa wants to begin her job search now to minimize the time during which she is not employed after her externship ends.

Lisa has participated in several volunteer activities while she has been attending school. She plans to list these experiences on her resume. She met many office managers and physicians while doing volunteer work, and she will be contacting those people in hopes of obtaining more job leads.

Lisa began saving for interview clothing when she first began school. She is on a strict budget, but she found several outfits appropriate for interviews at second-hand clothing shops and discount stores. Her best-looking suit cost only $20!

Not a person afraid to interview, Lisa looks forward to sharing her skills and experience with potential employers. She looks on each interview as a practice session for the next one, and this helps her to relax more and present a true picture of herself to the office manager. She has a great smile and projects a natural friendliness and positive attitude.

Lisa has given much thought to what she wants from her first job as a medical assistant. She knows that she may not start at a high salary, but she also realizes that there are benefits and perquisites ("perks") when working in a physician's office. She plans to commit to working for 2 years on her first job, gaining experience before looking for the next job at a higher salary.

Lisa is excited about her future as a medical assistant. She is ready to put the training she received to work with actual patients. She plans to perform exceptionally well at her externship site and to go above and beyond her designated duties to impress the staff in that facility, who will become references for her first paid position. Lisa is dedicated to becoming the best medical assistant possible and becoming indispensable to her employer.

Career Development and Life Skills

Learning Objectives

- Define and spell the terms listed in the vocabulary.
- Discuss the reasons that job search training is important to a medical assistant.
- List three expectations that employers have of employees.
- Explain the two best job search methods.
- Describe some of the errors that should be avoided on a resume.
- Explain the importance of having demographic information about former jobs before appearing for an interview.
- List the four phases of the interview process.
- Discuss the importance of the probationary period for a new employee.
- List some mistakes that should be avoided by a new employee.
- Explain why a performance appraisal's ratings are usually not perfect.

Vocabulary

appraisals   Act of giving an expert judgment of the value or merit of; also, evaluations of work performance.

counteroffer   Return offer made by one who has rejected an offer or job.

default   Failure to pay financial debts, such as a student loan.

deferment   Postponement, especially of a student loan.

genuineness   Expressing sincerity and honest feeling.

intolerable   Not tolerable or bearable.

mock   Simulated; intended for imitation or practice.

networking   Exchange of information or services among individuals, groups, or institutions; also, meeting and getting to know individuals in the same or similar career fields and sharing information about available opportunities.

pertinent   Having a clear, decisive relevance to the matter at hand.

proofread   To read and mark corrections.

ramifications   Consequence; outgrowth; something produced by a cause or necessarily following from a set of conditions.

rectify   To correct by removing errors.

subtle   Ingenious; artful; delicate.

succinct   Marked by compact, precise expression without wasted words.

synopsis   Condensed statement or outline.

vocation   The work in which a person is regularly employed.

Each day that a person exists is a small portion of a whole—in this case, the person's entire lifetime. The events that happen during a day, no matter how small, shape the future. In the same way, the events that happen in the life of a medical assistant play a role in shaping his or her career. Every day, he or she "writes a resume"—through actions that will reveal strengths, highlight skills, and summarize the accomplishments— that builds on the medical assistant's **vocation**. Each duty performed becomes a part of the medical assistant's sum of experience and is important in the overall growth of the individual. Each action taken can have an impact on the future for the medical assistant. If the actions are professional, accurate, and performed to his or her utmost ability, the resume that the medical assistant is writing through these actions will be one that will lead to greater opportunities. If the medical assistant performs poorly, the resume will be one that will not reflect trustworthiness and dependability. The small decisions that are made every day are those that greatly affect the overall impressions that the medical assistant makes in the workplace.

Approximately 85% of persons seeking employment have never had any type of formal training in the job search process. A newly graduated medical assistant should take advantage of job search training for three reasons:

1. The training will decrease the amount of time spent searching for a job.
2. The training will increase the chances of receiving better wages through negotiations.
3. The training will help to eliminate the fears of looking for work and interviewing.

What Does the Employer Want?

Employers have three basic desires when they are interviewing individuals for a job:

1. They want a person who has a neat appearance and looks as if he or she fits the job (Figure 25-1).
2. They want an individual who is dependable and can prove that he or she has been a reliable team member in other job positions.
3. They want a person with the skills to do the job.

From the beginning of the job search process, a medical assistant's attitude is the most critical part of his or her potential success in getting a job (Figure 25-2). A good attitude is not a trait that can be developed overnight. For this reason a medical assistant must have a positive

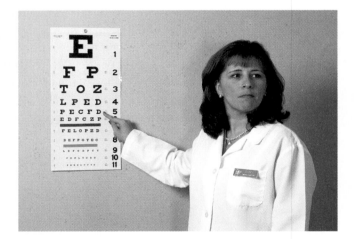

FIGURE 25-1   A professional appearance is mandatory in the medical office.

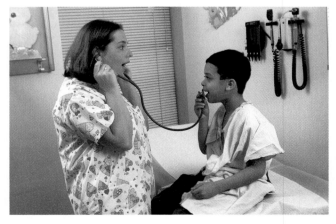

FIGURE 25-2   A great attitude is the best personal asset. Employers in the medical profession want medical assistants who will exhibit a positive attitude with the patients.

outlook in all situations, so the **genuineness** of his or her demeanor will be clear during job interviews.

Assessing Strengths

Before promoting himself or herself as a potential employee, a medical assistant must first determine the strengths that make him or her a valuable team member. There are three types of skill strengths: job skills, self-management skills, and transferable skills.

Job skills are the abilities that the medical assistant needs to perform the job. This includes such skills as venipuncture, filing insurance, answering the telephone, scheduling appointments, giving injections, and other tasks.

Self-management skills relate to the medical assistant's personality and character traits. They include such attributes as honesty, integrity, and enthusiasm.

Transferable skills can be taken from one job to another. For instance, if the medical assistant has the ability to communicate effectively, this skill can be used on every job. Leadership is a transferable skill, as are the ability to follow directions and the ability to manage people.

Developing Career Objectives

Each medical assistant has a reason for entering the healthcare field. This basic desire should influence decisions concerning his or her career choices. Because medical assisting is such a versatile profession, a medical assistant will have numerous options after graduation.

It is wise to take some time to think about what the medical assistant wants from his or her career. While he or she is attending school and subsequently completing an externship, ideas may surface about what specialty to enter.

When developing career objectives, the medical assistant should start by asking several questions:

- Where am I today?
- Where will I be in 5 years?
- Where will I be in 10 years?
- What additional skills do I need to get where I want to go?

Write down the questions and answers and go into specific detail. Set realistic goals and develop a plan as to how and when they will be reached. It is helpful to put a list of goals in a prominent place at home, where they will be seen every day. Some people use the front of the refrigerator, and some post the goals on the mirror in the area where they get dressed every day. Having the written goals in a visible place helps to keep them in mind even on the more difficult days, when the goals seem far from sight.

Knowing Personal Needs

A medical assistant must evaluate all of the needs that he or she requires in a work situation. Most people have a minimum salary that they require, as well as certain benefits. For example, if the medical assistant is a single mother, she may require a moderate salary and insist on health insurance benefits. We also have intrinsic needs, which are those internal desires that are important to us personally.

A helpful activity is to write a **synopsis** of a typical day on an ideal medical assisting job. Imagine the type of office, the job title, the daily duties, and the salary and benefits that would be a part of the ideal job (Figure 25-3). This will help to develop a focus and a goal to work toward as the medical assistant's career develops.

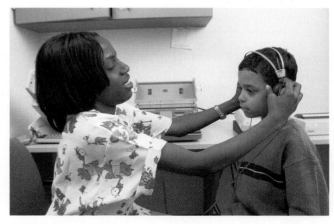

FIGURE 25-3 Enjoyment of the job is paramount. Medical assistants should enjoy their job and give compassionate, friendly care to all patients.

Finding a Job

Many people have misconceptions about the job market that exists today. Graduation from a medical assisting program does not guarantee that the student will obtain employment. Completion of the program will give the medical assistant the job skills needed to work, but a good attitude and positive outlook are essential for success in the job search.

Some job seekers assume that potential employers will not interact with students until they graduate. However, prospecting before graduation is a smart idea, and there are **subtle** ways of introducing oneself to a facility without bluntly asking for employment. Many also think that they must have work experience to be hired, but employers are more interested in attitude and teachability than a long resume full of experience. In fact, many physicians like hiring students fresh from school so that they can teach them how they want procedures done.

The Two Best Job Search Methods

Although there are many ways to find employment, two methods have proved to be the best and most effective. These are networking and direct contact with employers.

Networking is the exchange of information or services among individuals, groups, or institutions. When related to a job search, networking involves meeting and getting to know individuals in the same or similar career fields, and sharing information about available opportunities. A medical assistant should begin to form a network of friends, business associates, co-workers, and acquaintances early in training, and he or she should stay in contact with these people throughout the job search effort (Figure 25-4).

Networking is not limited to job searching, and many organizations are formed to develop networks of individuals or groups that assist each other and refer clients to each other. However, these groups are useful to the person who is looking for employment, and by attending meetings and get-togethers held for networking purposes, the medical assistant may happen into the ideal job he or she has been looking for.

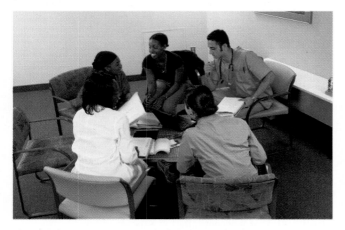

FIGURE 25-4 Stay in touch with classmates. Classmates are excellent networking contacts and may be able to provide job leads.

Direct contact with employers is also an effective method of job searching. Medical assistants often know of specific clinics or facilities that they would like to investigate as job possibilities. Compile a list of these places and learn as much about them as possible. If the facility has a website, read it thoroughly. Ask for brochures about the employer. Some have an annual report that lists details about the organization. All of this information will help the medical assistant get a good basic idea of why the facility exists and what it does for the community.

Contact with employers does not necessarily begin only after the student has graduated. Students can begin networking and contacting employers from the very start of their enrollment at school. The student may wish to keep a file on potential employers. Make a list of facilities that are good prospects for employment and then begin researching them. Call to find out who supervises medical assistants in the facility. In a physician's office, this is usually the office manager. Then call the office manager and ask to make an appointment to learn about the facility. Even the busiest people are usually willing to help a student investigate healthcare facilities in the area.

Do not express to the office manager that the objective of the appointment is a job offer. The goal at this point is to learn about the facility, what it offers the community, and what roles the medical assistants in the facility perform. Suggest that the appointment be set at his or her convenience. Then treat the appointment like an actual job interview, dressing appropriately and arriving on time. Have a list of questions about the facility prepared in advance, and do not take too much of the office manager's time. Take notes about what the office manager says about the facility, so that they can be referred to on graduation, during the actual job search.

After the appointment with the office manager, ask for a business card and always send a thank-you note or letter. *Do not fail to remember this critical point!* This helps the office manager to remember the name of the medical assistant and is a pleasant addition to the daily mail. Everyone enjoys being recognized for his or her efforts, and the office manager will appreciate the thank-you note.

Toward the time that he or she is to graduate, the medical assistant may wish to perform an externship at one of the facilities visited early in training. Check with school regulations to determine whether this is possible. Then the office manager can be approached about allowing the student to extern in the office. Be sure to follow school guidelines when investigating these possibilities.

Some schools allow students to secure their own externship sites, but this must be discussed with the externship supervisor at school. Performing an externship at a medical facility is usually the first practical experience the student will have in the medical field and can be used as a reference in building a resume.

After the externship is completed, the medical assistant may wish to send a resume to all of the office managers met through the direct contact efforts made earlier in his or her training. A professional resume with a cover letter that refers to the earlier meeting will prompt the office manager to remember the student. Ask in the cover letter whether any opportunities exist in the facility. Express that the facility and staff were impressive on the first meeting and that it would be an exciting place to begin a career. In the letter, request that if the office manager does not have any positions available at that time, the resume be kept on file or passed along to an acquaintance who is looking for an additional staff member.

Traditional Job Search Methods

The more traditional job search methods may be effective but are usually not as successful as networking and contacting employers directly.

Newspaper Ads. Newspaper ads normally produce a huge number of applicants and resumes for the employer. A resume or application will have to stand out in the crowd to be noticed when it arrives at the facility. Some applicants use clear envelopes, which draw attention to the resume quickly in a stack of mail.

Employment Agencies. Employment agencies usually charge a fee for their services. Even when the employer pays the fee, the medical assistant may be offered a lower wage to compensate for the fee. These agencies can be useful, however. In salary negotiation, the agency will know the salary range the employer is willing to pay. This means that medical assistants can command a salary within that range and not be short-changed by asking for a salary that is much lower than the employer was willing to pay.

CRITICAL THINKING APPLICATION

Lisa keeps an eye on the ads in local newspapers that mention a need for medical assistants. What current ads in local papers are interesting and would prompt sending a resume?

Professional Societies. Joining local chapters of medical assistant organizations helps the student in many ways. Not only will valuable information be exchanged at the meetings, but the medical assistant may also hear of positions that are coming available in various medical facilities. This is a form of networking.

Volunteering. By volunteering in medical offices or facilities, the medical assistant will meet other professionals who may be able to provide job leads. Volunteer activities should be added to the resume, because these valuable experiences can often be used in the physician's office as well. It does not matter that the position was not a paid job; experience counts, whether paid or not.

Mailing Resumes. Mailing a large number of resumes is not a very effective method of job search. Out of 100 resumes sent, one or two potential employers may respond with a request for an interview. It is much more effective to network first, and then follow up with a good cover letter and resume. Resumes can be used when contacting employers directly, and this approach allows the medical assistant to meet at least one employee of the facility when the document is delivered. Be sure to ask for a business card and write down the name of the person to whom the resume was delivered. For impressive facilities, send a note of thanks to the person who accepted the resume, asking to be considered for future positions.

Cold Calling. Cold calling is contacting employers by phone and prospecting for available positions. If the medical assistant asks, "Are you hiring?" at the beginning of the conversation, he or she should expect a negative answer and has just wasted the call. This is all but useless in the job search effort. However, an assistant who calls for information about the clinic and schedules an appointment with the office manager may have more success. Never attempt to get a job over the phone. Even when interested employers call and ask questions, attempt to set up an interview to discuss your qualifications in person.

Performing Well on Externships. Performing well on externships may be one of the best ways to secure a job. If an opening exists, the medical assistant extern is already oriented to the practice and may be the perfect fit for the job. Perform duties assigned on the externship as if they were final examinations at school. Even when the office does not have a position available at that time, there may be one soon, or the office manager or physician may know of an office that has an opening. Do the best job possible, and there may be an employment offer waiting at the conclusion of the externship.

Developing a Resume

A **resume** is a fact sheet that summarizes an applicant's qualifications, education, and experience. A medical assistant must determine what to include in the resume, remembering that he or she is "selling" himself or herself to an employer (Procedure 25-1).

There are many types of resumes. Three of the most common include the chronological resume, the functional resume, and the targeted resume. A chronological resume highlights the medical assistant's abilities in a logical order, such as most recent jobs back to the beginning of the individual's career (Figure 25-5). A functional resume highlights specific skill sets, emphasizing the most important abilities or the most valuable experiences that the medical assistant has performed (Figure 25-6). A targeted resume is perhaps the most effective: it emphasizes the skills that relate specifically to the job for which the medical assistant is applying (Figure 25-7).

PROCEDURE **25-1**

Preparing a Resume

GOAL: To write an effective resume for use as a tool in gaining employment.

EQUIPMENT AND SUPPLIES

- Scratch paper
- Pen or pencil
- Former job descriptions, if available
- List of addresses of former employers, schools, and names of supervisors
- Computer or word processor
- Quality stationery and envelopes

PROCEDURAL STEPS

1 Perform a self-evaluation by making notes about your strengths as a medical assistant. Consider job skills, self-management skills, and transferable skills.
Purpose: To determine the strongest aspects of your abilities so that they can be highlighted on the resume.

2 Explore formatting and decide on a professional resume appearance that best highlights your skills and experience. Use the templates available in word processing software or design your own.
Purpose: To construct an attractive document.

3 Place your name, address, and two telephone numbers where you can be contacted at the top of the resume.
Purpose: To make certain that potential employers have a means of contact.

4 Write a job objective that specifies your employment goals.
Purpose: To give the prospective employer an idea of what you are looking for in a medical assisting position.

5 Provide details about your educational experience. List degrees and/or certifications obtained.

6 Provide details about your work experience. Include all contact information and names of supervisors. Do not include salary expectations or reasons for leaving former jobs.
Purpose: No negative information should be put on the resume. Salaries should be discussed—if a certain salary is listed on the resume, it may limit the amount that the facility will offer the medical assistant.

7 Prepare a cover letter and a list of references. Send the references with the resume only when requested.

8 Type the resume carefully and make certain that there are no errors on the document.
Purpose: Resumes submitted with errors are often discarded without consideration.

9 Proofread the resume. Allow another person to read it as well and look for missed errors.
Purpose: To make certain that the resume is error free.

10 Print the resume on quality paper. Review the resume again for errors and to assure that it looks attractive on the printed page.

11 Target each resume to a specific person or position. Do not send generic resumes to each prospective employer.
Purpose: Targeted resumes get better results during the job search.

12 Follow up on all resumes that are distributed with a phone call to arrange an interview.
Purpose: A resume sent without follow-up is usually ineffective.

A medical assistant should target the resume toward the specific job that he or she is applying for. This means that the job requirements should be compared with the skills on the resume, and those skills should be highlighted in the document (Figure 25-8). Of course, to do this effectively, the medical assistant must actually know the job requirements. One can assume that clinical and administrative duties will be similar from place to place, but the ad for the position may provide further information about the scope of duties for the position. A medical assistant should read these carefully and emphasize that those are a part of his or her skill set on the resume.

A good way to approach the resume is to compose it on a computer and save it to the hard drive or a disk.

Then, as each job opportunity presents itself, the resume can be modified to fit the job. For instance, if the resume lists back-office skills first and the job is for an administrative position, the administrative skills should be moved to the top to draw more attention to them. This is easy to accomplish when the resume is on a computer, because the medical assistant can cut and paste where necessary to make changes and save several versions of the resume. Then an original can be printed on quality paper for every job for which he or she applies.

A resume is an important job search tool, but it should never be expected to get the medical assistant a job on its own merit. It is but one of many tools that should be used when looking for employment.

Ruby Dunham
9362 Caesar Creek Road
Mytown, OH 45458
(937) 555-1899

Education

• 1998: A.S. in Medical Assisting, Community College, Mytown, OH

Experience:

1995–present: Medical Transcriptionist, Community Hospital, Mytown, OH

• Transcribe 55 wpm
• Specialist in medical terminology
• Excellent attendance record
• Detail oriented
• Increased personal productivity each quarter

1990–1995: Secretary, State University School of Medicine, Mytown, OH

• Coordinated schedules of four full-time professors
• Maintained office supply and assistant budget
• Created final examination scheduling guidelines for department
• Developed excellent written communication skills
• Familiar with a variety of office machines

1986–1990: Shift Manager, Burger World, Mytown, OH

• Managed 10 employees, including hiring, training, evaluating, and firing
• Developed excellent oral communication skills and team player concept
• Improved inventory supply techniques, reducing losses by 10%
• Maintained cleanliness standards highest in chain
• Developed customer-focused service goals for store

FIGURE 25-5   Chronological resume.

Developing a professional resume takes some time and effort, and it will prove to be a good investment. Give the document some thought and follow generally accepted guidelines for its construction.

CRITICAL THINKING APPLICATION

Lisa has drafted her resume and given a copy to her placement director. She has recommended that Lisa remove the mention of her volunteer experience, because it was not in the medical field. Should Lisa do this? Why or why not?

Critical Resume Errors

The first error that should be avoided on a resume is just that—any error. There should be no errors at all on a resume. Many employers will automatically disqualify a job candidate if an error is found on a resume.

One medical assistant who was having a difficult time finding a job consulted her placement director at school. The director suggested that she come in for a **mock** interview. About halfway through the interview, the placement director realized the problem. The medical

Max Bryan
1234 Rolling View Court
Mytown, OH 45431
(937) 555-3137

OBJECTIVE

• An entry level position in medical assisting, with the opportunity to utilize and refine skills and training

EDUCATION

• 1998: A.S. in Medical Assisting, Community College, Mytown, OH. Dean's list senior year, cumulative GPA 3.5

STRENGTHS

• Possess excellent interpersonal and communication skills
• Demonstrate consistent positive attitude and high energy
• Caring and compassionate
• Responsible, self-motivated, precise in work
• Experienced in customer-focused service

ACCOMPLISHMENTS

• Tutored students in medical assisting and 12-lead EKG courses. Received excellent evaluations and positive results
• Certified Medical Assistant, active member of local AAMA
• Experienced in MS Office programs
• Consistent "excellent" ratings in clinical externships

COMMUNITY ACTIVITIES

• 1995–present: Organized, recruited, and trained 20 others for church hand bell choir, direct weekly practices and monthly performances
• 1996–present: Teach community CPR twice yearly to high school students
• Vice-President Student Government, Community College, Mytown, OH. Recruited members, organized fund-raisers, campaigned successfully for policy changes

EMPLOYMENT

• 1996–present: Tutor, Community College, Mytown, OH
• Waiter, Scott's Place, Mytown, OH

FIGURE 25-6   Functional resume.

assistant had worked for 2 years at a local grocery store and had misspelled the name of the store on the resume. Thinking from an employer's point of view, a person who cannot spell the name of a facility where she worked for 2 years, and cashed a paycheck with the name on it as well, might well make critical errors in charting or in other aspects of her duties. Within a week after this error was corrected, the medical assistant found a job.

Never list salary expectations on the resume. If the medical assistant lists a salary of $25,000 on the last job held, the future employer might not offer more than $26,000 to $27,000, realizing that this is a step up from the last salary. However, if they were willing to pay $32,000, the medical assistant has lost an opportunity for much higher wages.

Avoid using "I" or other personal pronouns on the resume. If abbreviations are used on the resume, be sure

Roscoe Patterson
3472 Vienna Woods Lane
Mytown, OH 45449
(937) 555-8874

Job Target:

• A long-term medical assistant position in a busy and
varied medical office

Education:

• 1992: BA in Art History, State University, Mytown, OH
• 1998: AS in Medical Assisting, Community College, Mytown, OH

Capabilities:

• Excellent interpersonal skills and caring attitude
• Detail oriented, with strong analytical and problem-solving abilities
• Utilize solid organizational and time-management abilities in
coordinating multiple projects
• Self-starter, take initiative to ensure jobs get done properly and
efficiently
• Upbeat, personable, and highly energetic
• Ability to communicate in Spanish and American Sign Language

Accomplishments/Achievements:

• Campaigned for and raised consistent 15% annual increase in
contributions and grants, allowing expansion of exhibits and needed
renovations to art museum
• Maintained museum budget with 100% accountability
• Organized annual "Art Ball" for 100 contributors under budget
• Museum employee of the year 1995
• Certificates in CPR and EKG; Certified Nursing Assistant; will sit for
CMA exam this November

Work History:

• 1998–present: Certified Nursing Assistant, Friendly Nursing Home,
Mytown, OH
• 1992–1998: Assistant to the Curator, Mytown Museum of Art,
Mytown, OH

FIGURE 25-7 Targeted resume.

USEFUL ACTION WORDS

Accelerated	Manage
Actively	Motivated
Adapted	Organized
Administered	Originate
Analyze	Participated
Approve	Perform
Completed	Pinpointed
Conceived conduct	Plan
Control	Proficient
Coordinate	Program
Created	Proposed
Delegate	Proved
Demonstrate	Provide
Develop	Recommended
Direct	Reduced
Effect	Reinforced
Eliminated	Reorganized
Established	Responsibilities
Evaluate	Revamped
Expanded	Review
Expedite	Revise
Founded	Schedule
Generated	Significantly
Improved	Simplify
Increased	Solve
Influence	Strategy
Implemented	Streamline
Interpret	Structure
Launched	Successfully
Lead	Supervise
Lecture	Support
Maintain	Teach

FIGURE 25-8 Use action words when describing skills on the resume.

to spell them out for clarity the first time they are used, if they are not well-known abbreviations. Never include personal information, such as height, weight, age, marital status, number of children, or any other information that is not **pertinent** to the job requirements.

Do not list dates along the left-hand side of the paper. This is distracting and draws attention away from the points that should be emphasized. A resume must be visually appealing and easy to read. The medical assistant should make good use of spacing, margins, indentions, capitalizing, and underlining to ensure an attractive document. **Proofread** the document several times to be sure there are no errors. It is helpful to have someone else proofread it, because many times the writer of a document misses errors when proofing.

Never include a photograph with the resume. Photographs can be a discriminatory factor in the hiring process, and the medical assistant should be wary of any employer who requests a photograph with the resume.

One of the most senseless errors common to resumes is not having the appropriate contact information, such as an address and telephone number. Two phone numbers are suggested, such as a cell phone and a home phone, so that there is a better chance of reaching the candidate when it is time to schedule an interview.

The Argument of Length

Professionals disagree about the acceptable length of a resume. One page may be considered the ideal length, but a person with 20 years' experience in the job market will never get all of his or her skills on one page. A medical assistant without previous work experience may easily fit the resume on one page.

Recent trends indicate that a good rule of thumb is to allow one page for every 6 years of experience. If a person has a 20-year career in healthcare, the resume would be approximately three pages long. This is a general guideline, however; the document should be as **succinct** as possible, while clearly communicating the strengths and experiences of the applicant.

The Purpose of a Resume

The purpose of a resume is *not* to get the medical assistant a job, although this is a commonly held belief. The purpose of the cover letter is to get the employer to look at the resume. The purpose of the resume is to get the applicant an interview. The purpose of the interview, of course, is to get the job. Remember this, and use the resume as a tool, along with other strategies for job searching.

The medical assistant should be the person to write the resume, or at the very least, have a hand in its composition. Professional resume services may be helpful, but the person who knows the most about the experience and education gained is the medical assistant.

CRITICAL THINKING APPLICATION

Lisa has been asked by a potential employer to email her resume. She has used an unusual font on her cover letter and the top of the resume. What concerns should Lisa have about emailing the document? How can Lisa make certain that her document arrives in a readable format when sending it electronically?

The Cover Letter

When sending a resume, always include a cover letter (Figure 25-9). This is the introduction to the resume and the person sending the document. A cover letter should always be sent to an individual, not to the facility or "to whom it may concern." A simple phone call will usually reveal the name of the person to whom the resume should be sent. Ask for the name of the office manager, or if this information is not obtained, address it specifically to the physician.

Make the cover letter brief and interesting. Use the same paper stock weight and color as the resume. Be sure to include contact information, such as an address and at least two phone numbers, even if these are on the attached resume. The supervisor may have separated the two documents, so there must be a method of contact on each one. Never start a cover letter with the sentence, "I saw your ad in the newspaper" or a similar phrase. Be creative with the opening line and try to capture the attention of the reader.

A cover letter should be one to three paragraphs long. The final section should include a call to action that will prompt an interview. If the document concludes with a request for a meeting, the medical assistant should state when he or she will call for a time and date.

Job Applications

Many facilities require a job application along with a resume (Figure 25-10). Arrive 15 minutes before the scheduled interview to allow time to fill out an application.

Brutis Walter
2345 Morrow Court
Mytown, OH 45310
(937) 555-7426

May 23, 1998

Andrea Foreman, CMA
Office Manager
Family Health, Inc.
123 Timberleaf Drive
Mytown, OH 45432

Ms. Foreman:

I will be graduating from Community College with an A.S. in Medical Assisting on June 9 and am interested in an entry-level medical assistant position in your office. I will consider part-time or temporary work to gain experience in a diverse office such as yours.

My training includes hands-on experience in pediatrics, cardiology, internal medicine, obstetrics, and geriatrics. My administrative training would allow me to fill in wherever needed in the office. I am highly motivated and have supported myself and paid my own way through college. I understand responsibility and am a true team player. Belinda Mallet, RN, a fellow church member, told me the office will be short-staffed this summer owing to vacations and a maternity leave. I believe I could help your office run smoothly this summer, and beyond.

I look forward to hearing from you. I am available Tuesday and Thursday afternoons and Friday mornings until graduation. I will call you next Tuesday to set up an appointment for an interview. Thank you for your consideration.

Very truly yours,

Brutis Walter

FIGURE 25-9   Cover letter.

Job applications can be considered a legal document if the person is hired. Therefore they should be neat and filled out correctly and completely. Always read the application before filling it out, so that directions make sense and information is not placed in the wrong area of the form. Carry a planner or address book to the interview so that former employers' and supervisors' names, addresses, and phone numbers are handy. The medical assistant should not be in a position that he or she must ask for a phone book to get an address. Have all of this information ready for the time that it is needed.

Applications often ask for a date that the medical assistant is available for work. Be careful with this question. If the applicant currently has a job, yet writes that he or she is "immediately available," it may indicate that the applicant intends to quit without notice. On the other hand, the current employer may be aware that the person is seeking other employment and may have granted him or her permission to quit immediately once a new job is found.

Be careful on the sections that ask the reason for leaving former positions. Think about the answers that are listed in those spaces, and try to put the information in as positive a light as possible. Ask the advice of the

APPLICATION FOR POSITION / Medical or Dental Office
AN EQUAL OPPORTUNITY EMPLOYER

(In answering questions, use extra blank sheet if necessary)

No employee, applicant, or candidate for promotion, training or other advantage shall be discriminated against (or given preference) because of race, color, religion, sex, age, physical handicap, veteran status, or national origin.

PLEASE READ CAREFULLY AND WRITE OR PRINT ANSWERS TO ALL QUESTIONS. DO NOT TYPE.

Date of Application

A. PERSONAL INFORMATION

| Name - Last | First | Middle | Social Security No. | Area Code/Phone No. ( ) |

| Present Address: - Street | (Apt #) | City | State | Zip | How Long At This Address?: |

| Previous Address: - Street | City | State | Zip | Person to notify in case of Emergency or Accident - Name: |
From: To: Address: Telephone:

B. EMPLOYMENT INFORMATION

| For What Position Are You Applying?: | ☐ Full-Time ☐ Part-Time ☐ Either | Date Available For Employment?: | Wage/Salary Expectations: |

| List Hrs./Days You Prefer To Work | List Any Hrs./Days You Are Not Available: (Except for times required for religious practices or observances) | Can You Work Overtime, If Necessary? ☐ Yes ☐ No |

| Are You Employed Now?: ☐ Yes ☐ No | If So, May We Inquire Of Your Present Employer?: ☐ No ☐ Yes, If Yes: Name Of Employer: Phone Number: ( ) |

| Have You Ever Been Bonded? ☐ Yes ☐ No | If Required For Position, Are You Bondable? ☐ Yes ☐ No ☐ Uncertain | Have You Applied For A Position With This Office Before? ☐ No ☐ Yes If Yes, When?: |

Referred By / Or Where Did You Learn Of This Job?:

| Can You, Upon Employment, Submit Verification Of Your Legal Right To Work In The United States?: ☐ Yes ☐ No Submit Proof That You Meet Legal Age Requirement For Employment? ☐ Yes ☐ No | Language(s) Applicant Speaks or Writes (If Use Of A Language Other Than English is Relevant To The Job For Which The Applicant Is Applying: |

C. EDUCATIONAL HISTORY

Name & Address Of Schools Attended (Include Current)	Dates From	Thru	Highest Grade/Level Completed	Diploma/Degree(s) Obtained/Areas of Study
High School				
College				Degree/Major
Post Graduate				Degree/Major
Other				Course/Diploma/License/Certificate

Specific Training, Education, Or Experiences Which Will Assist You In The Job For Which You Have Applied.

Future Educational Plans

D. SPECIAL SKILLS

CHECK BELOW THE KINDS OF WORK YOU HAVE DONE:

☐ BLOOD COUNTS	☐ DENTAL ASSISTANT	☐ MEDICAL INSURANCE FORMS	☐ RECEPTIONIST
☐ BOOKKEEPING	☐ DENTAL HYGIENIST	☐ MEDICAL TERMINOLOGY	☐ TELEPHONES
☐ COLLECTIONS	☐ FILING	☐ MEDICAL TRANSCRIPTION	☐ TYPING
☐ COMPOSING LETTERS	☐ INJECTIONS	☐ NURSING	☐ STENOGRAPHY
☐ COMPUTER INPUT	☐ INSTRUMENT STERILIZATION	☐ PHLEBOTOMY (Draw Blood)	☐ URINALYSIS
OFFICE EQUIPMENT USED: ☐ COMPUTER	☐ DICTATING EQUIPMENT	☐ POSTING	☐ X-RAY
		☐ WORD PROCESSOR	☐ OTHER:

| Other Kinds Of Tasks Performed Or Skills That May Be Applicable To Position: | Typing Speed | Shorthand Speed |

(PLEASE COMPLETE OTHER SIDE)

FIGURE 25-10   Application for employment. (Courtesy Bibbero Systems, Inc., Petaluma, Calif. 94654, (800) 242-2376, www.bibbero.com.)

E. EMPLOYMENT RECORD

LIST MOST RECENT EMPLOYMENT FIRST   May We Contact Your Previous Employer(s) For A Reference? ☐ Yes ☐ No

1) Employer   Work Performed. Be Specific:

Address   Street   City   State   Zip Code

Phone Number
(   )

Type of Business   Dates   Mo. Yr.   Mo. Yr.
                          From   To
Your Position   Hourly Rate/Salary
                          Starting   Final
Supervisor's Name

Reason For Leaving

2) Employer   Worked Performed. Be Specific:

Address   Street   City   State   Zip Code

Phone Number
(   )

Type of Business   Dates   Mo. Yr.   Mo. Yr.
                          From   To
Your Position   Hourly Rate/Salary
                          Starting   Final
Supervisor's Name

Reason For Leaving

3) Employer   Worked Performed. Be Specific:

Address   Street   City   State   Zip Code

Phone Number
(   )

Type of Business   Dates   Mo. Yr.   Mo. Yr.
                          From   To
Your Position   Hourly Rate/Salary
                          Starting   Final
Supervisor's Name

Reason For Leaving

F. REFERENCES — FRIENDS / ACQUAINTANCES NON-RELATED

(1) _____
    Name   Address   Telephone Number   (☐ Work ☐ Home) Occupation   Years Acquainted
(1) _____
    Name   Address   Telephone Number   (☐ Work ☐ Home) Occupation   Years Acquainted

Please Feel Free To Add Any Information Which You Feel Will Help Us Consider You For Employment

READ THE FOLLOWING CAREFULLY, THEN SIGN AND DATE THE APPLICATION

"I certify that all answers given by me on this application are true, correct and complete to the best of my knowledge. I acknowledge notice that the information contained in this application is subject to check. I agree that, if hired, my continued employment may be contingent upon the accuracy of that information. If employed, I further agree to comply with Company/Office rules and regulations."

Signature: _____   Date: _____

FIGURE 25-10, cont'd   For legend see previous page.

placement counselor if unsure what to say in these sections.

If there are sections available for listing special skills and qualifications, fill them out fully. Describe CPR and first aid certifications and any professional organizations joined. If references are requested, list the name, title, employer, and a means of contact. Be sure to get permission before using someone as a reference.

One of the most common mistakes on the job application is writing "see resume." This is an indication of laziness and must be avoided. Even if the exact information is found on the resume, the application must still be completed in its entirety. Additionally, most job applications include a disclaimer that states that if a false or incomplete statement is made on the application, the individual can be dismissed from any position for which he or she was hired.

The Job Interview

A medical assistant may interview with the office manager, the physician, or both. It is possible that other staff members may be brought in for a portion of the interview. This is especially true in offices that have a cohesive team of employees.

The interview is usually the most stressful of the job search steps. Some individuals dread job interviews and become extremely nervous at the prospect of interviewing. Others are very comfortable and consider the interview as much for their own purposes as for the employer's.

There are four phases to interviews. These are the preparation, the interview itself, the follow-up, and the negotiation.

Preparation for the Interview

When preparing for an interview, the medical assistant should learn everything possible about the employer. Look on the Internet for information about the facility. Practice answering potential interview questions. Prepare an outfit to wear to interviews. It is wise to drive to the interview site on a day preceding the interview date if the location is unfamiliar to avoid getting lost on the day of the important event. The better prepared the medical assistant is, the more comfortable he or she will be while interviewing.

When preparing on the day of the interview, be conservative with wardrobe choices. Be sure clothing is fresh and wrinkle free and shoes are shined. It is a good idea to carry a planner or other method of taking notes during the interview. This makes a good impression and indicates interest in the job. Always arrive 15 minutes early for the interview. Do not use heavy perfumes or colognes, do not chew gum, and avoid excessive jewelry. Never take anyone along on a job interview, especially children, even if they are older children.

Pay particular attention to other aspects of appearance (Figure 25-11). Be sure that the hair is clean and styled attractively, and that teeth are clean and breath is fresh. Nails are also important and should be clean and

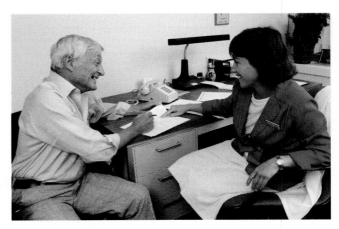

FIGURE 25-11 Present a professional appearance during the job interview and be sure to smile often!

well groomed, because the medical assistant will want to give the interviewer a firm handshake.

The Interview

During the actual interview, maintain good eye contact. Many supervisors refuse to hire people who seem uncomfortable with making strong eye contact. Never take control of the interview. Allow the supervisor to ask questions at his or her own pace. Do not fidget in the chair, and observe the interviewer's body language for clues as to how interested he or she might be. Do not volunteer any negative information, be honest, and do not exaggerate experience or lengths of employment. Never speak negatively about former employers.

Remember that the interview is centered on the medical assistant, so freely discuss the skills and attributes that will be brought to the job. The better prepared the medical assistant is, the smoother the interview will be. Be able to prove the skills claimed, and explain how they meet the needs of the company or facility. Avoid a "know-it-all" attitude, which indicates overconfidence and reluctance in taking direction. Always express an interest in the employer and its projects as opposed to what the employer can do for the employee. Ask intelligent questions at the end of the interview if given the opportunity (Figure 25-12).

Before the interview ends, the medical assistant should ask when a decision will be made, and if it would be acceptable to call to follow up.

CRITICAL THINKING APPLICATION

Lisa is enjoying a good interview when the supervisor, a man, asks her if she is married. When Lisa replies that she is not, he asks if she has a steady boyfriend. What might the supervisor's motive be with this line of questioning? How should Lisa respond? Are these questions inappropriate, or do they serve a purpose?

TOP 100 INTERVIEW QUESTIONS

1. Tell me about yourself.
2. Why do you want to work for this company?
3. Why should I hire you?
4. How do you work under pressure?
5. What type of job or salary do you expect to make in 5 years?
6. How do you handle criticism?
7. What do you think your co-workers think about you?
8. What is your opinion of the company you last worked for?
9. Describe your last supervisor.
10. What is your view of management?
11. What would you like to change about yourself and how would you do it?
12. What is your best asset?
13. What adjectives would you use to describe yourself?
14. What aspects of your life are you most happy with?
15. How would you describe the perfect job?
16. Why did you leave your last job?
17. Why did you choose this type of profession?
18. What salary do you expect?
19. What are your strongest and weakest personal qualities?
20. What motivates you?
21. What have you learned from some of your previous jobs?
22. What personal characteristics are necessary for success in your chosen field?
23. What do you know about this facility and our competitors?
24. What were your major courses of study in school?
25. Do you plan to continue your education?
26. Did school meet your expectations or were you disappointed?
27. How did you pay for your education?
28. Sell this pen to me.
29. To what extent do your grades reflect how much you have learned?
30. Do you feel your education was worthwhile?
31. What were the major responsibilities of your last job?
32. What has been your most rewarding experience at work?
33. What was your single most important accomplishment for the company on your last job?
34. What was the toughest problem you have ever solved and how did you do it?
35. How do you see yourself fitting in with our company?
36. What skills did you learn on your last job that can be used here?
37. What would you do if you were fired in two years?
38. What kinds of additional education do you think you need to meet your career goals?
39. How long do you plan to stay with our company?
40. What immediate contribution could you make if you came to work for us today?
41. Do you feel that you have received good general training?
42. If you were starting school all over again, what courses would you take?
43. How much money do you hope to earn in 5 years? 10 years?
44. Do you think that your extracurricular activities were worth the time spent?
45. Are you interested in making money or do you have other reasons for entering this career field?
46. Do you prefer working with others or by yourself?
47. Can you take instructions or criticism without being upset?
48. Tell me a story.
49. What do you know about the opportunities in the field in which you are trained?
50. How long do you expect to work?
51. Have you ever had any difficulty in getting along with a co-worker, classmate, or instructor?
52. Which of your school years was most difficult?
53. Do you like routine work?
54. Define cooperation.
55. Will you fight to get ahead?
56. Do you have an analytical mind?
57. Are you willing to go where the company sends you?
58. What job in this company would you choose if you could?
59. Do you think that employers should consider grades?
60. What have you done that shows initiative and willingness to work?
61. What benefits did you receive from your last employer?
62. What has been your most important accomplishment during your school years?
63. Have you ever helped to reduce operating costs, and how?
64. Have you ever developed or helped develop any programs, and how did you do this?
65. What do you think determines a person's progress in a company?
66. What would you do if a personal problem interfered with your work?
67. What would you do if you became bored with your job?
68. What would you do if you had a personality clash with a supervisor?
69. How will you be getting to work each day?
70. Do you have reliable transportation?
71. How do you feel about working with someone who is HIV positive?
72. What person has most influenced your life?
73. What is the last book you read?
74. Who do you most admire?
75. Who is your favorite relative?
76. What will previous supervisors say about you?
77. What makes a good supervisor?
78. Why would you be successful in this job?
79. Why have you held so many jobs?
80. Can you explain this gap in your employment history?
81. Have you ever been fired from a position?
82. Do you have adequate child care arrangements that will allow you to be at work when scheduled?
83. What is your philosophy of life?
84. How many other positions are you considering?
85. Why were your grades in school so low?
86. Are you a member of any professional organizations?
87. How old were you when you began to support yourself?
88. Do you participate in continuing education activities or seminars?
89. Have you had the hepatitis B injection series?
90. Where did you perform your externship?
91. How many days of school did you miss?
92. Why did you decide to attend the college/school you attended?
93. What kind of boss do you prefer?
94. How do you usually spend your weekends?
95. Why types of people seem to rub you the wrong way?
96. What planning procedures do you use?
97. What frustrates you about your current job?
98. What is unique about you?
99. What have you done that indicates you are qualified for this job?
100. Do you have any questions?

FIGURE 25-12 Top 100 interview questions.

Follow-Up After the Interview

Follow-up is critical after an interview. Always send a written thank-you letter to the person who conducted the interview. Many employers wait to see who sends a thank-you letter before making the final hiring decision. Limit follow-up calls to no more than once or twice a week. Most employers will give an indication of when the hiring decision will be made. The company should notify all those who interviewed once a decision has been made, unless there were specific protocols set during the interview in this area. For instance, if the office manager said that a decision will be made on Friday, and the final three candidates will be called for a second interview, then the medical assistant knows if a call is not received to continue the job search. Never place all your hopes on one job—continue to prospect until an offer is made.

REASONS PEOPLE DO NOT GET HIRED

Below is a rank order list of reasons that interviewers do not hire job candidates. The list is compiled from the results of a nationwide survey of 153 companies performed by North Central Technical Institute.

1. Poor personal appearance
2. Lack of interest or enthusiasm
3. Overemphasis on money
4. Poor voice, diction, grammar
5. Lack of planning
6. No purpose or goals
7. Condemnation of past employers
8. Poor eye contact
9. Limp, fishy handshake
10. Late to interview
11. Lack of tact
12. Lack of maturity
13. Lack of courtesy
14. Asking no questions
15. Overbearing "know-it-all"
16. Lack of confidence and poise
17. Failure to participate in activities
18. Making excuses, evading unfavorable factors on record
19. Indecisiveness
20. Just shopping around
21. No interest in company
22. Sloppy application blank
23. Wanting a job for a short time
24. Unwillingness to relocate
25. Cynical attitude
26. Low moral standards
27. Laziness
28. Intolerance or strong prejudices
29. No sense of humor
30. Narrow interests
31. Inability to take criticism
32. No appreciation for the value of experience
33. Radical ideas
34. Too aggressive during interview

The Negotiation

The negotiation stage of job acceptance can be as stressful as the actual interviews. A medical assistant should know the lowest salary he or she can afford and then ask for a little more than that figure. Bracket salary requests: instead of asking for $12.00 per hour, ask for a salary in the "mid to high twenties." Let the employer mention a figure first, or a range of salary. Usually the person who mentions a salary range first has the disadvantage. If the medical assistant requests $12.00 per hour and the facility was willing to pay $15.00 per hour, the medical assistant will probably get $12.00.

Never say "no" to a job offer on the spot. Request at least 24 hours to consider the offer. A medical assistant should not let the salary amount be the main factor in the decision to accept a position. Consider whether the position carries any authority, the benefits, the hours, the distance from home, and the potential for advancement before accepting or rejecting a job offer.

You Got the Job!

Once the job offer has been made and accepted, a start date will be determined (Figure 25-13). Before the first day, use the computer to map several ways to get to work. Because the medical assistant may be unsure of traffic flow, leave home extra early the first day so that arrival on time is guaranteed.

Most employees are placed on a 30- to 90-day probationary period, during which employment may be terminated if the employee's performance is not satisfactory. It is also an opportunity for the employer and employee to learn about each other. The medical

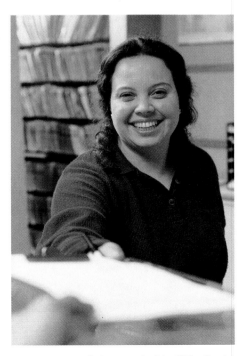

FIGURE 25-13   Congratulations, you're hired! The first job after school is an exciting experience for a medical assistant.

assistant will interact with other co-workers, with patients, and with providers. A new medical assistant should volunteer to help others and efficiently complete the duties assigned. Use the probationary period as a testing ground, carefully observing ways in which the office might run in a smoother manner. However, do not make numerous suggestions for change during this period. Discover why certain methods are used and make an effort to fit in with the rest of the team before suggesting that the routine of the office be changed. Remember, the people at the office may have been employed for substantially longer periods and may resent suggestions from a new staff member. Learn the office's rhythms, procedures, and culture first and demonstrate a team-oriented attitude.

Common Early Mistakes

Some medical assistants make mistakes early on a new job. Never be disruptive to the office by gossiping or complaining. A medical assistant must realize that there may be different ways of performing procedures and that the way he or she was taught in school is probably not the only correct way. Be open to learning new ideas, concepts, and procedures. Although some mistakes are to be expected, be certain that once a mistake is pointed out, it is corrected. Do not make the same mistakes over and over.

Supervisors may or may not work very closely with the medical assistants. Some will be expected to carry out orders on their own. Do not make too much supervision necessary or force the office manager to constantly check the work that is done. Finish all assigned duties in a timely manner and avoid procrastination. When problems arise, communicate them openly with the supervisor and attempt to find a quick resolution. Last, limit absences and tardy days to a minimum and miss work only when absolutely necessary—especially during the probationary period.

How to Be a Good Employee

There are several ways in which a medical assistant can be a better employee. First and foremost, arrive for the scheduled shift on time and do not leave early. Even the best medical assistant cannot benefit an office when he or she does not come to work. Be honest and demonstrate trustworthiness and professionalism. Get along with co-workers in the facility. A medical assistant should be able to resolve simple problems with others easily without involving the supervisor. Reflect a friendly attitude to others, even if they are difficult to get along with.

A medical assistant should constantly be performing assigned duties and not expect frequent breaks in the medical office. Most offices are fast paced, and the supervisor will expect the medical assistant to keep up with the activity. Even when there are slow periods, there is always a counter to clean or filing to do. Be supportive of the leadership in the facility and ask for more responsibility if necessary. Take initiative to perform duties that are cumbersome or repetitive, and get them done quickly.

It is vital to treat the patients with compassion. Remember that they are not always at their best when ill, so be kind and courteous to them and their families. The patients are the reason that the facility exists. Treat them with great respect and care.

CRITICAL THINKING APPLICATION

On Lisa's second day at the externship site, she clearly sees a co-worker taking and using a controlled drug from the storage area. What should Lisa do? What potential problems will this situation prompt? Who should Lisa report this incident to, if anyone?

Dealing With Supervisors

Supervisors appreciate employees who come to them when there are questions but who are able to handle minor decisions on their own. Never hesitate to approach supervisors when there is an issue at hand that needs their attention. Do not allow a situation to go unaddressed and then say, "I didn't want to bother you with that." It is the responsibility of the office manager to deal with difficult issues, and these should be handled immediately when they arise.

A medical assistant should never attempt to cover up a mistake; admitting the error is a much better approach to solving the problem. When talking with the supervisor, do not hesitate to speak or avoid the subject. State the problem clearly and explain what routes are available to **rectify** the situation. Work with the supervisor to resolve issues and accept the advice given with a positive attitude.

Performance Appraisals

Performance **appraisals** are usually done after the initial probationary period and annually after that. The performance appraisal is designed to inform the employee of his or her strengths and weaknesses on the job, according to the supervisor's point of view. Most of these appraisals offer a scale to rate the employee's performance, such as 1 to 5. Do not expect to receive a perfect appraisal, because employees are seldom perfect in all aspects of their jobs. If the supervisor gives perfect scores to an employee, there is no room for growth or improvement. It is the rare employee who completes all duties without any errors. When asked to sit down with your supervisor for a performance appraisal, go into the meeting open to addressing areas that may need improvement. Ask questions and work with the supervisor to improve in the areas that may need more effort or a different approach.

If the employee strongly disagrees with any area of the performance appraisal, discuss this with the supervisor. There may have been misunderstandings as to the duties involved. Clarify this and strive to do better next time.

Asking for a Raise

Most facilities have some type of schedule for pay increases. Some offer a cost of living increase on an annual basis; others use a merit system, offering raises only when earned and deserved based on performance.

There may come a time when the medical assistant feels the need to ask for a raise. Before doing so, do a little self-reflection to determine whether a raise is in order. Has attendance been exemplary? How many times was the medical assistant tardy? Does he or she work well with little supervision? Has he or she performed all the expected duties well and in a timely manner?

Approach the supervisor at a relatively calm part of the day, and ask how a salary raise might be earned in the near future. Do not expect a raise of more than 4% to 5% at any given time. If the supervisor is unable to grant a raise, determine whether the reasons are valid. If they are not, the medical assistant may wish to pursue other employment options. It is always easier to find a job if one already has a job, so do not quit outright unless the work environment is **intolerable**. Begin networking again and discover the options available.

Leaving A Job Professionally

Always offer at least a 2-week notice when resigning from a job. Give the supervisor a written notice of resignation, and take this to him or her in person. Do not just leave it on a desk or place it in the interoffice mail.

It is a dangerous practice to resign from a job just to attempt to get a salary increase. Once the employer doubts the employee's loyalty, the future is usually not bright for the employee at that facility. Resign only after a final decision has been made. If the medical assistant is resigning to take another position, expect the current employer to make a **counteroffer**. However, be wary about accepting counteroffers. What led to looking for a new job in the first place? Has the situation been resolved? Ask these questions before agreeing to stay with the current employer.

Life Skills

To be successful in the job search, the medical assistant must have the basic entry-level skills needed to perform in the workplace. Even more important, however, he or she must develop certain life skills that are essential to excel in any profession. If these skills are not developed and refined, the medical assistant may find fewer opportunities and advancements available, as well as less impressive salaries and benefits.

The most important life skill one can possess is the willingness to change. There are many employees who insist on doing things the same way they have always been done, and they resist any changes in policy or procedure. However, a medical assistant who does not welcome change and work hard at it is a failure waiting to happen.

Personal Growth

Personal growth is a comprehensive term that applies to many aspects of a person's mental, physical, and spiritual health. This growth is a result of goals that are set for self-improvement. Without clear goals, people rarely experience personal growth that is initiated from within. There may be growth that is a result of some outside influence, but a conscious effort toward personal growth is an innate decision.

No matter how great the training or how many opportunities are placed in front of a person, fear and doubt can sabotage efforts to improve the self-image, confidence, and future potential of an individual. Personal growth involves such traits as self-control, self-esteem, problem-solving skills, decision-making skills, and stress management.

STEPS FOR ACHIEVING GOALS

- Decide what you want.
- Write the goal down.
- Set the date of accomplishment.
- Read it three times daily.
- Think of the goal often.
- See yourself accomplishing the goal.
- Develop a plan of action for reaching the goal.
- Do not discuss the plan with others who might be discouraging.
- Be confident.
- Act successful, and you will be!

Self-Control. Self-control is a vital trait in the medical office. Some patients may not be at their best because of their illness, and this may make them less than cordial toward the staff. Remember that this is usually a temporary situation. A medical assistant must exercise self-control and not respond in kind to patients who are disagreeable.

Self-control is important in other areas of the medical office. Never remove drugs from the storage areas without permission, and be careful when dealing with petty cash. A medical assistant must get enough rest during the work week so that he or she can care for the patients in an enthusiastic manner.

Self-Esteem. Everyone has certain strengths and weaknesses. Good self-esteem is the result of knowing what those strengths are and overcoming the weaknesses. It is having a positive outlook about the self and others. A person with good self-esteem is motivated, able to express love, and capable of handling criticism. A person's self-esteem will improve if he or she has developed adaptive skills. Especially in the medical profession, one thing that is guaranteed in the workplace is change. Change can be positive or negative; this depends mostly on the way it is viewed by the individual.

A person is not doomed to live with poor self-esteem forever. With a degree of effort and open-mindedness, an individual can work toward better self-esteem, which can make a tremendous difference in the individual's future potential.

Problem-Solving Skills. For individuals to work together, they must have a degree of trust and be willing to make suggestions for the good of the group. The phrase "two heads are better than one" is still true when it comes to problem solving. Employees usually want to play a part in solving the problems in the workplace, and they appreciate knowing that their opinions make a difference. A medical assistant who can listen to the concerns of others and is willing to give and take will be an excellent problem-solver.

Decision-Making Skills. People who know how to make good decisions are usually successful. Thinking through a decision requires logic, and it is best to take some time to carefully think of all of the "pros and cons." Unfortunately, a medical assistant may not always have time to consider decisions in a leisurely fashion, especially when dealing with emergencies. A good decision-maker is honest when identifying the real problems and attempts to keep personal feelings isolated from the process.

There are several steps toward making a sound decision. The problem must be specifically defined and evaluated so that the individual understands clearly what needs to happen to resolve the situation at hand. Gather as much information as possible and consider all alternatives. It is sometimes helpful to choose an alternative, and then consider all of the **ramifications** of making a decision using that alternative. Then, when the best alternative is determined, the decision should be made and put into action. Care should be taken to avoid making a decision simply because it is easy and comfortable, because more problems could arise later as a result of not addressing the true problem in the beginning.

CRITICAL THINKING APPLICATION

Lisa has been on several interviews and likes the prospect of working for three different physicians. If an offer is made at each office, how can Lisa decide which to accept? What will help Lisa make this decision?

Stress Management. The demands of the medical profession make it a stressful environment at times. Stress is not always bad. In fact, some stress is a positive motivator toward a goal. A stressor is a stimulus that prompts a reaction from the body. Positive stress, or *eustress*, includes exhilarating activities or success, which often leads to higher expectations from the person experiencing the eustress. The opposite is distress, which includes disappointment, failure, or embarrassment. Stress management is a conscious effort toward controlling the stressors and resulting reactions so that the body and mind operate evenly, even when stress is present in an individual's life.

By learning to recognize the signs of stressful overload, a medical assistant can possibly ward off the negative reactions that are so physically and mentally draining to the body. Many people notice a headache or fatigue when overly stressed. Breathing correctly is one way to reduce stress. Often, an accelerated breathing pattern that is quick and shallow is a stress indicator. Breathing from the abdomen at a slower pace, inhaling through the nose, and exhaling through the mouth may help reduce tension. Taking time for relaxing activities and getting plenty of exercise are other methods of stress reduction.

Planning a Budget

A newly graduated medical assistant should formulate a simple budget and attempt to live within that budget. It is helpful to track spending with checkbook ledgers, bill stubs, receipts, and daily records for 3 months before developing a firm budget, so that there is a realistic accounting of where money goes when it leaves the checkbook. Use that information to design a spending plan for monthly income that accounts for monthly, quarterly, and annual expenses, as well as special activities.

Even when making only a small salary, building savings is important. A medical assistant should set aside 5% to 10% of the net income in a savings account. The money in savings should not be touched except in emergencies. It is even better to establish an emergency fund, which would ideally hold 3 months' salary. This way, there is enough cash to pay bills for 3 months in case of a sudden job loss or emergency. No one can do this immediately when beginning a new job, but it can be done over a period of time if one is committed to the effort.

Avoid going into debt whenever possible. If credit cards are used, they should be used conservatively and not for impulse purchases. Instead of using credit, set spending goals and save for a purchase or use lay-away programs. Make more than the minimum payment on credit cards to avoid excessive interest from accruing on the account. Everyone should work toward being debt free as soon as possible.

Limit housing and utilities to no more than 30% of the net income. Other monthly installment debt should total less than 15% of the net income. Many financial institutions figure a debt ratio when they consider loaning money to an individual. If that debt ratio is too high, the bank may not lend money, even to a person with stellar credit.

Student Loans. Student loans are extremely important. Loans are designed to provide the opportunity to obtain a good education. They must be paid back. If an individual allows a student loan to **default**, he or she becomes ineligible for future student loans until the original loan is paid back. There is never a reason for a student loan to default. The medical assistant should contact the company that services the student loan and explain any problems that are keeping him or her from repaying the debt. These companies want to work with students to clear their accounts. Often a deferment is available, which allows the student to postpone the payments for a period of time (Figure 25-14). Deferments may be

IN-SCHOOL DEFERMENT REQUEST
Federal Family Education Loan Program

SCH

WARNING: Any person who knowingly makes a false statement or misrepresentation on this form or on any accompanying documents shall be subject to penalties which may include fines, imprisonment or both, under the U.S. Criminal Code and 20 U.S.C. §1097.

OMB No. 1845-0005
Form Approved
Exp. Date 09/30/2005

SECTION 1: BORROWER IDENTIFICATION

Please enter or correct the following information.

SSN |___|___|___| - |___|___| - |___|___|___|___|

Name _____

Address _____

City, State, Zip _____

Telephone - Home (   ) _____

Telephone - Other (   ) _____

E-mail Address (optional) _____

SECTION 2: DEFERMENT REQUEST

Before answering any questions, carefully read the entire form, including the instructions and other information in Sections 5 and 6.

■ I meet the qualifications for the deferment checked below and request that my loan holder defer repayment of my loan(s):

❏ While I am enrolled at an eligible school as a **FULL-TIME STUDENT**. (For borrowers with a FFEL Program loan.)

❏ While I am enrolled at an eligible school as a **LESS THAN FULL-TIME BUT AT LEAST HALF-TIME STUDENT**. (For borrowers who, on the date they signed the promissory note, did not have an outstanding balance on a FFEL Program loan made **before July 1, 1987**.)

NOTE: *Your promissory note or other loan documents may state that a borrower with an outstanding balance on a FFEL Program loan made **prior to July 1, 1993**, must receive another loan in order to qualify for a half-time student deferment. This requirement was eliminated by the Higher Education Amendments of 1998. **Effective October 1, 1998**, no FFEL Program borrower who is eligible for a deferment based on enrollment as at least a half-time student is required to receive another loan in order to qualify for this deferment.*

SECTION 3: BORROWER UNDERSTANDINGS AND CERTIFICATIONS

■ **I understand that: (1)** I am not required to make payments of loan principal during my deferment. Interest will not be charged on my subsidized loan(s) during my deferment. However, interest will be charged on my unsubsidized loan(s). **(2)** I have the option of making interest payments on my unsubsidized loan(s) during my deferment. **(3)** I may choose to make interest payments by checking the box below. Interest that I do not pay during the deferment period will be capitalized by my loan holder.

❏ I wish to make interest payments on my unsubsidized loan(s) during my deferment.

(4) My deferment will begin on the date the condition that qualifies me for a deferment began, as certified by the authorized official who completes Section 4 of this form. **(5)** My deferment will end on the earlier of the date that I no longer meet the condition that qualifies me for the deferment, or the ending date of that condition as certified by the authorized official. **(6)** If my deferment does not cover all my past due payments, my loan holder may grant me a forbearance for all payments due before the begin date of my deferment or—if the period for which I am eligible for a deferment has ended—a forbearance for all payments due at the time my deferment request is processed. **(7)** If I am eligible for a post-deferment grace period on loans made before October 1, 1981, my loan holder may grant me a forbearance on my other loans for this period so that I can begin repayment of all my loans at the same time. I understand that my loan holder may capitalize the interest that accrues on my other loans during the six-month period and that this will increase the principal balance of my other loans. **(8)** My loan holder may grant me a forbearance on my loans for up to 60 days, if necessary, for the collection and processing of documentation related to my deferment request. Interest that accrues during the forbearance will not be capitalized.

■ **I certify that: (1)** The information I provided in Sections 1 and 2 above is true and correct. **(2)** I will provide additional documentation to my loan holder, as required, to support my deferment status. **(3)** I will notify my loan holder immediately when the condition(s) that qualified me for the deferment ends. **(4)** I have read, understand, and meet the eligibility criteria of the deferment for which I have applied.

Borrower's Signature _____ Date _____

SECTION 4: AUTHORIZED OFFICIAL'S CERTIFICATION

NOTE: As an alternative to completing this section, the school may attach its own enrollment certification report listing the required information.

I certify, to the best of my knowledge and belief, that the borrower named above:

(1) is/was enrolled as (check the appropriate box) ❏ a full-time student ❏ at least a half-time student

during the academic period from |___|___| - |___|___| - |___|___|___|___| to |___|___| - |___|___| - |___|___|___|___| and

(2) is reasonably expected to complete his/her program requirements on |___|___| - |___|___| - |___|___|___|___|.

Name of Institution _____ OPE-ID _____

Address _____ City, State, Zip _____

Name/Title of Authorized Official _____ Telephone (   ) _____

Authorized Official's Signature _____ **Date** _____

Page 1 of 2

FIGURE 25-14 In-school deferment form. Do not allow student loans to default. Contact the financial aid office at your educational institution for assistance and answers to questions about student loans.

SECTION 5: INSTRUCTIONS FOR COMPLETING THE FORM

Type or print using dark ink. Report dates as month-day-year (MM-DD-YYYY). For example, 'January 31, 2002' = '01-31-2002'. An authorized school official must either (A) complete Section 4, or (B) attach the school's own enrollment certification report listing the required information. If you need help completing this form, contact your loan holder.

Return the completed form and any required documentation to the address shown in Section 7.

SECTION 6: DEFINITIONS FOR IN-SCHOOL DEFERMENT REQUEST

■ The **Federal Family Education Loan (FFEL) Program** includes Federal Stafford Loans (both subsidized and unsubsidized), Federal Supplemental Loans for Students (SLS), Federal PLUS Loans, and Federal Consolidation Loans.

■ A **deferment** is a period during which I am entitled to postpone repayment of the principal balance of my loan(s). The federal government pays the interest that accrues during an eligible deferment for all subsidized Federal Stafford Loans and for Federal Consolidation Loans for which the Consolidation Loan application was received by my loan holder **(1)** on or after January 1, 1993, but before August 10, 1993, **(2)** on or after August 10, 1993, if it includes *only* Federal Stafford Loans that were eligible for federal interest subsidy, or **(3)** on or after November 13, 1997, for that portion of the consolidation loan that paid a subsidized FFEL Loan or a subsidized Federal Direct Loan. I am responsible for the interest that accrues during this period on all other FFEL Program loans.

■ **Forbearance** means permitting the temporary cessation of payments, allowing an extension of time for making payments, or temporarily accepting smaller payments than previously scheduled. I am responsible for the interest that accrues on my loan(s) during a forbearance. If I do not pay the interest that accrues, the interest may be capitalized.

■ The **holder** of my FFEL Program loan(s) may be a lender, guaranty agency, secondary market, or the U.S. Department of Education.

■ **Capitalization** is the addition of unpaid interest to the principal balance of my loan. This will increase the principal and the total cost of my loan.

■ An **authorized certifying official** for an In-School Deferment is an authorized official of the school where I am/was enrolled as a full-time or at least half-time student.

SECTION 7: WHERE TO SEND THE COMPLETED DEFERMENT REQUEST

RETURN THE COMPLETED DEFERMENT REQUEST AND ANY REQUIRED DOCUMENTATION TO:
(IF NO ADDRESS IS SHOWN, RETURN TO YOUR LOAN HOLDER)

SECTION 8: IMPORTANT NOTICES

Privacy Act Notice

The Privacy Act of 1974 (5 U.S.C. 552a) requires that the following notice be provided to you:

The authority for collecting the requested information from and about you is §428(b)(2)(A) et seq. of the Higher Education Act of 1965, as amended (20 U.S.C. 1078(b)(2)(A) et seq.) and the authority for collecting and using your Social Security Number (SSN) is §484(a)(4) of the HEA (20 U.S.C. 1091(a)(4)). Participating in the Federal Family Education Loan (FFEL) Program and giving us your SSN are voluntary, but you must provide the requested information, including your SSN, to participate.

The principal purposes for collecting the information on this form, including your SSN, are to verify your identity, to determine your eligibility to receive a loan or a benefit on a loan (such as a deferment, forbearance, discharge, or forgiveness) under the FFEL program, to permit the servicing of your loan(s), and, if it becomes necessary, to locate you and to collect on your loan(s) if your loan(s) become delinquent or in default. We also use your SSN as an account identifier and to permit you to access your account information electronically.

The information in your file may be disclosed to third parties as authorized under routine uses in the appropriate systems of records. The routine uses of this information include its disclosure to federal, state, or local agencies, to other federal agencies under computer matching programs, to agencies that we authorize to assist us in administering our loan programs, to private parties such as relatives, present and former employers, business and personal associates, to credit bureau organizations, to educational institutions, and to contractors in order to verify your identity, to determine your eligibility to receive a loan or a benefit on a loan, to permit the servicing or collection of your loan(s), to enforce the terms of the loan(s), to investigate possible fraud and to verify compliance with federal student financial aid program regulations, to locate you if you become delinquent in your loan payments or if you default, to provide default rate calculations, to provide financial aid history information, to assist program administrators with tracking refunds and cancellations, or to provide a standardized method for educational institutions efficiently to submit student enrollment status.

In the event of litigation, we may send records to the Department of Justice, a court, adjudicative body, counsel, party, or witness if the disclosure is relevant and necessary to the litigation. If this information, either alone or with other information, indicates a potential violation of law, we may send it to the appropriate authority for action. We may send information to members of Congress if you ask them to help you with federal student aid questions. In circumstances involving employment complaints, grievances, or disciplinary actions, we may disclose relevant records to adjudicate or investigate the issues. If provided for by a collective bargaining agreement, we may disclose records to a labor organization recognized under 5 U.S.C. Chapter 71. Disclosures may also be made to qualified researchers under Privacy Act safeguards.

Paperwork Reduction Notice

According to the Paperwork Reduction Act of 1995, no persons are required to respond to a collection of information unless it displays a currently valid OMB control number. The valid OMB control number for this information collection is 1845-0005. The time required to complete this information collection is estimated to average 0.16 hours (10 minutes) per response, including the time to review instructions, search existing data resources, gather and maintain the data needed, and complete and review the information collection. ***If you have any comments concerning the accuracy of the time estimate(s) or suggestions for improving this form, please write to:***

U.S. Department of Education, Washington, DC 20202-4651

If you have any comments or concerns regarding the status of your individual submission of this form, write directly to the address shown in Section 7.

Page 2 of 2

FIGURE 25-14, cont'd   For legend see previous page.

available when the student is unemployed, attending school to continue his or her education, suffering economic hardship, completing a graduate fellowship, completing rehabilitation training, or in other situations. Contact the lender to find out whether a deferment is in order.

TOP TEN WAYS TO AVOID DEFAULT ON A STUDENT LOAN

1. Understand your rights and responsibilities regarding your repayment obligation as well as your repayment options.
2. Borrow for college expenses only. Borrow only the amount you need and only what you can reasonably expect to be able to repay.
3. Keep all records regarding your loan. Make copies of all letters, canceled checks, and any forms you sign.
4. Notify your lender or servicer when you have a change of address, phone number, or name, or if you change schools or your enrollment status.
5. Seek help as early as possible if you have any difficulty maintaining your student loan repayment arrangement.
6. If you have any questions, talk to your lender or student loan guarantor about the particular terms of your loan.
7. Keep credit card debt to a minimum or avoid credit card debt completely.
8. Create and maintain a budget that is within your monthly income.
9. Consider making nominal student loan payments while in school. This will reduce the amount you owe after graduation.
10. Make loan payments on time.

Courtesy Texas Guaranteed Student Loan Corporation, http://www.tgslc.org.

The Guideline Budget

Dealing with personal finances can be a stressor. Developing a realistic budget will assist a medical assistant in planning his or her spending. When careful planning is implemented, more can be accomplished with less money if a commitment has been made to staying on budget and resisting the temptation to spend.

Dangerous Habits. Some individuals practice dangerous habits related to finances. For instance, if this month's bills are arriving and last month's have not been paid, frustration and depression may result. Some people may even avoid opening letters or bills just so they do not have to deal with seeing the balance due. Writing checks on funds that are not in the checking account is not only unwise—it is also illegal. All states

have laws related to insufficient fund checks, and most legislation considers this a form of theft. It is possible to be arrested for writing "hot" checks. People headed for financial disaster also purchase daily items, such as bread and milk, with a credit card. All of these behaviors are signs of financial trouble.

A sample budget outline is shown in Figure 25-15. Take an honest look at each item listed and determine what amount is spent monthly in each category. Compare these amounts with the monthly income and see if the current budget is positive or negative. Remember that the gross salary is the amount earned before taxes and other deductions. The net salary is the take-home pay. Adjustments may be needed to bring the budget into balance.

Closing Comments

The period surrounding graduation will be a celebration, but also a busy time for which much planning is required. Cooperate with the school when securing externship sites and make an effort to obtain a site that will be of the most benefit to the career desired. Do not take an externship just because it is close to home. Think about the skills that will be offered and learn as much as possible. Then perform well, so that the staff and physicians are happy to offer a good reference to potential employers.

Even though this educational experience has ended, remember that there is constantly something new to learn in the medical profession. Join professional societies and participate in as many educational seminars and continuing education classes as possible. Remain in a continual state of learning and be determined to be the best medical assistant you can be.

Patient Education

Some patients assume that the people who assist the physician in the office are all nurses. The medical assistant should always specify that he or she is a medical assistant, especially when making initial introductions. There should never be any representation that the medical assistant is the "office nurse." If a patient uses that term, he or she should be corrected in a friendly manner.

A medical assistant may find it necessary to educate the patient as to the definition of a medical assistant. An occasional rare patient may not have heard of the term. Explain the type of training that was completed, emphasizing that medical assistants are trained specifically for working in a physician's office. If patients have any questions about the medical assistant's qualifications, refer them to the office manager or physician.

Legal and Ethical Issues

Remember to be completely honest when completing a job application and offering information on a resume.

MONTHLY INCOME	AMOUNT
Net Income	
Spouse Net Income	
Child Support	
Other Income	

MONTHLY EXPENSES	AMOUNT
Rent	
Gas	
Electric	
Home/Renters Insurance	
Water/Sewage	
Trash	
Home Telephone	
Cell Telephone	
Pager	
Cable TV/Satellite	
Internet/DSL	
Child Care	
Lawn Care	
Clothing	
Food - Home	
Food - Work or School	
Food - Eating Out	
Laundry/Dry Cleaning	
Medical Expenses	
Dental Expenses	
Life Insurance	
Medical Insurance	
Dental Insurance	
Eyeglasses	
Prescriptions	
Automobile Payment	
Automobile Insurance	
Repairs	
Gas/Oil	
Furniture	
Beauty/Barber Shop	
Pet Expenses	
Student Loan	
Other Loans	
Credit Cards	
Church/Charities	
Birthdays	
Anniversaries	
Christmas	
Vacation Planning	
Entertainment	

FIGURE 25-15 The guideline budget.

Most facilities stipulate that if an individual is not truthful on these documents, his or her employment can be terminated once the deception is discovered. Employers are more interested in honesty and a forthright explanation than in minor problems that affect the job performance.

If a medical assistant has had some brush with the law that requires disclosure on the job application, the best policy is to be honest and deal with the ramifi-

cations of telling the truth. Most businesses can verify whether a potential employee has any type of criminal record. A solid explanation of the facts, admission of a past mistake, and excellent, current references will often prompt an employer to have faith and make a positive decision about extending employment.

SUMMARY OF SCENARIO

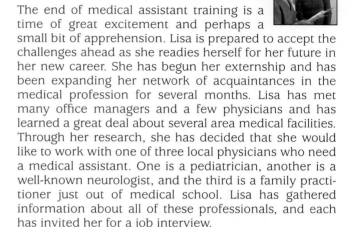

The end of medical assistant training is a time of great excitement and perhaps a small bit of apprehension. Lisa is prepared to accept the challenges ahead as she readies herself for her future in her new career. She has begun her externship and has been expanding her network of acquaintances in the medical profession for several months. Lisa has met many office managers and a few physicians and has learned a great deal about several area medical facilities. Through her research, she has decided that she would like to work with one of three local physicians who need a medical assistant. One is a pediatrician, another is a well-known neurologist, and the third is a family practitioner just out of medical school. Lisa has gathered information about all of these professionals, and each has invited her for a job interview.

Lisa knows that she will need to be at her best, so she takes care of herself and gets plenty of rest. She has a long list of interview questions and has taken the time to write out answers to the questions in preparation for her interviews. She is careful about her grooming every day that she reports to the externship, because she knows that the physician at her site is her first reference in the medical field. In addition, she knows that she may be called for an interview any day that might be scheduled just after her workday ends. Looking professional prepares her for this each day.

Lisa is comfortable during her interviews because she is well prepared. She has identified her strengths and can share them with a potential employer. She is focused on her objectives and knows what the minimum requirements will be for her to accept a position. She has a healthy self-esteem, and her good decision-making skills will help her to determine which position will be right for her. Her enthusiasm and excitement show in her eyes, and she is dedicated to making a difference in the lives of her patients and co-workers.

SUMMARY OF LEARNING OBJECTIVES

■ Because approximately 85% of individuals do not have any formal training in job search skills, taking the time to learn the best methods will place the medical assistant at an advantage. Training decreases the time spent looking for work and increases the benefits and salary offered when using good negotiating skills. The medical assistant will also be more comfortable during interviews and throughout the job search process.

- Employers have three basic expectations of their medical assistant employees. They want an employee with a good appearance, who looks as if he or she fits in the medical profession. A medical assistant should also be dependable and have the skills to do the job for which he or she was hired.

- There are three types of skill strengths that may be used by employees. Job skills are those used to actually perform a job, such as venipunctures or scheduling appointments. Self-management skills are usually a part of the medical assistant's personality; these include honesty and dependability. Transferable skills are those that can be taken from one job to another or used on any job. Examples include the ability to communicate effectively and lead and manage individuals.

- Networking and contacting employers directly are the two best methods of job searching. Networking involves developing a network of individuals that can assist in finding employment. This group may include co-workers, other students, relatives, or friends who provide leads to potential employers. Contacting employers directly includes taking resumes to specific offices or setting appointments to gain knowledge about the facility, then later using that knowledge during the job search. These two methods are more effective than most traditional means of finding a job.

- Any error on a resume should be avoided. Be sure that everything is spelled correctly, but do not rely on the computer's spell-check feature alone. Proofread the document and have someone else proofread it to catch errors that may be overlooked. Salary expectations should never be stated on the resume, and a photograph should not be included. Do not include personal information, such as height and weight.

- Demographic information on other employers should be taken to interviews and kept handy when filling out job applications. A medical assistant should never have to ask for a phone book to look up the address of a former employer. This demonstrates a lack of preparation and planning on the part of the potential employee.

- The four phases of the interview process include the preparation, the actual interview, the follow-up, and the negotiation. The preparation includes all efforts made before the actual interview in obtaining information about the company, deciding on the wardrobe, and making sure nails are groomed and shoes are shined. The interview itself is designed to help the employer and potential employee get to know each other and discover whether they are compatible. The follow-up is perhaps the most critical stage, wherein the medical assistant should send a thank-you letter and continue to stay in touch with the facility until the job is filled. The negotiation includes discussion of the salary and benefits that will be offered to the new employee.

- The probationary period is a time for the new medical assistant to become oriented to the facility. It also allows the employer to assess whether the medical assistant fits with the team and performs the duties of the job in a satisfactory way. During this time, the medical assistant should demonstrate that he or she is a productive team member with an excellent attitude. There should never be idle time; instead, look for ways to assist others when all duties are completed.

- A new employee in the medical office should avoid arriving late or any absences, especially during the probationary period. Never participate in office gossip, and make a good attempt to get along with

APPENDIX A

Procedure A-1

PROCEDURE **A-1**

Obtaining a Medical History

This procedure is to be done on another student. To make the experience more realistic, choose a student about whom you know very little.

GOAL: To obtain an acceptable written background from the patient to help the physician determine the cause and effects of the present illness. This includes the chief complaint (CC), present illness (PI), past history (PH), family history (FH), and social history (SH).

EQUIPMENT AND SUPPLIES
- History form
- Two pens—a red pen for recording patient allergies and a black pen to meet legal documentation guidelines
- A quiet, private area

PROCEDURAL STEPS

1 Greet and identify the patient in a pleasant manner. Introduce yourself and explain your role.
  Purpose: To make the patient feel comfortable and at ease.

2 Take the patient to a quiet, private area for the interview and explain to the patient why the information is needed.
  Purpose: A quiet, private area is necessary to protect confidentiality and prevent interruptions. An informed patient is more cooperative and thus more likely to contribute useful information.

3 Complete the history form by using therapeutic communication techniques. Make sure that all medical terminology is adequately explained. A self-history may have been mailed to the patient before the visit. If so, review the self-history for completeness.
  Purpose: Therapeutic communication techniques will assist the medical assistant in gathering complete information while the self-history is designed to save time and to involve the patient in the process.

4 Speak in a pleasant, distinct manner, remembering to maintain eye contact with your patient.

  Purpose: Positive nonverbal behaviors create a friendly atmosphere.

5 Record the following statistical information on the patient information form:
  Patient's full name, including middle initial
  Address, including apartment number and ZIP code
  Marital status
  Sex (gender)
  Age and date of birth
  Telephone number for home and work
  Insurance information if not already available
  Employer's name, address, telephone number

6 Record the following medical history on the patient history (PH) form:

Chief complaint (CC)	Present illness
Past history	Family history
Social history	

  Purpose: This is information that the physician needs to know to make an accurate assessment and diagnosis. The physician usually completes the review of systems (ROS) during the preexamination interview.

7 Ask about allergies to drugs and any other substances, and record any allergies in red ink on every page of the history form, on the front of the chart, and on each progress note page. Some practices apply allergy alert labels to the front of each chart.
  Purpose: The presence of an allergy may alter medication and treatment procedures.

8 Record all information legibly and neatly and spell words correctly. Print rather than write in longhand. Do not erase, scribble, or use whiteout. If you make an error, draw a single line through the error, write "error" above it, add the correction, and initial and date the entry.

Purpose: To maintain a medical record that is understandable and defensible in a court of law.

9 Thank the patient for cooperating and direct him or her back to the reception area.

10 Review the record for errors before you pass it to the physician.

11 Use the information on the record to complete the patient's chart. Keep the information confidential.

Purpose: All information concerning the patient must remain in the office. This information may be legally and ethically discussed with only the physician.

Documentation Practice: Your patient's CC is dizziness for 2 weeks. She denies headaches, Hx of ear infections, or Hx of hypertension. Her BP is 172/94, T 97.6, P 88, R 22. Document pertinent patient findings using the SOAPE method.

S: _____

O: _____

_____

APPENDIX B

A Patient's Bill of Rights*

1. The patient has the right to considerate and respectful care.

2. The patient has the right to and is encouraged to obtain from physicians and other direct caregivers relevant, current, and understandable information concerning diagnosis, treatment, and prognosis.

Except in emergencies when the patient lacks decision-making capacity and the need for treatment is urgent, the patient is entitled to the opportunity to discuss and request information related to the specific procedures and/or treatments, the risks involved, the possible length of recuperation, and the medically reasonable alternatives and their accompanying risks and benefits.

Patients have the right to know the identity of physicians, nurses, and others involved in their care, as well as when those involved are students, residents, or other trainees. The patient also has the right to know the immediate and long-term financial implications of treatment choices, insofar as they are known.

3. The patient has the right to make decisions about the plan of care prior to and during the course of treatment and to refuse a recommended treatment or plan of care to the extent permitted by law and hospital policy and to be informed of the medical consequences of this action. In case of such refusal, the patient is entitled to other appropriate care and services that the hospital provides or transfer to another hospital. The hospital should notify patients of any policy that might affect patient choice within the institution.

4. The patient has the right to have an advance directive (such as a living will, health care proxy, or durable power of attorney for health care) concerning treatment or designating a surrogate decision maker with the expectation that the hospital will honor the intent of that directive to the extent permitted by law and hospital policy.

Health care institutions must advise patients of their rights under state law and hospital policy to make informed medical choices, ask if the patient has an advance directive, and include that information in patient records. The patient has the right to timely information about hospital policy that may limit its ability to implement fully a legally valid advance directive.

5. The patient has the right to every consideration of privacy. Case discussion, consultation, examination, and treatment should be conducted so as to protect each patient's privacy.

6. The patient has the right to expect that all communications and records pertaining to his/her care will be treated as confidential by the hospital, except in cases such as suspected abuse and public health hazards when reporting is permitted or required by law. The patient has the right to expect that the hospital will emphasize the confidentiality of this information when it releases it to any other parties entitled to review information in these records.

7. The patient has the right to review the records pertaining to his/her medical care and to have the information explained or interpreted as necessary, except when restricted by law.

8. The patient has the right to expect that, within its capacity and policies, a hospital will make reasonable response to the request of a patient for appropriate and medically indicated care and services. The hospital must provide evaluation, service, and/or referral as indicated by the urgency of the case. When medically appropriate and legally permissible, or when a patient has so requested, a patient may be transferred to another facility. The institution to which the patient is to be transferred must first have accepted the patient for transfer. The patient must also have the benefit of complete information and explanation concerning the

need for, risks, benefits, and alternatives to such a transfer.

9. The patient has the right to ask and to be informed of the existence of business relationships among the hospital, educational institutions, other health care providers, or payers that may influence the patient's treatment and care.

10. The patient has the right to consent to or decline to participate in proposed research studies or human experimentation affecting care and treatment or requiring direct patient involvement, and to have those studies fully explained prior to consent. A patient who declines to participate in research or experimentation is entitled to the most effective care that the hospital can otherwise provide.

11. The patient has the right to expect reasonable continuity of care when appropriate and to be informed by physicians and other caregivers of available and realistic patient care options when hospital care is no longer appropriate.

12. The patient has the right to be informed of hospital policies and practices that relate to patient care, treatment, and responsibilities. The patient has the right to be informed of available resources for resolving disputes, grievances, and conflicts, such as ethics committees, patient representatives, or other mechanisms available in the institution. The patient has the right to be informed of the hospital's charges for services and available payment methods.

A Patient's Bill of Rights © 1992 by the American Hospital Association.
These rights can be exercised on the patient's behalf by a designated surrogate or proxy decision maker if the patient lacks decision-making capacity, is legally incompetent, or is a minor.

APPENDIX C

Claim Form Comparison Charts

Appendix C lists and compares the CMS-1500 form requirements for each type of payor. The large table covers every box of the CMS-1500 form for common payors. Special considerations for other, less common payors are covered in smaller tables at the end of this appendix.

Claim Form Comparison Chart

Block	Commercial	BC/BS*	Medicare	Medicaid	TRICARE	Workers' Compensation
1	Enter X in "Other" box	Enter X in "Other" box	Enter X in Medicare box	Enter X in Medicaid box	Enter X in CHAMPUS box	Enter X in FECA box
1A	Insurance ID number—omit dashes	BCBS ID number, 2sp, group identification number if provided	Enter Medicare ID number from health insurance card	Enter insured's Medicaid ID number	Enter sponsor's SSN	Enter patient's SSN
2	Enter FULL name of patient (all CAPS no punctuation)	FULL name of patient—for case studies all CAPS no punctuation	Enter patient's name as appears on card (all CAPS no punctuation)	Enter patient's name as it appears on card (all CAPS no punctuation)	Enter FULL name of patient (all CAPS no punctuation)	Enter FULL name of patient (all CAPS no punctuation)
3	Birth date using eight digits MM DD YYYY (use spaces)	Birth date using eight digits MM DD YYYY and X sex block	Birth date using eight digits MM DD YYYY (use spaces)	Birth date using eight digits MM DD YYYY	Enter patient's birth date MM DD YYYY and sex	Enter patient's birth date—MM DD YYYY and sex
4	Enter SAME (if patient and policyholder are same person)	Enter SAME (if patient and policyholder are same person)	Leave blank	Leave blank	Sponsor's name if other than patient, enter SAME if patient is sponsor	Enter employer's name if known
5	Enter patient's mailing address, ZIP, phone number—spaces—no (), -, or punctuation	Enter patient's mailing address, ZIP, phone number—spaces—no (), -, or punctuation	Enter patient's mailing address, ZIP, phone number—spaces—no (), -, or punctuation	Enter patient's mailing address, ZIP, phone number—spaces—no (), -, or punctuation	Enter patient's mailing address, ZIP, phone number—spaces—no (), -, or punctuation	Enter patient's mailing address, ZIP, phone number—spaces—no (), -, or punctuation
6	Enter X in appropriate box—relationship to policyholder	Enter X in appropriate box—relationship to policyholder	Leave blank	Leave blank	Enter X in appropriate box	Enter X in OTHER box
7	If policyholder's address same as in block 5, enter SAME	If policyholder's address same as in block 5, enter SAME	Leave blank	Leave blank	Enter sponsor's duty station/mailing address; if same as patient's—SAME	Enter address and phone number of employer if known
8	Enter X in appropriate box	Enter X in appropriate box	Enter X in appropriate box	Leave blank	Enter X in appropriate box	Enter X in EMPLOYED box
9	Enter NONE (leave 9A-9D blank)	9-9D leave blank	Leave 9-9D blank	Leave 9-9D blank	Enter NONE/9A-9D blank	9-9D leave blank
10A	Enter X in NO box if visit is not related to an on-the-job injury	Enter X in NO box if visit is not related to an on-the-job injury	Enter X in NO box if visit is not related to an on-the-job injury	Enter X in No box	If YES selected, sponsor must complete DD 2527	Enter X in YES box
10B	Enter X in appropriate box; yes indicates possible third party liability	Enter X in appropriate box; yes indicates possible third party liability	Enter X in appropriate box; yes indicates possible third party liability	Enter X in No box	If YES selected, sponsor must complete DD 2527	Enter X in appropriate box
10C	Enter X in appropriate box; yes indicates possible third party liability	Enter X in appropriate box; yes indicates possible third party liability	Enter X in appropriate box; yes indicates possible third party liability	Enter X in No box	If YES selected, sponsor must complete DD 2527	Enter X in appropriate box
10D	Leave blank for case study purposes	Leave blank for case study purposes	Leave blank unless eligible for Medicaid	Leave blank	Leave blank	Leave blank
11	Enter group policy name of number if on patient's card	Leave blank	NONE unless change from Medicare secondary to Medicare primary status	Leave blank	Enter NONE	Leave blank

Claim Form Comparison Chart—Cont'd

Block	Commercial	BC/BS*	Medicare	Medicaid	TRICARE	Workers' Compensation
11A	Enter birth date and sex of person, if other than patient (policyholder/subscriber)	Enter birth date and sex of person, if other than patient (policyholder/subscriber)	Leave blank	Leave blank	Leave blank	Leave blank
11B	Enter name of employer, if identified on patient's ID card	Enter name of employer, if identified on patient's ID card	If applicable, enter description of change from Medicare secondary to primary and date effective	Leave blank	Leave blank	Enter name of patient's employer
11C	Enter name of carrier for patient's policy	Enter name of carrier	Leave blank	Leave blank	Leave blank	Enter name of workers' compensation carrier
11D	Enter X in NO box if covered by only one insurance policy	Enter X in NO box if covered by only one insurance policy	Leave blank	Leave blank	Enter X in appropriate box	Leave blank
12	Enter "SIGNATURE ON FILE" if patient has signed an Authorization for Release; case studies assume one has been signed	Enter "SIGNATURE ON FILE" if patient has signed an Authorization for Release; do not enter date	Enter "SIGNATURE ON FILE" if patient has signed an Authorization for Release; case studies — assume one has been signed	Leave blank	Enter "SIGNATURE ON FILE"	Leave blank
13	Enter "SIGNATURE ON FILE"	Leave blank	PAR-SOF/nonPar—leave blank	Leave blank	Leave blank	Leave blank
14	Enter date of first symptom—MM DD YYYY	Enter date of first symptom—MM DD YYYY	Enter date of first symptom—MM DD YYYY	Leave blank	Information appreciated but not required	Enter date symptoms/injury occurred
15	Enter date of prior episode of same illness if documented in patient's record	Leave blank	Leave blank	Leave blank	Information appreciated but not required	Enter date if in patient's documentation
16	Enter dates patient unable to work if documented in patient's record	Leave blank	Leave blank	Leave blank	Information appreciated but not required	Enter dates if available
17	Enter full name and credentials of referring physician	Enter full name and credentials of referring physician	Enter full name, NOT credentials of referring/ordering etc, physician	Enter full name and credentials of referring/ordering physician, etc.	Enter referring provider; if referred from a military facility, enter name of facility	Enter name and title of referring health care provider, if applicable
17A	PAR providers—enter PIN/nonPAR SSN	Enter UPIN of any provider named in block 17	Enter UPIN of physician in block 17	Enter Medicaid number of provider in block 17	Enter referring physician's EIN	Enter SSN (no spaces or hyphens) of block 17
18	Enter admission/discharge dates if inpatient status	Enter admission/discharge dates if inpatient status	Enter admission/discharge dates if inpatient status	Enter admission/discharge dates if inpatient status	Enter admission/discharge dates if inpatient status	Enter admission/discharge dates if inpatient status
19	Local use; for case studies leave blank	For case studies leave blank or X in NO box	Various information	Local use	Leave blank	Leave blank

Claim Form Comparison Chart—Cont'd

Block	Commercial	BC/BS*	Medicare	Medicaid	TRICARE	Workers' Compensation
20	Enter X in NO box if all laboratory tests performed in provider's office; for case studies—NO	Enter X in NO box if all laboratory tests performed in provider's office; for case studies—NO	Enter X in NO box if all laboratory tests performed in provider's office; for case studies—NO	Enter X in appropriate box	Enter X in NO box	Enter X in appropriate box
21	Enter ICD-9 codes—no decimals	Enter ICD-9 codes—no decimals	Enter ICD-9 codes—no decimals	Enter ICD-9 codes—no decimals	Enter ICD-9 codes	Enter ICD-9 codes
22	Leave blank	Leave blank	Leave blank	For case studies leave blank	Leave blank	Leave blank
23	Enter authorization number when required by patient's insurance plan	Enter authorization number when required by patient's insurance plan	Enter authorization number if one assigned	Enter authorization number if one assigned	Enter prior authorization number	Enter preauthorization number
24A	Enter FROM date MMDDYYYY—no spaces TO not filled in if for single procedure entry	Enter FROM and TO date MMDDYYYY—no spaces TO not filled in if for single procedure entry	Enter FROM date MMDDYYYY—no spaces TO not filled in if for single procedure entry	Enter FROM date MMDDYYYY—no spaces TO not filled in for Medicaid	Enter eight-digit date with no spaces in FROM column, no TO if single procedure entry	Enter eight-digit date with no spaces in FROM column, no TO if single procedure entry
24B	Enter Place of Service code	Enter Place of Service code	Enter Place of Service code	Enter Place of Service code	Use appropriate two-digit code	Use appropriate two-digit code
24C	Enter Type of Service code	Leave blank	Leave blank	Enter Type of Service code	Use appropriate code	Use appropriate code
24D	Enter CPT or HCPCS number	Enter CPT or HCPCS number	Enter CPT or HCPCS number	Enter CPT or HCPCS number	Enter CPT code or HCPCS number	Enter CPT or HCPCS number
24E	Enter reference number (1-4) from block 24D For case studies enter only one number	Enter reference number (1-4) from block 24D For case studies enter only one number	Enter reference number (1-4) from block 24D For case studies enter only one number	Enter reference number (1-4) from block 24D For case studies enter only one number	Enter reference number (1-4) from block 24D For case studies enter only one number	Enter reference number (1-4) from block 24D For case studies enter only one number
24F	Enter fee charged	Enter fee charged	Enter fee charged/ nonPAR limiting fee	Enter fee charged	Enter fee for procedure	Enter fee for procedure
24G	Enter number of units/ days of service or procedures reported in 24D	Enter number of units/ days of service or procedures—use 3 digits: 1 = 001 10 = 010	Enter number of units/ days of service or procedures reported in 24D	Enter number of units/ days of service or procedures reported in 24D	Enter number of units/ days reported in 24D	Enter number of units/ days reported in 24D
24H	Leave blank	Leave blank	Leave blank	Enter E, F, B as appropriate	Leave blank	Leave blank
24I	Enter X if documentation indicates a medical emergency existed	Leave blank	Leave blank	Enter X or E if appropriate	Enter X if services provided in emergency department	Enter X if patient given emergency care
24J	Leave blank	Leave blank	Solo—blank/Group-NPI	Leave blank	Leave blank if services performed by 2 providers	Leave blank
24K	Leave blank	Leave blank	Solo—blank/Group-PIN	Leave blank	Leave blank if services performed by 2 providers	Leave blank

Claim Form Comparison Chart—Cont'd

Block	Commercial	BC/BS*	Medicare	Medicaid	TRICARE	Workers' Compensation
25	Enter EIN and X in appropriate box Be sure to enter hyphen	Enter EIN and X in appropriate box Be sure to enter hyphen	Enter EIN and X in appropriate box Be sure to enter hyphen	Enter Tax ID number if available; enter X in appropriate box	Enter billing's entity Tax ID Number	Enter billing's entity Tax ID Number
26	Enter number for patient's account	Enter number for patient's account	Enter number for patient's account	Enter number for patient's account	Enter patient's account number	Enter patient's account number
27	For case studies enter case study number For case studies enter X in NO box	For case studies enter case study number Enter X in YES if PAR; NO if nonPAR	For case studies enter case study number Enter YES or NO to accept assignment	For case studies enter case study number Enter X in YES box	Enter X in appropriate box/NO for case study	Leave blank
28	Enter total charges	Enter total charges	Enter total charges	Enter total charges	Enter total charges	Enter total charges
29	Enter amount patient has paid/blank if 0	Leave blank	Enter amount patient has paid/blank if 0	Leave blank	Amount received from other health insurance	Leave blank
30	Enter balance	Leave blank	Leave blank	Leave blank	Enter balance due	Leave blank
31	For case studies enter provider's full name, credentials, and date completed—MMDDYYYY	For case studies enter provider's full name, credentials, and date completed—MMDDYYYY	For case studies enter provider's full name, credentials, and date completed—MMDDYYYY	For case studies enter provider's full name, credentials, and date completed—MMDDYYYY	TRICARE requires provider/supplier personally sign claim	For case studies enter provider's full name, credentials, and date completed—MMDDYYYY
32	Enter data if services performed were not in provider's office or patient's home	Enter data if services performed were not in provider's office or patient's home	Enter data if services performed were not in provider's office or patient's home	Enter data if services performed were not in provider's office or patient's home	Enter information if services performed were not in provider's office or patient's home	Enter information if services performed at a site other than provider's office
33	Enter information	Enter information	Enter information	Enter information and Medicaid number in PIN box	Enter information and TRICARE provider number	Enter information; leave PIN and GRP blank—study

Other Payors

Block	Medicare With Medigap
1–8	Same as for Medicare
9	Enter name of enrollee in Medigap if different from block 2
9a	Enter word Medigap and policy/group number
9b	Enter Medigap enrollee's birth date and sex
9c	Leave blank if Medigap PlanID is known; if PlanID not known, enter abbreviated mail address
9d	Enter Medigap PlanID number; if number not available, enter plan name
13	Enter "SIGNATURE ON FILE"

Block	Medicare-Medicaid Crossover
1a	Enter X in both Medicare and Medicaid boxes
10d	Enter abbv "MCD" followed by ID number
27	NonPAR must accept assignment

Block	Medicare–Secondary Payor
1	Enter X in Medicare and Other boxes
4	Enter primary policyholder's name; if policyholder is patient enter SAME
6	If block 4 is completed, enter relationship
7	Enter address and phone number of policyholder in block 4; if same as block 5, enter SAME
11	Enter policy/group number of primary plan; blocks 4 and 7 must be filled out
11a	Primary policyholder's birth date and sex if patient not policyholder
11b	Employer's name for group plan
11c	Primary plan name or PlanID; primary EOB must be attached to claim
16	Enter dates if patient is employed and unable to work
29	Enter patient payment for service on form EOB from primary; will show payments

Block	TRICARE With Supplemental Policy
9a	Policy or group number of other policy
9b	Enter other insured's date of birth, X in appropriate box for sex
9c	Enter name of employer/school
9d	Enter name of insurance plan or program, name of other insurance coverage

Block	TRICARE As Secondary Payor
11	Insured policy group, FECA number if insurance primary; to TRICARE/enter Medicare if appropriate
11a	If different from block 3 enter information
11b	Enter employer/school if applicable
11c	Enter insurance plan or program
11d	Enter X in appropriate box
29	Enter only payments from other insurances

APPENDIX D

English-Spanish Phrases

Are you having pain? Where?
¿Siente usted dolor? ¿Dónde?

What does the pain feel like?
¿Qué tipo de dolor es?

How long have you had problems with this?
¿Desde cuándo tiene este tipo de problemas?

When did it start?
¿Cuándo comenzó?

Does your child have a temperature?
¿Tiene fiebre su hijo?

Have you given your child any medication?
¿Le ha dado alguna medicina a su hijo?

Are you allergic to any medication?
¿Es usted alérgico a algo?

How did your child get hurt?
¿Cómo se lastimó su hijo?

What is your name?
¿Cómo se llama usted?

How old are you?
¿Qué edad tiene?

Do you take any medication regularly?
¿Toma usted alguna medicación con regularidad?

How many times have you been pregnant?
¿Cuántas veces ha estado embarazada?

How many children were born alive?
¿Cuántos niños sanos ha dado usted a luz?

Who is your closest relative?
¿Quién es su familiar más cercano?

Do you speak English?
¿Habla usted inglés?

Can someone come with you the next time who does speak English?
¿Puede acompañarle alguien que hable inglés la próxima vez?

Can you read English?
¿Sabe usted leer en inglés?

Does someone in your family read English?
¿Alguien de su familiar sabe leer en inglés?

My name is...You are...
Yo soy... Usted es...

Please put the gown on.
Por favor, póngase la bata.

Your blood pressure is...
Su presión arterial es de...

Your blood sugar is...
Su nivel de azúcar en la sangre es de...

The doctor recommends a low fat diet.
El médico recomienda una dieta baja en grasa.

Does this hurt?
¿Le duele esto?

Do you have medical insurance?
¿Tiene usted seguro médico?

Please point to where it hurts.
Por favor, indíqueme dónde le duele.

Where do you work?
¿Dónde trabaja usted?

Have you seen blood in your urine?
¿Ha visto algo de sangre en su orina?

Do you have pain when urinating?
¿Siente algún dolor al orinar?

Please fill out this form.
Por favor, llene este formulario.

Do you have an insurance card?
¿Tiene usted una tarjeta del seguro?

Do you have a telephone? What is the number?
¿Tiene usted teléfono? ¿Cuál es el número?

Please come back to see the doctor on...
Por favor, regrese para ver al médico el...

All days of the week.
Todos los días de la semana.

All months of the year.
Todos los meses del año.

All times.
A todas horas.

All numbers (to 31).
Todos los números (hasta el 31).

The doctor wants you to see another doctor.
El médico quiere que la vea otro médico.

Go to the hospital.
Vaya al hospital.

Call the ambulance now.
Pida una ambulancia ahora mismo.

Take your medication as ordered.
Tómese la medicación tal como se le indicó.

These are the side effects of your medication.
Su medicación tiene algunos efectos secundarios.

Thank you.
Gracias.

You are welcome.
De nada.

Please.
Por favor.

Please come this way.
Venga por aquí, por favor.

Please come with me.
Acompáñeme, por favor.

Please wait here to see the doctor.
Por favor, espere aquí para ver al médico.

You may leave now.
Ya puede marcharse.

We need to get a blood sample.
Necesitamos una muestra de su sangre.

We need to get a urine sample.
Necesitamos una muestra de su orina.

You owe "xxx" today.
Hoy debe abonar "xxx".

Who should we call to pick you up?
¿A quién debemos contactar para que lo recojan?

Please go to the lab at this address.
Por favor, vaya al laboratorio que está en este lugar.

When did you last eat?
¿Cuándo comió por última vez?

Have you had nausea?
¿Ha tenido náuseas?

Have you vomited?
¿Ha vomitado?

Please sign your name here.
Por favor, firme aquí.

Take this medicine (3) times a day.
Tómese esta medicina (3) veces al día.

This paper allows us to file your insurance.
Este papel nos permite presentarle su caso al seguro.

This paper allows the insurance company to pay the doctor.
Este papel es para que el seguro le pague al médico.

The doctor will see you now.
El médico le puede ver ahora.

Good morning.
Buenos días.

Good afternoon.
Buenas tardes.

Here is information (written) about your illness.
Aquí se incluye información (escrita) sobre su enfermedad.

Please follow these directions.
Por favor, siga estas instrucciones.

It is nice to meet you.
Es un placer conocerle.

Thank you for coming.
Gracias por su visita.

Take care of yourself.
¡Cuídese!

Do you drink?
¿Toma usted alcohol?

Do you smoke? How much?
¿Fuma? ¿Cuántos cigarrillos al día?

Have you had this problem before?
¿Ha tenido antes este problema?

Glossary

academic degree A title conferred by a college, university, or professional school on completion of a program of study.

account A statement of transactions during a fiscal period and the resulting balance.

account balance The amount owed on an account.

accounts payable Debts incurred and not yet paid.

accounts receivable Amounts owed to the physician.

accounts receivable ledger A record of the charges and payments posted on an account.

accounts receivable trial balance A method of determining that the journal and the ledger are in balance.

accreditation The process through which an organization is recognized for adherence to a group of standards that meet or exceed expectations of the accrediting agency.

accrual basis of accounting Method of accounting in which income is recorded when earned, and expenses are recorded when incurred.

act The formal action of a legislative body; a decision or determination of a sovereign state, a legislative council, or a court of justice.

adage A saying, often in metaphorical form, that embodies a common observation.

advent A coming into being or use.

advocate One who pleads the cause of another; one who defends or maintains a cause or proposal.

affable Being pleasant and at ease in talking to others; characterized by ease and friendliness.

agenda A list or outline of things to be considered or done.

aggression A forceful action or procedure intended to dominate; hostile, injurious, or destructive behavior, especially when caused by frustration.

allegation A statement by a party to a legal action of what the party undertakes to prove, an assertion made without proof.

allied health fields Occupational disciplines in which professionals involved with the delivery of healthcare or related services assist physicians with the diagnosis, treatment, and care of patients in many different specialty areas.

allocating Apportioning for a specific purpose or to particular persons or things.

allopathy A word coined by Samuel Christian Hahnemann to contrast homeopathic medicine with mainstream medicine; medicine supposedly characterized by an effort to counteract the symptoms of a disease by administration of treatments that produce an opposite effect from the symptoms.

allowed charge The maximum amount of money that many third-party payors allow for a specific procedure or service.

alphabetical filing Any system that arranges names or topics according to the sequence of the letters in the alphabet.

alphanumeric Systems made up of combinations of letters and numbers.

ambiguous Capable of being understood in two or more possible senses or ways; unclear.

ambulatory Able to walk about and not be bedridden.

amenities Something that contributes to comfort, enjoyment, or convenience.

amenity Something conducive to comfort, convenience, or enjoyment.

ancillary Subordinate; auxiliary.

ancillary diagnostic services Services that support patient diagnoses (e.g., laboratory or radiology services).

ancillary therapeutic services Services that support patient treatment (specialists or surgery).

"and" In the context of ICD-9-CM, the word "and" should be interpreted as "and/or."

animate Full of life; to give spirit and support to expressions.

annotating To furnish with notes, which are usually critical or explanatory.

annotation A note added by way of comment or explanation.

appeal A legal proceeding by which a case is brought before a higher court for review of the decision of a lower court.

appellate Having the power to review the judgment of another tribunal or body of jurisdiction, such as an appellate court.

applications software Software programs designed to perform specific tasks.

appraisal To give an expert judgment of the value or merit of; judging as to quality.

appraisals Act of giving an expert judgment of the value or merit of; also, evaluations of work performance.

arbitration The hearing and determination of a cause in controversy by a person or persons either chosen by the parties involved or appointed under statutory authority.

arbitrator A neutral person chosen to settle differences between two parties in a controversy.

archaic Of, relating to, or characteristic of an earlier or more primitive time.

archived To have filed or collected records or documents.

artificial intelligence The aspect of computer science that deals with computers taking on the attributes of humans. One such example is expert systems, which are capable of making decisions, such as software that is designed to help a physician diagnose a patient, given a set of symptoms. Game-playing programs and programs that are designed to recognize human speech are other examples.

ASCII codes Acronym for American Standard Code for Information Interchange; a code representing English characters as numbers where each is given a number from 0 to 127.

assault An intentional, unlawful attempt of bodily injury to another by force.

assent To agree to something, especially after thoughtful consideration.

assets The entire property of a person, association, corporation, or estate applicable or subject to the payment of debts.

assignment of benefits The transfer of the patient's legal right to collect benefits for medical expenses to the provider of those services, authorizing the payment to be sent directly to the provider.

asystole The absence of a heartbeat.

audit A formal examination of an organization's or individual's accounts or financial situation; a methodical examination and review.

audit trail The path left by a transaction when it has been completed, often referred to when tracking medical services used by patients or researching claims.

augment To make greater, more numerous, larger, or more intense.

authenticated Proof of; with regard to medical records, it applies to a signature, initials, or computer keystroke by the maker of the record who verifies that the record is correct.

authorization A term used in managed care for an approved referral.

backup Any type of storage of files to prevent their loss in the event of hard disk failure.

bailiff An officer of some U.S. courts usually serving as a messenger or usher, who keeps order at the request of the judge.

balance sheet A financial statement for a specific date that shows the total assets, liabilities, and capital of the business.

bank reconciliation The process of proving that a bank statement and checkbook balance are in agreement.

banners Advertisements often found on a web page that can be animated to attract the user's attention in hopes that he or she will click on the ad, be redirected to the advertiser's home page, and purchase from the site or gain information from the site.

battery A willful and unlawful use of force or violence on the person of another; an offensive touching or use of force on a person without his or her consent.

beneficence The act of doing or producing good, especially performing acts of charity or kindness.

beneficiary Individual entitled to receive benefits from an insurance policy or program, or a governmental entitlement program offering healthcare benefits. Also called a *participant*, *subscriber*, *dependent*, *enrollee*, or *member*.

benefits Services or payments provided under a health plan, employee plan, or some other agreement, including programs such as health insurance, pensions, retirement planning, and many other options that may be offered to employees of a company or organization; the amount payable by an insurance company for a monetary loss to an individual insured by that company, under each coverage.

birthday rule Under law, when an individual is covered under two insurance policies, the insurance plan of the policyholder whose birthday comes first in the calendar year (month and day—not year) becomes the primary insurance.

bit The smallest unit of information inside the computer, represented by either the digit "0" or "1"; eight bits equal one byte.

blatant Completely obvious, conspicuous, or obtrusive, especially in a crass or offensive manner; brazen.

bond A durable, formal paper used for documents.

bookkeeping The recording of business and accounting transactions.

bundled codes Procedures or services that are grouped together and paid as one.

burnout Exhaustion of physical or emotional strength or motivation, usually as a result of prolonged stress or frustration.

byte A unit of data that contains eight binary digits, or bits.

cache A special high-speed storage that can either be a part of the computer's main memory or can be a separate storage device. One function of a cache is to store websites visited in the computer memory for faster recall the next time the website is requested.

capitation Payment method used by many managed care organizations wherein a fixed amount of money is reimbursed to the provider for patients enrolled during a specific period of time, no matter what services received or number of visits made.

caption A heading, title, or subtitle under which records are filed.

cardiac arrhythmias Irregular heartbeat resulting from a malfunction of the electrical system of the heart.

carrier As related to insurance, a company that assumes the risk of an insurance policy.

carrier-direct system A system for electronic data submission in which the medical facility has a computer system designed to transmit claims to a specific carrier directly, without first passing through a clearinghouse.

case management The process of assessing and planning patient care, including referral and follow-up to ensure continuity of care and quality management.

cash basis of accounting Method of accounting in which income is recorded when received, and expenses are recorded when paid.

cash flow statement A financial summary for a specific period that shows the beginning balance on hand, the receipts and disbursements during the period, and the balance on hand at the end of the period.

categorically Placed in a specific division of a system of classification.

caustic A remark or phrase marked by sarcasm.

CD burner A device that is capable of "writing" data onto a blank compact disk (CD) or copying data from one CD to a blank CD.

certification To attest as being true, as represented, or as meeting a standard; to have been tested, usually by a third party, and awarded a certificate based on proven knowledge.

chain of command A series of executive positions in order of authority.

channels Means of communication or expression; courses or directions of thought.

characteristics Distinguishing traits, qualities, or properties.

chiropractic A medical discipline in which chiropractic physicians focus on the nervous system and painlessly, manually adjust the vertebral column to affect the nervous system, resulting in healthier patients.

chronological order Of, relating to, or arranged in or according to the order of time.

circumvent To manage to get around, especially by ingenuity or stratagem.

circumvention To manage to get around, especially by ingenuity or stratagem.

cited Quoted by way of example, authority, or proof or mentioned formally in commendation or praise.

Civilian Health and Medical Program of the Uniformed Services (CHAMPUS) A government-sponsored program wherein authorized dependents of military personnel receive medical care. This program is now referred to as TRICARE.

Civilian Health and Medical Program of the Veterans Administration (CHAMPVA) A health benefits program run by the Department of Veterans Affairs (VA) that helps eligible beneficiaries pay the cost of specific healthcare services/supplies.

clarity The quality or state of being clear.

clauses A group of words containing a subject and predicate and functioning as a member of a complex or compound sentence.

clean claim An insurance claim form that has been completed correctly (no errors or omissions) and can be processed and paid promptly if the claim meets the restrictions on covered services and items.

clearinghouse A centralized facility, sometimes called a *third-party administrator* (TPA), to whom insurance claims are transmitted. Clearinghouses separate, check, and redistribute claims electronically to various insurance carriers, and may offer additional services to the physician; networks of banks that exchange checks with each other.

clinical trials Research studies that test how well new medical treatments or other interventions work in the subjects, usually human beings.

"code also" When more than one code is necessary to fully identify a given condition, "code also" or "use additional code" is used.

"code if applicable" Notation meaning that the designated code may be principal if no casual condition is applicable or known.

Code of Federal Regulations (CFR) A coded delineation of the rules and regulations published in the Federal Register by the various departments and agencies of the federal government. The CFR is divided into 50 titles that represent broad subject areas, and then chapters that provide specific detail.

coding Converting verbal or written descriptions into numerical and alphanumerical designations.

cohesive The state of sticking together tightly; exhibiting or producing the cohesion.

coinsurance A policy provision frequently found in medical insurance whereby the policyholder and the insurance company share the cost of *covered* losses in a specified ratio (i.e., 80/20 means 80% is covered by the insurer and 20% by the insured).

collect on delivery (COD) Method of payment used when an article or item is delivered and payment is expected before it is released.

comfort zone A place in the mind where an individual feels safe and confident.

commensurate Corresponding in size, amount, extent, or degree; equal in measure.

commercial insurance Plans (sometimes called *private insurance*) that reimburse the insured for expenses resulting from illness or injury according to a specific fee schedule as outlined in the insurance policy and on a fee-for-service basis.

comorbidities Preexisting conditions that will, because of their presence with a specific principal diagnosis, cause an increase in length of an inpatient hospital stay by at least 1 day in approximately 75% of cases.

competence The quality or state of being competent; having adequate or requisite capabilities.

competent Having adequate abilities or qualities; having the capacity to function or perform in a certain way.

complications Conditions that arise during a hospital stay that prolong the length of stay by at least 1 day in approximately 75% of cases.

component A constituent part; a part of a larger group.

computer A machine that is designed to accept, store, process, and give out information.

concise Expressing much in brief form.

concurrently Occurring at the same time.

congruent Being in agreement, harmony, or correspondence; conforming to the circumstances or requirements of a situation.

connotation An implication; something suggested by a word or thing.

contamination A process by which something is made impure, unclean, or unfit for use by the introduction of unwholesome or undesirable elements.

continuation pages The second and following pages of a letter.

continuing education units (CEUs) Credits for courses, classes, or seminars related to an individual's profession, designed to promote education and to keep the professional up-to-date on current procedures and trends in their field; often required for licensing.

continuity of care Care that continues smoothly from one provider to another, so that the patient receives the most benefit and no interruption in care.

contraindication Something, as a symptom or condition, that makes a particular treatment or procedure inadvisable.

contributory negligence Statutes in some states that may prevent a party from recovering damages if he or she contributed in any way to the injury or condition.

cookies Messages sent to a web browser from a web server that identify users and can prepare custom web pages for them, possibly displaying their name on return to the site.

coordination of benefits (COB) The mechanism used in group health insurance to designate the order in which multiple carriers are to pay benefits to prevent duplicate payments.

copayment A sum of money that is paid at the time of medical service; a form of coinsurance.

counteroffer Return offer made by one who has rejected an offer or job.

credentialing The act of extending professional or medical privileges to an individual; the process of verifying and evaluating that person's credentials.

credibility The quality or power of inspiring belief.

credit An entry on an account constituting an addition to a revenue, net worth, or liability account; the balance in a person's favor in an account.

critical thinking The constant practice of considering all aspects of a situation when deciding what to believe or what to do.

cross-training Training in more than one area, so that a multitude of duties may be performed by one person, or so that substitutions of personnel may be made when necessary or in emergencies.

cultivate To foster the growth of; to improve by labor, care, or study.

cursor A symbol appearing on the monitor that shows where the next character to be typed will appear.

curt Marked by rude or peremptory shortness.

cyanosis Blue color of the mucous membranes and body extremities caused by lack of oxygen.

cyberspace Describes the nonphysical space of the online world of computer networks in which communication takes place.

damages Loss or harm resulting from injury to person, property, or reputation; compensation in money imposed by law for losses or injuries.

database A collection of related files that serves as a foundation for retrieving information.

debit An entry on an account constituting an addition to an expense or asset account or a deduction from a revenue, a net worth, or a liability account.

debit cards A card that looks like a credit card and by which money may be withdrawn or the cost of purchases paid directly from the holder's bank account without the payment of interest.

decedent A legal term for a deceased person.

decode To convert, as in a message, into intelligible form; to recognize and interpret.

deductible A specific amount of money a patient must pay out-of-pocket before the insurance carrier begins paying. Usually this amount ranges from $100 to $500. This deductible amount is met on a yearly or per-incident basis.

default Failure to pay financial debts, such as a student loan.

defense mechanisms Psychological methods of dealing with stressful situations that are encountered in day-to-day living.

deferment Postponement, especially of a student loan.

demeanor Behavior toward others; outward manner.

demographic The statistical characteristics of human populations (as in age or income) used especially to identify markets.

dependents The spouse, children, and sometimes domestic partner or other individuals designated by the insured who are covered under a healthcare plan.

depleted To lessen markedly in quantity, content, power, or value.

detrimental Obviously harmful or damaging.

device driver The program or commands given to a device connected to a computer that enable the device to function. For instance, a printer may come equipped with a software program that must be loaded onto the computer first, so that the printer will work.

"diagnosis" The determination of the nature of a disease, injury, or congenital defect.

dictation The act or manner of uttering words to be transcribed.

diction The choice of words especially with regard to clearness, correctness, or effectiveness.

digital signature A signature used for electronic claims; it consists of lines of text or a text box and is attached through a software application.

digital subscriber line (DSL) High-speed, sophisticated modulation scheme that operates over existing copper telephone wiring systems; often referred to as "last-mile technologies," because DSL is used for connections from a telephone switching station to a home or office, and not from between switching stations.

digital versatile disk or digital video disk (DVD) An optical disk that holds approximately 28 times more information than a CD; a DVD is most commonly used to hold full-length movies. Compared with a CD, which holds approximately 600 megabytes, a DVD has the capacity to hold approximately 4.7 gigabytes.

dingy claim A claim that is delayed because it cannot be processed, usually because the software used to transfer the claim or system changes make it incompatible with the receiving system.

direct filing system A filing system in which materials can be located without consulting an intermediary source of reference.

dirty claim Claims that contain errors or omissions that cannot be processed or must be processed by hand because of OCR scanner rejection.

disability income insurance   Insurance that provides periodic payments to replace income when an insured person is unable to work as a result of illness, injury, or disease.

disbursements   Money (funds) paid out.

disbursements journal   A summary of accounts paid out.

discretion   The quality of being discrete; having or showing good judgment or conduct, especially in speech.

disk   A removable device with a magnetic surface that is capable of storing computer programs, stored in a hard plastic square; also called diskettes, and early versions were called "floppy disks."

disk drives   Devices that load a program or data stored on a disk into the computer.

disparaging   Speak slightingly about, with a negative or degrading tone.

disparities   Containing or made up of fundamentally different and often incongruous elements; markedly distinct in quality or character.

disposition   The tendency of something or someone to act in a certain manner under given circumstances.

disruption   An unexpected event that throws a plan into disorder; an interruption that prevents a system or process from continuing as usual or as expected.

dissection   Separation into pieces and exposure of parts for scientific examination.

disseminate   To disperse throughout; to spread around.

docket   A formal record of judicial proceedings; a list of legal causes to be tried.

domestic mail   Mail that is sent within the boundaries of the United States and its territories.

downcoding   A change in code done by the insurance company that receives a claim resulting in a lesser reimbursement. The change will usually be the code closest to the one submitted on the claim, because the code does not match in some way to the specifications of the insurance company.

drawee   Bank or facility on whom a check is drawn or written.

drawer   Person who writes a check.

due process   A fundamental constitutional guarantee that all legal proceedings will be fair; that one will be given notice of the proceedings and given an opportunity to be heard before the government acts to take away life, liberty, or property; a constitutional guarantee that a law will not be unreasonable or arbitrary.

duty   Obligatory tasks, conduct, service, or functions that arise from one's position, as in life or in a group.

dyspnea   Difficult or painful breathing.

e-banking   Electronic banking via computer modem or over the Internet.

ecchymosis   A hemorrhagic skin discoloration commonly called bruising.

ecommerce   An abbreviation for *electronic commerce*; used to describe the sale and purchase of goods and services over the Internet; doing business over the Internet.

effective date   The date on which an insurance policy or plan takes effect so that benefits are payable.

electronic claims   Claims that are submitted to insurance processing facilities using a computerized medium, such as direct data entry, direct wire, dial-in telephone digital fax, or personal computer download/upload.

electronic data interchange   The transfer of data back and forth between two or more entities using an electronic medium.

electronic signature   A scanned signature or other such mark that is accepted as proof of approval and/or responsibility for the content of an electronic document.

email   Communications transmitted via computer using a modem.

emancipated minor   A person under legal age who is self-supporting and living apart from parents or guardian; a mature minor considered to possess a sufficient understanding of self-care and responsibility.

embezzlement   Stealing from an employer; to appropriate goods, services, or funds for personal use without permission.

emetic   A substance that causes vomiting.

empathy   Sensitivity to the individual needs and reactions of patients.

employer identification number (EIN)   The number used by the Internal Revenue Service that identifies a business or individual functioning as a business entity for income tax reporting.

encode   To convert from one system of communication to another; to convert a message into code.

encounter   Any contact between a healthcare provider and a patient that results in treatment or evaluation of the patient's condition; not limited to in-person contact.

encroachments   That which advances beyond the usual or proper limits.

encrypt   To convert from one system of communication to another; encode.

endorser   Person who signs his or her name on the back of a check for the purpose of transferring title to another person.

enunciate   To utter articulate sounds; the act of being very distinct in speech.

enunciation   Utterance of articulate, clear sounds.

environment   The state of a computer, usually determined by the programs that are running as well as hardware and software characteristics.

equities   The money value of a property or of an interest in a property in excess of claims or liens against it.

erroneous   Containing or characterized by error or assumption.

established patients   Patients who are returning to the office who have previously been seen by the physician.

etiology   The cause of the disorder; a claim may be classified according to etiology.

euthanasia   The act or practice of killing or permitting the death of hopelessly sick or injured individuals in a relatively painless way for reasons of mercy.

"excludes"   Exclusion terms are always written in italics, and the word "excludes" is often enclosed in a box to draw particular attention to these instructions. Exclusion terms may apply to a chapter, a section, a category, or subcategory. The applicable code number usually follows the exclusion term.

exclusions Limitations on an insurance contract for which benefits are not payable.

expediency A means of achieving a particular end, as in a situation requiring haste or caution.

expert witness A person who provides testimony to a court as an expert in a certain field or subject to verify facts presented by one or both sides in a lawsuit, often compensated and used to refute or disprove the claims of one party.

external noise Sounds or factors outside the brain that interfere with the communication process.

externalization To attribute an event or occurrence to causes outside the self.

externship/internship A training program that is part of a course of study of an educational institution and is taken in the actual business setting in that field of study; these terms are often interchanged in reference to medical assisting.

extrinsic External to a thing, its essential nature, or its original character.

fax Abbreviation for *facsimile*; also, a document sent using a facsimile (fax) machine.

fee for service An established schedule of fees set for services performed by providers and paid by the patient.

fee profile A compilation or average of physician fees over a given period of time.

fee schedule A compilation of preestablished fee allowances for given services or procedures.

feedback The transmission of evaluative or corrective information to the original or controlling source about an action, event, or process.

felony A major crime, such as murder, rape, or burglary; punishable by a more stringent sentence than that given for a misdemeanor.

fermentation An enzymatically controlled transformation of an organic compound.

fervent Exhibiting or marked by great intensity of feeling.

fibrillation Rapid, random, ineffective contractions of the heart.

fidelity Faithfulness to something to which one is bound by pledge or duty.

fine A sum imposed as punishment for an offense; a forfeiture or penalty paid to an injured party or the government in a civil or criminal action.

fiscal agent An organization under contract to the government as well as some private plans to act as financial representatives in handling insurance claims from providers of health care; also referred to as *fiscal intermediary*.

fiscal intermediary An organization that contracts with the government to handle and mediate insurance claims from medical facilities, home health agencies, or providers of medical services or supplies.

fiscal year An accounting period of 12 months.

flagged Marked in some way as to remind or remember that specific action needs to be taken.

flash Animation technology often used on the opening page of a website to draw attention, excite, and impress the user.

flush Directly abutting or immediately adjacent, as set even with an edge of a type page or column; having no indention.

font A design for a set of type characters; a combination of typeface, spacing, pitch, and other qualities. Fonts are named; examples include Times Roman, Arial, and Garamond.

format To magnetically create tracks on a disk where information will be stored, usually done by the manufacturer of the disk.

gametes Mature male or female germ cells usually possessing a haploid chromosome set and capable of initiating formation of a new diploid individual.

genome The genetic material of an organism.

genuineness Expressing sincerity and honest feeling.

gigabyte Approximately 1 billion bytes; abbreviated GB.

girth A measure around a body or item.

gleaned Gathered bit by bit (e.g., information or material); picked over in search of relevant material.

government plan An entitlement program or healthcare plan that is sponsored and/or subsidized by the state or federal government, such as Medicaid and Medicare.

gradient A change in response with distance from the stimulus.

grammar The study of the classes of words, their inflections, and their functions and relations in the sentence; a study of what is to be preferred and what avoided in inflection and syntax.

grief An unfortunate outcome; a deep distress caused by bereavement.

group policy Insurance written under a policy that covers a number of people under a single master contract issued to their employer or to an association with which they are affiliated.

guarantor The person who is responsible for paying a medical bill; a person who makes or gives a guarantee of payment for a bill.

guardian ad litem Legal representative for a minor.

hard copy The readable paper copy or printout of information.

harmonious Marked by accord in sentiment or action; having the parts agreeably related.

health insurance Protection in return for periodic *premium* payments, which provides reimbursement of expenses resulting from illness or injury. Includes these forms of insurance: accident, disability income, medical expense, and accidental death and dismemberment. Also known as *accident* and *health insurance* or *disability income insurance*.

Health Insurance Portability and Accountability Act (HIPAA) The Kassebaum-Kennedy Act designed to improve portability and continuity of health insurance coverage; to combat waste, fraud, and abuse in health insurance and healthcare delivery; to promote the use of medical savings accounts; to improve access to long-term care services and coverage; to simplify the administration of health insurance; and for other purposes.

health maintenance organization (HMO) An organization that provides a wide range of comprehensive healthcare services for a specified group at a fixed periodic payment. HMOs can be sponsored by the government, medical schools, hospitals, employers, labor unions, consumer groups, insurance companies, and hospital-medical plans.

hematuria Blood in the urine.

holder Person presenting a check for payment.

holistic Related to or concerned with all of the systems of the body, rather than breaking it down into parts.

HTML Acronym for HyperText Markup Language, which is the language used to create documents for use on the Internet.

HTTP Acronym for HyperText Transfer Protocol, which defines how messages are formatted and transmitted over the Internet. When a URL is entered into the computer, an HTTP command tells the web server to retrieve the requested web page.

hub A common connection point for devices in a network containing multiple ports, often used to connect segments of a LAN.

icon A picture, often on the desktop of a computer, that represents a program or an object. By clicking on the icon, the user is directed to the program.

idealism The practice of forming ideas or living under the influence of ideas.

immigrant A person who comes to a country to take up permanent residence.

impenetrable Incapable of being penetrated or pierced; not capable of being damaged or harmed.

implied consent Presumed consent, such as when a patient offers an arm for a phlebotomy procedure.

in balance The total ending balances of patient ledgers equal total of accounts receivable control.

incentives Something that incites or spurs to action; a reward or reason for performing a task.

"includes" This term appearing under a subdivision, such as a category (three-digit code) or two-digit procedure code, indicates that the code and title include these terms. Other terms also classified to that particular code and title are listed in the Alphabetic Indexes.

incomplete claim A claim that is missing information and is returned to the provider for correction and resubmission.

indemnity plan Traditional health insurance plan that pays for all or a share of the cost of covered services, regardless of which physician, hospital, or other licensed healthcare provider is used. Policyholders of indemnity plans and their dependents choose when and where to get healthcare services.

indicators An important point or group of statistical values that, when evaluated, indicate the quality of care provided in a healthcare institution.

indicted Charged with a crime by the finding or presentment of a jury with due process of law.

indigent Totally lacking in something of need.

indirect filing system A filing system in which an intermediary source of reference, such as a card file, must be consulted to locate specific files.

individual policy An insurance policy designed specifically for the use of one person (and his or her dependents), not associated with the amenities of a group policy, namely higher premiums. Often called *personal insurance*.

infertile Not fertile or productive; not capable of reproducing.

inflection A change in pitch or loudness of the voice.

informed consent A consent in which there is understanding of what treatment is to be undertaken and of the risks involved, why it should be done, and alternative methods of treatment available (including no treatment) and their attendant risks.

infraction Breaking the law; a minor offense of the rules.

initiative To cause or facilitate the beginning of; to initiate something into happening.

innate Existing in, belonging to, or determined by factors present in an individual since birth.

input Information entered into and used by the computer.

instigate To goad or urge forward; to provoke.

insubordination Disobedient to authority.

insured An individual or organization who is covered by an insurance policy according to the policy terms, usually the individual or group who pays the premiums. Blue Cross/Blue Shield refers to this person or group as the *subscriber*.

intangibles Incapable of being perceived, especially by touch; incapable of being precisely identified or realized by the mind.

integral Essential; being an indispensable part of a whole.

interaction A two-way communication; mutual or reciprocal action or influence.

intercom A two-way communication system with a microphone and loudspeaker at each station for localized use.

intermittent Coming and going at intervals; not continuous.

internal noise Factors inside the brain that interfere with the communication process.

***International Classification of Diseases, Ninth Revision, Clinical Modification* (ICD-9-CM)** System for classifying disease to facilitate collection of uniform and comparable health information, for statistical purposes and indexing medical records for data storage and retrieval.

***International Classification of Diseases, Tenth Revision* (ICD-10)** System containing the greatest number of changes in ICD's history. To allow more specific reporting of disease and newly recognized conditions, the ICD-10 contains approximately 5500 more codes than ICD-9.

international mail Mail that is sent outside the boundaries of the United States and its territories.

interval Space of time between events.

intolerable Not tolerable or bearable.

intrinsic Belonging to the essential nature or constitution of a thing; indwelling, inward.

intrinsic Originating or due to causes within a body, organ, or part.

introspection An inward, reflective examination of one's own thoughts and feelings.

invalid claim A claim that is incorrect in some manner or does not present a logical picture of the patient's situation.

invariably Consistent; not changing or capable of change.

invasive Involving entry into the living body, as by incision or insertion of an instrument.

invoice A paper describing a purchase and the amount due.

jargon The technical terminology or characteristic idiom of a particular group or special activity.

Java A commonly used object-oriented high-level programming language that is well suited for the Internet.

judicial Of or relating to a judgment, the function of judging, the administration of justice, or the judiciary.

jurisdiction A power constitutionally conferred on a judge or magistrate to decide cases according to law and to carry sentence into execution; jurisdiction is original when it is conferred on the court in the first instance, called original jurisdiction; or it is appellate, which is when an appeal is given from the judgment of another court.

jurisprudence The science or philosophy of law; a system or body of law or the course of court decisions.

language barrier Any type of interference that inhibits the communication process that is related to languages spoken by the people attempting to communicate.

law A binding custom or practice of a community; a rule of conduct or action prescribed or formally recognized as binding or enforceable by a controlling authority.

learning style The way that an individual perceives and processes information to learn new material.

liabilities Something that is owed; a debt.

liable Obligated according to law or equity; responsible for an act or circumstance.

libel A written defamatory statement or representation that conveys an unjustly unfavorable impression.

litigious Prone to engage in lawsuits.

maker (of a check) Any individual, corporation, or legal party who signs a check or any type of negotiable instrument.

malediction To speak evil of or curse.

managed care plans An umbrella term for all healthcare plans that provide healthcare in return for preset monthly payments and coordinated care through a defined network of primary care physicians and hospitals.

mandated Required by an authority or law.

mandatory Containing or constituting a command.

manifestation Something that is easily understood or recognized by the mind.

marketing The process or technique of promoting, selling, and distributing a product or service.

matrix Something in which a thing originates, develops, takes shape, or is contained; a base on which to build.

m-banking Banking through the use of wireless devices, such as cellular phones and wireless Internet services.

media Term applied to agencies of mass communication, such as newspapers, magazines, and telecommunications.

mediastinum Space in the center of the chest under the sternum.

medical savings account A tax-deferred bank or savings account combined with a low-premium/high-deductible insurance policy, designed for individuals or families who choose to fund their own healthcare expenses and medical insurance.

medically indigent An individual who may be able to afford to pay for his or her normal daily living expenses but cannot afford adequate healthcare.

medically necessary Phrase indicating that the patient's symptoms and diagnosis justify or support specific medical services or procedures, as determined through a decision-making process used by third-party payors. Also known as *medical necessity*.

Medigap A term sometimes applied to private insurance products that supplement Medicare insurance benefits.

megabyte Approximately 1 million bytes; abbreviated MB.

megahertz The measuring device for microprocessors, abbreviated MHz. A megahertz is 1 million cycles of electromagnetic currency alternation per second and is used as a unit of measure for the clock speed of computer microprocessors. The hertz is a unit of measure named after Heinrich Hertz, a German physicist.

mentor A trusted counselor or guide.

meticulous Marked by extreme or excessive care in the consideration or treatment of details.

microfilm A film bearing a photographic record on a reduced scale of printed or other graphic matter.

micromanage To manage with great or excessive control or attention to details.

MIDI Acronym for Musical Instrument Digital Interface; a MIDI interface allows computers to record and manipulate sound.

misdemeanor A minor crime, as opposed to a felony, punishable by fine or imprisonment in a city or county jail rather than in a penitentiary.

mnemonic A device, such as a sentence or rhyme, used as a memory aid (e.g., Roy G. Biv for remembering the colors of the spectrum: red-orange-yellow-green-blue-indigo-violet).

mock Simulated; intended for imitation or practice.

modem A device that allows information to be transmitted over telephone lines, at speeds measured in bits per second (bps); short for modulator-demodulator.

modifiers Code additions that explain circumstances that alter a service that has been provided and clarify exactly what was done to the patient.

monochromatic Having or consisting of one color or hue.

monotone A succession of syllables, words, or sentences in one unvaried key or pitch.

morale   The mental and emotional condition, such as enthusiasm, confidence, or loyalty, of an individual or group with regard to the function or tasks at hand.

morbidity   The relative incidence of disease.

mortality   The number of deaths in a given time or place.

motivation   The process of inciting a person to some action or behavior.

multimedia   The presentation of graphics, animation, video, sound, and text on a computer in an integrated way, or all at once. CD-ROMs are the most effective multimedia devices.

multitasking   Performing multiple tasks at the same time.

municipal   A court that sits in some cities and larger towns and that usually has civil and criminal jurisdiction over cases arising within the municipality.

myocardium   The muscular lining of the heart.

mysticism   The experience of seeming to have direct communication with God or ultimate reality.

national provider identifier (NPI)   A lifetime number consisting of 10 digits that Medicare will use to replace the provider identification number (PIN) and the unique physician identification number (UPIN).

naturopathy   An alternative to conventional medicine in which holistic methods are used, as well as herbs and natural supplements, with the belief that the body will heal itself. Naturopathic physicians can currently be licensed in 12 states.

necrosis   Pertaining to the death of cells or tissue.

negligence   Failure to exercise the care that a prudent person usually exercises; implies inattention to one's duty or business; implies want of due or necessary diligence or care.

negotiable   Legally transferable to another party.

networking   Exchange of information or services among individuals, groups, or institutions; also, meeting and getting to know individuals in the same or similar career fields and sharing information about available opportunities.

nonmaleficence   Refraining from the act of harming or committing evil.

no-show   A person who fails to keep an appointment without giving advance notice.

nosocomial   Originating or taking place in a hospital.

"note"   Notes are found in both the Alphabetic Index and the Tabular List as instructions or guides in classification assignments, defining category content or the use of subdivision codes.

numeric filing   The filing of records, correspondence, or cards by number.

objective information   Information that is gathered by watching or observation of a patient.

objectives   Something toward which effort is directed; an aim, goal, or end of action.

obliteration   Act of making undecipherable or imperceptible by obscuring or wearing away.

"omit code"   Term used primarily in Volume 3 of the ICD-9-CM when the procedure is the method of approach for an operation.

opinion   A formal expression of judgment or advice by an expert; the formal expression of the legal reasons and principles on which a legal decision is based.

optical character recognition (OCR)   The electronic scanning of printed items as images and use of special software to recognize these images (or characters) as ASCII text.

ordinance   An authoritative decree or direction; a law set forth by a governmental authority, specifically a municipal regulation.

osteopathy   A medical discipline based primarily on the manual diagnosis and holistic treatment of impaired function resulting from loss of movement of all kinds of tissues.

other potentially infectious material (OPIM)   Substances or material other than blood that has the potential to carry infectious pathogens, such as body fluid, urine, semen, and others.

OUTfolder   A folder used to provide space for the temporary filing of materials.

OUTguide   A heavy guide that is used to replace a folder that has been temporarily moved from the filing space.

output   Information that is processed by the computer and transmitted to a monitor, printer, or other device.

outreach   The process of using marketing and education strategies to reach and involve diverse audiences through the use of key messages and effective programs.

packing slip   An itemized list of objects in a package.

pandemic   Affecting the majority of the people in a country or a number of countries.

paper claims   Hard copies of insurance claims that have been completed and sent by surface mail.

paraphrased   A restatement of a text, passage, or work giving the meaning in another form.

paraphrasing   To express an idea in different wording in an effort to enhance communication and clarify meaning.

participating provider (PAR)   A physician or other healthcare provider who enters into a contract with a specific insurance company or program, and by doing so, agrees to abide by certain rules and regulations set forth by that particular third-party payor.

payables   The balance due to a creditor on an account.

payee   Person named on a draft or check as the recipient of the amount shown.

payor   Person who writes a check in favor of the payee.

peer review organizations   A group of medical reviewers contracted by the Centers for Medicare and Medicaid Services (CMS) (formerly HCFA) to ensure quality control and medical necessity of services provided by a facility.

pegboard system   Also called the *write-it-once system*; a method of tracking patient accounts that allows the figures to be proved accurate through mathematical formulas.

perceiving   How an individual looks at information and sees it as real.

perception   A quick, acute, and intuitive cognition; a capacity for comprehension; an awareness of the elements of the environment.

perjured testimony   The voluntary violation of an oath or vow either by swearing to what is untrue or by omission to do what has been promised under oath; false testimony.

perks   Extra advantages or benefits from working in a specific job that may or may not be commonplace in that particular profession; a shortened form of *perquisites*.

persona   An individual's social facade or front that reflects the role in life the individual is playing; the personality that a person projects in public.

pertinent   Having a clear, decisive relevance to the matter at hand.

petty cash fund   A fund maintained to pay small unpredictable cash expenditures.

philanthropist   An individual who makes an active effort to promote human welfare.

philosopher   A person who seeks wisdom or enlightenment; an expounder of a theory in a certain area of experience.

phlebotomy   The invasive procedure used to obtain a blood specimen for testing, experimentation, or diagnosis of disease.

phonetic   Constituting an alteration of ordinary spelling that better represents the spoken language, that employs only characters of the regular alphabet, and that is used in a context of conventional spelling.

photophobia   Visual sensitivity to light.

physician office laboratories (POLs)   Laboratories owned by a private physician or corporation, such as the lab inside a physician's office or a free-standing laboratory.

physiological noise   Physiological interferences with the communication process.

pitch   Highness or lowness of a sound; the relative level, intensity, or extent of some quality or state.

pitch   The property of a sound, especially a musical tone, that is determined by the frequency of the waves producing it; the highness or lowness of sound.

policyholder   A person who pays a premium to an insurance company and in whose name the policy is written in exchange for the insurance protection provided by a policy of insurance, usually applicable to an automobile policy; thus the "holder" of the policy.

polydipsia   Excessive thirst.

polyuria   Excreting large amounts of urine.

portfolio   A set of pictures, drawings, documents, or photographs either bound in book form or loose in a folder.

posting   Transferring or carrying from a book of original entry to a ledger; entering figures in an accounting system.

postmortem   Done, collected, or occurring after death.

power of attorney   A legal statement in which a person authorizes another person to act as his or her attorney or agent. The authority may be limited to the handling of specific procedures. The person authorized to act as the agent is known as the *attorney in fact*.

precedence   To surpass in rank, dignity, or importance; to be, go, or come ahead or in front of.

precedents   A person or thing that serves as a model; something done or said that may serve as an example or rule to authorize or justify a subsequent act of the same kind.

preexisting condition   Physical condition of an insured person that existed before the issuance of the insurance policy.

premium   The periodic (monthly, quarterly, or annual) payment of a specific sum of money to an insurance company for which the insurer, in return, agrees to provide certain benefits.

preponderance   A superiority or excess in number or quantity; a majority.

preponderance of the evidence   Evidence that is of greater weight or more convincing than the evidence offered in opposition to it; evidence that as a whole shows that the fact sought to be proven is more probable than not.

prerequisite   Something that is necessary to an end or to carry out a function.

pressboard   A strong, highly glazed composition board resembling vulcanized fiber; heavy card stock.

primary diagnosis   The condition or chief complaint for which a patient is treated in an outpatient (physician's office or clinic) medical care setting.

principal   A capital sum of money due as a debt or used as a fund for which interest is either charged or paid.

principal diagnosis   A condition established after study that is chiefly responsible for the admission of a patient to the hospital. Used in coding inpatient hospital insurance claims.

processing   How an individual internalizes new information and makes it his or her own.

procrastination   Intentionally putting off doing something that should be done.

professional behaviors   Those actions that identify the medical assistant as a member of a healthcare profession including dependability, respectful patient care, initiative, positive attitude, and teamwork.

professional courtesy   Reduction or absence of fees to professional associates.

professionalism   The conduct or qualities characterized by or conforming to the technical or ethical standards of a profession; exhibiting a courteous, conscientious, and generally businesslike manner in the workplace.

proficiency   Competency as a result of training or practice.

profit sharing   Offer of a part of the company's profits to employees or other designated individuals or groups.

progress notes   Notes used in the patient chart to track the progress and condition of the patient.

proofread   To read and mark corrections.

prosthetic   The surgical or dental specialty concerned with the design, construction, and fitting of prostheses, which are artificial devices that replace missing parts of the body.

provider   The company, individual, or group that provides medical services to a patient.

provider identification number (PIN) A number assigned to providers by carriers for use in submission of claims.

provisional diagnosis A temporary diagnosis made prior to receiving all test results.

proxemics The study of the nature, degree, and effect of the spatial separation individuals naturally maintain.

prudent Marked by wisdom or judiciousness; shrewd in the management of practical affairs.

public domain The realm embracing property rights that belong to the community at large, are unprotected by copyright or patent, and are subject to use or appropriation by anyone.

putrefaction Decomposition of animal matter that results in a foul smell.

quackery The pretense of curing disease.

quality assurance Activities designed to increase the quality of a product or service through process or system changes that increase efficiency or effectiveness.

quality control An aggregate of activities designed to ensure adequate quality, especially in manufactured products or in the service industries.

queries Requests for information from a database.

ramifications Consequence; outgrowth; something produced by a cause or necessarily following from a set of conditions.

ream A quantity of paper being 20 pounds or, variously, 480, 500, or 516 sheets.

reasonable doubt Doubt based on reason and arising from evidence or lack of evidence; it is not doubt that is imagined or conjured up, but doubt that would cause reasonable persons to hesitate before acting.

receipts Amounts paid on patient accounts.

receivables Total monies received on accounts.

recipient The receiver of some thing or item.

rectify To correct by removing errors.

reflection The process of considering new information and internalizing it to create new ways of examining information.

rejected claim A claim returned to the provider for clarification of any question and that must be corrected prior to resubmission.

relevant Having significant and demonstrable bearing on the matter at hand.

reparations The act of making amends, offering atonement, or giving satisfaction from a wrong or injury.

reprimands Criticisms for a fault; a severe or formal reproof.

reproach An expression of rebuke or disapproval; a cause or occasion of blame, discredit, or disgrace.

requisites Something considered essential or necessary.

resource-based relative value system (RBRVS) A fee schedule designed to provide national uniform payment of Medicare benefits after being adjusted to reflect the differences in practice costs across geographic areas.

retention To keep in possession or use; to keep in one's pay or service.

retention schedule A method or plan for retaining or keeping medical records, and their movement from active, to inactive, to closed filing.

revenue The total income produced by a given source.

rider A special provision or group of provisions that may be added to a policy to expand or limit the benefits otherwise payable. It may increase or decrease benefits, waive a condition or coverage, or in any other way amend the original contract.

robotics Technology dealing with the design, construction, and operation of robots in automation.

router A device used to connect any number of LANs, which communicate with other routers and determine the best route between any two hosts.

salutation An expression of greeting, goodwill, or courtesy by words or gestures.

sarcasm A sharp and often satirical response or ironic utterance designed to cut or give pain.

scanner Device that reads text or illustrations on a printed page and can translate the information on that page into a form that the computer can understand.

screen Something that shields, protects, or hides; to select or eliminate through a screening process.

search engines Programs that search documents for keywords and return a list of documents containing those words.

"see" A direction given to the coder to look in another place. This term must always be followed and is found in the Alphabetic Index, Volumes 2 and 3.

"see also" A direction given to the coder to look elsewhere if the main term or subterm (or subterms) for that entry are not sufficient for coding the information. If a code number follows, "see also" is enclosed in parentheses. If there is no code number, "see also" is preceded by a dash.

"see category" A direction given to the coder to see a specific category (three-digit code). This must always be followed.

self-insured plan An insurance plan funded by an organization having a large enough employee base that they can afford to fund their own insurance program.

self-referral The act of a patient or insured individual who refers himself or herself to a specialist without requesting the referral to the primary provider, such as a woman seeking an annual gynecological examination. Managed care guidelines may require the patient to report the self-referral.

sentinel event An unexpected occurrence involving death or serious physical or psychologic injury, or the risk thereof.

sequentially Of, relating to, or arranged in a sequence.

server A computer or device on a network that manages shared network resources.

service benefit plan Plan that provides its benefits in the form of certain surgical and medical services rendered, rather than cash. A service benefit plan is not restricted to a fee schedule.

shelf filing A system that uses open shelves rather than cabinets for storing records.

shingling A method of filing whereby one report is laid on top of the older report, resembling the shingles of a roof.

socioeconomic Relating to a combination of social and economic factors.

sociological Oriented or directed toward social needs and problems.

sound card Device that allows a computer to output sound through speakers that are connected to the main circuitry board, or motherboard.

staff privileges Allowance of a healthcare professional to practice within a specific facility.

standards Established by authority, custom, or general consent as a model or example; something set up and established by authority as a rule for the measure of quantity, weight, extent, value, or quality.

standards Item or indicator used as a measure of quality or compliance with a statutory or accrediting body's policies and regulations.

stat Medical abbreviation for immediately; at this moment.

statement A request for payment.

statement of income and expense A summary of all income and expenses for a given period.

stationers Sellers of stationery.

statute A law enacted by the legislative branch of a government.

stereotype Something conforming to a fixed or general pattern; a standardized mental picture that is held in common by many and represents an over-simplified opinion, prejudiced attitude, or uncritical judgment.

stipulate To specify as a condition or requirement of an agreement or offer; to make an agreement or covenant to do or forbear something.

stock option Offer of stocks for purchase to a certain group of individuals or certain groups, such as employees of a for-profit hospital.

stressors Stimulus that causes stress.

subjective information Information that is gained by questioning the patient or taken from a form.

subluxations Slight misalignments of the vertebrae or a partial dislocation.

subordinate Submissive to or controlled by authority; placed in or occupying a lower class, rank, or position.

subpoena A writ or document commanding a person to appear in court under a penalty for failure to appear.

substance number A number based on the weight of a ream of paper containing 500 sheets.

subtle Difficult to understand or perceive; having or marked by keen insight and ability to penetrate deeply and thoroughly.

subtle Ingenious; artful; delicate.

succinct Marked by compact, precise expression without wasted words.

superbill A form on which to list procedures and ICD-9-CM codes most frequently used in a specific practice. The encounter is marked off on this form at the time of patient checkout and utilized for billing purposes. This is usually called an encounter form.

superfluous Exceeding what is sufficient or necessary.

surrogate A substitute; to put in place of another.

switch In networks, a device that filters information between LAN segments and decreases overall network traffic and increases speed and bandwidth usage efficiency.

synopsis Condensed statement or outline.

systems software The operating system and all utility programs that allow the computer to function and perform operations.

tactful Having a keen sense of what to do or say to maintain good relations with others or to avoid offense.

tangible Capable of being appraised at an actual or approximate value; capable of being precisely identified or realized by the mind.

target market A specific group of individuals to whom the marketing plan is focused.

targeted Directed or used toward a target; directed toward a specific desire or position.

TCP/IP Acronym for Transmission Control Protocol/Internet Protocol; a suite of communications protocols used to connect users or hosts to the Internet.

tedious Tiresome because of length or dullness.

telecommunication The science and technology of communication by transmission of information from one location to another via telephone, television, telegraph, or satellite.

telemedicine The use of telecommunications in the practice of medicine, in which great distances can exist between healthcare professionals, colleagues, patients, and students.

teleradiology The use of telecommunications devices to enhance and improve the results of radiological procedures.

testimony A solemn declaration usually made orally by a witness under oath in response to interrogation by a lawyer or authorized public official.

thanatology The description of the study of the phenomena of death and of psychological methods of coping with death.

third-party administrator An organization that processes claims and performs other business-related functions for a health plan.

third-party payor Someone other than the patient, spouse, or parent who is responsible for paying all or part of the patient's medical costs; an entity that makes a payment on an obligation or debt but is not a party of the contract that created the debt.

tickler file A chronological file used as a reminder that something must be taken care of on a certain date.

transaction An exchange or transfer of goods, services, or funds.

transcription To make a written copy of, either in longhand or by machine.

transient ischemic attack Temporary neurological symptoms because of a gradual or partial occlusion of a cerebral blood vessel.

transpose To change the relative place or normal order of; to alter the sequence.

treatises Systematic expositions or arguments in writing including a methodical discussion of the facts and principles involved and the conclusions reached.

triage The sorting of and allocation of treatment to patients according to a system of priorities designed to maximize the number of survivors and treat the sickest patients first.

trial balance   A method of checking the accuracy of accounts.

TRICARE   See CHAMPUS.

unbundled codes   Separating the components of a procedure and reporting them separately.

Uniform Commercial Code (UCC)   A series of laws (regulations), adopted by most states, that regulate the fields of sales of goods; commercial paper, such as checks; secured transactions in personal property; and particular aspects of banking, letters of credit, warehouse receipts, bills of lading, and investment securities; a unified set of rules covering many business transactions; it has been adopted in all 50 states, the District of Columbia, and most U.S. territories.

unique identifiers   Codes used instead of names to protect the confidentiality of the patient in a method of anonymous HIV testing.

unique provider identification number (UPIN)   A number assigned by fiscal intermediaries to identify providers on claims for services.

universal claim form   The form developed by the Health Care Financing Administration (HCFA) (now known as the Centers for Medicare and Medicaid Services [CMS]) and approved by the AMA for use in submitting all government-sponsored claims.

upcoding   A deliberate increase in a CPT code to receive higher reimbursements.

URL   Acronym for Uniform Resource Locator; specifies the global address of documents or information on the Internet. The URL provides the IP address and the domain name for the web page, such as *microsoft.com*.

"use additional code"   This term appears only in volume 1 in those subdivisions in which the user should add further information by means of an additional code to give a more complete picture of the diagnosis. In some cases you will find "if desired" following the term. For the purpose of coding, the "if desired" phrase will not be used. When the term "use additional code…if desired" appears, you will disregard "if desired" and assign the appropriate additional code.

utilization   Related to the process of reviewing procedures and services for medical necessity.

utilization review   A review of individual cases by a committee to make sure that services are medically necessary and to study how providers use medical care resources.

vehemently   Marked by forceful energy; intensely emotional.

veracity   A devotion to or conformity with the truth.

verdict   The finding or decision of a jury on a matter submitted to it in trial.

versatile   Embracing a variety of subjects, fields, or skills; having a wide range of abilities.

vested   Granted or endowed with a particular authority, right, or property; to have a special interest in.

virtual reality   An artificial environment presented to a computer user that feels as if it were a real environment, often using special gloves, earphones, and goggles to enhance the experience.

vocation   The work in which a person is regularly employed.

volatile   Easily aroused; tending to erupt in violence.

watermark   A marking in paper resulting from differences in thickness usually produced by the pressure of a projecting design in the mold or on a processing roll and visible when the paper is held up to the light.

"with"   In the context of ICD-9-CM, the terms "with," "with mention of," and "associated with" in a title dictate that both parts of the title be present in the statement of the diagnosis order to assign the particular code.

workers' compensation   Insurance against liability imposed on certain employers to pay benefits and furnish care to employees who are injured and to pay benefits to dependents of employees killed in the course of or arising out of their employment.

Zip drive   A small, portable disk drive that is primarily used for backing up information and archiving computer files. A 100-megabyte Zip disk will hold the equivalent of about 70 floppy disks.

Index

Page references followed by "*f*" indicate figures and by "*t*" indicate tables.

I-1

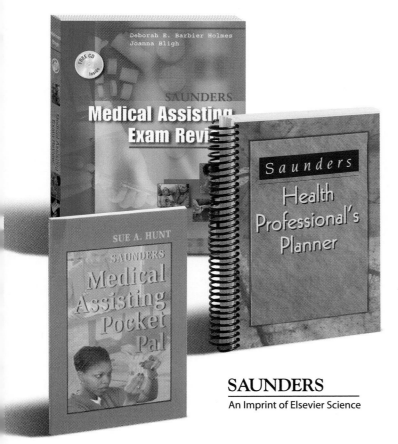

AAMA Entry-Level Competencies for the Medical Assistant

From the 1999 *Standards and Guidelines*

Competency content in all areas (administrative, clinical, and transdisciplinary) should be presented utilizing manual and state-of-the-art methods.
Invasive procedures must be taught to clinical competency.

Patient care **instructions** should encompass all phases of the life cycle: pediatric, adult, and geriatric.
Adaptations for special needs patients should be addressed.

ADMINISTRATIVE

(1) Perform Clerical Functions
   a. Schedule and manage appointments
   b. Schedule inpatient and outpatient admissions
   c. Perform medical transcription
   d. Organize a patient's medical record
   e. File medical records
(2) Perform Bookkeeping Procedures
   a. Prepare a bank deposit
   b. Reconcile a bank statement
   c. Post entries on a daysheet
   d. Perform accounts receivable procedures
   e. Perform accounts payable procedures
   f. Perform billing and collection procedures
   g. Prepare a check
   h. Establish and maintain a petty cash fund
(3) Prepare Special Accounting Entries
   a. Post adjustments
   b. Process a credit balance
   c. Process refunds
   d. Post nonsufficient (NSF) checks
   e. Post collection agency payments
(4) Process Insurance Claims
   a. Apply managed care policies and procedures
   b. Apply third party guidelines
   c. Obtain managed care referrals and precertifications
   d. Perform procedural coding
   e. Perform diagnostic coding
   f. Complete insurance claim form
   g. Use a physician's fee schedule

CLINICAL COMPETENCIES

(1) Fundamental Principles
   a. Perform hand washing
   b. Wrap items for autoclaving
   c. Perform sterilization techniques
   d. Dispose of biohazardous materials
   e. Practice standard precautions
(2) Specimen Collection
   a. Perform venipuncture
   b. Perform capillary puncture
   c. Obtain throat specimen for microbiological testing
   d. Perform wound collection procedure for microbiological testing
   e. Instruct patients in the collection of a clean-catch, midstream urine specimen
   f. Instruct patients in the collection of a fecal specimen

(3) Diagnostic Testing
   a. Use methods of quality control
   b. Perform urinalysis
   c. Perform hematology testing
   d. Perform chemistry testing
   e. Perform immunology testing
   f. Perform microbiology testing
   g. Screen and follow-up test results
   h. Perform electrocardiograms
   i. Perform respiratory testing
(4) Patient Care
   a. Perform telephone and in-person screening
   b. Obtain vital signs
   c. Obtain and record patient history
   d. Prepare and maintain examination and treatment area
   e. Prepare patients for and assist with routine and specialty examinations
   f. Prepare patients for and assist with procedures, treatments, and minor office surgery
   g. Apply pharmacology principles to prepare and administer oral and parenteral medications
   h. Maintain medication and immunization records
   i. Obtain CPR certification and first aid training

TRANSDISCIPLINARY COMPETENCIES*

(1) Communication
   a. Respond to and initiate written communication
   b. Recognize and respond to verbal communication
   c. Recognize and respond to nonverbal communication
   d. Demonstrate telephone techniques
(2) Legal Concepts
   a. Identify and respond to issue of confidentiality
   b. Perform within legal and ethical boundaries
   c. Establish and maintain the medical record
   d. Document appropriately
   e. Perform risk-management procedures
(3) Patient Instruction
   a. Explain general office procedures
   b. Instruct individuals according to their needs
   c. Instruct and demonstrate the use and care of patient equipment
   d. Provide instruction for health maintenance and disease prevention
   e. Identify community resources
(4) Operational Functions
   a. Perform an inventory of supplies and equipment
   b. Perform routine maintenance of administrative and clinical equipment
   c. Utilize computer software to maintain office systems

May be addressed in clinical, administrative, or both areas.

(Courtesy of the American Association of Medical Assistants)